Challenging Cases in Urological Surgery

Published and forthcoming titles in the Challenging Cases in series

Anaesthesia (Edited by Dr Phoebe Syme, Dr Robert Jackson, and Dr Timothy Cook)

Cardiovascular Medicine (Edited by Dr Aung Myat, Dr Shouvik Haldar, and Professor Simon Redwood)

Critical Care (Edited by Dr Christopher Gough, Dr Justine Barnett, Professor Tim Cook, and Professor Jerry Nolan)

Emergency Medicine (Edited by Dr Sam Thenabadu, Dr Fleur Cantle, and Dr Chris Lacy)

Infectious Diseases and Clinical Microbiology (Edited by Dr Amber Arnold and Professor George E. Griffin)

Interventional Radiology (Edited by Dr Irfan Ahmed, Dr Miltiadis Krokidis, and Dr Tarun Sabharwal)

Neurology (Edited by Dr Krishna Chinthapalli, Dr Nadia Magdalinou, and Professor Nicholas Wood)

Neurosurgery (Edited by Mr Robin Bhatia and Mr Ian Sabin)

Obstetrics and Gynaecology (Edited by Dr Natasha Hezelgrave, Dr Danielle Abbott, and Professor Andrew Shennan)

Oncology (Edited by Dr Madhumita Bhattacharyya, Dr Sarah Payne, and Professor Iain McNeish)

Oral and Maxillofacial Surgery (Edited by Mr Matthew Idle and Group Captain Andrew Monaghan)

Paediatric Critical Care (Edited by Hari Krishnan, Miriam R. Fine-Goulden, Sainath Raman, and Akash Deep)

Respiratory Medicine (Edited by Dr Lucy Schomberg, Dr Elizabeth Sage, and Dr Nick Hart)

Challenging Cases in Urological Surgery

Cases with Expert Commentary

Edited by

Karl H. Pang MBChB, BSc(Hons), MSc, PhD, FRCS(Urol), FEBU, AFHEA

Post-CCT Clinical Fellow in Andrology, Institute of Andrology, University College London Hospitals NHS Foundation Trust; Honorary Clinical Lecturer, University College London; Honorary Clinical Lecturer, Department of Oncology and Metabolism and Academic Urology Unit, University of Sheffield, UK

James W.F. Catto MBChB, PhD, FRCS(Urol)

Professor in Urological Surgery, Department of Oncology and Metabolism and Academic Urology Unit, University of Sheffield, UK; Honorary Consultant Urological Surgeon, Royal Hallamshire Hospital, Sheffield Teaching Hospitals NHS Foundation Trust
European Urology Editor-in-Chief

Series editors

Aung Myat

Medical Director for Cardiology and Academic Interventional Cardiologist, Medpace Inc., London, UK

Shouvik Haldar

Consultant Cardiologist and Electrophysiologist, Heart Rhythm Centre, Royal Brompton and Harefield NHS Foundation Trust, and Honorary Clinical Senior Lecturer, Imperial College London, London, UK

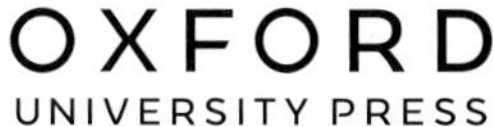
OXFORD
UNIVERSITY PRESS

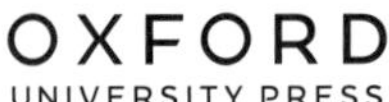

Great Clarendon Street, Oxford, OX2 6DP,
United Kingdom

Oxford University Press is a department of the University of Oxford. It furthers the University's objective of excellence in research, scholarship, and education by publishing worldwide. Oxford is a registered trade mark of Oxford University Press in the UK and in certain other countries

First Edition published in 2023

Impression: 1

Published in the United States of America by Oxford University Press
198 Madison Avenue, New York, NY 10016, United States of America

British Library Cataloguing in Publication Data

Data available

Library of Congress Control Number: 2022930152

ISBN 978–0–19–885437–1

DOI: 10.1093/med/9780198854371.001.0001

Printed in the UK by
Bell & Bain Ltd., Glasgow

FOREWORD

At any national or international urology congress, the sessions delegates most enjoy are those where experts debate the management of complex cases and in so doing dissect the evidence base and show how it should be applied. This book looks to do the same, and a urologist who reads it will acquire a lot of knowledge and save an airfare, a conference registration fee and a hotel bill! It's a new concept and I think it works.

The list of subjects covered is broad ranging and very interesting; challenging in every way. The views expressed by the authors and the experts will, I am sure, generate much debate. I'm a retroperitoneal surgeon and certainly found much to debate in case 7 (renal oncocytoma), case 16 (upper urinary tract urothelial carcinoma) and case 19 (growing teratoma syndrome in testis cancer). That though I think is the point, in a challenging case there may not be a right or a wrong answer but understanding how experts reach their decisions can be a very valuable way of learning. The book should be a very good primer for board exams or the FRCS (Urol) examination.

So, well done to the editors, Karl Pang and Jim Catto, on pulling it all together. The book reminded me once again of the staggering breadth of the specialty we practise and I'm looking forward to debating with specialist registrars, fellows, and consultants at Guy's all 48 of the cases.

Tim S. O'Brien MA, DM, FRCS(Urol)
Consultant Urological Surgeon
Immediate past-President of BAUS

PREFACE

This is the first urological surgery book added to the Challenging Cases series. Common cases, challenges, and controversial topics are discussed in a format utilizing boxes to highlight learning points, evidence bases, and future directions. Using case examples, experts provide clinical tips and personal comments on how they manage specific presentations. Expert commentary is provided throughout each chapter with a concluding 'Final word' from the expert at the end of each case. This book includes a variety of cases covering most sections outlined in the Intercollegiate Surgical Curriculum for Urological Surgery including oncology, endourology, functional and female urology, neurourology, andrology, trauma, transplantation, and paediatric urology. This book is a highly valuable resource for all those interested in urological surgery, allied health professionals, trainees in the field and those sitting postgraduate urology examinations. We thank all authors and experts for their hard work and hope you enjoy reading this text.

Karl H. Pang and James W.F. Catto

CONTENTS

ABBREVIATIONS

5-FU	5-fluorouracil
AAST	American Association for the Surgery of Trauma
ABP	acute bacterial prostatitis
ADT	androgen deprivation therapy
AFP	alpha-fetoprotein
AFS	autologous fascial sling
AML	angiomyolipoma
AMR	antimicrobial resistance
ANH	antenatal hydronephrosis
APD	anterior–posterior diameter
AS	active surveillance
ATLS®	Advanced Trauma Life Support®
AUA	American Urological Association
AUR	acute urinary retention
AUS	artificial urethral sphincter
BAUS	British Association of Urological Surgeons
BC	bladder cancer
BCD	bell clapper deformity
BEP	bleomycin, etoposide, and cisplatin
BMD	bone mineral density
BMG	buccal mucosal graft
BMI	body mass index
BN	bladder neck
BOO	bladder outlet obstruction
BPH	benign prostate hyperplasia
BPO	benign prostate obstruction
BPS	bladder pain syndrome
BTX	botulinum toxin
BXO	balanitis xerotica obliterans
CAD	coronary artery disease
CAP	continuous antibiotic prophylaxis
CBP	chronic bacterial prostatitis
CCH	collagenase *Clostridium histolyticum*
ccRCC	clear cell renal cell carcinoma
CES	cauda equina syndrome
CI	confidence interval
CIS	carcinoma-*in situ*
CISC	clean intermittent self-catheterization
CIT	cold ischaemic time
CKD	chronic kidney disease
CP	chronic prostatitis
CPPS	chronic pelvic pain syndrome
CRP	C-reactive protein *or* cytoreductive radical prostatectomy
CT	computed tomography
CTU	computed tomography urogram/urography
CUR	chronic urinary retention
DBD	donation after brain death
DCD	donation after circulatory death
DE	delayed ejaculation
DM	diabetes mellitus
DMSA	dimercaptosuccinic acid
DOA	detrusor overactivity
DRE	digital rectal examination
DSD	disorder of sex development
DVIU	direct visual internal urethrotomy
EAU	European Association of Urology
ECIRS	endoscopic combined intrarenal surgery
ECOG	Eastern Cooperative Oncology Group
ED	Erectile dysfunction
eGFR	estimated glomerular filtration rate
EORTC	European Organisation for Research and Treatment of Cancer
ePLND	extended pelvic lymph node dissection
EPS	expressed prostatic secretions
ERAS®	Enhanced Recovery After Surgery
ESWL	extracorporeal shock wave lithotripsy
FDG	fluorodeoxyglucose
Fr	French (gauge)
FSH	follicle-stimulating hormone
GCNIS	germ cell neoplasia *in situ*
GCT	germ cell tumour
GnRH	gonadotropin-releasing hormone
GP	general practitioner
GTS	growing teratoma syndrome
hCG	human chorionic gonadotropin
HGNMIBC	high-grade non-muscle-invasive bladder cancer
HIV	human immunodeficiency virus
HLA	human leukocyte antigen
HoLEP	holmium laser enucleation of the prostate
HPCR	high-pressure chronic retention
HPV	human papillomavirus
HR	hazard ratio
HRR	homologous recombination repair
HTN	hypertension

IC	interstitial cystitis
ICIQ	International Consultation on Incontinence Questionnaire
ICS	International Continence Society
ICSI	intracytoplasmic sperm injection
IFNα	interferon alpha
IIEF	International Index of Erectile Function
IPSS	International Prostate Symptom Score
ISC	intermittent self-catheterization
ISD	intermittent self-dilatation
IVC	inferior vena cava
KS	Klinefelter syndrome
KUB	kidneys, ureters, and bladder
LATP	local anaesthetic transperineal
LDH	lactate dehydrogenase
LH	luteinizing hormone
LN	lymph node
LND	lymph node dissection
LPCR	low-pressure chronic retention
LUTS	lower urinary tract symptoms
MAG3	mercaptoacetyltriglycine
mCRPC	metastatic castration-resistant prostate cancer
MCUG	micturating cystourethrogram
MDT	multidisciplinary team
MET	medical expulsion therapy
MFI	male factor infertility
MHRA	Medicines and Healthcare products Regulatory Agency
MI	myocardial infarction
MIBC	muscle-invasive bladder cancer
MMC	mitomycin C
mpMRI	multiparametric magnetic resonance imaging
MRI	magnetic resonance imaging
mTESE	microdissection testicular sperm extraction
mTOR	mammalian target of rapamycin
MUL	membranous urethral length
MUT	mid-urethral tape
MVAC	methotrexate, vinblastine, Adriamycin® (doxorubicin), and cisplatin
NAC	neoadjuvant chemotherapy
NICE	National Institute for Health and Care Excellence
NIDDK	National Institute of Diabetes and Digestive and Kidney Diseases
NMIBC	non-muscle-invasive bladder cancer
NNNB	non-neurogenic neurogenic bladder
NOA	non-obstructive azoospermia
NSAID	non-steroidal anti-inflammatory drug
NSGCT	non-seminomatous germ cell tumour
NVB	neurovascular bundle
NYHA	New York Heart Association
OA	obstructive azoospermia
OAB	overactive bladder
OAT	oligoasthenoteratospermia
onco-TESE	onco-testicular sperm extraction
OR	odds ratio
PCCL	percutaneous nephrostomy cystolitholapaxy
PCN	percutaneous nephrostomy
PCNL	percutaneous nephrolithotomy
PD	Peyronie's disease
PDE5	phosphodiesterase type 5
PDE5i	phosphodiesterase type 5 inhibitor
PE	premature ejaculation
PET	positron emission tomography
PFMT	pelvic floor muscle training
PI-RADS	Prostate Imaging Reporting and Data System
PLND	pelvic lymph node dissection
POD	post-obstructive diuresis
POP	pelvic organ prolapse
PSA	prostate-specific antigen
PSM	positive surgical margin
PTNS	percutaneous tibial nerve stimulation
PUV	posterior urethral valves
qSOFA	quick Sepsis-related Organ Failure Assessment
RARP	robotic-assisted radical prostatectomy
RC	radical cystectomy
RCC	renal cell carcinoma
RCT	randomized control trial
RNU	radical nephroureterectomy
RPLND	retroperitoneal lymph node dissection
RR	risk ratio
RRT	renal replacement therapy
SCC	squamous cell carcinoma
SCD	sickle-cell disease
SFA	semen fluid analysis
SFR	stone-free rate
SNM	sacral neuromodulation
SNS	sacral nerve stimulation
SPC	suprapubic catheter
SRE	skeletal-related event
SSRI	selective serotonin reuptake inhibitor

SUI	stress urinary incontinence
SWL	shockwave lithotripsy
TA	tunica albuginea
TC	testicular cancer
TCC	transitional cell carcinoma
TESE	testicular sperm extraction
TKI	tyrosine kinase inhibitor
TNM	tumour, node, and metastasis
TRUS	transrectal ultrasound
TS	tuberous sclerosis
TUC	transurethral catheter
TUCL	transurethral cystolitholapaxy
TURBT	transurethral resection of a bladder tumour
TURP	transurethral resection of the prostate
TV	tunica vaginalis
UCC	urothelial cell carcinoma
UDS	urodynamic studies
UDT	undescended testis
UI	urinary incontinence
UISS	University of California Integrated Staging System
UO	ureteric orifice
UPJO	ureteropelvic junction obstruction
UR	urinary retention
URS	ureteroscopy
USS	ultrasound scan
UTI	urinary tract infection
UTUC	upper tract urothelial carcinoma
UUI	urge urinary incontinence
VCMG	video cystometrography
VTT	venous tumour thrombus
VUDS	video urodynamic studies
VUJ	vesicoureteric junction
VUR	vesicoureteral reflux
VVF	vesicovaginal fistula
WCC	white cell count
WHO	World Health Organization

EXPERTS

Ased Ali
Consultant Urological Surgeon, Department of Urology, Mid Yorkshire Hospitals NHS Trust, Wakefield, UK

Christopher Anderson
Consultant Urological Surgeon, Department of Urology, St George's University Hospitals NHS Foundation Trust, London, UK

Mohammed Belal
Consultant Urological Surgeon, Department of Urology, University Hospitals Birmingham NHS Foundation Trust, Birmingham, UK

Axel Bex
Consultant Urological Surgeon, Specialist Centre for Kidney Cancer, Royal Free London NHS Foundation Trust, London; Honorary Associate Professor, UCL Division of Surgical and Interventional Science, UK

Suzanne Biers
Consultant Urological Surgeon, Department of Urology, Cambridge University Hospitals NHS Foundation Trust, Cambridge, UK

Anthony Browning
Consultant Urological Surgeon, Department of Urology, Mid Yorkshire Hospitals NHS Trust, Wakefield, UK

Richard J. Bryant
Associate Professor of Urological Surgery and Honorary Consultant Urological Surgeon, Nuffield Department of Surgical Sciences, Oxford Cancer Research Centre, University of Oxford; Department of Urology, Oxford University Hospitals NHS Foundation Trust, Oxford, UK

James W.F. Catto
Professor of Urological Surgery and Honorary Consultant Urological Surgeon, Department of Oncology and Metabolism, University of Sheffield; Department of Urology, Sheffield Teaching Hospitals NHS Foundation Trust, UK

Christopher R. Chapple
Professor and Consultant Urological Surgeon, Section of Functional and Reconstructive Urology, Department of Urology, Sheffield Teaching Hospitals NHS Foundation Trust, Sheffield, UK

Noel W. Clarke
Consultant Urological Surgeon, Department of Urology, The Christie NHS Foundation Trust; Honorary Professor of Urological Oncology, University of Manchester, UK

Peter Cuckow
Professor of Paediatric Urological Surgery, Department of Paediatric Urology, Great Ormond Street Hospital for Children NHS Foundation Trust, London, UK

Marcus Drake
Professor of Physiological Urology, Translational Health Sciences, Bristol Medical School, University of Bristol, Bristol, UK

Ian Eardley
Consultant Urological Surgeon, Department of Urology, Leeds Teaching Hospitals NHS Trust, Leeds, UK

Archie Fernando
Consultant Urological Surgeon, Department of Urology, Guy's and St Thomas' NHS Foundation Trust, London, UK

James A. Gilbert
Consultant in Transplantation and Vascular Access Surgery, Oxford Transplant Centre, Oxford University Hospitals NHS Foundation Trust, Oxford, UK

Jonathan Glass
Consultant Urological Surgeon, Department of Urology, Guy's and St Thomas' NHS Foundation Trust, London, UK

Freddie C. Hamdy
Nuffield Professor of Surgery and Professor of Urology, Department of Urology, Churchill Hospital, Oxford University Hospitals NHS Trust; Nuffield Department of Surgical Sciences, University of Oxford, Oxford, UK

Christopher K. Harding
Consultant Urological Surgeon and Honorary Professor of Urology, Department of Urology, The Newcastle upon Tyne Hospitals NHS Foundation Trust; University of Newcastle, Newcastle, UK

Hashim Hashim
Consultant Urological Surgeon and Honorary Professor of Urology, Bristol Urological Institute, Southmead Hospital, Bristol, UK

Swati Jha
Consultant in Urogynaecology, Department of Urogynaecology, Sheffield Teaching Hospitals NHS Foundation Trust, Sheffield, UK

Jose A. Karam
Assistant Professor of Urological Surgery, Department of Urology, The University of Texas MD Anderson Cancer Center, Houston, TX, USA

Oliver Kayes
Consultant Urological Surgeon and Honorary Senior Lecturer, Department of Urology, University of Leeds, Leeds, UK

Steven Kennish
Consultant Radiologist, Department of Clinical Radiology, Sheffield Teaching Hospitals NHS Foundation Trust, Sheffield, UK

Andrea Lavinio
Consultant in Intensive Care, Department of Anaesthesia, Cambridge University Hospitals NHS Foundation Trust, Cambridge, UK

James Lenton
Consultant in Interventional Radiology, Department of Radiology, Leeds Teaching Hospitals NHS Trust, Leeds; Mid Yorkshire Hospitals NHS Trust, Wakefield, UK

Altaf Mangera
Consultant Urological Surgeon, Department of Urology, Sheffield Teaching Hospitals NHS Foundation Trust, Sheffield, UK

Suks Minhas
Professor and Consultant Urological Surgeon, Department of Urology, Imperial College Healthcare NHS Trust, London, UK

Asif Muneer
Professor and Consultant Urological Surgeon, Institute of Andrology, University College London Hospitals NHS Foundation Trust; NIHR Biomedical Research Centre University College London Hospital; Division of Surgery and Interventional Science, University College London, London, UK

Imran Mushtaq
Professor and Consultant Paediatric Urological Surgeon, Department of Paediatric Urology, Great Ormond Street Hospital for Children NHS Trust, London, UK

Aidan P. Noon
Consultant Urological Surgeon, Department of Urology, Sheffield Teaching Hospitals NHS Foundation Trust, Sheffield, UK

Neil Oakley
Consultant Urological Surgeon, Department of Urology, Sheffield Teaching Hospitals NHS Foundation Trust, Sheffield, UK

Jeremy Ockrim
Consultant Urological Surgeon, Department of Urology, University College London Hospitals NHS Foundation Trust, London, UK

Richard Parkinson
Consultant Urological Surgeon, Department of Urology, Nottingham University Hospitals NHS Trust, Nottingham, UK

Andrew Protheroe
Associate Professor and Consultant in Medical Oncology, Department of Oncology, Oxford University Hospitals NHS Foundation Trust, Oxford, UK

David Ralph
Professor in Urological Surgery, Institute of Andrology, University College London Hospitals NHS Foundation Trust, London, UK

Vijay A.C. Ramani
Consultant Urological Oncological and Robotic Surgeon, Department of Urology, The Christie and Manchester University Hospitals NHS Foundation Trust, Manchester, UK

Georgina Reall
Consultant in Histopathology, Department of Histopathology, Mid Yorkshire Hospitals NHS Trust, Wakefield, UK

Rowland Rees
Consultant Urological Surgeon, Department of Urology, University Hospital Southampton NHS Foundation Trust, Southampton, UK

Arun Sahai
Consultant Urological Surgeon and Reader in Urology, Department of Urology, Guy's and St Thomas' NHS Foundation Trust; King's College London, London, UK

Christian Seipp
Consultant Urological Surgeon, The Alan De Bolla Wrexham Urology Department, Wrexham Maelor Hospital, Wrexham, UK

Majid Shabbir
Consultant Urological Surgeon and Honorary Senior Lecturer, Department of Urology, Guy's and St Thomas' NHS Foundation Trust, London, UK

Julian Shah
Consultant Urological Surgeon, King Edward VII's Hospital and London Spinal Cord Injury Unit, Royal National Orthopaedic Hospital NHS Trust, London, UK

Davendra M. Sharma
Consultant Urological Surgeon, Department of Urology, St George's University Hospitals NHS Foundation Trust, London, UK

Daron Smith
Consultant Endoluminal Endourologist, Endourology and Stone Unit, Department of Urology, University College London Hospitals NHS Foundation Trust, London, UK

Prasanna Sooriakumaran
Lead for Urology, Digestive Disease and Surgery Institute, Cleveland Clinic London, London, UK; Consultant Urological Surgeon, Department of Urology, University College London Hospitals NHS Foundation Trust, UK

Mark Sullivan
Consultant Urological Surgeon and Honorary Senior Lecturer, Department of Urology, Oxford University Hospitals NHS Foundation Trust, Oxford, UK

Nikesh Thiruchelvam
Consultant Urological Surgeon, Department of Urology, Cambridge University Hospitals NHS Foundation Trust, Cambridge, UK

André Van der Merwe
Professor in Urological Surgery, Division of Urology, Faculty of Medicine and Healthcare Sciences, Stellenbosch University; Tygerberg Academic Hospital, Cape Town, South Africa

Andrew Winterbottom
Consultant in Interventional Radiology, Department of Interventional Radiology, Cambridge University Hospitals NHS Foundation Trust, Cambridge, UK

Oliver Wiseman
Consultant Urological Surgeon, Department of Urology, Cambridge University Hospitals NHS Foundation Trust, Cambridge, UK

Ayman Younis
Consultant Urological Surgeon, Department of Urology, Swansea Bay University Health Board, Swansea, UK

CONTRIBUTORS

Kimberly Aikins
Specialist Registrar in Paediatric Surgery, Department of Paediatric Surgery and Urology, Starship Children's Hospital, Auckland, New Zealand

Adnan Ali
Clinical Research Fellow in Urological Surgery, Genito-Urinary Cancer Research Group, Division of Cancer Sciences, The University of Manchester; FASTMAN Centre of Prostate Cancer Excellence, Manchester Cancer Research Centre; Department of Surgery, The Christie NHS Foundation Trust, Manchester, UK

Siân Allen
Consultant Urological Surgeon, Department of Urology, University College London Hospitals NHS Foundation Trust, London, UK

Hussain Alnajjar
Consultant Urological Surgeon and Andrologist, Institute of Andrology, University College London Hospitals NHS Foundation Trust, London, UK

Omer Altan
Consultant Urological Surgeon, Department of Urology, University Hospitals Coventry and Warwickshire NHS Trust, Coventry, UK

Rachel Barratt
Post-CCT Clinical Fellow in Urology, Department of Urology, University College London Hospitals NHS Foundation Trust, London, UK

Lisa Bibby
Urology Registrar, Department of Urology, Addenbrookes Hospital, Cambridge, UK

Nicholas Bullock
Welsh Clinical Academic Track Fellow and Urology Registrar, Division of Cancer and Genetics, Cardiff University School of Medicine, Cardiff, UK

Kevin Cao
Paediatric Urology Registrar, Department of Paediatric Urology, Great Ormond Street Hospital for Children NHS Foundation Trust, London, UK

Alexander Cho
Consultant Paediatric Urological Surgeon, Department of Paediatric Urology, Great Ormond Street Hospital for Children NHS Foundation Trust, London, UK

Francesco Claps
Urology Registrar, Urology Clinic, Department of Medical, Surgical and Health Science, University of Trieste, Trieste, Italy

Jennifer Clark
Urology Registrar, Department of Urology, The Christie NHS Foundation Trust; Manchester University Hospitals Foundation Trust, Manchester, UK

Samantha Conroy
Clinical Research Fellow, Academic Unit of Urology, Department of Oncology and Metabolism, University of Sheffield, Sheffield, UK

Emily Decker
Clinical Fellow in Paediatric Urological Surgery, Department of Paediatric Urology, Great Ormond Street Hospital for Children NHS Foundation Trust, London, UK

Andrew Deytrikh
Urology Registrar, Department of Urology, Sheffield Teaching Hospitals, Sheffield, UK

Hazel Ecclestone
Consultant Urological Surgeon, London North West University Healthcare NHS Trust, London, UK

Thomas Ellul
Urology Registrar, Department of Urology, Royal Gwent University Hospital, Newport, UK

María S. Figueroa-Díaz
Consultant Paediatric Urological Surgeon, Department of Pediatric Urology, Hospital San Borja Arriarán, Santiago, Chile

Huw Garrod
Urology Registrar, Department of Urology, Royal Liverpool University Hospital, Liverpool

Tamsin Greenwell
Consultant Urological Surgeon, Department of Urology, University College London Hospitals NHS Foundation Trust, London, UK

Rizwan Hamid
Honorary Assistant Professor and Consultant Urological Surgeon, Department of Urology, University College London Hospitals NHS Foundation Trust; Spinal Cord Injury Unit, Royal National Orthopaedic Hospital NHS Trust, London, UK

Cherrie Ho
Urology Registrar, Bristol Urological Institute, North Bristol NHS Trust, Bristol, UK

Joseph Jelski
Consultant Urological Surgeon, Department of Urology, Gloucestershire Hospitals NHS Foundation Trust, UK

James Jenkins
Urology Registrar, Bristol Urological Institute, North Bristol NHS Trust, Bristol, UK

Tobias Klatte
Consultant Urological Surgeon, Department of Urology, Royal Bournemouth and Christchurch Hospitals NHS Foundation Trust, Bournemouth, UK; Department of Surgery, University of Cambridge, Cambridge, UK

Jamie V. Krishnan
Urology Registrar, Section of Functional and Reconstructive Urology, Department of Urology, Sheffield Teaching Hospitals NHS Foundation Trust, Sheffield, UK

Priyanka H. Krishnaswamy
Subspecialty Registrar in Urogynaecology, Department of Urogynaecology, Queen Elizabeth University Hospital, NHS Greater Glasgow and Clyde, Glasgow, UK

Alastair Lamb
Senior Fellow in Robotic Surgery and Honorary Consultant Urological Surgeon, Nuffield Department of Surgical Sciences, University of Oxford, Oxford, UK

Hack Jae Lee
Urology Registrar, Department of Urology, St George's University Hospitals NHS Foundation Trust, London, UK

Thomas A. Lee
Urology Registrar, Department of Urology, The Christie NHS Foundation Trust and Manchester University Hospitals Foundation Trust, Manchester, UK

Sara Lobo
Paediatric Urology Senior Fellow, Department of Paediatric Urology, Great Ormond Street Hospital, London, UK

Findlay MacAskill
Urology Registrar, Department of Urology, Guy's and St Thomas' NHS Foundation Trust, London, UK

Sachin Malde
Consultant Urological Surgeon, Pelvic Floor Unit, Department of Urology, Guy's and St Thomas' NHS Foundation Trust, London, UK

Guglielmo Mantica
Consultant Urological Surgeon, Department of Urology, Policlinico San Martino Hospital, University of Genova, Genova, Italy

Sacha Moore
Academic Foundation Trainee, The Alan De Bolla Wrexham Urology Department, Wrexham Maelor Hospital, Wrexham, UK

Uwais Mufti
Post-CCT Clinical Fellow in Robotic Pelvic Urological Surgery, Department of Urology, Leeds Teaching Hospital NHS Trust, Leeds, UK

Naomi L. Neal
Consultant Urological Surgeon, Department of Urology, Hampshire Hospitals NHS Foundation Trust, UK

Joana B. Neves
Clinical Research Fellow, Division of Surgery and Interventional Science, University College London, London, UK

Richard Nobrega
Consultant Urological Surgeon, Department of Urology, University College London Hospitals NHS Foundation Trust, London, UK

Mohamed Noureldin
Clinical Fellow in Urological Surgery, Department of Urology, Imperial College Healthcare NHS Trust, London, UK

John M. O'Callaghan
Consultant Transplant Surgeon, University Hospitals Coventry and Warwickshire NHS Trust, Coventry, UK

Nadir I. Osman
Consultant Urological Surgeon, Section of Functional and Reconstructive Urology, Department of Urology, Sheffield Teaching Hospitals NHS Foundation Trust, Sheffield, UK

Emma Papworth
Urology Registrar, Department of Urology, North Bristol NHS Trust, Bristol, UK

Sanjeev Pathak
Consultant Urological Surgeon, Department of Urology, Sheffield Teaching Hospitals NHS Foundation Trust, Sheffield, UK

Nicola Pavan
Consultant Urological Surgeon, Department of Medical, Surgical and Health Science, University of Trieste, Trieste, Italy

Sarah Prattley
Clinical Fellow in Urological Surgery, Department of Urology, University Hospital Southampton NHS Foundation Trust, Southampton, UK

Anudini Ranasinghe
Female Functional Reconstructive Fellow, Department of Urology, University College London Hospitals NHS Foundation Trust, London, UK

Pravisha Ravindra
Consultant Urological Surgeon, Department of Urology, University Hospitals of Leicester NHS Trust, Leicester, UK

Antony C.P. Riddick
Consultant Urological Surgeon and Lead Clinician for Renal Cancer, Department of Urology, Cambridge University Hospitals NHS Foundation Trust, Cambridge, UK

Ishtiakul G. Rizvi
Urology Registrar, Department of Urology, Queen Elizabeth Hospital Birmingham, University Hospitals Birmingham NHS Foundation Trust, Birmingham, UK

Maria Satchi
Consultant Urological Surgeon, Department of Urology, Dartford and Gravesham NHS Trust, Kent, UK

Yousef Shahin
Academic Clinical Lecturer and Interventional Radiology Fellow, Department of Academic Unit of Radiology, University of Sheffield and Sheffield Teaching Hospitals, Sheffield, UK

Mostafa Sheba
Urology Registrar, Department of Urology, Cambridge University Hospitals NHS Foundation Trust, Cambridge, UK

Iqbal Shergill
Consultant Urological Surgeon, The Alan De Bolla Wrexham Urology Unit, Wrexham Maelor Hospital, Wrexham, UK

Martin Skott
Peadiatric Urology, Deparment of Urology, Aarhus University Hospital, Aarhus, Denmark

Pieter V. Spies
Senior Consultant and Lecturer, Division of Urology, Department of Surgical Sciences, Stellenbosch University and Tygerberg Academic Hospital, Cape Town, South Africa

Grant D. Stewart
Professor of Surgical Oncology, Department of Surgery, University of Cambridge, Cambridge, UK

Kiarash Taghavi
Consultant Paediatric Urological Surgeon, Department of Paediatric Urology, Monash Children's Hospital, Melbourne, Victoria, Australia

James Tracey
Clinical Fellow in Urological Surgery, Department of Urology, Guy's and St Thomas' NHS Foundation Trust, London, UK

Maxine G. B. Tran
Professor and Consultant Urological Surgeon, Division of Surgery and Interventional Science, University College London, London, UK

Fabio Traunero
Urology Registrar, Urology Clinic, Department of Medical, Surgical and Health Science, University of Trieste, Trieste, Italy

Lona Vyas
Consultant Urological Surgeon with Specialist Interest in Andrology, Department of Urology, Chelsea and Westminster Hospital NHS Foundation Trust, London, UK

Matthew Young
Consultant Urological Surgeon, Department of Urology, Mid Yorkshire Hospitals NHS Trust, Wakefield, UK

CURRICULUM MAP

Chapter	1	2	3	4	5	6	7	8	9	10	11	12	13	14	15	16
	Recurrent urinary tract infection	Prostatitis	Renal stones	Ureteric stones	Bladder stone management	Ureteropelvic junction obstruction	Oncocytoma	Localized prostate cancer	Oligometastatic prostate cancer	Newly diagnosed metastatic prostate cancer	Non-muscle-invasive bladder cancer	Muscle invasive bladder cancer	High grade non-muscle invasive bladder cancer	Renal cancer (inferior vena cava tumour)	Metastatic renal cancer	Upper urinary tract urothelial carcinoma
Final stage topics for all trainees																
Basic science						✓	✓			✓	✓	✓	✓	✓	✓	
Clinical pharmacology	✓			✓						✓	✓	✓	✓	✓	✓	
Stone disease			✓	✓	✓	✓										
Urinary tract obstruction				✓		✓						✓				✓

Chapter	17	18	19	20	21	22	23	24	25	26	27	28	29	30	31	32
	Localized penile cancer	Advanced and metastatic penile cancer	Growing teratoma syndrome in testis cancer	Metastatic testicular cancer	Benign prostatic enlargement and acute urinary retention	Chronic retention, renal failure, and diuresis	Urge urinary incontinence	Stress urinary incontinence	Bladder pain syndrome/interstitial cystitis	Female urinary retention	Neurogenic bladder	Genitourinary prolapse	Urethral stricture disease	Urethral diverticulum	Ketamine induced upper-UTI	Vesicovaginal fistula
Final stage topics for all trainees																
Basic science				✓		✓	✓	✓	✓	✓	✓	✓	✓			
Clinical pharmacology			✓	✓	✓	✓	✓	✓	✓	✓						
Stone disease																
Urinary tract obstruction					✓	✓				✓	✓		✓		✓	

Chapter	33	34	35	36	37	38	39	40	41	42	43	44	45	46	47	48
	Male factor infertility	Erectile dysfunction	Peyronie's disease	Ejaculatory orgasmic disorders	Testicular torsion controversies	Priapism	Renal trauma	Bladder and ureteric trauma	Penile fracture	Renal transplantation	Recurrent UTIs/Non-neurogenic bladder in children	Undescended testis	Neurogenic bladder in children	Haemorrhagic eschar of the glans	Vesicoureterel reflux in children	Acute interventional radiology procedures in urology
Final stage topics for all trainees																
Basic science	✓	✓	✓	✓	✓	✓			✓	✓	✓	✓		✓		
Clinical pharmacology		✓	✓	✓		✓				✓	✓			✓		
Stone disease																
Urinary tract obstruction											✓				✓	✓

Urinary tract infections	✓		✓	✓	✓						✓										✓		✓	✓	✓	✓	✓		✓	✓													✓		✓	✓	✓	✓
Urinary incontinence								✓													✓		✓	✓			✓	✓		✓		✓											✓		✓			
Urological oncology									✓		✓	✓	✓	✓	✓	✓		✓	✓	✓																												✓
Andrology																																	✓	✓	✓	✓		✓			✓							
Paediatric urology																																											✓	✓	✓	✓	✓	
Renal function/ nephrology				✓		✓						✓				✓						✓					✓				✓											✓	✓				✓	
Emergency urology			✓	✓						✓																✓											✓	✓	✓	✓	✓							✓
Urinary tract trauma			✓																									✓				✓							✓	✓								
Urological radiology			✓	✓	✓	✓	✓	✓		✓		✓	✓	✓	✓	✓			✓	✓		✓		✓			✓		✓	✓	✓						✓	✓	✓	✓	✓		✓		✓		✓	✓
Urinary tract stone disease																																																
Renal calculi			✓			✓																																										
Ureteric calculi				✓																																												
Bladder calculi					✓																																											
Benign disease of the upper urinary tract																																																
Upper tract obstruction						✓																									✓																	
Pelviureteric junction obstruction						✓																									✓																	
Ureteric strictures																															✓																	✓
Renal failure																						✓									✓																	
Prostate cancer																																																
Locally confined prostate cancer (T1a–T2c)								✓																																								
Locally advanced (T3–T4) N0 M0								✓	✓																																							
Metastatic disease (any T, and N, M1)									✓	✓																																						
Hormone-refractory disease										✓																																						
Bladder cancer																																																
Superficial bladder cancer (pTis and pTa-1 G1–G3)											✓		✓																																			

Chapter	1	2	3	4	5	6	7	8	9	10	11	12	13	14	15	16	17	18	19	20	21	22	23	24	25	26	27	28	29	30	31	32	33	34	35	36	37	38	39	40	41	42	43	44	45	46	47	48
Muscle invasive bladder cancer (pT2–4)												✓	✓																																			
Metastatic bladder cancer													✓																																			
Renal cancer																																																
Localized renal cancer														✓																																		
Metastatic renal cancer															✓																																	
Upper tract transitional cell carcinoma																✓																																
Penile cancer																																																
Management of the primary cancer																		✓																														
Management of the lymph nodes																		✓																														
Metastatic penile cancer																		✓																														
Testicular cancer																																																
Management of the primary cancer																			✓	✓																												
Metastatic testis cancer																			✓	✓																												
Female urology																																																
Management of continence problems in the elderly and the cognitively impaired																							✓																									
Urinary frequency/ urgency syndrome and urinary urge incontinence																							✓					✓		✓																		
Bladder and pelvic pain syndromes																							✓		✓																							

Stress urinary incontinence and mixed urinary incontinence																						✓	✓																								
Female urinary retention																									✓																						
Genitourinary prolapse																									✓		✓																				
Urinary fistula																															✓																
Urethral diverticulum																									✓				✓																		
Trauma to the genitourinary tract in women																											✓				✓																
Bladder and upper urinary tract reconstruction																																																
Assessment and follow-up of patients requiring urinary tract reconstruction																										✓				✓																	
Urethral reconstruction																																																
Male urethral reconstruction																												✓																			
Neurourology																																																
Neurogenic bladder or sexual dysfunction			✓																						✓	✓																✓					
Male factor infertility																																																
Male factor infertility																		✓														✓															
Benign disorders of male sexual dysfunction																																																
Erectile dysfunction																																	✓	✓													
Penile deformity																																		✓													
Prolonged erection																																					✓										
Rapid ejaculation, retrograde ejaculation, delayed ejaculation, orgasmic disorders, desire disorders																			✓																✓												
Penile fracture																																								✓							

Chapter	1	2	3	4	5	6	7	8	9	10	11	12	13	14	15	16	17	18	19	20	21	22	23	24	25	26	27	28	29	30	31	32	33	34	35	36	37	38	39	40	41	42	43	44	45	46	47	48
Paediatric urology																																																
Congenital disorders affecting the urinary tract																																												✓	✓	✓	✓	
Urinary tract infections																																											✓		✓	✓	✓	
The acute scrotum																																					✓											
Upper urinary tract obstruction																																											✓		✓		✓	
Radiology																																											✓		✓		✓	
Urinary incontinence and neuropathic bladder																																											✓		✓		✓	
Assessment of children requiring urinary tract reconstruction																																													✓	✓	✓	
Assessment and management of boys requiring urethral reconstruction																																														✓		
Renal transplantation																																																
Renal transplantation																✓																										✓						

SECTION 1

Urinary tract infection

CASE

Recurrent urinary tract infection

Christopher K. Harding

Expert commentary Christopher K. Harding

Case history

A 55-year-old postmenopausal woman was referred from primary care following a 3-year history of recurrent urinary tract infections (rUTIs). These episodes often presented as infective cystitis with dysuria, increased urinary frequency (including new-onset nocturia), and offensive smelling cloudy urine[1] and were usually without any systemic symptoms. She described these infections as occurring approximately six times per year and informed that they were previously responsive to short-course narrow-spectrum antibiotic therapy with either nitrofurantoin or trimethoprim. More recently, she had been requiring longer or multiple antibiotic courses to resolve her symptoms. She had been referred to another hospital 2 years ago with non-visible haematuria and had a full urinary tract evaluation via a renal ultrasound scan, a flexible cystoscopy, and a urine flow study which revealed no structural or functional abnormalities. Her estimated glomerular filtration rate was normal. Serial urine cultures obtained over the preceding 12–18 months had shown a variety of uropathogenic organisms but most often *Escherichia coli* was isolated. Over the preceding 6 months, the episodes had increased in frequency and the patient reported the feeling of having 'an almost constant' urinary tract infection (UTI). Her last two urine cultures had again shown evidence of *E. coli* exhibiting antimicrobial resistance (AMR) to nitrofurantoin and amoxycillin. She was referred to a specialist rUTI clinic for consideration of preventative treatment.

Learning point Definitions and statistics

- UTI is described as complicated or uncomplicated with the latter referring to occurrence in a structurally and functionally normal urinary tract. The vast majority of rUTIs are uncomplicated.
- Most national and international guidelines[2–4] do not recommend routine investigation of women with rUTIs because the diagnostic yield is low.
- rUTI can occur due to either bacterial persistence or reinfection. Persistence is suspected if there is infection with the same bacterial species within a short time frame after clinical resolution of a previous episode.
- Most clinicians would classify rUTI as being two episodes of infection in 6 months, or three episodes in 1 year.
- The annual incidence of a single UTI is approximately 30 per 1000 women, with almost half of affected women experiencing recurrence within 12 months.
- rUTI is associated with significant morbidity, studies estimate an average of 6 days of symptoms, 2 days of restricted activity, and 1 day of time off work per episode.

Expert comment Diagnosis of UTI

- UTI is the inflammatory response of the urothelium to microbial pathogens.
- Traditionally, diagnosis has required the demonstration of bacteria at concentrations $\geq 10^5$ colony-forming units/mL using culture methods that were developed in the 1950s—a time when urine was thought to be a sterile fluid.
- Recent work has demonstrated that the urinary tract has its own microbiome.
- Some research studies are moving away from microbiological confirmation of UTI and are recommending a clinical diagnosis based on symptoms and antibiotic requirement.[6]
- Despite this, the current guideline recommendation is that UTI should be diagnosed by urine culture.[4]
- The challenge for future diagnostic tests is to define the pathogen from the large numbers of bacteria that may colonize the urinary tract.[5]

The patient herself had expressed a concern regarding her recent (necessary) antibiotic consumption and wanted to explore prophylactic options, especially non-antibiotic alternatives. In line with the European Association of Urology guidelines on urological infections[4] which state that 'prevention of rUTI includes counselling regarding avoidance of risk factors, non-antimicrobial measures and antimicrobial prophylaxis', the patient's initial consultations were structured sequentially in this manner.

Expert comment AMR

Central to the discussion regarding UTI prevention should be an exploration with the patient of the dangers of AMR, which is an emerging global problem. In 2018, the UK National Institute for Health and Care Excellence (NICE) released a guideline entitled 'Urinary tract infection (recurrent): antimicrobial prescribing'.[7] One of the aims of this guideline was to 'optimise antibiotic use and reduce antibiotic resistance'. The UK AMR strategy and action plan highlights the fact that 'no new classes of antibiotic have been discovered since the 1980s' and states 'inappropriate use of the drugs we already have, means we are heading rapidly towards a world in which our antibiotics no longer work'.[8] It is postulated that AMR represents adaptive selection by microorganisms which is in part secondary to the overuse of antimicrobial agents. Statistics taken from this document reveal that resistant infections are estimated to cause 700,000 deaths each year and highlight that the World Bank estimates an extra 28 million people could be forced into extreme poverty by 2050 unless AMR is contained. The extent of AMR in nosocomial UTIs has been described in a recent 8-year study which reported overall global and regional resistance rates as >20% for all antibiotics studied (which included trimethoprim, cefuroxime, amoxicillin, gentamicin, and piperacillin–tazobactam) with the single exception of imipenem.[9]

It was pointed out to the patient that lifestyle measures such as regular voiding, immediate postcoital urination, wiping from front to back, douching, and avoiding occlusive underwear have previously been believed to reduce the risk of rUTI but several studies have 'consistently documented the lack of association with rUTI'.[10] A study showing high-level evidence of benefit from increasing oral fluid intake in women who admit to poor hydration and suffer with rUTIs was discussed with the patient as she volunteered that she 'didn't drink a lot of fluid'. This randomized controlled trial (RCT) involved 140 premenopausal women with rUTIs who reported drinking < 1.5 L of total fluid daily. In this trial, UTI episodes were reduced by 47% in women who drank an extra 1.5 L of water per day over a 12-month period compared with women who maintained their usual fluid intake.[11] The evidence for the association of UTI and recent sexual intercourse, the use of spermicide, and the use of condoms was highlighted.[3] None of this was applicable to our patient as she had been celibate for 5 years. The patient reported some previous symptomatic relief with over-the-counter cystitis remedies and the role of changing urinary pH was debated. The evidence from the Cochrane review on urinary alkalinization was highlighted.[12] Despite reviewing 172 studies on the subject, the review concluded that not a single report was suitable for inclusion in a meta-analysis due to various factors and hence no recommendation could be made. The clinical advice was that these remedies were reasonable to try if the patient had previously achieved benefit but it was pointed out that alkalinization of the urine would not be recommended if the patient elected to try the urinary antiseptic methenamine hippurate as a prophylactic agent because its efficacy is dependent on acid urine.

Non-antibiotic options for rUTI prevention were then outlined and discussions centred around the treatments with high-level evidence to evaluate their effect: probiotics, methenamine hippurate, cranberry supplements, and topical vaginal oestrogen. Probiotics are microorganisms introduced into the body for their beneficial qualities and have been well studied in the context of rUTI. A meta-analysis including nine RCTs comprising 735 patients, with significant risks of selection and attrition bias, showed benefits were not statistically significant versus placebo (risk ratio (RR) = 0.82) or antibiotics (RR = 1.12).[13] However, it was commented that 'benefit cannot be ruled out as the number of patients was small and the trials had poor methodological reporting'. The patient was told that there was insufficient current evidence to say how effective probiotics could be in her case, but the low reported incidence of side effects was highlighted, and so she may wish to try them. These adverse events included vaginal discharge, genital irritation, and diarrhoea and were quantified as affecting 3% of patients in this meta-analysis.

Methenamine hippurate is a urinary antiseptic that is licensed for prevention of rUTI using a dose of 1 g twice daily. It is hydrolysed to formaldehyde in the distal convoluted tubule of the kidney in the presence of acidic urine. Formaldehyde is bactericidal and probably acts via denaturation of bacterial proteins. The evidence for methenamine has been collated in a meta-analysis which included 2032 patients from 13 RCTs, with one of the included trials reporting a significant reduction in UTI frequency when women with uncomplicated rUTIs were studied (RR = 0.46).[14] Contraindications for the use of methenamine include gout, hepatic impairment, and renal impairment. The patient had a past medical history of gout and therefore this treatment was not considered.

The discussion then moved on to cranberry supplements as these had been recommended to the patient by one of her friends. The best evidence for cranberries comes from a meta-analysis including 24 studies and comprising 4473 participants which showed no significant reduction in symptomatic UTI for women with rUTIs and hence this treatment was not recommended.[15] The patient had given a history of vulvodynia and clinical examination had confirmed vaginal atrophy, so she was interested to hear about topical vaginal oestrogen as a preventative treatment against rUTI. A meta-analysis which included three RCTs comparing vaginal oestrogen to placebo (RR = 0.25) reported benefit in terms of UTI reduction but highlighted that this benefit was not seen with oral hormone replacement therapy.[6] The included trials contained only small patient numbers with differing results. Current guidelines reflect this and only make a weak recommendation for its use. Adverse events such as breast tenderness, vaginal bleeding, non-physiological vaginal discharge, and vaginal irritation/burning were detailed but these are reported in a minority of participants only. The consultation was concluded with an exploration of current promising treatments; D-mannose, immunostimulants/vaccines, and intravesical preparations. However, the patient opted to try a regimen of increased fluid intake and topical oestrogen with a planned review in 4 months.

Evidence base Reviews from Cochrane evaluating preventative non-antibiotic options for rUTI

Urinary alkalinization

Urinary alkalinization achieved using oral medications, such as potassium citrate, to reduce the acidity of urine is postulated to reduce the severity of dysuria. No recommendations were possible given the low quality of existing evidence, but the authors concluded that larger, well-designed RCTs are necessary and should include symptomatic rUTI as a primary outcome.[12]

Probiotics

Probiotics refers to the use of medicines containing live bacteria or yeast that supplements normal gastrointestinal flora. These organisms (e.g. *Lactobacillus* spp.) are thought to modulate host defences by reducing pathogen adherence, growth, and colonization. The Cochrane review failed to show any benefit from the use of probiotics as prophylaxis against rUTI.[13]

Methenamine hippurate

Methenamine hippurate is hydrolysed to formaldehyde in the presence of acidic urine and has a bactericidal effect on *E. coli*. The conclusion of the Cochrane meta-analysis was that it may be useful in reducing symptomatic UTI in patients with uncomplicated UTIs.[14]

Cranberry supplements

It is postulated that cranberries (active ingredient: proanthocyanidin) prevent bacteria (particularly *E. coli*) from adhering to the urothelium and create an acidic urine which impedes bacterial colonization of the urinary tract. The conclusions of the Cochrane review were that cranberry supplements did not significantly reduce UTI incidence when compared with placebo or no treatment.[15]

Topical oestrogen

Topical application of vaginal oestrogen lowers vaginal pH, improves vaginal atrophy, and increases vaginal lactobacilli colonization which is protective against uropathogenic *E. coli*. The meta-analysis demonstrated a benefit of topical oestrogen in terms of UTI reduction but included trials contained only small numbers and no firm recommendations were possible.[16]

Future directions Emerging preventative treatments

D-mannose

D-mannose is a naturally occurring sugar postulated to prevent bacterial adhesion to urothelium via direct binding to bacterial fimbriae. A single good-quality RCT has shown its effect was comparable to daily low-dose antibiotics (nitrofurantoin).[17] The rate of symptomatic infections was significantly reduced (when compared to placebo) by D-mannose in this study (RR = 0.24) which used a daily dose of 2 g taken as 1 g twice a day.

Immunostimulants

Immunostimulants contain heat-killed/inert uropathogens designed to upregulate the patient's immune response to infection. They are not true vaccines as they do not confer acquired immunity to a specific pathogen. The oral immunostimulant OM-89 is an immunologically active bacterial lysate of 18 *E. coli* strains and has been shown in a meta-analysis of 891 patients from four RCTs to confer significant benefit in women with rUTIs in terms of reducing recurrent episodes (RR = 0.61).[18]

Intravesical preparations

Intravesical treatment is in two main forms. Firstly, substances aimed at replacing the glycosaminoglycan layer which is superficial to urothelial umbrella cells and hence is putatively protective against bacterial adherence and secondly, antibiotics which are administered directly into the bladder. A meta-analysis examining the use of hyaluronic acid as a glycosaminoglycan replacement substance included two randomized studies showing an improvement in the rates of rUTI which equated to improved prevention of over three episodes per patient year.[19] Intravesical antibiotics are not as well studied but a meta-analysis consisting mainly of case series reported a 71% success rate (poorly defined) and a low (8%) discontinuation rate.[20]

At the 4-month review appointment, the patient reported two discrete episodes of UTI since starting the regimen of increased fluid intake and topical oestrogen. She stated that the increase in her fluid intake made her feel better in general and she intended to continue with her current daily fluid intake which was estimated at 2.5–3 L. However, she did not feel that these changes had been effective in reducing the frequency of her infections and was seeking further treatment for these episodes. It was pointed out that the use of low-dose daily antibiotics was considered the most evidence-based therapy for her condition and that they were strongly recommended by international guidelines.[4] The Cochrane systematic review and meta-analysis of the effect of prophylactic antibiotics on recurrence rates was summarized for the patient.[21] It included 19 RCTs with data from > 1000 patients. A reduction in the incidence of symptomatic infection with daily antibiotics compared to placebo of 85% is reported (RR = 0.15). This review calculated that the number needed to treat with prophylactic antibiotics to prevent recurrence over a 6–12-month period was 1.85. Side effects including vaginal and oral candidiasis and gastrointestinal symptoms were outlined but the rates were low in the meta-analysis and severe side effects were thought to be rare. The patient elected to try the low-dose antibiotics and, in line with NICE recommendations, a narrow-spectrum agent, trimethoprim, was chosen and a dose of 100 mg per day recommended.[7] The patient was told of the significant rate of relapse following completion of the low-dose antibiotic treatment in that only a risk reduction of 0.82 was reported following treatment completion (compared to 0.15 during therapy). A 9-month review was scheduled, and the patient was instructed to take the daily antibiotics for the first 6-months. At review, the patient reported zero episodes of UTI while on the treatment. During the subsequent 3 months without treatment she had suffered very short-lived periods of dysuria but none of these required therapeutic antibiotics and resolved with increasing fluid intake only. She was discharged at this stage with advice to consider a further 6-month period of low-dose antibiotics if the infections became recurrent again.

A final word from the expert

The presentation described is very common and one which most urologists would encounter regularly. Although it is widely accepted that the majority of these patients do not require extensive investigation, arriving at a diagnosis of rUTI is not always straightforward. Reliance on urine culture results has been called into question recently and it is not unusual to see patients with a series of negative culture results who report resolution of symptoms from courses of therapeutic antibiotics. The effect of previous antibiotic treatment is important to elicit when taking a history and this must be considered alongside the fact that standard urine culture is not 100% accurate for UTI diagnosis. It is probably reasonable to assume that a patient with episodic urinary symptoms and bladder pain who responds to antibiotics has rUTIs, in spite of urine culture results. Patients presenting with serial negative cultures do, however, merit more in the way of investigations and a cystoscopy, renal tract ultrasound, and urine flow study are often indicated in these cases.

The range of available treatments necessitates a lengthy discussion with the patient as outlined above. It is important when managing patients with rUTIs to ensure they understand the importance of simple measures such as increasing fluid intake but that these are often not enough to control the frequency of infections, the effect of which can be very debilitating. There are several non-antibiotic alternatives for rUTI but the evidence for them is generally weak with several meta-analyses all identifying studies of poor methodological quality. Fortunately, most of the non-antibiotic agents currently in use have a favourable side effect profile and therefore a trial of any of these agents can be considered low risk. Long-term, low-dose prophylactic antibiotics remain the treatment with the most supportive evidence to recommend their use, but this has to be balanced against the theoretical risk of AMR both within the individual and within the community. AMR has received a lot of publicity in recent years and is recognized as a significant global threat. As a consequence, the patient may (as in this case) prefer to try non-antibiotic options first. If it is decided, by clinician and patient together, that low-dose antibiotics are preferred then it is important to keep the patient under close review with any symptom exacerbations or breakthrough infections carefully recorded. This will allow the time spent on antibiotic treatment to be kept to a minimum and enable prompt discontinuation when appropriate. It may be necessary in very severe cases to use a combination of prophylactic therapies such as antibiotics plus methenamine alongside the simple lifestyle modifications described.

It is evident from a review of the currently available literature that there is a paucity of high-quality studies in this topic area. Future research should concentrate not only on improving the speed and accuracy of UTI diagnosis but ensure that meaningful comparative treatments are included in trials. Given that long-term, low-dose narrow-spectrum antibiotics are widely accepted as the gold-standard treatment for this condition, any novel treatments should be compared to them in order for an accurate assessment of relative efficacy to be achieved. Finally, development of a bespoke patient-reported outcome measure for rUTI patients would allow for easier pooling of trial results in future meta-analyses.

References

1. Public Health England. Urinary tract infection: diagnostic tools for primary care. GOV.UK. 19 October 2020. https://www.gov.uk/government/publications/urinary-tract-infection-diagnosis
2. Barclay J, Veeratterapillay R, Harding C. Non-antibiotic options for recurrent urinary tract infections in women. *BMJ.* 2017;359:j5193.
3. Sihra N, Goodman A, Zakri R, Sahai A, Malde S. Nonantibiotic prevention and management of recurrent urinary tract infection. *Nat Rev Urol.* 2018;15(12):750–776.
4. Bonkat G, Bartoletti RR, Bruyère F, et al. EAU guidelines on urological infections. European Association of Urology. March 2019. https://uroweb.org/wp-content/uploads/EAU-Guidelines-on-Urological-infections-2019.pdf
5. Harding C, Rantell A, Cardozo L, et al. How can we improve investigation, prevention and treatment for recurrent urinary tract infections—ICI-RS 2018. *Neurourol Urodyn.* 2019;38(Suppl 5):S90–S97.

6. Forbes R, Ali, A, Abouhajar A. et al. ALternatives To prophylactic Antibiotics for the treatment of Recurrent urinary tract infection in women (ALTAR): study protocol for a multicentre, pragmatic, patient-randomised, non-inferiority trial. *Trials.* 2018;19:616.
7. National Institute for Health and Care Excellence. Urinary tract infection (recurrent): antimicrobial prescribing. NICE guideline [NG112]. National Institute for Health and Care Excellence. 31 October 2018. https://www.nice.org.uk/guidance/ng112
8. Department of Health and Social Care. Tackling antimicrobial resistance 2019–2024: the UK's five-year national action plan. HM Government. 24 January 2019. https://assets.publishing.service.gov.uk/government/uploads/system/uploads/attachment_data/file/784894/UK_AMR_5_year_national_action_plan.pdf
9. Tandogdu Z, Cek M, Wagenlehner F, et al. Resistance patterns of nosocomial urinary tract infections in urology departments: 8-year results of the global prevalence of infections in urology study. *World J Urol.* 2014;32(3):791–801.
10. Hooton TM. Recurrent urinary tract infection in women. *Int J Antimicrob Agents.* 2001;17(4):259–268.
11. Hooton TM, Vecchio M, Iroz A, et al. Effect of increased daily water intake in premenopausal women with recurrent urinary tract infections: a randomized clinical trial. *JAMA Intern Med.* 2018;178(11):1509–1515.
12. O'Kane DB, Dave SK, Gore N, et al. Urinary alkalisation for symptomatic uncomplicated urinary tract infection in women. *Cochrane Database Syst Rev.* 2016;4(4):CD010745.
13. Schwenger EM, Tejani AM, Loewen PS. Probiotics for preventing urinary tract infections in adults and children. *Cochrane Database Syst Rev.* 2015;15(12):CD008772.
14. Lee BSB, Bhuta T, Simpson JM, Craig JC. Methenamine hippurate for preventing urinary tract infections. *Cochrane Database Syst Rev.* 2012;10(10):CD003265.
15. Jepson RG, Williams G, Craig JC. Cranberries for preventing urinary tract infections. *Cochrane Database Syst Rev.* 2012;10(10):CD001321.
16. Perrotta C, Aznar M, Mejia R, Albert X, Ng CW. Oestrogens for preventing recurrent urinary tract infection in postmenopausal women. *Cochrane Database Syst Rev.* 2008;2:CD005131.
17. Kranjcec B, Papeš D, Altarac S. D-mannose powder for prophylaxis of recurrent urinary tract infections in women: a randomized clinical trial. *World J Urol.* 2014;32(1):79–84.
18. Naber KG, Cho YH, Matsumoto T, Schaeffer AJ. Immunoactive prophylaxis of recurrent urinary tract infections: a meta-analysis. *Int J Antimicrob Agents.* 2009;33(2):111–119.
19. De Vita D, Antell H, Giordano S. Effectiveness of intravesical hyaluronic acid with or without chondroitin sulfate for recurrent bacterial cystitis in adult women: a meta-analysis. *Int Urogynecol J.* 2013;24(4):545–552.
20. Pietropaolo A, Jones P, Moors M, et al. Use and effectiveness of antimicrobial intravesical treatment for prophylaxis and treatment of recurrent urinary tract infections (UTIs): a systematic review. *Curr Urol Rep.* 2018;19(10):78.
21. Albert X, Huertas I, Pereiró II, Sanfélix J, Gosalbes V, Perrota C. Antibiotics for preventing recurrent urinary tract infection in non-pregnant women. *Cochrane Database Syst Rev.* 2004;3:CD001209.

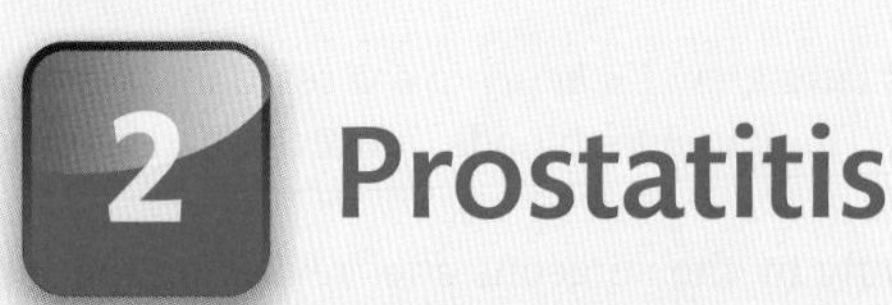

Prostatitis

Uwais Mufti and Ased Ali

Expert commentary Ased Ali

Case history

A 65-year-old male was admitted under the acute medical team through the accident and emergency department with a short history of difficulty passing urine. He felt slightly unwell and had saturation of 92% on air with associated decreased air entry into the left lung base. He gave a history of smoking. He denied any preceding lower urinary tract symptoms (LUTS).

A chest X-ray ruled out a lower respiratory tract infection but he was found to be in urinary retention. He was catheterized and a residual of around 835 mL drained. A urine dipstick test showed glucose 2 +, leucocytes 2 +, and nitrites. A urine specimen was sent for microscopy, culture, and sensitivity. His white cell count was 16.7 × 10^9/L, estimated glomerular filtration rate had decreased to 22 mL/min/1.73 m^2 from a baseline of 84 mL/min/1.73 m^2, and creatinine concentration had increased from a baseline of 83 μmol/L to 253 μmol/L. An ultrasound scan of the urinary tract showed no abnormalities in the kidneys and in particular, there was no hydronephrosis. The patient was given a stat dose of 1.2 g of intravenous co-amoxiclav in the emergency department but this was not continued. He had also reported a history of weight loss and was asked to see his general practitioner about this.

Learning point Risk factors, presentation, and treatment

Acute bacterial prostatitis (ABP) is an ascending urinary tract infection (UTI). The risk factors include benign prostatic enlargement, genitourinary infections including sexually transmitted infections, immunocompromised state, urethral stricture, and prostatic manipulations such as prostatic massage, prostate biopsy, and urethral catheterization.

Patients usually report a sudden onset or worsening of existing LUTS (storage or voiding). Systemic symptoms such as fever and malaise are not infrequent.

In this case, the risk was higher owing to factors like benign prostatic enlargement, urethral catheterization, and a history of diabetes. The patient was not treated with a course of antibiotics despite a strong suspicion of UTI on the urine dipstick. In ABP, urine dipstick testing has a positive predictive value of 95% and a negative predictive value of 70%. Unsurprisingly the urine culture was subsequently positive.

A urology consultation was requested and a diagnosis of 'high-pressure chronic retention' (interactive obstructive uropathy) was made. DRE suggested a moderately enlarged smooth prostate. A plan to discharge the patient with an indwelling catheter and review in a urology clinic to discuss options was suggested.

The urine culture reported a few days later grew *Escherichia coli* resistant to amoxicillin, trimethoprim, and pivmecillinam. The patient's bloods, however, had returned to baseline.

Ten days later he was admitted urgently by the surgeons after reviewing the findings of a computed tomography (CT) scan done for a short history of general deterioration and weight loss of around two stones (about 13 kg). The CT scan had suggested a primary sigmoid tumour later proven to be a poorly differentiated adenocarcinoma pT3N1cR0. A prostatic abscess was also noted on the CT scan and hence a urology opinion was sought at that time (Figure 2.1).

Clinical tip Evaluation

Digital rectal examination (DRE) in patients is performed gently due to the risk of bacteraemia and sepsis if done vigorously. For this reason, prostatic massage is contraindicated.

The Meares–Stamey four-glass or modified two-glass test (described below) is used in the diagnosis of chronic bacterial prostatitis (CBP) but this test is contraindicated in ABP as it involves a prostatic massage.

Learning point Aetiology of bacterial prostatitis

Being an ascending UTI, ABP has similar microbial aetiology. Enterobacteriaceae are the commonest pathogens. *E. coli* as was seen in this case accounts for 67% of cases while *Pseudomonas aeruginosa* is seen in 16% and *Klebsiella* spp. in 6%. *Proteus* and *Serratia* have been implicated as well. *Neisseria gonorrhoeae* and *Chlamydia trachomatis* should be considered in young sexually active men. Atypical organisms such as *Salmonella*, *Candida*, and *Cryptococcus* can be a cause in immunocompromised patients.

Only about 5–10% cases of ABP progress to CBP. In CBP, the microbiological spectrum is wider. Although *E. coli* is the most common organism implicated, Gram-positive cocci were most common isolates in patients with CBP. These include coagulase-negative *Staphylococcus*, *Enterococcus faecalis*, *Streptococcus* spp., and *Staph. aureus*.[1] Some studies have shown that majority of cases of CBP are monomicrobial but a significant percentage may be polymicrobial.

The patient was haemodynamically stable and apyrexial. On DRE, the prostate felt tender and abnormal. He was started on ciprofloxacin 500 mg twice daily with a plan to intervene if he showed signs of sepsis based on change in clinical parameters or increase in inflammatory markers.

As the patient started spiking a fever, he was switched to intravenous co-amoxiclav and a transrectal drainage was arranged. Seven millilitres of thick pus were aspirated to dryness. This specimen grew *E. coli* on culture.

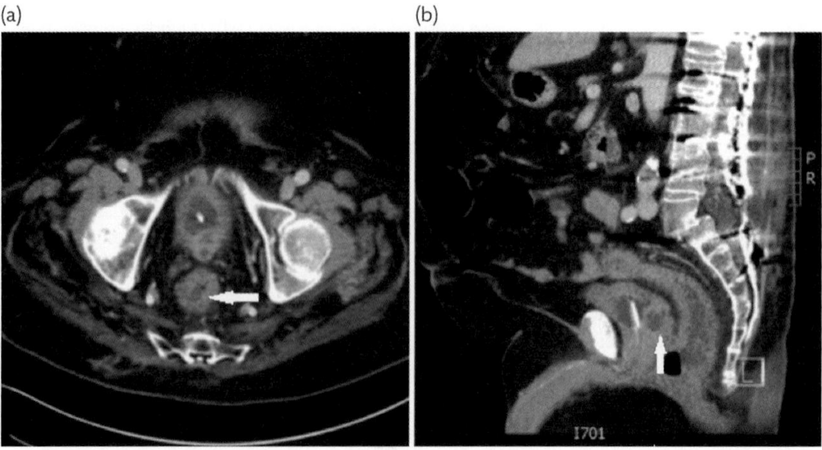

Figure 2.1 Abdomen–pelvis cross-sectional imaging with CT. (a) Transverse section and (b) sagittal section showing a prostatic abscess (red arrow) in a catheterized patient.

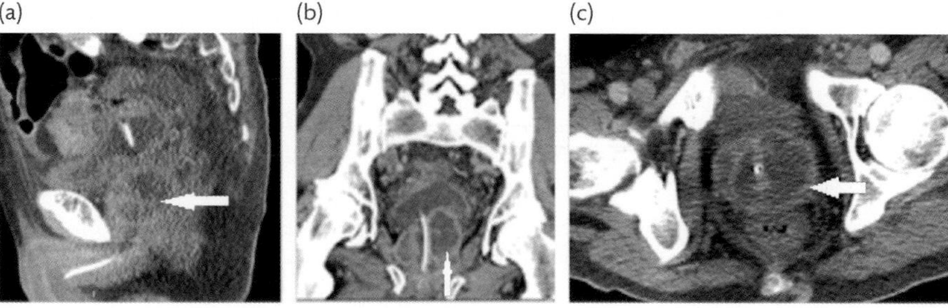

Figure 2.2 Cross-sectional imaging of the pelvis. (a) Coronal section, (b) sagittal section, and (c) transverse section showing progression in appearances of the known prostatic abscess (red arrow) despite transrectal drainage.

The patient initially showed signs of recovery but thereafter had further episodes of pyrexia and his inflammatory markers worsened. A repeat CT scan was carried out and this demonstrated multifocal prostatic abscesses (Figure 2.2).

Learning point Imaging in prostatic abscess

Transrectal ultrasound (TRUS) is a reliable and accurate method to diagnose prostatic abscess[2] and is the most commonly used one as it is readily available. However, some patients with prostatic abscess may find the TRUS probe in the rectum too painful. CT can selectively be used in cases where TRUS is not tolerated and also in cases where extra-prostatic spread or necrotising infection is suspected.[3] Magnetic resonance imaging (MRI) provides better resolution than CT and can even diagnose early stages of abscess formation where TRUS can be inconclusive.[4] However, as MRI availability is often more limited, it is less widely used.

At this point, a decision to carry out a transurethral drainage of the prostatic abscess was made. On cystoscopy no obvious abnormality was seen in the prostatic urethra but on incising the prostatic urethra at the 6 o'clock position, an abscess cavity proximal to the verumontanum opened up and a significant volume of pus discharge was seen. A three-way catheter was introduced over a guidewire to allow drainage of any residual pus. The planned catheter removal was carried out 3 weeks later.

Expert comment Management of prostatic abscess

In this patient a diagnosis of prostatic abscess was made and this most likely was a complication of untreated UTI at the time of urethral instrumentation leading to ABP. The patient was initially treated conservatively as per guidelines as a complicated UTI. As he failed to improve, the management interventions were escalated. Both conservative and drainage interventions are feasible strategies in prostatic abscess cases. However, conservative management is more likely to succeed if the abscess cavity is <1 cm in size. Larger abscesses require either a single aspiration or continuous drainage for a successful outcome. A flow chart adapted from Abdelmoteleb et al.[5] depicting management of patients with prostatic abscess is depicted in Figure 2.3.

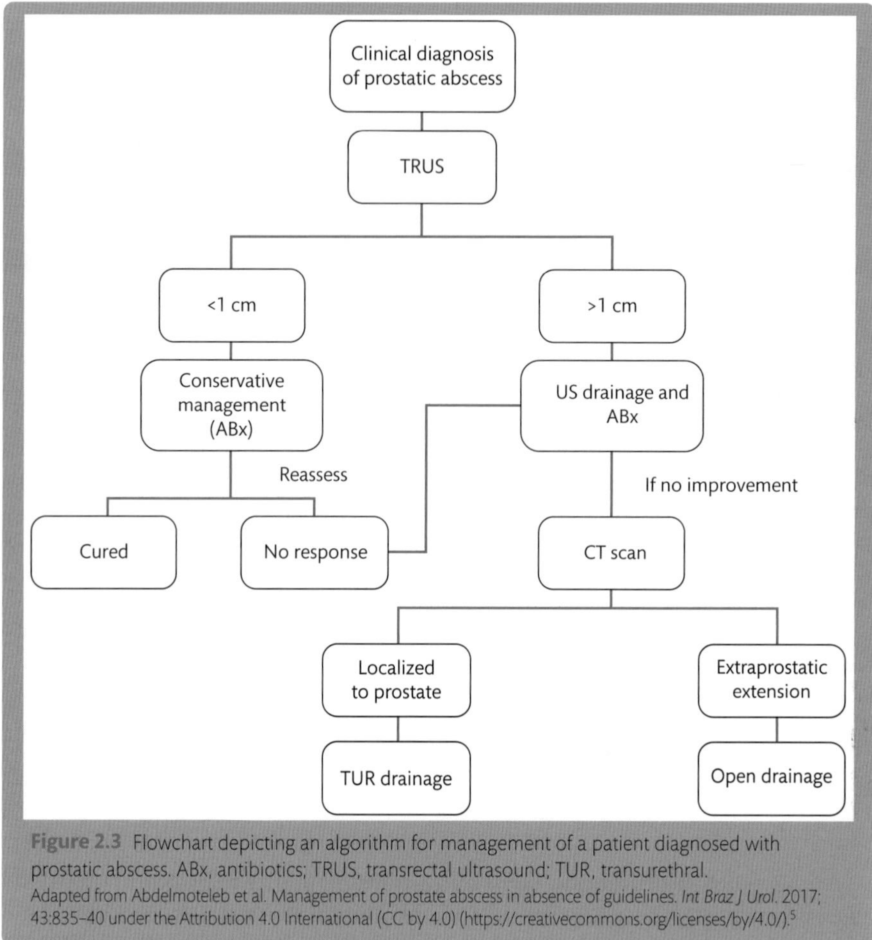

Figure 2.3 Flowchart depicting an algorithm for management of a patient diagnosed with prostatic abscess. ABx, antibiotics; TRUS, transrectal ultrasound; TUR, transurethral.
Adapted from Abdelmoteleb et al. Management of prostate abscess in absence of guidelines. *Int Braz J Urol*. 2017; 43:835–40 under the Attribution 4.0 International (CC by 4.0) (https://creativecommons.org/licenses/by/4.0/).[5]

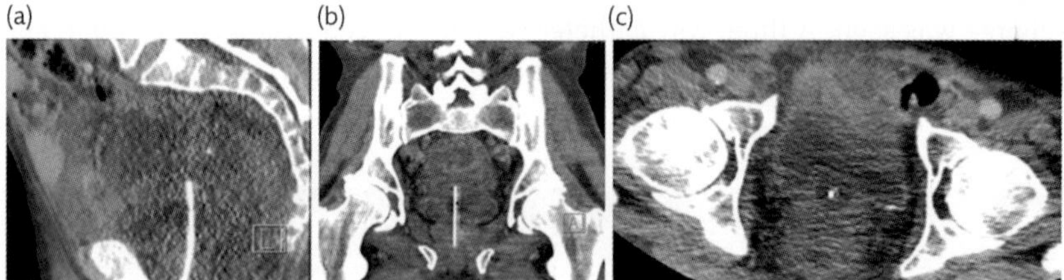

Figure 2.4 Cross-sectional imaging of the pelvis. (a) Coronal section, (b) sagittal section, and (c) transverse section showing resolution of prostatic abscess following transurethral drainage.

The patient recovered thereafter and a CT scan done by the colorectal team suggested resolution of the prostatic abscess as seen in Figure 2.4.

Learning point Classification of prostatitis

Prostatitis is one of the common urinary tract problems found especially in men younger than 50 years of age. It is a group of disorders with a wide spectrum of symptoms and ranges from a clinically straightforward entity to a more complex-to-treat presentation. The disease was traditionally classified into acute bacterial, chronic bacterial, chronic non-bacterial, and prostatodynia.[6] However, in 1995 the National Institute of Diabetes and Digestive and Kidney Diseases (NIDDK) of the US National Institutes of Health (NIH) adopted a new working definition[7] which is currently applied in clinical practice (Table 2.1).

Table 2.1 NIH classification of prostatitis

Category	Designation	Status of infection
I	Acute bacterial prostatitis	Acute infection of prostatitis
II	Chronic bacterial prostatitis	Recurrent infection of prostate
III	Chronic non-bacterial prostatitis/ chronic pelvic pain syndrome	No demonstrable infection
IIIA	Inflammatory	WBC in semen/EPS/post-prostatic massage urine
IIIB	Non-inflammatory	No WBC in semen/EPS/post-prostatic massage urine
IV	Asymptomatic inflammatory prostatitis	Asymptomatic

EPS, expressed prostatic secretion; WBC, white blood cell.

Clinical tip Meares–Stamey test

Stamey et al. described a test in 1965 to help localize UTIs.[8] It enables separation of voided urinary stream into urethral (voided bladder one or VB1), midstream urine (voided bladder two or VB2), and post-prostatic massage urine (voided bladder three or VB3) in order to distinguish urethral and prostatic infection in the presence of sterile midstream urine. In 1968, Meares and Stamey introduced the concept and value of direct culture of expressed prostatic secretions (EPS) when VB1 and VB3 were equivocal. In simpler terms, the VB1 is the first 10 mL of voided urine and represents the urethral specimen; the next 150–200 mL is VB2 and represents the bladder specimen. EPS is collected while carrying out a vigorous prostatic massage and represents prostatic fluid. Finally, VB3 is the first 10 mL of urine after prostatic massage and represents EPS trapped in prostatic urethra. This information continues to be relevant with the new classification system of prostatitis as shown in Table 2.2 below.

Although the four-glass (specimen) Meares–Stamey test is the standard method of assessing men with symptoms of chronic pelvic pain syndrome (CPPS) or chronic prostatitis (CP), it can be quite cumbersome and thus a simplified two-glass pre- and post-massage test is being widely used. The results from a two-glass test have been shown to have a strong concordance with results from a four-glass Meares–Stamey test and thus offers a reasonable alternative that is simple and cost-effective.[9]

Semen culture has also been proposed as a simpler test than the gold standard four-glass test. The sensitivity of semen cultures for diagnosing CBP is very variable, therefore the diagnostic value remains controversial and further studies are needed.

Table 2.2 Diagnostic criteria used for the classification of prostatitis

Type	White blood cell count/ high-power field (400 ×)	VBI	VB2	EPS	VB3
I	>10	+	+	X	+
II	>10	–	–	+	+
IIIA	>10	–	–	–	–
IIIB	<10	–	–	–	–
IV	>10	–	–	–	–

Expert comment Bacterial prostatitis (types I and II)

Type 1 prostatitis presents acutely either in the outpatient or emergency setting. The diagnosis is mainly clinical and treatment with antibiotics usually resolves the problem. The symptoms initially are storage or voiding LUTS associated with suprapubic rectal or perineal pain. If untreated or inadequately treated, ABP can progress to prostatic abscess and one needs to have an index of suspicion for prostatic abscess if the patient has systemic symptoms like fever, chills, nausea, vomiting, and malaise. Some patients may develop urinary retention as a complication of prostatic abscess.

Ten per cent of patients diagnosed with ABP may progress to CBP and this diagnosis is made if the patient is symptomatic for at least 3 months or has recurrent prostatitis. The aetiology of the bacterial types of prostatitis has been described earlier and for successful treatment, use of appropriate antibiotics is important.

Antibiotic penetration into the prostate depends upon their lipid solubility, dissociation constant (pKa), and protein binding. Beta lactam antibiotics due to their low pKa and low lipid solubility penetrate poorly into prostate. However good to excellent penetration is seen with quinolones, tetracyclines, macrolides, sulphonamides, nitrofurantoin, and aminoglycosides like tobramycin and netilmicin.[10]

In CBP, oral antibiotic therapy can achieve cure rates of 70–90% at 6 months but a systematic review did not identify any randomized controlled trials to compare it with a placebo or no treatment.[11] There are some studies showing the effectiveness of anal submucosal[12] or prostatic antimicrobial injections,[13] but the evidence is limited and such treatment is not standard and mostly experimental. Interventions like transurethral resection of the prostate (TURP) for treatment of CBP have not been studied in a randomized controlled setting but some retrospective studies have suggested a role for TURP in patients with CBP and obstructive symptoms.[14] There are some reports of surgical options like TURP and radical prostatectomy performed in extreme cases of CBP.

Future directions

Treatment with phage therapy has been explored recently due to the role of phage strains in bacterial elimination and local immunomodulation.[15] However, further research needs to be done to establish its effectiveness as a future tool in treatment of bacterial prostatitis.

Learning point Aetiology and symptoms in CP/CPPS

CP/CPPS is the most common form of prostatitis and also the most poorly understood one. Ten per cent of patients with CP progress to CP/CPPS. However, the aetiology is unclear in most of the cases. Non-infectious factors that have been implicated include inflammation, autoimmunity, hormonal imbalances, pelvic floor tension myalgia, intraprostatic urinary reflux, and psychological disturbances.[16] A case–control study by Pontari et al. showed that the lifetime prevalence of non-specific urethritis, cardiovascular disease, neurological disease, psychiatric conditions, and haematopoietic, lymphatic, and infectious disease was significantly greater in men with CP/CPPS.[17] CP/CPPS shares multiple demographic, clinical, and psychosocial aspects with chronic pain conditions like fibromyalgia and chronic fatigue syndrome and thus may have a similar primary pathophysiology.[18]

The patients experience chronic pelvic pain and LUTS but there may also be associated sexual dysfunction. Some patients may complain of unusual symptoms like the sensation of a foreign body in the rectum, rectal pain during and after defecation, premature ejaculation, spontaneous sexual stimulation, or alteration of orgasms.[19] Owing to the heterogeneous nature of this condition, the diagnosis is based on symptoms; absence of any diagnostic biomarkers makes its diagnosis and treatment approaches variable and thus outcomes relatively poor. As a result of this, there is high disease burden and patient as well as physician dissatisfaction.

Clinical tip Clinical evaluation of CP/CPPS

Clinical evaluation to assess the severity of CP/CPPS can be carried out using the 13-point validated National Institute of Health Chronic Prostatitis Symptoms Index (NIH-CPSI) (Figure 2.5).[20] An alternative classification system using the UPOINT system categorizes the severity of patients' symptoms based on the predominant symptom group.[21] This UPOINT system in CP/CPPS originally encompassed Urinary, Psychosocial, Organ specific, Infective, Neurological, and Tenderness as different symptom phenotypes but the aspect of Sexual dysfunction was added later on (Table 2.3).[22]

NIH-Chronic Prostatitis Symptom Index (NIH-CPSI)

Pain or Discomfort

1. **In the last week, have you experienced any pain or discomfort in the following areas? Yes/ No**

a. Area between rectum and ☐1 ❑0 testicles (perineum)   b. Testicles ❑1 ❑0

c. Tip of the penis (not related to ❑1 ❑0 urination)   d. Below your waist, in your ❑1 ❑0 pubic or bladder area

2. In the last week, have you experienced: Yes/ No

a. Pain or burning during ❑1 ❑0 urination   b. Pain or discomfort during or ❑1 ❑0 after sexual climax (ejaculation)?

3. How often have you had pain or discomfort in any of these areas over the last week?

❑0 Never ❑1 Rarely ❑2 Sometimes ❑3 Often ❑4 Usually ❑5 Always

4. **Which number best describes your AVERAGE pain or discomfort on the days that you had it, over the last week?**

❑	❑	❑	❑	❑	❑	❑	❑	❑	❑	❑
0	1	2	3	4	5	6	7	8	9	10

NO PAIN   AS PAIN BAD AS YOU CAN IMAGINE

Urination

5. How often have you had a sensation of not emptying your bladder completely after you finished urinating, over the last week?

❑0 Not at all   ❑1 Less than 1 time in 5   ❑2 Less than half the time

❑3 About half the time   ❑4 More than half the time   ❑5 Almost always

6. How often have you had to urinate again less than two hours after you finished urinating, over the last week?

❑0 Not at all   ❑1 Less than 1 time in 5   ❑2 Less than half the time

❑3 About half the time   ❑4 More than half the time   ❑5 Almost always

Impact of Symptoms

7. How much have your symptoms kept you from doing the kinds of things you would usually do, over the last week?

❑0 None   ❑1 Only a little   ❑2 Some   ❑3 A lot

8. How much did you think about your symptoms, over the last week?

❑0 None   ❑1 Only a little   ❑2 Some   ❑3 A lot Quality of Life

9. If you were to spend the rest of your life with your symptoms just the way they have been during the last week, how would you feel about that?

❑0 Delighted   ❑1 Pleased   ❑2 Mostly satisfied   ❑3 Mixed (equally satisfied and dissatisfied)

❑4 Mostly dissatisfied   ❑5 Unhappy   ❑6 Terrible

Scoring the NIH-Chronic Prostatitis

Symptom Index Domains

Pain: Total of items 1a, 1b, 1c,1d, 2a, 2b, 3, and 4 = -----------

Urinary Symptoms: Total of items 5 and 6 = ------------------

Figure 2.5 The NIH-CPSI.

Table 2.3 UPOINT classification phenotypes in CP/CPPS

U	**Urinary**	NIH-CPSI score >4, obstructive and storage LUTS, high post-void residuals
P	**Psychosocial**	Clinical depression, anxiety, stress, maladaptive coping, etc.
O	**Organ specific**	Prostate tenderness, leucocytes in prostatic fluid, haematospermia, prostatic calcification
I	**Infective**	Gram-negative bacilli or enterococci in prostatic fluid, documented successful response to antimicrobial therapy
N	**Neurological**	Clinical evidence of central neuropathy, pain beyond pelvis, irritable bowel syndrome, fibromyalgia, chronic fatigue syndrome, etc.
T	**Tenderness**	Painful tenderness and/or painful muscle spasm or trigger points in abdomen and/or pelvic floor
S	**Sexual**	Sexual and ejaculatory dysfunction

Treatment is aimed to alleviate symptoms using strategies targeting the predominant phenotype of symptom. Interventions include identification and avoidance of risk factors[23] which include aspects of lifestyle (sedentary, fatigue, high stress), diet (alcohol, coffee, pepper, spicy foods, excessive dieting), sexual habits (delaying ejaculation, extremes in frequency of sexual activity, coitus interruptus), and perineal trauma (sitting position, sports, tight clothing). Education and clear communication with the patient and his sexual partner providing information about the nature of disorder, chronic pain cycle, treatment options, and clinical outcomes is important.[24]

Expert comment Patients with CP/CPPS

CP/CPPS is a complex and poorly understood condition with a huge impact on the quality of life of the affected person and treating the condition needs effective communication with the patient and a shift away from a traditional approach to management towards a more pragmatic multimodal approach. Communication not only between the physician and the patient but also between the multidisciplinary team looking after the patient, including their general practitioner, is the key element of this. Education of patients and their sexual partners to understand the current concepts, the chronic pain cycles, and the challenging nature of this disease can level expectations and help focus on achievable objectives. Social support helps gain the much-needed adjustments that might need to be made at work or elsewhere to help the patient manage his condition.

Learning point Therapeutic and evidence base in CP/CPPS

A combined approach addressing risk factors, promoting a healthy lifestyle and diet, and pharmacological, psychological, and neuromodulatory interventions improve outcomes. Pharmacological interventions include the use of alpha blockers, antimicrobials, anti-inflammatory and other pain medications, antidepressants, and neuroleptics. By reducing voiding pressures and improving voiding flow patterns, alpha blockers alleviate discomfort. A randomized placebo-controlled study, however, did not show any benefit and hence these are reserved for the subset of patients with voiding symptoms. There is no clear-cut role for 5-alpha reductase inhibitors but they reduce NIH-CPSI scores; the same is true for phosphodiesterase type 5 inhibitors.[25]

There is only moderate to low-quality evidence for benefit from short-term use of anti-inflammatory medications (non-steroidal anti-inflammatory drugs and steroids), antibiotics, and phytotherapy (quercetin, pollen extract (Cernilton®), cranberry, etc.). Intraprostatic botulinum toxin A has been shown to have benefit in improving NIH-CPSI scores and pain scores but the benefit is short term and treatment may need to be repeated. Pelvic floor botulinum toxin A did not show much benefit. In a recent Cochrane review, allopurinol, anticholinergics, antidepressants, pentosan polysulfate, pregabalin, and mepartricin were ineffective.[25]

There is moderate quality evidence for non-pharmacological interventions like acupuncture, extracorporeal shockwave therapy, circumcision, and tibial nerve stimulation in improving prostatitis symptoms, but the quality of evidence is weak for other interventions like lifestyle modifications, physical activity, prostatic massage, electromagnetic chair, thermotherapy, sonoelectromagnetic therapy, ultrasound therapy, biofeedback, external radiofrequency, laser therapy, myofascial trigger point release, osteopathy, trans-electrical nerve stimulation, transurethral needle ablation, and so on.[26] However, lifestyle modifications and physical activity have an overall benefit on health and are frequently recommended.

Future directions

Further research to study the effect of various proven and unproven interventions on various different parameters of this symptom complex is needed as most studies have so far focused on urinary and pain symptoms. Cannabinoids such as *N*-palmitoylethanolamide and flavonoid polydatin are currently being studied.[27]

Psychological distress evaluation should be carried out by a dedicated psychologist or mental health practitioner such that at-risk patients can be identified and interventions introduced as an integrative therapy and as part of a multimodal approach.[28] Such evaluation would provide an insight into patients' internal beliefs, perception of chronic pain, social support and interactions, relationships, and so on. This would not only help understand possible psychological causes of physical manifestations but also help plan adjustment and coping strategies.

Expert comment Asymptomatic inflammatory prostatitis

Asymptomatic inflammatory prostatitis is usually a histological diagnosis and is frequently an incidental finding in men undergoing investigations for prostate cancer or in men undergoing infertility investigations. Its prevalence ranges between 11% and 42%.[29] As the name suggests, it is asymptomatic and only presents clinical issues in the context of unnecessary biopsies for raised prostate-specific antigen or abnormal findings on MRI related to it. There are suggestions of a role in development of benign prostate hyperplasia and prostate cancer[30] but this unproven. It is usually left untreated but when seen in conjunction with leucocytospermia, it can be associated with male infertility.

A final word from the expert

Inflammation of the prostate gland has been recognized as an entity for around two centuries but remains essentially a clinical diagnosis with the use of other investigations primarily to provide supportive evidence of either inflammation or infection localized to the prostate. The term 'prostatitis' itself can cover a wide range of clinical conditions and it is therefore important that, whenever possible, this is also qualified with type and the 1995 NIDDK/NIH classification is useful for this purpose.

Acute prostatitis (category I) has the clearest treatment pathway, and the majority of patients have infection from Gram-negative bacteria which usually responds well to antibiotic treatment with only a small proportion developing an abscess which can be readily identified on imaging and drained via the transrectal or transurethral route. As for any acute infection, a high index of suspicion and early diagnosis is critical to avoid systemic involvement and improve outcomes.

Unfortunately, CP (categories II and III) is an altogether more difficult entity both to characterize and treat. The role of the Meares–Stamey test and/or semen culture should not be underestimated as it is important to establish early on in the management whether bacteria are involved in causing symptoms. Where this is the case, that is, CBP (category II), treatment with extended courses of antibiotics can lead to a satisfactory resolution in much the same manner as acute prostatitis. However, it is more commonly the case that bacteria are not detected and chronic non-bacterial CP/CPPS (category III) is therefore the most common form of prostatitis.

The treatment of CP/CPPS is difficult, often unsatisfactory for patients, and should not be regarded as the purview of the urologist alone. Its effective management frequently requires the use of multiple modalities and multiple clinical disciplines with the primary focus being on symptomatic management. Early recognition of the need for a multimodality approach is perhaps the most important aspect of the modern-day management of this still very poorly understood condition.

References

1. Stamatiou K, Magri V, Perletti G, et al. Chronic prostatic infection: microbiological findings in two Mediterranean populations. *Arch Ital Urol Androl.* 2019;91(3):177–181.
2. Barozzi L, Pavlica P, Menchi I, et al. Prostatic abscess: diagnosis and treatment. *AJR Am J Roentgenol.* 1998;170(3):753–757.
3. Wen SC, Juan YS, Wang CJ, et al. Emphysematous prostatic abscess: case series study and review. *Int J Infect Dis.* 2012;16(5):e344–e349.
4. Papanicolaou N, Pfister RC, Stafford SA, Parkhurst EC. Prostatic abscess: imaging with transrectal sonography and MR. *AJR Am J Roentgenol.* 1987;149(5):981–982.
5. Abdelmoteleb H, Rashed F, Hawary A. Management of prostate abscess in the absence of guidelines. *Int Braz J Urol.* 2017;43(5):835–840.
6. Stamey TA. Prostatitis. *J. R Soc Med.* 1981;74(1):22–40.
7. Krieger JN, Nyberg L Jr, Nickel JC. NIH consensus definition and classification of prostatitis. *JAMA.* 1999;282(3):236–237.
8. Stamey TA, Govan DE, Palmer JM. The localisation and treatment of urinary tract infections: the role of bactericidal urine levels as opposed to serum levels. *Medicine (Baltimore).* 1965;44:1–36.
9. Nickel JC, Shoskes D, Wang Y, et al. How does the pre-massage and post-massage 2-glass test compare to the Meares-Stamey 4-glass test in men with chronic prostatitis/chronic pelvic pain syndrome? *J Urol.* 2006;176(1):119–124.
10. Charalabopoulos K, Karachalios G, Baltogiannis D, Charalabopoulos A, Giannakopoulos X, Sofikitis N. Penetration of antimicrobial agents into the prostate. *Chemotherapy.* 2003;49(6):269–279.
11. Perletti G, Marras E, Wagenlehner FM, et al. Antimicrobial therapy for chronic bacterial prostatitis. *Cochrane Database Syst Rev.* 2013;8:CD009071.
12. Hu WL, Zhong SZ, He HX. Treatment of chronic bacterial prostatitis with amikacin through anal submucosal injection. *Asian J Androl.* 2002;4(3):163–167.
13. Baert L, Leonard A. Chronic bacterial prostatitis: 10 years of experience with local antibiotics. *J Urol.* 1988;140:755–757.
14. Smart CJ, Jenkins JD, Lloyd RS. The painful prostate. *Br J Urol.* 1975;47(7):861–869.
15. Górski A, Jończyk-Matysiak E, Łusiak-Szelachowska M, et al. Phage therapy in prostatitis: recent prospects. *Front Microbiol.* 2018;9:1434.
16. Bowen DK, Dielubanza E, Schaeffer AJ. Chronic bacterial prostatitis and chronic pelvic pain syndrome. *BMJ Clin Evid.* 2015;2015:1802.
17. PontarI MA, Ruggieri MR. Mechanisms in prostatitis/chronic pelvic pain syndrome. *J Urol.* 2004;172:839–845.
18. Bullones Rodríguez MÁ, Afari N, Buchwald DS; National Institute of Diabetes and Digestive and Kidney Diseases Working Group on Urological Chronic Pelvic Pain. Evidence for overlap between urological and nonurological unexplained clinical conditions. *J Urol.* 2013;189(1 Suppl):S66–S74.

19. Roberts RO, Jacobson DJ, Girman CJ, Rhodes T, Lieber MM, Jacobsen SJ. Prevalence of prostatitis-like symptoms in a community based cohort of older men. *J Urol.* 2002;168(6):2467–2471.
20. Litwin MS, McNaughton-Collins M, Fowler FJ Jr, et al. The National Institutes of Health chronic prostatitis symptom index: development and validation of a new outcome measure. Chronic Prostatitis Collaborative Research Network. *J Urol.* 1999;162(2):369–375.
21. Shoskes DA, Nickel JC, Dolinga R, Prots D. Clinical phenotyping of patients with chronic prostatitis/chronic pelvic pain syndrome and correlation with symptom severity. *Urology.* 2009;73(3):538–542.
22. Magri V, Wagenlehner F, Perletti G, et al. Use of the UPOINT chronic prostatitis/chronic pelvic pain syndrome classification in European patient cohorts: sexual function domain improves correlations. *J Urol.* 2010;184(6):2339–2345.
23. Gallo L. Effectiveness of diet, sexual habits and lifestyle modifications on treatment of chronic pelvic pain syndrome. *Prostate Cancer Prostatic Dis.* 2014;17(3):238–245.
24. Rees J, Abrahams M, Doble A, Cooper A. Diagnosis and treatment of chronic bacterial prostatitis and chronic prostatitis/chronic pelvic pain syndrome: a consensus guideline. *BJU Int.* 2015;116(4):509–525.
25. Franco JVA, Turk T, Jung JH, et al. Pharmacological interventions for treating chronic prostatitis/chronic pelvic pain syndrome: a Cochrane systematic review. *BJU Int.* 2020;125(4):490–496.
26. Franco JV, Turk T, Jung JH, et al. Non-pharmacological interventions for treating chronic prostatitis/chronic pelvic pain syndrome. *Cochrane Database Syst Rev.* 2018;5(5):CD012551.
27. Magri V, Boltri M, Cai T, et al. Multidisciplinary approach to prostatitis. *Arch Ital Urol Androl.* 2019;90(4):227–248.
28. Nickel JC, Mullins C, Tripp DA. Development of an evidence-based cognitive behavioural treatment program for men with chronic prostatitis/chronic pelvic pain syndrome. *World J Urol.* 2008;26(2):167–172.
29. Wu C, Zhang Z, Lu Z, et al. Prevalence of and risk factors for asymptomatic inflammatory (NIH-IV) prostatitis in Chinese men. *PLoS One.* 2013;8(8):e71298.
30. Krušlin B, Tomas D, Džombeta T, Milković-Periša M, Ulamec M. Inflammation in prostatic hyperplasia and carcinoma—basic scientific approach. *Front Oncol.* 2017;7:77.

SECTION 2

Urinary tract stones

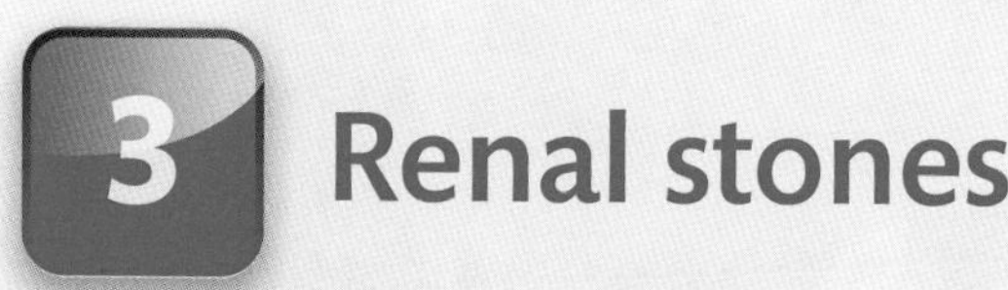

Renal stones

Jonathan Glass

Expert commentary Jonathan Glass

Case history

A 32-year-old woman presented with recurrent urinary tract infections (UTIs). She had very little in the way of past medical history but started developing UTIs over the previous 18 months and after initial treatment with antibiotics by her general practitioner, a decision was taken to refer her on for urological investigation. Her body mass index was slightly high at 27 kg/m^2.

Her mid-stream urine specimens all grew a *Klebsiella* sp. with multiple sensitivities. She was imaged initially with an ultrasound scan (USS). This showed a normal left kidney, a right kidney with evidence of multiple stones within it, and a normal bladder. Her haemoglobin (Hb) level at the time of her initial presentation was 143 g/L, and the creatinine was normal at 74 μmol/L.

A computed tomography (CT) scan (Figure 3.1) was performed that showed what had looked like multiple stones on the USS was in fact a single staghorn stone occupying the whole of the collecting system of the right kidney (Guy's stone score 4; Table 3.1).[1] After discussion with the patient, consent was taken for a right percutaneous nephrolithotomy (PCNL).

Clinical tip PCNL consent

The patient was informed that it was possible that not all the stone would be cleared with a single procedure, that she would have a nephrostomy and urinary catheter on waking, and consent included injury to other organs. A 25% chance of postoperative fever and a chance of sepsis was described and bleeding requiring embolization was discussed. A 1% chance of needing a blood transfusion was given to the patient. A risk of significant bleeding of between 1 in 50 and 1 in 100 is described on the British Association of Urological Surgeons (BAUS) website,[2] with a 1 in 1000 risk of the bleeding being so severe that it might require a nephrectomy. In the experience of the surgeon, the risk of bleeding was rarer, and the individual surgeon's risk was discussed with the patient.

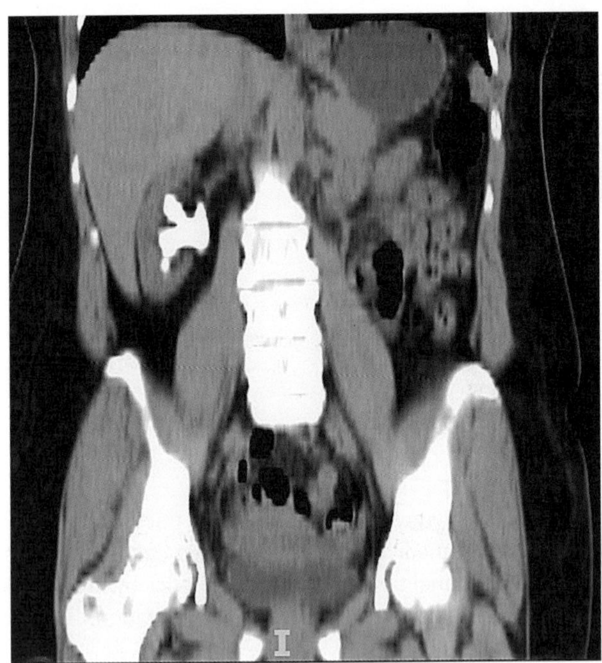

Figure 3.1 A CT scan demonstrating a right staghorn calculus.

Table 3.1 The Guy's stone score

Grade	Description
1	Solitary stone in mid/lower pole *or* Solitary stone in the pelvis with simple anatomy 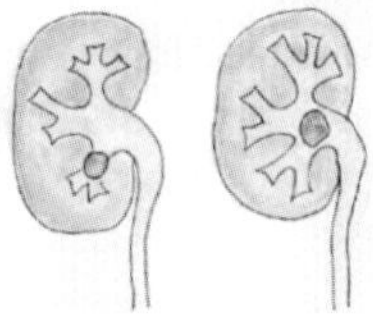
2	Solitary stone in upper pole *or* Multiple stones in a patient with simple anatomy *or* Any solitary stone in a patient with abnormal anatomy 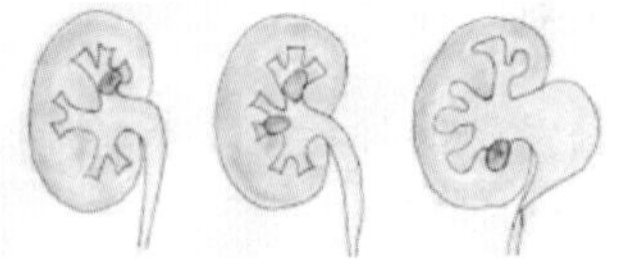
3	Multiple stones in a patient with abnormal anatomy *or* Stones in a caliceal diverticulum *or* A partial staghorn calculus 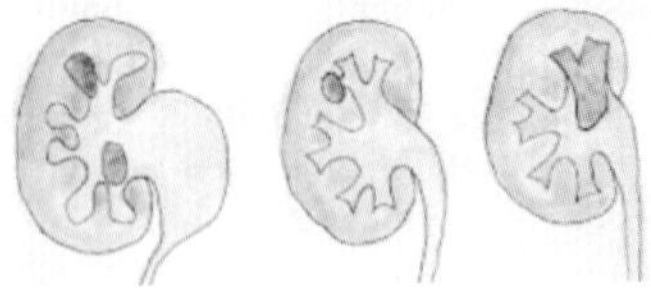
4	Staghorn calculus *or* Any stone in a patient with spina bifida or spinal injury 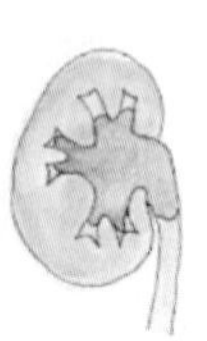

The Guy's stone score was developed through a combination of expert opinion, published data review, and iterative testing. It comprises four grades to grade the complexity of PCNL.
Adapted from Thomas K et al.[1]

Expert comment PCNL operative note

The patient underwent a right PCNL. She was given prophylactic gentamicin and co-amoxiclav on induction of anaesthesia. The PCNL was performed in a standard method with a urologist performing the whole procedure. A cystoscopy was performed, a ureteric balloon occlusion catheter was placed into the right kidney at the pelviureteric junction, and a urethral catheter was placed. The patient was then positioned prone and a Mitty–Pollack needle used to gain access to a lower pole posterior calyx and the track secured with the placement of two guidewires into the collecting system. The track was dilated to 26 French (Fr) (Figure 3.2), and on placement of the nephroscope an infected stone was seen and cleared using a combined ultrasonic and pneumatic device. Progress was made rapidly to clear the stone with a path made through to the renal pelvis. Further stone clearance of the upper pole stones was only possible using a flexible cystoscope; the excellent access through the posterior calyx facilitated this possibility and a flexible cystoscope was used to clear the stone from the upper pole with stone fragmentation being achieved using a holmium laser.

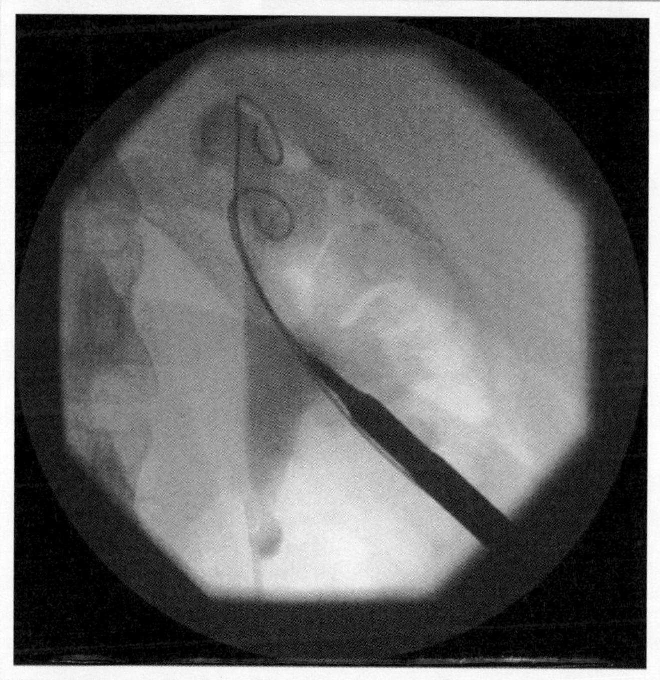

Figure 3.2 Intraoperative image showing placement of serial metal dilators to dilate the tract to 26 Fr.

There was minimal bleeding at the time of the procedure allowing good views throughout the length of the operation; at the end of the procedure a 10 Fr nephrostomy was placed.

The nephrostomy drained some blood-stained urine in the first 48 hours but the patient remained apyrexial postoperatively so the nephrostomy was removed on the second postoperative day and the patient was discharged.

Intraoperative and postoperative imaging showed a single remaining stone sitting in the lower pole for which the patient was to be booked for a flexible ureteroscopy.

On day 10, the patient was readmitted to the hospital with heavy haematuria. Her Hb level was 12.7 g/L on admission but the bleeding was heavy and the patient went into clot retention requiring placement of a urinary catheter and a bladder washout. A USS showed no significant perinephric haematoma. Although the patient remained haemodynamically stable, the Hb level continued to fall, reaching 10.0 g/L with ongoing bleeding. No transfusion was necessary but it was felt further imaging was appropriate.

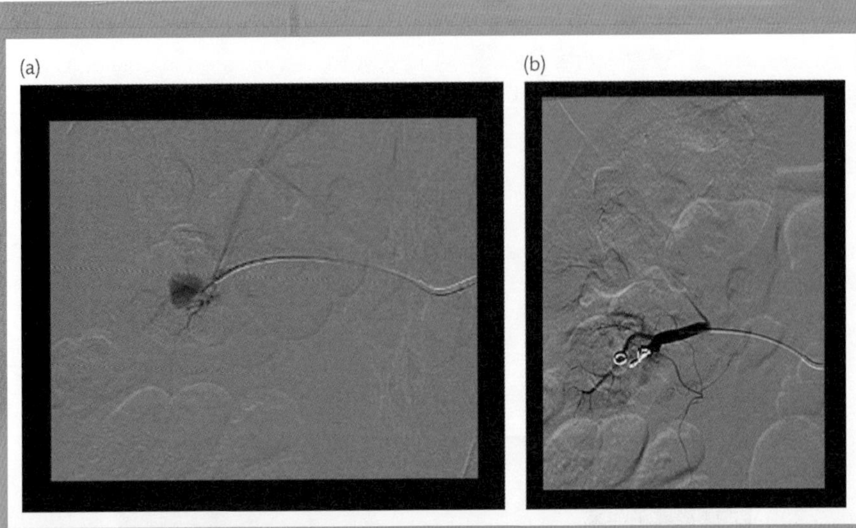

Figure 3.3 Super-selective arteriogram showing (a) pseudoaneurysm and (b) embolization clips.

The patient went on to have a CT angiogram. This showed an obvious pseudoaneurysm in the lower pole of the right kidney. After appropriate counselling, the patient was taken to the interventional radiology suite and a right renal angiogram was performed through a right-sided femoral puncture. A pseudoaneurysm with arteriovenous shunting was seen in the lower pole of the right kidney and a highly selective embolization was performed with the deployment of two embolization coils (Figure 3.3). The patient returned to the ward, the urine colour changed almost immediately, the Hb level stabilized, and the patient was fit for discharge 48 hours after the embolization.

The remaining stone required treatment. After some delay to allow the patient to recover after the embolization, the patient was readmitted for a right ureterorenoscopy.

Expert comment Ureterorenoscopy operative note

Under general anaesthesia, a cystoscopy was performed and a sensor wire placed into the right kidney. A rigid ureteroscopy was performed with a 7.5 Fr short rigid ureteroscope alongside the guidewire. No stone was seen along the length of the ureter. A flexible ureteroscope was passed over the guidewire and into the right kidney. The remaining single stone was seen in the lower pole calyx and fragmented completely with a holmium laser, initially on settings of 0.6 J at 6 Hz and then after initial fragmentation had been achieved, dusting was achieved with settings of 0.2 J and 25 Hz. A 6 Fr, 24 cm stent was placed at the end of the procedure. This was removed after 10 days.

On subsequent follow-up, the patient has been free of infection and subsequent imaging with kidney, ureter, and bladder X-ray and USS has shown the patient to be stone free.

Discussion

First described and popularized by Alken et al. in 1982,[3] percutaneous surgery remains the intervention of choice in the treatment of large and staghorn stones of the kidney. This case highlights a number of issues in the management of renal stones by percutaneous surgery.

Staghorn stones are very frequently associated with colonization with a urease producing organism such as a *Proteus* sp. or *Klebsiella* sp. as in this case.

A 26 Fr sheath was used to access the kidney and a single track was performed. The development of the use of smaller tracks has occurred in the last 10 years with smaller tracks predominantly being used to extend the role of percutaneous surgery in the treatment of intrarenal stones.[5,6] Some practitioners are using smaller tracks to treat large stones using high-power laser settings. There is some evidence that these smaller tract sizes are associated with a lower complication rate, particularly a lower transfusion rate. In the most part, tracts of 26–30 Fr are being used to treat staghorn stones. A single track was performed. Again, placement of a second track might have led to clearance of the remaining piece of stone. The use of a greater number of tracks can facilitate higher rates of stone clearance but are associated with increased rates of blood transfusion and bleeding complications. Minimally invasive surgery does allow for safe surgery with the lowest risk to the patient being performed and then a further procedure performed to complete stone clearance as in this case.[7]

Expert comment Nephrostomy post PCNL

A nephrostomy was placed at the end of the procedure. This was indicated as the patient was at risk of postoperative sepsis. There is a vogue to perform 'tubeless' PCNLs although often when authors refer to a tubeless procedure, in fact a ureteric stent is placed instead of a nephrostomy.[8] This may facilitate earlier discharge from hospital but it does leave the patient with a stent in place that requires removal. In the author's opinion, there is little to gain by placing a stent rather than a nephrostomy in most cases, but in the context of a staghorn calculus, a nephrostomy is preferable. Bernard Shaw stated in the foreword to his play 'The Doctor's Dilemma' that 'There is a fashion in operations as there is in sleeves and skirts'.[9] I am wary that a tubeless PCNL is a trend, but it may be judged unwise in some cases.

Another option would have been to consider the combined use of transurethral flexible ureteroscopy at the time of the PCNL—termed endoscopic combined intrarenal surgery (ECIRS).[10] This is being utilized increasingly in the treatment of complex stones in the kidney, particularly when there are multiple stones in a number of calyces and there is a desire to keep the number of percutaneous tracks to a single track. The procedure requires appropriate expertise in the theatre, with a second endourologist and a theatre team able to coordinate the use of two endoscopic imaging stacks, and so on.

Learning point Prone and supine PCNL

The procedure described was performed with the patient positioned prone. Valdivia, in the 1990s, was the first to popularize the performance of PCNL with the patient positioned supine.[11] There are undoubtedly pros and cons for both positions. The supine position does facilitate the easier use of ECIRS and is becoming increasingly popular although there is evidence that stone clearance rates for staghorn stones may be better with the patient prone. In my view, the best position for the patient having percutaneous surgery is determined by the anatomy of the patient and the position of the kidney. Currently, I perform approximately 10% of my PCNLs with the patient lying supine.

Stone clearance was achieved using a device that combines ultrasonic and mechanical stone fragmentation. Percutaneous surgery, though increasingly being used for smaller stones when the laser is an excellent stone fragmentation device, should be performed with a minimum of an ultrasonic device when treating staghorn stones. These stones are often soft, and a mechanical lithotripter such as the Swiss LithoClast® is an inefficient device for clearing these stones. A number of new devices are available including the Swiss Lithoclast® Master, the ShockPulse-SE®, and the Swiss Lithoclast® Trilogy devices, all of which offer very rapid clearance of renal stones.

Clinical tip Mid-stream urine specimen prior to surgery

A preoperative mid-stream urine specimen is essential before considering PCNL and consideration should be given to pretreating the patient with appropriate antibiotics. Despite this, a fever in the immediate postoperative period is common, with the BAUS advice sheet giving a risk of sepsis of between 2% and 10%.[2] The surgeon should also know local microorganism resistance and ensue prophylactic antibiotics are given at the time of the surgery.

Evidence base PCNL puncture

In this patient, the whole procedure, the puncture, and the stone retrieval was performed by a urologist. We know from the BAUS registry data that in the UK currently 40% of punctures are performed by a urologist, the remainder being performed by a radiologist.[4] There is no evidence that outcome is determined by who makes the puncture.

Clinical tip Recognition of intra/postoperative bleeding

Intraoperatively, it is important that the surgeon has an impression of the significance of any bleeding. Postoperative bleeding associated with a decreasing Hb level may be associated with the development of an arteriovenous malformation or a pseudoaneurysm. If this is suspected, a CT angiogram or formal CT scan should be performed and any vascular anomaly treated ideally with super-selective embolization to reduce the loss of renal parenchyma to a minimum.

Bleeding as a consequence of percutaneous surgery is well recognized.[7] The percutaneous surgeon is dilating a track into an organ that receives 10% of cardiac output. Some practitioners suggest that the puncture can be untargeted,[12] although a targeted calyceal puncture is likely to be associated with a lower rate of bleeding complications.

The benefit of the minimally invasive approach to stone surgery that has been increasingly utilized over the last 30 years, such that open stone surgery is really a thing of the past, is that each procedure is generally well tolerated. The compromise is repeated procedures. This patient underwent a flexible ureterorenoscopy 1 month postoperatively. A reusable fibreoptic scope was used. There has been a move in the last few years to the use of initially reusable and now disposable digital endoscopes. These have the advantage of a clearer image than the fibreoptic scopes and the proponents of the reusable scopes argue that they offer safety against the risk of cross contamination with failed sterilization processes. Such failures have been documented but they are rare. Against this is the environmental cost of using a single-use scope. My suspicion is that in the developed world there will be increased utilization of disposable endoscopes in the years ahead.

The laser settings used in this case were first a setting to achieve fragmentation and second a setting used to achieve dusting. The holmium laser is a solid-state, 2100 nm wavelength laser (in the infrared part of the spectrum, not visible to the human eye) that has been used in the treatment of stones since the mid 1990s. As a device, they are workhorses, very easy to maintain, and able to fragment any urinary tract stone. In the last 5 years, some manipulations to the settings have been developed to achieve quicker stone fragmentation and more effective dusting of the stone. This may allow for lower rates of postoperative stenting (see 'Expert comment' box on postoperative stenting).

Holmium achieves stone fragmentation by photothermal energy, this was defined in a series of experiments defined by Chan.[13] The three factors that can be altered in the use of the laser are laser power (measured in joules), the frequency (measured in hertz), and the pulse width. Most lasers can alter the first two factors, some newer lasers allow alteration of the third as well. There is a new technology whereby a double firing of the laser is achieved. This is believed to create an air bubble such that the second laser pulse passes through air and this is thought to get more energy to the stone, achieving a higher rate of stone fragmentation. The holmium laser has been around for > 20 years and, unlike many lasers that were developed in the 1980s, has stood the test of time. Further developments of its use will enhance its utilization in the years ahead.[14]

Expert comment Postoperative stenting

The use of postoperative stenting is controversial with the recently published National Institute for Health and Care Excellence (NICE) guidelines on urinary tract stone disease suggesting stents should not be routinely used following an uncomplicated ureteroscopy.[15] The definition of an uncomplicated ureteroscopy is, in itself, complicated. Defining whether a ureteroscopy is uncomplicated is difficult, but this patient has had a history of UTIs so it was felt that there was a significant risk of infection after the ureteroscopy that placement of a stent was prudent.

The NICE guidelines entitled 'Urinary tract stone disease: assessment and management' recently been published in the UK. Unlike guidelines developed by the American Urological Association and the European Urological Association, the UK guidelines make recommendations only when there is thought to be evidence from well-conducted studies and do not accept expert opinion evidence. This produces a rather unusual set of recommendations, some of which are controversial in particular aspects. With respect to staghorn stones, they are uncontroversial in recommending that PCNL be offered as first-line treatment, and stating that ureteroscopy be considered in patients where percutaneous surgery is not an option. UK practitioners should be aware of the UK guidelines. A critique of them has been published in the *British Journal of Urology International*.[16]

The complication rate of percutaneous surgery has been defined in the UK following the nationwide collection of data by the BAUS. This has enabled contemporary complication rates from a real-life series by true subspecialists and the occasional percutaneous surgeon.[17–19] The mean number of cases performed by a practitioner per year is only ten cases. Subgroup analysis of percutaneous surgery has been possible in the elderly, in those with neurological pathology, and so on. This has allowed public access to individual surgeons' procedure numbers and transfusion rates. A number of publications have been produced based on this series which have increased our knowledge of percutaneous surgery which are listed in 'Further reading'. The UK is the only country with nationwide data on complication rates and other data on a large number of urological procedures.

A final word from the expert

Richard Tiptaft, my predecessor as the senior surgeon in the stone unit at Guy's Hospital, London, suggested to me when I joined him in 1999 that with respect to percutaneous surgery, I'll make mistakes with my first 1000 cases and then I'll get the hang of it. John Denstedt, a percutaneous surgeon from Canada similarly said he was a better percutaneous surgeon after 3000 cases then he was after 2000 cases. This paints a picture of the challenge faced by the percutaneous surgeon. It is a procedure from which one continues to learn and technically improve even after many procedures under one's belt. At the time of writing, I have performed 825 PCNLs so Tiptaft and Denstedt would suggest I am still on my learning curve!

It is a challenging procedure with a transfusion rate in the UK of just >2%. It is also a procedure associated with high rates of postoperative sepsis as PCNLs are performed on patients with UTI, and in whom there is no chance of clearing the infection until the stone has been cleared. A fever on the first postoperative night has been recorded in up to 25% of patients undergoing a PCNL.

Endourology is a specialty that embraces change and new developments. The most significant change in percutaneous surgery in the past 5–10 years has been the development of smaller and smaller nephroscopes, from the standard sheath size of 28–30 Fr to sheath sizes of 16 Fr, referred to as a mini-PCNL, and 8–11 Fr, termed an ultra-mini-PCNL. The smaller tracts do appear to be associated with lower transfusion rates but they have also resulted in extending the indication for PCNL, where, particularly in the developing world, it is being utilized to treat smaller stones in markets where liquid sterilization of flexible instruments is less available. As flexible ureteroscopy is being used to treat larger and larger stones with the development of new settings when using a holmium laser, resulting in better stone destruction to dust, percutaneous surgery is being used to treat smaller and smaller stones. The more techniques a stone surgeon has in their armamentarium, the better, and these developments are giving patients more choice in how to have their intrarenal stone managed.

The dataset produced by the data collection under the auspices of the BAUS has resulted in a unique set of current, up-to-date information on the approaches to percutaneous surgery and the complication rate of the procedure. The dataset currently includes >10,000 cases and it means that patients can now be given information about the risks and outcomes of the procedure in the UK. These are very powerful data to give to a patient. Indeed, the patient is able to look up the dataset of the surgeon who is going to operate on them. This is surely what patients are entitled to know about their surgeon.

References

1. Thomas K, Smith NC, Hegarty N, Glass JM. The Guy's stone score—grading the complexity of percutaneous nephrolithotomy procedures. *Urology.* 2011;78(2):277–281.
2. British Association of Urological Surgeons. Percutaneous nephrolithotomy (keyhole surgery for kidney stones). British Association of Urological Surgeons. June 2021. https://www.baus.org.uk/_userfiles/pages/files/Patients/Leaflets/PCNL.pdf
3. Alken P, Hutschenreiter G, Gunther R. Percutaneous kidney stone removal. *Eur Urol.* 1982;8(5):304–311.
4. Armitage JN, Withington J, Fowler S, et al. Percutaneous nephrolithotomy access by urologist or interventional radiologist: practice and outcomes in the UK. *BJU Int.* 2017;119(6):913–918.
5. Jones P, Elmussareh M, Aboumarzouk OM, Mucksavage P, Somani BK. Role of minimally invasive (micro and ultra-mini) PCNL for adult urinary stone disease in the modern era: evidence from a systematic review. *Curr Urol Rep.* 2018;19(4):27.
6. Lahme S. Miniaturisation of PCNL. *Urolithiasis.* 2018;46(1):99–106.
7. Kamphuis GM, Baard J, Westendarp M, de la Rosette JJ. Lessons learned from the CROES percutaneous nephrolithotomy global study. *World J Urol.* 2015;33(2):223–233.
8. Tailly T, Denstedt J. Innovations in percutaneous nephrolithotomy. *Int J Surg.* 2016;36(Pt D):665–672.
9. Shaw GB. *The Doctor's Dilemma.* New York: Brentano's; 1909.
10. Scoffone CM, Cracco CM. The tale of ECIRS (Endoscopic Combined IntraRenal Surgery) in the Galdakao-modified supine Valdivia position. *Urolithiasis.* 2018;46(1):115–123.
11. Valdivia JG, Scarpa RM, Duvdevani M, et al. Supine versus prone position during percutaneous nephrolithotomy: a report from the clinical research office of the endourological society percutaneous nephrolithotomy global study. *J Endourol.* 2011;25(10):1619–1625.
12. Kalidonis P, Kyriazis I, Kotsiris D, Koutava A, Kamal W, Liatsikos E. Papillary vs nonpapillary puncture in percutaneous nephrolithotomy: a prospective randomized trial. *J Endourol.* 2017;31(S1):S4–S9.
13. Vassar GJ, Chan KF, Teichman JM, et al. Holmium: YAG lithotripsy: photothermal mechanism. *J Endourol.* 1999;13(3):181–190.
14. Aldoukhi AH, Roberts WW, Hall TL, Teichman JMH, Ghani KR. Understanding the popcorn effect during holmium laser lithotripsy for dusting. *Urology.* 2018;122:52–57.
15. NICE guideline—renal and ureteric stones: assessment and management. *BJU Int.* 2019;123(2):220–232.
16. Smith D, Glass J. NICE stone guidelines 2019. BJU International. 16 January 2019. http://www.bjuinternational.com/bjui-blog/nice-stone-guidelines-2019/
17. Withington J, Armitage J, Finch W, Wiseman O, Glass J, Burgess N. Assessment of stone complexity for PCNL: a systematic review of the literature, how best can we record stone complexity in PCNL? *J Endourol.* 2016;30(1):13–23.
18. Armitage JN, Withington J, van der Meulen J, et al. Percutaneous nephrolithotomy in England: practice and outcomes described in the Hospital Episode Statistics database. *BJU Int.* 2014;113(5):777–782.

19. Withington JM, Charman SC, Armitage JN, et al. Hospital volume does not influence the safety of percutaneous nephrolithotomy in England: a population-based cohort study. *J Endourol.* 2015;29(8):899–906.

Further reading

Davis NF, Quinlan MR, Poyet C, et al. Miniaturised percutaneous nephrolithotomy versus flexible ureteropyeloscopy: a systematic review and meta-analysis comparing clinical efficacy and safety profile. *World J Urol.* 2018;36(7):1127–1138.

Knoll T, Daels F, Desai J, et al. Percutaneous nephrolithotomy: technique. *World J Urol.* 2017;35(9):1361–1368.

Proietti S, Giusti G, Desai M, Ganpule AP. A critical review of miniaturised percutaneous nephrolithotomy: is smaller better? *Eur Urol Focus.* 2017;3(1):56–61.

Rivera M, Viers B, Cockerill P, Agarwal D, Mehta R, Krambeck A. Pre- and postoperative predictors of infection-related complications in patients undergoing percutaneous nephrolithotomy. *J Endourol.* 2016;30(9):982–986.

Rivera ME, Bhojani N, Heinsimer K, et al. A survey regarding preference in the management of bilateral stone disease and a comparison of Clavien complication rates in bilateral vs unilateral percutaneous nephrolithotomy. *Urology.* 2018;111:48–53.

Tailly T, Denstedt J. Innovations in percutaneous nephrolithotomy. *Int J Surg.* 2016;36(Pt D):665–672.

Usawachintachit M, Masic S, Allen IE, Li J, Chi T. Adopting ultrasound guidance for prone percutaneous nephrolithotomy: evaluating the learning curve for the experienced surgeon. *J Endourol.* 2016;30(8):856–863.

Yarimoglu S, Bozkurt IH, Aydogdu O, Yonguc T, Gunlusoy B, Degirmenci T. External validation and comparisons of the scoring systems for predicting percutaneous nephrolithotomy outcomes: a single center experience with 506 cases. *J Laparoendosc Adv Surg Tech A.* 2017;27(12):1284–1289.

Yarimoglu S, Polat S, Bozkurt IH, et al. Comparison of S.T.O.N.E and CROES nephrolithometry scoring systems for predicting stone-free status and complication rates after percutaneous nephrolithotomy: a single center study with 262 cases. *Urolithiasis.* 2017;45(5):489–494.

York NE, Borofsky MS, Chew BH, et al. Randomized controlled trial comparing three different modalities of lithotrites for intracorporeal lithotripsy in percutaneous nephrolithotomy. *J Endourol.* 2017;31(11):1145–1151.

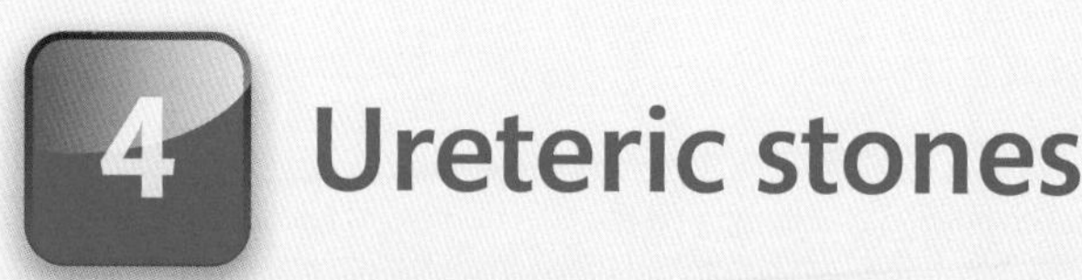

4 Ureteric stones

Lisa Bibby and Mostafa Sheba

Expert commentary Andrea Lavinio, Andrew Winterbottom, and Oliver Wiseman

Case history

A 74-year-old male presented with a 2-day history of right loin pain. The pain was of gradual onset over 24 hours. On presentation, the pain radiated from the right loin to right groin. It was associated with nausea. He was assessed by the urology team in the accident and emergency department. Initial investigations included urinalysis which was positive for blood.

Learning point Presentation, investigation, and management

Ureteric stones are a common cause for emergency presentation to hospital. Urinary stones affect 2–3% of the population and have a male predominance. The peak age of presentation is between 40 and 60 years in males and the late 20s in females. Once a patient has a urinary stone, they have a 50% chance of recurrence, of which 10% reoccur within the first year.[1–3]

While patients can be asymptomatic, the typical presenting history is of loin to groin pain which is colicky in nature. It is normally of sudden onset. Stones tend to obstruct at the three narrowest points in the ureter: the pelviureteric junction, the point at which they cross with the iliac vessels near the pelvic brim, and the vesicoureteric junction (VUJ). Stones at the VUJ can cause storage symptoms of urinary frequency and urgency, as well as dysuria and strangury. Furthermore, they can cause pain which radiates to the tip of the penis or vulva. Renal colic associated with a fever or signs of sepsis should raise alarms for an infected obstructed system, a pyonephrosis, which is a urological emergency.[4]

Urinalysis is positive for blood (including trace of blood) in 92.9% of patients and hence not all patients with renal colic will have a haematuria, either visible or non-visible, on presentation.[5] Likewise, blood in the urine can be caused by other presentations of the acute abdomen such as appendicitis or diverticulitis.

In the acute setting, initial management of suspected renal colic aims to control the pain. National Institute for Health and Care Excellence (NICE) guidance recommends non-steroidal anti-inflammatory drugs (NSAIDs) by any route as first-line treatment.[6] Diclofenac suppositories are commonly used as renal colic often presents with vomiting and so an oral route is less effective. Paracetamol can be offered first line if there is a contraindication to NSAIDs (such as history of asthma, gastric ulceration with oral use, or proctitis when using suppositories) or as an adjunct to NSAIDs if pain is not controlled. NSAIDs should be avoided in renal impairment. If the pain is still not sufficiently controlled or if both paracetamol and NSAIDs are contraindicated, opioids can be considered.[6,7] The exact mechanism of action which enables NSAIDs to exert their analgesic effect in renal colic is unknown. It is thought to be due to the inhibitory effect on the production of prostaglandins, which leads to a reduction in diuresis, ureteric wall oedema, and ureteric smooth muscle stimulation.[8]

Evidence base NSAIDs

There have been two Cochrane reviews looking at the use of NSAIDs for the management of acute renal colic. The first was undertaken in 2005 and compared the effectiveness of NSAIDs to opioids for analgesia. The review included 29 randomized controlled trials which looked at a total of 1613 patients from nine different countries. Both NSAIDs and opioids were found to reduce patient-reported pain scores. Ten of 13 studies reported reduced pain scores when treated with NSAIDs compared to opioids. There was a significant reduction in the need for rescue medication with treatment ($p < 0.00001$). Opioids were associated with high rates of vomiting and hence had a greater side effect risk.[9]

The second Cochrane review was published in 2015. This compared NSAIDs with antispasmodics. A total of 50 studies were included in the review of which 37 contributed to the meta-analysis. NSAIDs significantly reduced pain compared to antispasmodics. Pain recurrence within 24 hours had a higher incidence in those treated with diclofenac compared to piroxicam.[10]

A non-contrast computed tomography (CT) scan of the kidneys, ureters, and bladder (KUB) was undertaken to investigate the cause of symptoms. It showed a 6 mm right mid-ureteric calculus with hydroureteronephrosis to that level (Figure 4.1). The blood results showed a white cell count (WCC) of 13 × 10^9/L, C-reactive protein (CRP) level of 6 mg/dL, and creatinine level of 68 µmol/L.

The pain was well controlled with diclofenac suppositories. The patient was discharged with NSAID analgesia for trial of spontaneous passage and booked for the stone clinic 2 weeks later. An abdominal X-ray was performed to see if the stone was visible on X-ray for monitoring purposes. It was not.

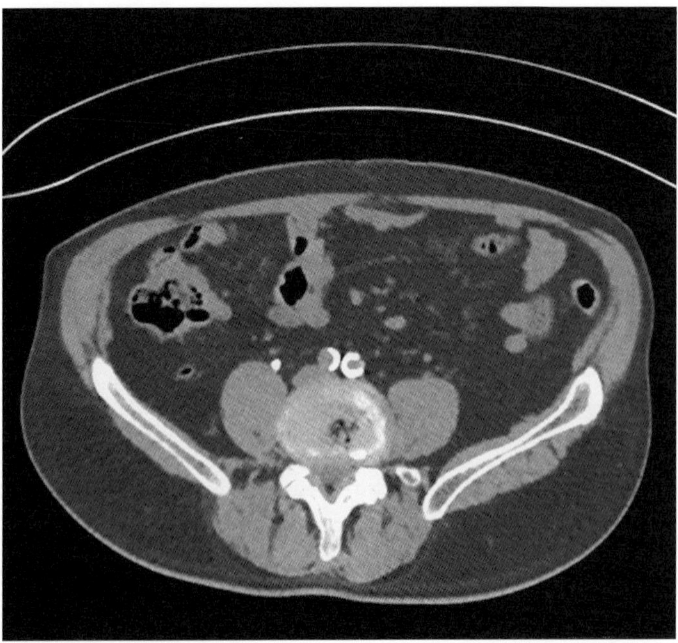

Figure 4.1 A CT KUB scan showing a 6 mm right mid-ureteric stone.

Evidence base The use of CT imaging, ultrasound scanning, and magnetic resonance imaging

A study of 4000 patients presenting with acute flank pain found a urinary stone on the CT scan of 78% of patients; 10.5% were found to have an entirely normal CT scan. The alternative diagnoses on the CT scans of patients presenting with acute flank pain included appendicitis, pancreatitis, renal abscess, diverticulitis, uterine fibroids, and ovarian masses among many others, including a leaking abdominal aortic aneurysm.[11] Ten per cent of abdominal aortic aneurysms present with symptoms compatible with renal colic. This is more frequently the case in men over the age of 50 years but also applies to females.[12] These patients tend to present with left-sided pain. CT can also infer a diagnosis of recent spontaneous passage of a ureteric stone, due to the secondary phenomena of ureteric dilatation and perinephric stranding or the presence of the stone in the bladder.[13]

Non-contrast CT of the abdomen and pelvis (10–12 mSv) is the gold standard imaging modality for diagnosis of renal and ureteric stones. NICE guidance recommends this to be undertaken within the first 24 hours of presentation.[6,14] CT imaging is particularly advantageous as not only can it identify most ureteric stones, it can provide additional information on size, location, associated hydronephrosis, fat stranding suggesting inflammation or infection, and the Hounsfield units which give an indication as to how hard the stone is.

Non-contrast CT has been quoted to have a sensitivity and specificity of 96% and 97% respectively.[14] Increasing awareness of exposure to radiation doses has led to the use of low-dose CT (1–3 mSv). This has been found to have a high sensitivity and specificity of 97% and 95% respectively.[15]

In cases where radiation doses need to be limited, such as in children and younger patients, the use of ultrasound scanning (USS) as first-line imaging is recommended.[6] The benefit of USS is that it does not use ionizing radiation and is relatively inexpensive. USS can show the secondary features of renal colic such as hydronephrosis as well as showing some renal stones and VUJ stones in the presence of a filled bladder. It is less sensitive than CT but has a similar specificity (45% and 94% respectively for ureteric stones and 45% and 88% for renal stones).[16] USS can have limited usefulness in patients with a high body mass index or in cases where intestinal gas overlies the area of interest.

In pregnant women, NICE guidance advises USS as the first-line imaging technique.[6] Renal colic is the most common non-obstetric cause for abdominal pain in pregnancy. However, USS in pregnancy is unable to differentiate physiological hydronephrosis from hydronephrosis secondary to an obstructing ureteric stone. Therefore, USS in pregnancy is reported to have a sensitivity of 34% and specificity of 86%.[17] If there is ongoing diagnostic uncertainty, European Association of Urology (EAU) guidance suggests magnetic resonance imaging as second line and low-dose CT as a last line. Of these three imaging modalities, CT has the higher positive predictive value (95.8%) compared to magnetic resonance imaging (80%) and USS (77%) but is last line due to concerns over exposure to ionizing radiation in pregnancy.[18]

Evidence base Important clinical studies

A large multicentre UK study (Multi-centre cohort study evaluating the role of Inflammatory Markers In patients presenting with acute ureteric Colic (MIMIC)) was undertaken over 71 hospitals in four countries. CT images of 4170 patients with acute ureteric colic were reviewed to confirm a single ureteric stone. The MIMIC study investigated the role of biochemical makers (including creatinine, CRP, and WCC) in predicting which patients would benefit from intervention and those who would not. The study was unable to demonstrate a single biomarker which would enable clinicians to identify patients who would spontaneously pass their stones from those who would require intervention. It found a spontaneous passage rate of 84% of stones <5 mm in diameter.[19]

Medical expulsion therapy (MET) has been used in the past as it was thought to aid spontaneous passage of ureteric stones. Its use was recommended in the 2007 joint EAU/American Urological Association guideline for the management of ureteral calculi. However, more recently there have been randomized controlled trials aimed at evaluating the effectiveness of MET.[20]

The Spontaneous Urinary Stone Passage Enabled by Drugs (SUSPEND) study is the largest double-blind, multicentre randomized controlled trial to date comparing the rate of spontaneous ureteric stone expulsion in patients treated with tamsulosin, nifedipine, or placebo. This study took data from 24 different hospitals and included 1136 patients with a CT-proven single ureteric stone. Patients were randomized to daily tamsulosin, nifedipine, or placebo for 4 weeks. Eighty per cent of patients receiving placebo did not require any further intervention. This compared to 81% of patients taking tamsulosin (p-value 0.73) and 80% of patients taking nifedipine (p-value 0.88). They therefore demonstrated no statistically or clinically significant difference between the three interventions on rate of spontaneous stone passage.[21]

There has been some criticism of this study. One limiting factor is that the majority of patients had stones <5 mm which are more likely to be passed spontaneously. Approximately 75% of the patients had stones <5 mm and 65% were in the lower third of the ureter. The placebo group had a high rate of no need for further intervention at 80%, which could mask the effects of MET. Furthermore, the primary endpoint was defined as no need for further intervention rather than CT-proven stone clearance and so the actual spontaneous passage rate is unknown.[22]

MET was routinely used to aid spontaneous passage of ureteric stones prior to 2015. However, following the publication of the SUSPEND trial which was unable to demonstrate a significant difference, this changed. Many clinicians, especially in the UK, have ceased to prescribe MET. Recent NICE guidance has reviewed all of the evidence surrounding MET including trials more recent than the SUSPEND trial. It concluded that both calcium channel blockers and alpha blockers can aid the passage of small stones and be a useful pain management adjunct. Alpha blockers were found to be more effective than calcium channel blockers and NICE recommends their use for distal ureteric stones <10 mm. NICE guidance states 'MET is low cost, and the savings from interventions avoided because of this therapy, are likely to offset the cost of the therapy'. EAU guidance advises that MET agents can also reduce the frequency of episodes of colic until stone expulsion.[6,18]

The patient returned 3 days later to the emergency department with a fever of 38.5°C, a tachycardia of 120 beats per minute, and blood pressure of 95/60 mmHg. His WCC was 23 × 10^9/L, and his CRP level was >250 mg/dL. The on-call urology team were called, and the Sepsis Six protocol instituted. A repeat CT KUB scan showed the stone in the same location as previously, and hydronephrosis and hydroureter above the stone (Figure 4.2). The team contacted the interventional radiology team for urgent nephrostomy tube insertion.

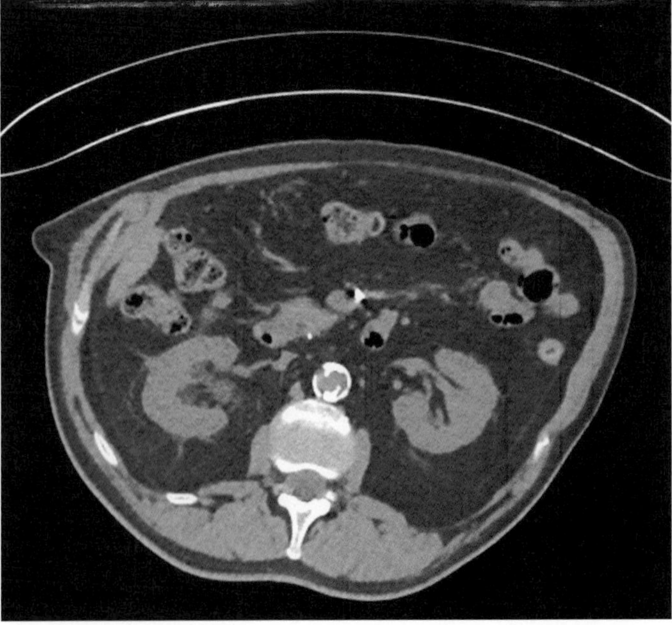

Figure 4.2 A CT KUB scan showing right hydronephrosis and associated fat stranding.

Expert comment Sepsis

Urosepsis is defined as 'life-threatening organ dysfunction caused by a dysregulated host response to infection of the urinary tract'. Septic shock includes circulatory and metabolic dysfunction and is by definition associated with significantly higher mortality.[23] Urosepsis is estimated to affect >6 million people worldwide, leading to >1 million deaths globally every year.[24]

Early diagnosis and prompt establishment of treatment are essential. The diagnosis of sepsis is based on suspicion of infection (i.e. abnormal temperature, leucocytosis, or leucopoenia) and the presence of organ dysfunction, including (1) abnormal mentation (agitation, drowsiness, confusion or coma (Glasgow Coma Scale score <15)), (2) increased respiratory rate (≥22 breaths per minute), and (3) reduced systolic blood pressure (≤100 mmHg). The presence or absence of these three simple clinical features is used to calculate the quick Sepsis-related Organ Failure Assessment (qSOFA) and to stratify risk. Mortality is approximately 20% in patients who present with all three features (qSOFA score of 3). NHS England endorses the latest version of the National Early Warning Score (NEWS, last updated in 2017) to identify deteriorating patients in a standardized fashion based on simple physiological parameters. A NEWS score >5 should trigger urgent or emergency clinical review.

The clinical diagnosis of urinary tract infection can be confirmed by urinalysis demonstrating the presence of bacteriuria, pyuria, and nitrites in the urine. Bacteriuria and the presence of nitrites are highly specific but poorly sensitive tests. The absence of pyuria virtually excludes a urinary tract infection. The most commonly isolated pathogen is *Escherichia coli*, followed by other Enterobacteriaceae. Antibiotic-resistant extended spectrum beta-lactamase bacteria are becoming more prevalent. Inflammatory markers such as CRP and procalcitonin are commonly used to confirm the diagnosis of sepsis and response to treatment.

Treatment and monitoring should be initiated as soon as possible. The **Sepsis Six** bundle is designed to facilitate early intervention with three diagnostic and three therapeutic steps to be delivered within 1 hour ('golden hour') to patients with suspected sepsis, irrespective of CRP or procalcitonin values. The six steps are:

1. Administer oxygen, targeting saturations >94%.
2. Take blood cultures and urinary cultures.
3. Give intravenous antibiotics.
4. Administer intravenous fluids up to 30 mL per kg.
5. Check serial lactates and refer to critical care if lactate >4 mmol/L.
6. Measure urine output.

If the patient remains hypotensive, drowsy, tachypnoeic or acidotic despite delivering the Sepsis Six bundle, an urgent referral should be made to critical care outreach.[25]

Evidence base Retrograde ureteric stent versus percutaneous nephrostomy

The infected obstructed kidney is a urological emergency and after urgent decompression carries a risk of septic shock and mortality. A 2018 study found the risk of septic shock and mortality post emergency decompression to be 15% and 5% respectively.[26] Initial management includes the Sepsis Six which involves starting empirical antibiotics immediately and fluid resuscitation. EAU guidance recommends urgent decompression to prevent further complications. Decompression can be achieved either by cystoscopic insertion of a retrograde ureteric stent or a percutaneous nephrostomy (PCN). They have been found to be of equal effectiveness with a similar rate of complications. These patients are often very sick and may require management in an intensive therapy unit (ITU) and so early involvement with the ITU team is often recommended.[18]

An early randomized controlled study comparing ureteric stents and PCN was undertaken in 1998. Data were obtained from 42 patients. The time between randomization and intervention was similar between the two groups. However, procedure time including use of fluoroscopy was less in the ureteric stent group compared to the PCN group. No statistically significant difference was observed in length of stay and time for WCC and temperature to normalize. Positive urine cultures were obtained in 62.9% of patients with a PCN compared to 19.1% of patients with a ureteric stent which was statistically significant ($p = 0.001$). Collection of urine for microscopy and sensitivity testing following decompression is important for guiding antibiotic treatment. Empirical antibiotics need to be re-evaluated as culture results and sensitivities become available. Patients undergoing PCN experienced greater back pain following the procedure when compared to ureteric stenting ($p < 0.05$). This study concluded that the decision between one decompressive intervention over another is based upon surgeon preference, logistical factors, and stone characteristics. Logistical factors to consider include the stability of the patient, whether the patient can tolerate lying flat, clotting function and anticoagulant medications, access to fluoroscopy in emergency theatre, space on emergency theatre lists, access to interventional radiology, and fitness for anaesthetic.[27]

A more recent retrospective non-randomized study in 2015 looked at 130 patients. Of these patients, two failed ureteric stent insertion and one failed nephrostomy insertion. The study found patients who underwent PCN were more likely to have larger stones and be more unwell than patients selected for ureteric stenting. It found no difference between time from septic event to definitive treatment. The PCN group had a greater length of stay ($p = 0.0001$), higher rate of ITU admission ($p = 0.006$), and were more unwell than patients selected for ureteric stenting. PCN and ureteric stents were both found to be equally effective.[28]

Definitive management of the obstructing stone is recommended to be delayed until the sepsis has resolved and the course of antibiotics has been completed.[18]

Expert comment Percutaneous nephrostomy placement

Expert tip

CT KUB is often performed in a prone position to differentiate between a VUJ stone and a stone that has passed and sits in the bladder at the VUJ.

Nephrostomy insertion

Indications for nephrostomy insertion include urinary tract obstruction (e.g. stone, tumour, ureteric stricture, and pregnancy), urine diversion (fistula), and access (percutaneous nephrolithotomy, ureteric stent, stone retrieval).

Contraindications are few and relative including bleeding disorders, an uncooperative patient, hyperkalaemia causing cardiac dysfunction, and no percutaneous access to the kidney due to adjacent organs (e.g. spina bifida).

A nephrostomy is usually performed with the patient lying in a prone position but can also be performed in a lateral and modified supine position depending on the position of the kidney with respect to adjacent organs. The procedure is performed as a sterile procedure under local anaesthesia. Ultrasound is used to guide a needle into the kidney. Access is ideally through the tip of a calyx avoiding the main blood vessels through Brodel's avascular plane. Once inside the collecting system, X-rays are used to monitor a Seldinger technique to place a wire, dilate the tract, and place a pigtail-type drainage catheter that gets connected to a catheter bag.

Major complications are infrequent, including bleeding (5%), sepsis (1–3%), and perforation of adjacent organ (e.g. bowel or pleura) (0.2%).

A nephrostomy tube was inserted and pus was drained. This was sent for culture. The patient recovered over the next 72 hours, and was discharged on a further course of oral antibiotics. He was then scheduled to undergo an urgent ureteroscopy (URS) and laser stone fragmentation.

Evidence base Extracorporeal shock wave lithotripsy and ureteroscopy

NICE guidance recommends extracorporeal shockwave lithotripsy (ESWL) as first-line treatment of ureteric stones <10 mm. In cases where ESWL is technically possible, URS can be considered if ESWL does not clear stones within 4 weeks, previous ESWL courses have failed, the stone cannot be targeted with ESWL, or there are contraindications to ESWL. The effectiveness of ESWL is affected by the efficiency of the lithotripter, patient body habitus, the stone itself (size, location, composition), and renal anatomy (e.g. infundibulopelvic angle, and infundibular length and width of the lower pole calix) which can be determined radiographically. A wide infundibulopelvic angle or short infundibular length and broad infundibular width are favourable for stone clearance following ESWL.[29] For stones >10 mm, URS is suggested as first line as the risk of loss of renal function is higher. Percutaneous nephrolithotomy and antegrade URS can be considered in large proximal impacted stones, especially where URS has failed.[6,18]

In situations where there is no pyonephrosis, guidance recommends active treatment of renal colic within 48 hours of diagnosis or readmission if pain is ongoing and not tolerated or the stone is unlikely to pass. The rationale behind this is that ureteric colic can be extremely painful and can lead to loss of renal function.[6]

Ureteroscopy has a small benefit over ESWL for stone-free rates, number of repeat treatments required, and quality of life. However, ESWL offers a shorter hospital stay, associated with less pain and fewer major adverse effects. ESWL is significantly more cost-effective than URS which is why it is first line for stones <10 mm. For those larger than 10 mm, URS is recommended due to concerns that delay in their management can lead to renal obstruction and subsequent permanent damage. This risk is present with smaller stones but is even greater with stones >10 mm.[6]

The patient underwent an elective URS 4 weeks later. At URS, the stone was visualized, and was well fragmented with a holmium laser fibre. All the fragments were removed with a zero-tip basket and sent for analysis. A JJ stent was placed after the procedure, and the nephrostomy tube was removed.

Expert comment Operative note

The patient was consented and marked appropriately. The patient was placed in the lithotomy position, and was prepped and draped. Intravenous gentamicin and co-amoxiclav were given in accordance with local antibiotic guidance. A sensor guidewire was passed up to the right kidney under X-ray guidance. A 7-French (Fr) rigid ureteroscope was passed alongside the guidewire, and the stone was visualized with some ureteric oedema around the stone. Irrigation was minimized. A 200 μm holmium laser fibre was passed, and fragmentation of the stone was commenced. The stone was soft, and was well fragmented with settings of 0.4 J and 20 Hz. One small piece of stone was seen to remain at the end of the procedure, and this was grasped with a 1.9 Fr tipless basket, and sent for stone analysis. A 26 cm, 6 Fr stent was placed. The nephrostomy tube was removed using X-ray control, and the stent was seen to remain in a good position after nephrostomy tube removal.

Postoperative plan

The patient was sent home later when able to pass urine. Stent removal in 2 weeks with flexible cystoscope was planned.

Expert comment Clinical surgical tip

In elderly men, accessing the ureteric orifice (UO) can be difficult, due to the size of the prostate. If there is a median lobe of the prostate, then entry to the bladder in the groove on the left side should be undertaken, and the tip of the cystoscope gently pressed down to reveal the UO. It is important to minimize the number of times the cystoscope comes over the bladder neck, due to increased risk of contact bleeding which may make the UO harder to find. If the wire which is passed does not come out of the tip of the cystoscope at the 6 o' clock position, then a retrograde catheter can be placed through the cystoscope and the wire passed through this. While spending time trying to intubate the UO, it is important that the surgeon does not overfill the bladder, which may also cause bleeding, and therefore the irrigation used should be minimized and the bladder should be regularly emptied.

Preventing retropulsion is important when dealing with ureteric stones. While many units do possess flexible ureteroscopes to retrieve a ureteric stone which has been retropulsed to the kidney, there are costs associated with this, and the skills and/or equipment may not always be readily available. Therefore, minimizing irrigation through the rigid ureteroscope is important. The choice of laser settings can also help to minimize retropulsion. Settings which involve having a low energy and, if possible, a longer pulse width will help to do this, as will the use of a smaller (200 μm) laser fibre. There are a number of anti-retropulsion devices available, but these are not often used unless the stone is larger and in the upper ureter, in which case some surgeons find them useful.

Fragmentation of a ureteric stone should start at the middle of the stone, to minimize the risk of ureteric trauma. With a softer stone, the decision to mostly dust the stone will help minimize retropulsion, and will also mean that there are fewer fragments to remove. It is important to try and have a fragment to send for analysis if one has not been sent previously, and the fragment must be made small enough to extract without the risk of traumatizing the ureter or getting the basket stuck with a stone fragment that is too large. If there is any doubt that the fragment may be too large to extract, it should be further lasered. If a stone is captured in the basket and then basket extraction becomes difficult because of a tight ureter, then if a 1.9 Fr basket is used, a 200 μm laser fibre can be passed alongside the basket, and the stone fragment further lasered to be made small enough to allow removal of the basket. Occasionally the basket itself may be lasered in this scenario, and if this happens the stone will be released, making the situation safe, and can then be further lasered to dust, or another basket used to remove stone fragments once the stone fragment has been further fragmented.

While routine ureteric stenting is not recommended after URS, in this situation, where there was a history of urosepsis and significant ureteric oedema below the stone, the decision was made to place a stent for 2 weeks.

Evidence base Ureteric stenting post URS

Routine retrograde ureteric stenting post URS is not recommended after uncomplicated complete stone removal.[18] A review paper looking at ureteric stenting post URS reviewed nine randomized controlled trials. Patients with stents inserted post URS experienced a higher incidence of lower urinary tract symptoms such as dysuria, frequency, and urgency than those who had not been stented. No benefit was elicited in terms of analgesia, urinary tract infections, stone-free rate, or ureteric strictures. However, ureteric stents did reduce the likelihood of acute admissions to hospital post URS but this difference was not statistically significant.[30] There is a role for ureteric stents post URS in patients who are at increased risk of complications due to ureteric trauma, residual stone fragments, and bleeding, for example.[18]

The EAU 2019 guidelines[18] recommend JJ stent insertion in the following circumstances:

- Ureteric trauma during the procedure.
- Residual stone fragments >2 mm remaining in ureter.
- Bleeding (potential for clot colic).
- Pregnancy.
- If treating an impacted stone (usually ureter very oedematous at site of impaction).
- Prolonged manipulation within ureter, particularly upper one-third.
- After flexible ureteroscopy and use of an access sheath.
- All doubtful cases, to avoid stressful emergencies.

NICE guidance similarly does not recommend routine stenting post URS for stones <20 mm. It recognized that ureteric stents are associated with numerous adverse effects such as pain, haematuria, and storage urinary symptoms which impact on quality of life and provide no benefit. Stenting could be considered where repeat treatment is required, solitary kidney cases, or if there is evidence of infection or obstruction. No recommendation was made on stones >20 mm because this is a small group of patients who would undergo variable treatments and the decision to stent would be made on clinical judgement. There is also a lack of evidence about stenting in this group of patients.[6]

The patient was reviewed in the outpatient clinic following removal of his stent. He was well. The stone was identified as a uric acid stone (94%). The patient underwent a basic metabolic screen.

Learning point Medical management of stones

EAU guidance advises a biochemical analysis of urine and blood in all patients presenting as an emergency with renal colic.[18] All patients should have a urine dipstick and serum blood samples sent for creatinine, uric acid, calcium, sodium, potassium, WCC, and CRP (and a clotting screen if intervention is required). Furthermore, first-time stone formers should have their stones sent for analysis by infrared spectroscopy or X-ray diffraction. In addition, patients on pharmacological stone prevention, or who have early or late recurrence following complete stone clearance, should also undergo a stone analysis. Patients who are managed conservatively are advised to sieve their urine in order to collect the stone when passed, so that it can be brought to their follow-up clinic and sent for analysis.

Following on from the acute setting, patients are classified as high or low risk for stone recurrence based on a number of factors including their stone history, the results of the basic blood tests, and stone analysis performed in the acute setting. Those with risk factors for recurrence are classified as high risk and therefore require a full metabolic workup at least 20 days after being stone free.[18]

There are many risk factors which increase the risk of stone recurrence. Certain medical conditions associated with an increased risk include hyperparathyroidism, polycystic kidney disease, and gastrointestinal diseases such as Crohn's disease to name but a few. Patients with anatomical variations of the urinary tract such as ureteral strictures, horseshoe kidneys, and ureteroceles are also at risk. Furthermore, stone formation in childhood and in teenagers, a family history of stone formation, and the composition of the stone itself including brushite containing stones, uric acid stones, and infection stones all increase the risk. A full list of these risk factor can be found in the EAU guidelines.[18]

Full metabolic testing should consist of one or two 24-hour urine collections obtained on a random diet and analysed at minimum for total volume, pH, calcium, oxalate, uric acid, citrate, sodium, potassium, and creatinine.[31]

Due to the high risk of recurrence (approximately 50%), all patients should be counselled on addressing risk factors. Generic advice includes drinking between 2.5 and 3 L of water daily, eating a balanced diet with limited salt and animal protein intake, maintaining a heathy body mass index, and exercising regularly.[18]

Uric acid stones are the only type of stone which can be dissolved by oral alkalinizing agents which act by raising the urinary pH. Ten per cent of urinary tract stones are composed of uric acid and are associated with a low urine pH and sometimes hypouricosuria. In patients with a low urinary pH, oral alkaline citrate such as potassium citrate or sodium bicarbonate can be used to raise the pH of the urine and dissolve the stone by chemolysis. The target pH is 7.0–7.2. Patients with uric acid stones are at high risk of recurrence and can be taught to monitor the pH of their urine with urine dipsticks and thus adjust the dose of their alkalizing agent according to their urine pH as prophylaxis.[18] No good-quality evidence is available for this therapy, but it has been used for some time. The principles behind this management and guidance for its clinical use have been provided by Rodman et al.[32] and supported by Becker.[33] Monitoring of radiolucent stones during therapy is usually undertaken by USS, but repeat non-contrast CT might be necessary in some situations.[32,33]

If they are found to have hyperuricosuria, patients should be treated with allopurinol to reduce the risk of recurrence.[18]

A final word from the expert

Ureteric colic is one of the commonest surgical emergencies. It is also one which can present with a broad range of morbidity, from the patient who has a small stone that has caused some transient pain, to the moribund patient with urosepsis who needs urgent intervention and time on the critical care unit. Developing a logical approach to the management of these patients, many of who will pass their stone spontaneously, while trying to avoid complications of urosepsis and kidney damage is important, and available guidelines help us to do this. There is no one-size-fits-all approach, however, and management options will be dependent upon local infrastructure and skill set, and be guided by patient factors such as occupation and social circumstances. The key in this group of patients is to intervene immediately for those who are sick and drain the kidney, to intervene early and definitively for those whose symptoms dictate or who are unlikely to pass their stone, and to manage the remainder of patients expectantly. In those patients who undergo surgical intervention, reducing the stenting rate and minimizing the indwell time of a stent if it is placed will help limit the morbidity experienced.

References

1. Menon M, Resnick MI. Urinary lithiasis: etiology, diagnosis, and medical and management. In: Walsh PC, Retik AB, Vaughan ED Jr, Wein AJ, eds. *Campbell's Urology*. 8th ed. Philadelphia, PA: WB Saunders Co; 2002:3229–3305.
2. Wilkinson H. Clinical investigation and management of patients with renal stones. *Ann Clin Biochem*. 2001;38:180–187.
3. Bihl G, Meyers A. Recurrent renal stone disease—advances in pathogenesis and clinical management. *Lancet*. 2001;358:651–656.
4. Serinken M, Karcioglu O, Turkcuer I, Ozkan H, Keysan M, Bukiran A. Analysis of clinical and demographic characteristics of patients presenting with renal colic in the emergency department. *BMC Res Notes*. 2008;1:79.
5. Argyropoulos A, Farmakis A, Doumas K, Lykourinas M. The presence of microscopic hematuria detected by urine dipstick test in the evaluation of patients with renal colic. *Urol Res*. 2004;32(4):294–297.
6. National Institute for Health and Care Excellence. Renal and ureteric stones: assessment and management [NG118]. National Institute for Health and Care Excellence. 2019. Available at: https://www.nice.org.uk/guidance/ng118
7. Joint Formulary Committee. British National Formulary (online). BMJ Group and Pharmaceutical Press. 2019. http://www.medicinescomplete.com
8. Teichman JMH. Acute renal colic from ureteral calculus. *N Engl J Med*. 2004;350(7):684–693.
9. Holdgate A, Pollock T. Nonsteroidal anti-inflammatory drugs (NSAIDs) versus opioids for acute renal colic. *Cochrane Database Syst Rev*. 2005;2:CD004137.
10. Afshar K, Jafari S, Marks AJ, Eftekhari A, MacNeily AE. Nonsteroidal anti-inflammatory drugs (NSAIDs) and non-opioids for acute renal colic. *Cochrane Database Syst Rev*. 2015;6:CD006027.
11. Ather M, Faizullah K, Achakzai I, Siwani R, Irani F. Alternate and incidental diagnoses on noncontrast-enhanced spiral computed tomography for acute flank Pain. *Urol J*. 2009;6(1):14–18.
12. Culp O, Bersatz P. Urologic aspects of lesions in the abdominal aorta. *J Urol*. 1961;86:189–195.
13. Greenwell T, Woodhams S, Denton E, Mackenzie A, Rankin S, Popert R. One year's clinical experience with unenhanced spiral computed tomography for the assessment of acute loin pain suggestive of renal colic. *BJU Int*. 2000;85(6):632–636.
14. Smith R, Verga M, McCarthy S, Rosenfield AT. Diagnosis of acute flank pain: value of unenhanced helical CT. *Am J Roentgenol*. 1996;166(1):97–101.
15. Niemann T, Kollmann T, Bongartz G. Diagnostic performance of low-dose CT for the detection of urolithiasis: a meta-analysis. *Am J Roentgenol*. 2008;191(2):396–401.

16. Smith-Bindman R, Aubin C, Bailitz J, et al. Ultrasonography versus computed tomography for suspected nephrolithiasis. *N Engl J Med*. 2014;371(12):1100–1110.
17. Masselli G, Weston M, Spencer J. The role of imaging in the diagnosis and management of renal stone disease in pregnancy. *Clin Radiol*. 2015;70(12):1462–1471.
18. European Association of Urology. Guidelines on urolithiasis. European Association of Urology. 2019. http://uroweb.org/guideline/urolithiasis/
19. Shah TT, Gao C, Peters M, et al. Factors associated with spontaneous stone passage in a contemporary cohort of patients presenting with acute ureteric colic: results from the Multi-centre cohort study evaluating the role of Inflammatory Markers In patients presenting with acute ureteric Colic (MIMIC) study. *BJU Int*. 2019; 124(3):504–513.
20. Preminger GM, Tiselius HG, Assimos DG, et al. 2007 guideline for the management of ureteral calculi. *Eur Urol*. 2007;52(6):1610–1631.
21. Pickard R, Starr K, MacLennan G, et al. Medical expulsive therapy in adults with ureteric colic: a multicentre, randomised, placebo-controlled trial. *Lancet*. 2015;386(9991):341–349.
22. Dauw CA, Hollingsworth JM. Medical expulsive therapy: PRO position. *Int J Surg*. 2016;36:655–656.
23. Singer M, Deutschman CS, Seymour CW, et al. The Third International Consensus Definitions for Sepsis and Septic Shock (Sepsis-3). *JAMA*. 2016; 315(8):801–810.
24. Fleischmann C, Scherag A, Adhikari NK, et al. Assessment of global incidence and mortality of hospital-treated sepsis. Current estimates and limitations. *Am J Respir Crit Care Med*. 2016;193(3):259–272.
25. Robson WP, Daniel R. The Sepsis Six: helping patients to survive sepsis. *Br J Nurs*. 2008;17(1):16–21.
26. Srougi V, Moscardi PR, Marchini GS, et al. Septic shock following surgical decompression of obstructing ureteral stones: a prospective analysis. *J Endourol*. 2008;32(5):446–450.
27. Pearle MS, Pierce HL, Miller GL, et al. Optimal method of urgent decompression of the collecting system for obstruction and infection due to ureteral calculi. *J Urol*. 1998;160(4):1260–1264.
28. Goldsmith ZG, Oredein-McCoy O, Gerber L, et al. Emergency ureteric stent vs percutaneous nephrostomy for obstructive urolithiasis with sepsis: patterns of use and outcomes from a 15-year experience. *BJU Int*. 2013;112(2):122–128.
29. Elbahnasy AM, Shalhav AL, Hoenig DM, et al. Lower caliceal stone clearance after shock wave lithotripsy or ureteroscopy: the impact of lower pole radiographic anatomy. *J Urol*. 1998;159(3):676–682.
30. Nabi G, Cook J, N'Dow J, McClinton S. Outcomes of stenting after uncomplicated ureteroscopy: systematic review and meta-analysis. *BMJ*. 2007;334(7593):572.
31. Pearle MS, Goldfarb DS, Assimos DG, et al. Medical management of kidney stones. AUA guideline. *J Urol*. 2014;192(2):316–324.
32. Rodman JS, Williams JJ, Peterson CM. Dissolution of uric acid calculi. *J Urol*. 1984;131(6):1039–1044.
33. Becker G. Uric acid stones. *Nephrology*. 2007;12(Suppl 1):S21.

Bladder stone management

Siân Allen and Daron Smith

Expert commentary Daron Smith

Case history 1: acute urinary retention, catheter, and stone

A 67-year-old man with a previous history of ureteric colic developed painful acute urinary retention secondary to bladder outlet obstruction from an 80 cc benign enlarged prostate. A computed tomography (CT) scan of the kidneys, ureters, and bladder (KUB) showed a catheter *in situ* with a 15 × 13 × 11 mm bladder stone (Figure 5.1). Following a failed trial of voiding and re-catheterization, a transurethral resection of the prostate (TURP) and cystolitholapaxy with a stone punch was performed; follow-up showed a good improvement in flow rate and resolution of his lower urinary tract symptoms.

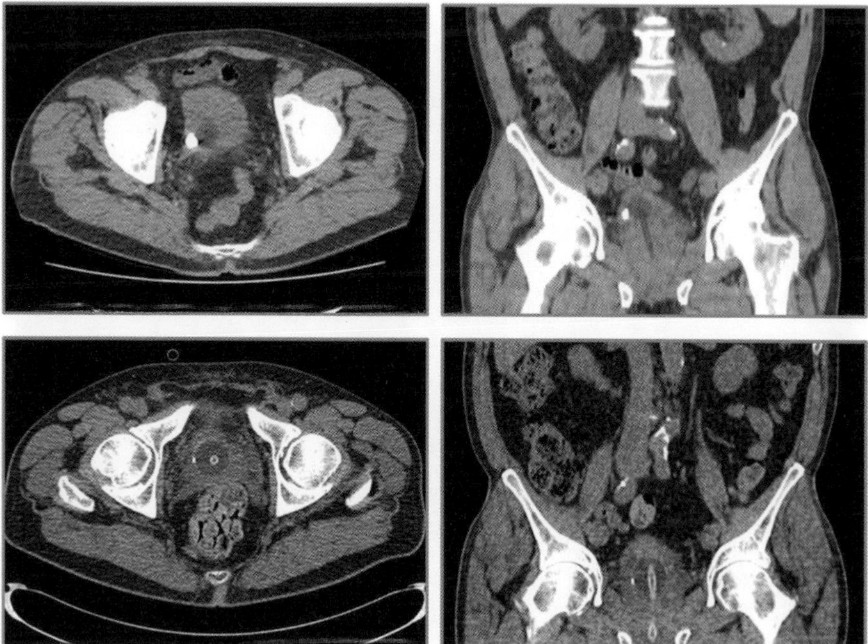

Figure 5.1 Acute urinary retention, catheter, and stone. This CT KUB scan shows a 15 × 13 × 11 mm bladder stone with a catheter *in situ* and an enlarged prostate. There is a tiny residual fragment next to the catheter on a CT scan performed after mechanical fragmentation with a stone punch followed by TURP.

Learning point Clinical features and risk factors

Bladder stones are one of the oldest known diagnoses, and urolithiasis is one of the most common urological conditions, but bladder stone formation is currently relatively uncommon. In fact, bladder calculi account for just 5% of urinary calculi, and are more common in men than women (who represent approximately 5% of bladder stone formers).

Bladder stones can present with haematuria, recurrent urinary tract infections, and/or voiding symptoms, and can be formally diagnosed on imaging studies such as KUB X-ray, ultrasound, or abdominal CT or identified during diagnostic cystoscopy. They may also be asymptomatic, and detected as an incidental finding during investigations for other conditions.

Risk factors for bladder stone formation include bladder outlet obstruction, neuropathic voiding dysfunction, bladder augmentation/reconstructions, recurrent infection and foreign bodies. As such, adult men with bladder outlet obstruction account for most cases of bladder stones, raising the question of whether bladder outlet surgery is also needed, and if this should be performed at the time the stones are treated. In females, the identification of a bladder stone raises the possibility of a foreign body (sutures, synthetic tapes, or mesh) from previous continence surgery. Considering this from an alternative perspective, investigations to identify or exclude a bladder stone should be considered in women who have storage bladder symptoms or recurrent urinary infections following reconstructive pelvic floor surgery where synthetic material has been used. The same applies to men with similar symptoms who have undergone radical prostatectomy where a bladder stone may have occurred on a clip.

Learning point Bladder stone treatment options

The treatment of bladder stones has evolved from open surgical removal through blind transurethral stone crushing to endourological 'natural orifice' surgery via the urethra or as 'minimally invasive surgery' via a percutaneous approach. As long ago as 1993, John Wickham noted that 'nearly all bladder stones can be treated by transurethral endoscopy' (at that time using an electrohydraulic probe) and that 'only the largest renal tract stones still require open surgery'.

The aim of bladder stone treatment is to achieve a completely stone-free bladder with a short hospital stay and minimal risk of postoperative complications. The treatment options are extracorporeal shockwave lithotripsy (SWL), transurethral cystolitholapaxy (TUCL), percutaneous cystolitholapaxy (PCCL), and open surgical removal by cystolithotomy. The endourological treatments use a variety of energy sources to fragment/disintegrate the stones including mechanical cystolitholapaxy with a 'stone punch', ultrasound, electrohydraulic lithotripsy, pneumatic/ballistic LithoClast®, and holmium:yttrium aluminium-garnet (HoYAG) laser. Each treatment option has advantages and disadvantages; as such, the characteristics of the stone (size, number, consistency), ease of access to the bladder, and the general health of the patient need to be considered before determining the best choice of treatment. In addition, the likely underlying cause for the stone formation should be borne in mind, such that relieving bladder outlet obstruction, eliminating infection, and removing foreign bodies are important in bladder stone management, particularly for reducing the likelihood of recurrent stone formation.

Clinical tip SWL

SWL is an easy, simple, and well-tolerated procedure for bladder stones, but has the lowest stone clearance rate of the treatment options. It is therefore generally reserved to avoid anaesthesia in high-risk patients with small-volume stones, and without significant bladder outflow obstruction such that the stone fragments can be passed satisfactorily.

Expert comment Benign prostate hyperplasia and stones

While it has long been recognized that bladder stones are associated with bladder outlet obstruction secondary to benign prostatic enlargement, for many years it was considered high risk to combine cystolitholapaxy and TURP in a single operation. This created a conflicting treatment rationale that lower urinary tract symptoms due to bladder stones are due to bladder outlet obstruction and therefore an outflow procedure is also needed, while recommending that bladder stone treatment and relief of outflow obstruction should not be performed at the same time due to increased surgical morbidity, including of postoperative infection.

However, as technology has developed, so has the feasibility of combining these procedures safely and effectively. Over the last 30 years, simultaneous treatment has evolved from SWL therapy with a Dornier HM3 lithotripter in patients with small stones undergoing TURP for small to medium prostates through pneumatic lithotripsy and TURP for larger stones and prostates to laser cystolitholapaxy combined with holmium laser enucleation of the prostate for those with still larger stone burdens and prostate sizes.

The key to a successful outcome is to complete the stone treatment in reasonable time before the prostate surgery. If stone treatment via the urethra would add too much time to the overall operation, it is possible to combine percutaneous stone surgery with TURP, either as sequential or even simultaneous procedures. In the sequential approach, the suprapubic sheath can be left *in situ* following PCCL to provide continuous drainage during TURP, followed by a suprapubic catheter for additional postoperative drainage/monitoring. A simultaneous approach has also been described whereby PCCL can be performed on the stone(s) in a laparoscopic entrapment bag while the TURP is performed concurrently by a second surgeon.

Case history 2: stone on mesh

A 67-year-old lady who had undergone a transvaginal tape procedure 10 years previously had recurrent bladder stones treated three times over a 4-year period in another hospital. Further stones were identified at CT KUB—a larger oval stone measuring 30 × 28 × 18 mm and a smaller spherical 10 mm stone that appeared adherent to the right anterolateral bladder wall (Figure 5.2a). At cystoscopy, during which both stones were treated by laser cystolitholapaxy, the 10 mm stone was adherent to eroded mesh, which was lasered to just beneath the urothelium. A follow-up CT a year and a half postoperatively showed a curvilinear calcification where the adherent stone had been previously (Figure 5.2b). A cystoscopy showed some eroded mesh with surface calcification. A transvaginal/laparoscopic mesh excision was scheduled, but a repeat cystoscopy prior to that procedure 4 months later showed no stone or eroded mesh, and she has remained stone free at further follow-up CT imaging 2 years after the cystolitholapaxy and mesh lasering.

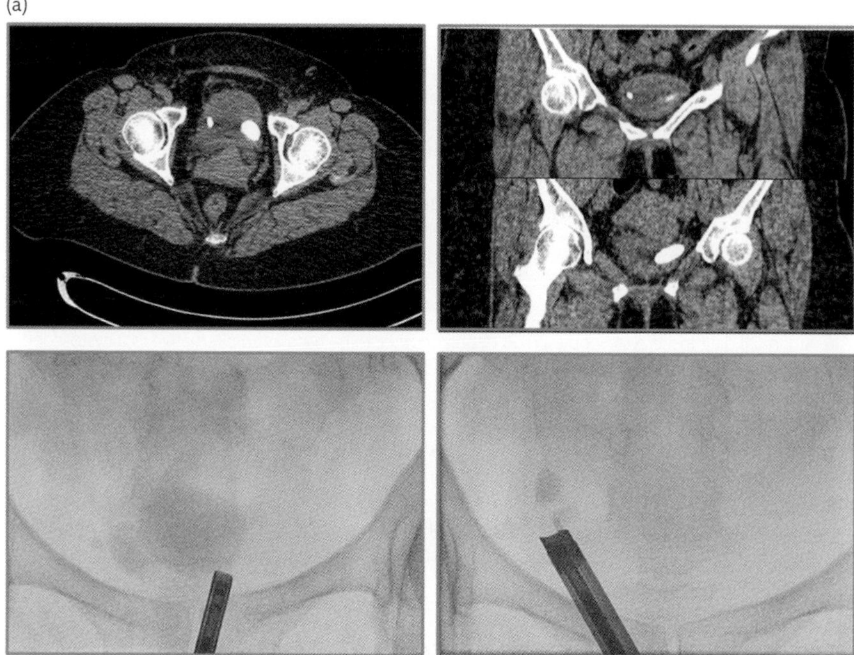

Figure 5.2 Stone on mesh. (a) This CT KUB scan shows a free-floating 30 × 28 × 18 mm and a 10 mm stone adherent to eroded mesh. An initial 22 Fr cystoscopy was followed by laser cystolitholapaxy and laser to intravesical mesh using a resectoscope to allow larger fragments to be washed out than possible via a cystoscope. (b) A follow-up CT scan 18 months after her cystolitholapaxy/showed curvilinear calcification where the adherent stone had been previously, which had fully resolved at further follow-up after 2 years.

(b)

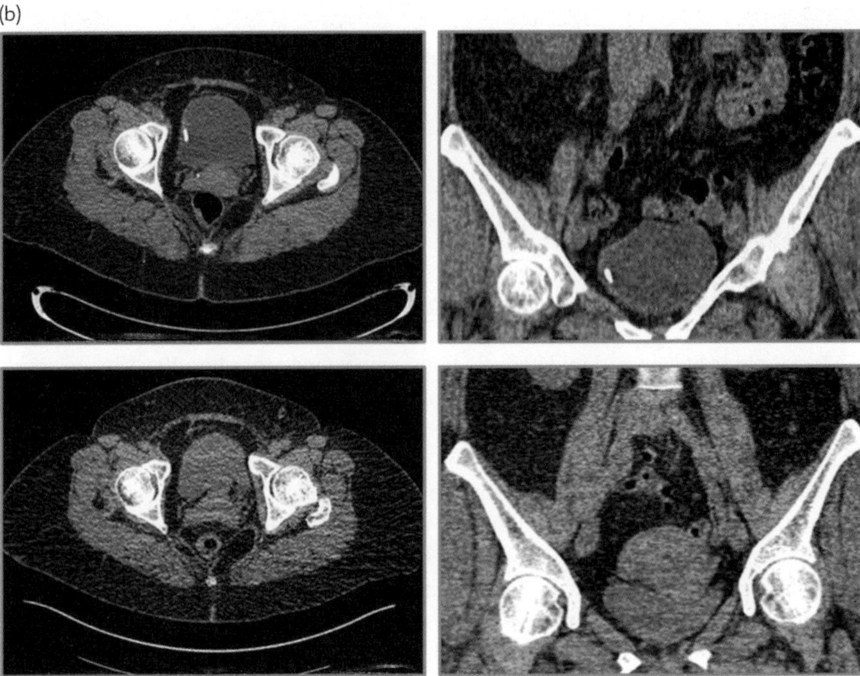

Figure 5.2 Continued

Learning point TUCL

Cystoscopic treatment

A standard 22 French (Fr) cystoscope allows an initial assessment of the urethra, prostate/bladder neck, as well as the bladder urothelium and the stone burden itself. After treating the stone with an energy source (most commonly a laser), the fragments and dust can be washed out using an Ellik evacuator. Small fragments can also be retrieved directly via the cystoscope sheath using biopsy/stent removal forceps. A short-term postoperative catheter may be inserted, including the use of a 'three-way' catheter to irrigate stone dust and tiny fragments, and avoid the potential for clot formation from associated bleeding from a prominent prostate middle lobe.

Nephroscopic treatment

After an initial diagnostic cystoscopy, a rigid nephroscope can be used as an alternative to a cystoscope for treating the stone. Having a wider lumen than a cystoscope, a nephroscope offers better irrigation, and therefore improved vision, as well as the opportunity to use larger calibre lithotripters, such as a combined pneumatic/ultrasound lithotripsy device. This has the advantage over laser fragmentation as stone dust and small fragments can be actively suctioned via the probe, improving vision and reducing the time required to wash out or remove small fragments with forceps. When the stones have been fully treated, the cystoscope can be re-inserted to identify and remove any small remaining fragments, whereas larger fragments may require re-insertion of the nephroscope and further disintegration with the energy source. As for cystoscopic treatment, a postoperative urethral catheter will usually be required.

Expert comment

Mesh/synthetic material

Suture or synthetic mesh associated with bladder stone formation can be laser ablated until just below the bladder mucosa to reduce the risk of recurrent stone formation. Preoperative cross-sectional imaging should be reviewed to assess the proximity of neighbouring structures which may have become tethered to the bladder to avoid inadvertent fistula creation following lasering. If this technique fails, surgical resection of the mesh should be considered.

Case history 3: stone and urethral stricture

A 24-year-old male, who had a 2 year-history of prior urethral stricture disease requiring regular urethral dilatations, was referred for a urethroplasty. A large bladder stone was identified on the urethrogram, for which a non-contrast CT KUB was

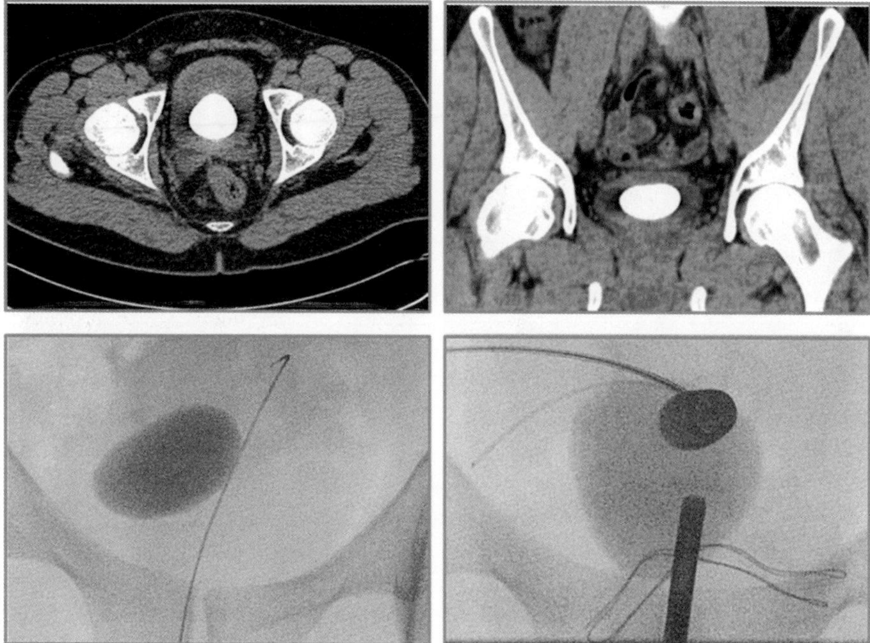

Figure 5.3 Stone and urethral stricture. This CT scan shows a 38 × 37 × 21 mm bladder stone with intraoperative PCCL images showing a guidewire in the bladder to safely negotiate a 22 Fr cystoscope via a narrow urethra to the bladder. An Amplatz sheath is seen 'end on' via which the stone was fragmented and cleared.

performed, confirming a 38 × 37 × 21 mm bladder stone. To avoid exacerbating his urethral stricture, this was treated percutaneously, and was confirmed to be stone free on postoperative CT KUB. His lower urinary tract symptoms improved such that he did not keep further urological follow-up appointments and the anticipated urethroplasty has not been required (Figure 5.3).

Case history 4: small-volume neobladder

A 53-year-old man who had undergone a radical cystectomy with an orthotopic neobladder formation 3 years previously reported increasing difficulty performing clean intermittent self-catheterization and recurrent urinary tract infections. He was diagnosed with two rapidly enlarging bladder stones (17 × 14 × 13 mm and 14 × 13 × 13 mm) on CT abdomen and pelvis imaging performed as part of his oncological follow-up (Figure 5.4). A laser cystolitholapaxy was scheduled, including the possibility of percutaneous access to the right kidney to pass an antegrade guidewire to help identify the Studer extension of his neobladder to facilitate accessing that part of the neobladder with a flexible cystoscope. Following a urethral dilatation, both stones were successfully identified and cleared; the biochemistry was pure calcium magnesium ammonium phosphate with a positive bacterial culture of both *Escherichia coli* and *Proteus mirabilis*. The rapid stone growth was therefore likely to have been the consequence of urinary stasis and recurrent infections, as opposed to the cause of them, with an increase in the urinary pH causing increased calcium phosphate and magnesium ammonium phosphate crystalluria and stone formation.

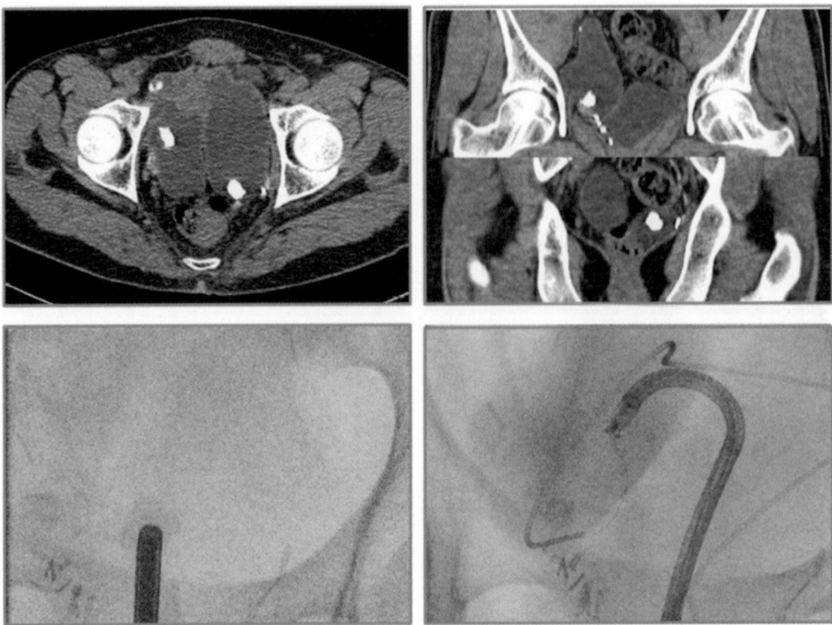

Figure 5.4 Small-volume neobladder. This CT KUB scan shows a 17 × 14 × 13 mm and 14 × 13 × 13 mm stone in a Studer neobladder reconstruction. The first stone was treated straightforwardly with a laser via a 22 Fr cystoscope. A flexible cystoscope was used to direct a wire and ureteric catheter to the Studer extension of the neobladder, where the second stone was identified, grasped in a Nitinol basket, and retrieved to the main bladder lumen, where it was treated using the rigid cystoscope.

Case history 5: small-volume neobladder and artificial urinary sphincter

A 23-year-old woman with spina bifida, requiring a wheelchair to mobilize, had an augmentation cystoplasty and Mitrofanoff channel for neuropathic detrusor over-activity and incontinence. She had formed bladder stones previously, and although she still had urethral access to her bladder, there was an artificial urinary sphincter *in situ*, such that these were treated percutaneously. Follow-up imaging 2 years later showed two new spiculated bladder stones measuring 20 × 16 × 16 mm and 10 × 9 × 9 mm for which a further PCCL was performed. The stone biochemistry was 75% magnesium ammonium phosphate/25% ammonium urate, with a positive culture of *Corynebacterium*, which is a urease-producing organism generating an alkaline urine consistent with the stone biochemistry (Figure 5.5).

Learning point PCCL

A percutaneous suprapubic approach to the bladder offers a minimally invasive option for larger bladder calculi, or where the urethral approach would be challenging or impossible. As stones enlarge, the time taken to treat them and the number of fragments generated increase (see 'Expert comment' box on stone size). The percutaneous approach allows high flow rates via a nephroscope, with efflux of irrigation fluid and stone dust via the Amplatz sheath offering excellent visualization during stone fragmentation. Furthermore, it avoids prolonged urethral instrumentation and thereby reduces the risk of a subsequent urethral stricture.

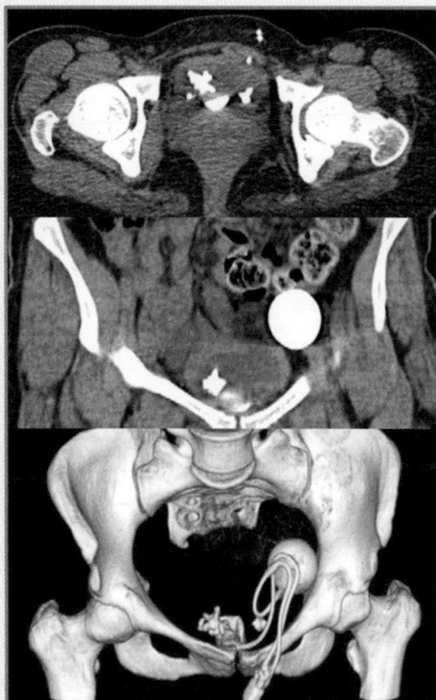

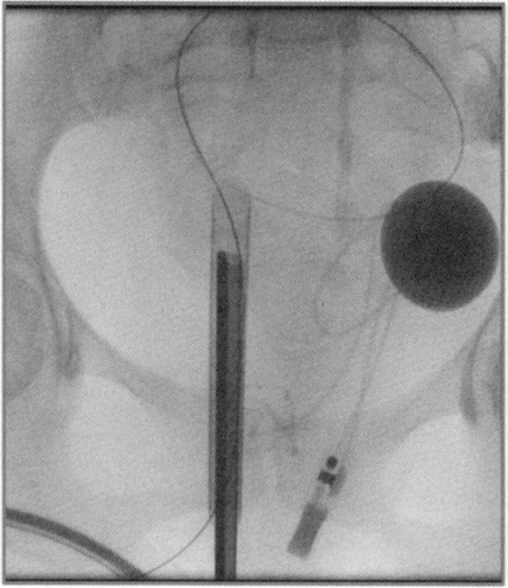

Figure 5.5 Small-volume neobladder and artificial urinary sphincter. This CT KUB scan and rendered reconstruction image shows two spiculated bladder stones measuring 20 × 16 × 16 mm and 10 × 9 × 9 mm with an artificial urinary sphincter *in situ* (reservoir, pump, cuff and tubing). The stones were treated with a nephroscope via a 30 Fr Amplatz sheath.

The bladder/neobladder is filled with saline though a catheter or endoscope via the urethra or Mitrofanoff catheterizable stoma. When adequately distended, guidewire access can be achieved via a needle puncture or through an existing suprapubic catheter tract with any combination of cystoscopic, ultrasound, or fluoroscopic guidance. A tract is dilated over the wire, often using a balloon dilator, to allow insertion of an Amplatz sheath via which a nephroscope is placed and the stone fragmented and retrieved percutaneously through the sheath.

Access can also be obtained directly via a Mitrofanoff channel, although care has to be taken to make sure that this does not affect the continence mechanism or ease for the patient to catheterize postoperatively. For this reason, it is often advisable to gain separate percutaneous access away from the Mitrofanoff stoma.

Postoperatively, the patient may be left with both a suprapubic and urethral catheter; the former can be used for irrigation and the latter for drainage.

Expert comment PCCL technical tweaks

- A bladder evacuator can be attached to the Amplatz sheath to wash out large quantities of stone fragments more rapidly than they can be aspirated through the nephroscope probe, or removed under vision with forceps (Figure 5.6). This should be performed with the bladder underfilled to avoid high intravesical pressures, especially in reconstructed bladders, where there is a risk of bladder rupture.
- The use of a 12 mm self-retaining laparoscopic trocar has been described to allow the use of large-calibre nephroscopes for rapid stone fragmentation and extraction.
- Laparoscopic entrapment sacs have also been used to manipulate calculi into for ease of subsequent fragmentation. After the initial laparoscopic trocar has been removed over the

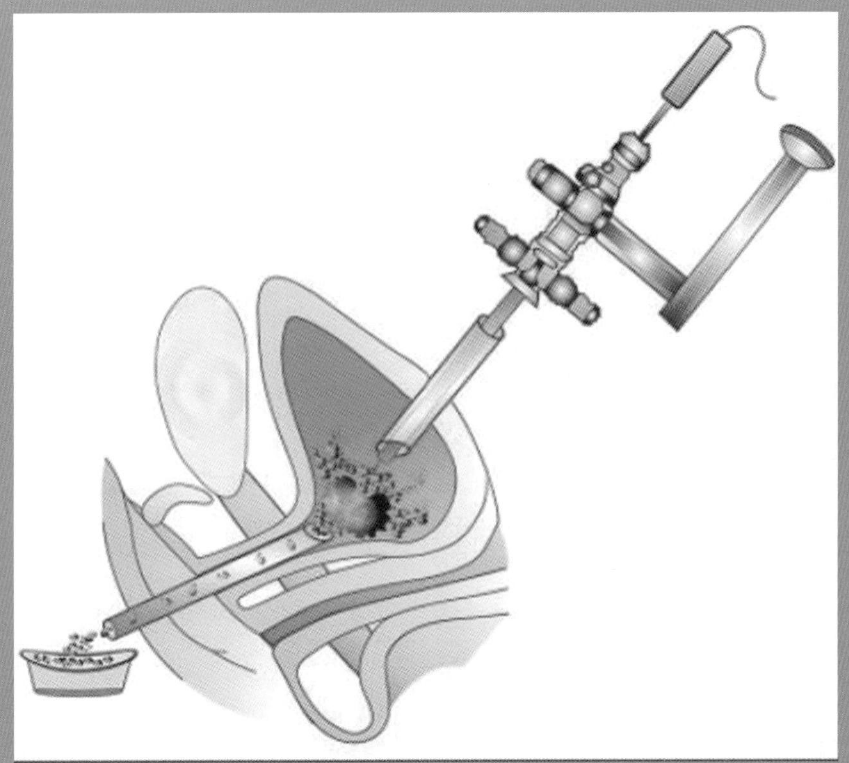

Figure 5.6 Fragmented stone particles slide out through the urethral Amplatz.
From Kumar et al. *J Surg Tech Case Rep*. 2013 Jul;5(2):109–111.

entrapment sac, an Amplatz sheath can be inserted into the bag; the nephroscope and lithotripsy device can then fragment and evacuate the calculi without the need to 'chase' fragments around the bladder.

- A 'twin Amplatz sheath' technique has been described in females with bladder stones >5 cm. The stone fragmentation is performed via a suprapubic 30 Fr Amplatz sheath, while a second 28 Fr sheath is placed via the urethra. With the patient positioned at 20° 'feet down', the bevelled end of the sheath is placed at the bladder neck to act like a 'water slide' so that fragments wash out passively via the urethral Amplatz tube.

Expert comment Stone size

Stone size is crucial in determining the operative approach.

Assuming a stone is a sphere, its volume can be calculated according to the formula $V = 4/3 \times \pi \times r^3$. Figure 5.7 shows the exponential increase in stone volume as the diameter increases in 5 mm increments, such that a 40 mm stone has a volume eight times as much as a 20 mm stone and a 50 mm stone has a volume nearly 16 times as much.

Assuming the stone is purely fragmented (as opposed to 'dusted' and washed out), Figure 5.7 also shows the number of fragments that need to be created to be retrieved via scopes of different diameter, that is, a 22 Fr cystoscope, 26 Fr resectoscope, or removed with grasping forceps via a 30 Fr Amplatz sheath. These values help demonstrate why a PCCL may be a better choice than a urethral approach for a 35–40 mm stone (particularly if the urethra would not accommodate a scope with a larger calibre), and why an open cystolithotomy and lifting out a single stone >60 mm (which has a volume 27 times as much as a 20 mm stone) is likely to be a faster operation, and guaranteed to be totally stone free, than a PCCL for this size of stone.

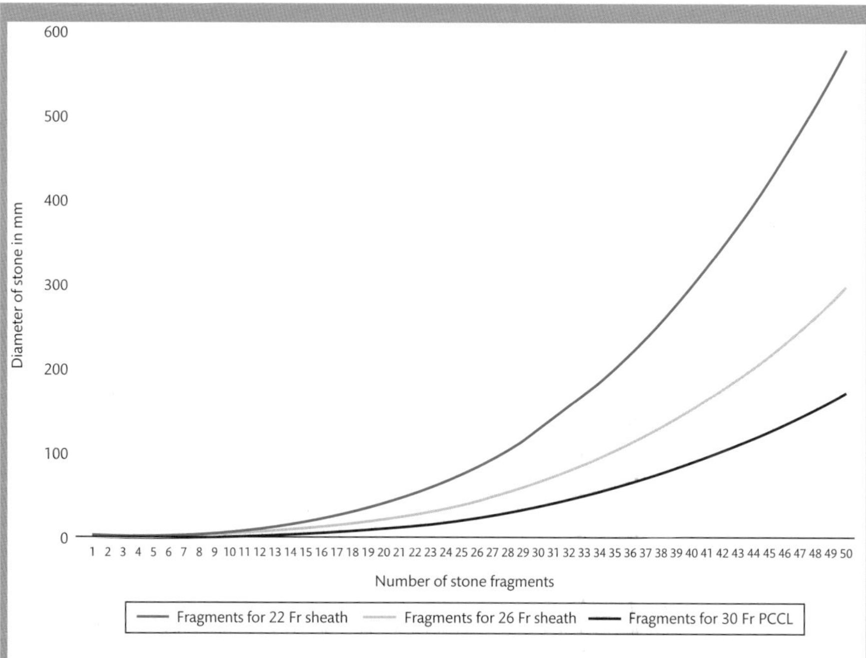

Stone diameter (mm)	Volume (cc)	No. of fragments for 22 Fr sheath	No. of fragments for 26 Fr sheath	No. of fragments for 30 Fr PCCL
5	63	1	1	1
10	500	5	2	1
15	1688	16	8	5
20	4000	37	19	11
25	7813	72	37	21
30	13,500	125	64	37
35	21,438	198	102	59
40	32,000	296	152	88
45	45,563	422	216	125
50	62,500	579	296	171

Figure 5.7 Stone diameter, volume, and fragments. The calculated stone volume as a spherical stone increases in 5 mm diameter increments, with the number of fragments this would generate to be removed via sheaths of increasing calibre from 22Fr cystoscope to 26Fr resectoscope to a 30 Fr Amplatz sheath. The curves for number of fragments show divergence around 30–40 mm (i.e. where PCCL may be faster and more effective than a urethral approach) and are widely separated by 50 mm (i.e. where open cystolithotomy and removal of whole stones in single figures is likely to be the preferred treatment).

Expert comment Neobladders and neuropaths

Augmented bladders

- Patients with augmented/neobladder formation are at increased risk of urinary tract infections due to poor drainage and the presence of mucus. All three of these factors predispose to stone formation, which are often large or complex requiring percutaneous or open stone removal.
- After stone removal, bladder drainage should be optimized, which may include more frequent self-catheterization and/or saline bladder washouts. Metabolic assessment including the stone

biochemistry and urine pH may help with preventative advice (e.g. calcium phosphate stones in association with alkaline urine may benefit from urinary acidification).

Neuropaths

- Patients with a high (i.e. cervical) level injury and those undergoing procedures with more than one modality have been shown to be more likely to have a postoperative complication and longer length of stay than lower level cord injury or stone burdens that can be treated with a single modality.

Clinical tip Treatment tips and tricks

- Stone treatment is a balance between sufficient irrigation to afford good vision for fragmentation while avoiding overdistension of the bladder, particularly in a thin-walled neobladder.
- The inflow of saline should be as slow as vision permits, and can even be stopped and the drainage outflow opened on the cystoscope to allow the bladder to empty and dust to drain while continuing to treat the stone. This requires care not to empty the bladder fully, risking laser damage to the urothelium. as vision will be lost as the bladder collapses around the scope.
- The use of an Amplatz working sheath via the urethra to facilitate access, irrigation and drainage, and fragment removal has been described in both male and female patients after prior urethral dilatation. This allows small stone fragments to drain with the irrigating fluid while larger fragments can be retrieved using grasping forceps in an analogous fashion to PCNL.
- Balloon dilatation for PCCL offers a rapid single-step method to create the track, but may not work if there is significant fibrosis (e.g. a pre-existing suprapubic track). If so, alternative approaches include metal dilators via the existing track, or a separate percutaneous puncture and creation of a new track.
- Following PCCL, the timing of suprapubic catheter removal depends on the circumstances—if neobladder remove suprapubic catheter first, let the wound site heal, and then remove the urethral catheter. If stones are likely secondary to bladder outlet obstruction, and this has not been treated during the procedure, the urethral would be removed first for a trial of voiding, leaving the suprapubic catheter clamped as a 'fail safe'.

Case history 6: large-volume neobladder

A 57-year-old man who had undergone a radical cystoprostatectomy and neobladder reconstruction 4 years previously had haematuria following performing self-intermittent catheterization per urethram. A CT scan showed seven spherical/tetrahedral bladder stones 20–30 mm in maximum diameter (Figure 5.8). These were considered too large a stone burden to manage endoscopically due to the potential for multiple procedures or injury to the neobladder wall from a stone fragment. As such, an open surgical removal was performed, extracting all seven stones whole. A postoperative cystogram showed all stones had been removed and confirmed no leak from the neobladder before removing the urethral catheter and resuming clean intermittent self-catheterization.

Clinical tip Open stone removal

Patients with large bladder calculi (perhaps 5 cm or larger) have traditionally been managed with open cystolithotomy. Endoscopic management with cystolitholapaxy or electrohydraulic lithotripsy can be more challenging for stones this size and above—procedures take longer and views are poorer owing to the higher volume of stone fragments and dust. In turn, this means a greater chance of bleeding and bladder damage (especially in the case of a thin-walled neobladder). Stone-free rates are therefore lower for endoscopic management of large stones so it is often preferable to lift out the stones whole through an open cystotomy, and thereby ensure a stone-free bladder in a single procedure.

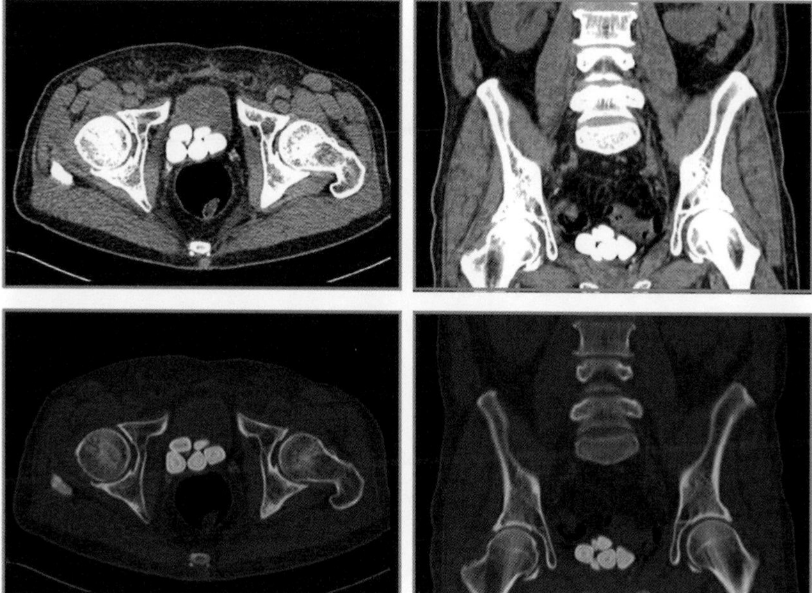

Figure 5.8 Large-volume neobladder. This CT KUB scan shows seven spherical/tetrahedral bladder stones between 20 and 30 mm in maximum diameter in a neobladder. The 'bone windows' images underneath show their laminated structure. These were removed whole by open cystolithotomy.

Learning point Choice of treatment

- If the appropriate modality of treatment is chosen, stones should be fully cleared in a single sitting.
- Nephroscopic stone treatment (either transurethrally or percutaneously) with combined pneumatic/ultrasound fragmentation allows suction via the treatment probe, improving the endoscopic vision and the ease of removing small stones/stone dust.
- Transurethral nephroscopic treatment for larger stones is usually faster than treatment with a laser via a cystoscope, but is associated with a greater number of urethral passages of the scope (including an initial and final cystoscopy to assessment the stone burden).
- The percutaneous approach is more effective for patients with larger stones, especially if these are in a neobladder, and has a lower risk of urethral trauma/postoperative stricture than the urethral approach. It is therefore particularly useful if the urethral route is difficult or impossible (urethral stricture, artificial urinary sphincter, bladder neck closure).
- The disadvantage of PCCL is the added risk from suprapubic access compared with 'natural orifice' urethral surgery, which increases the morbidity of the procedure. Accordingly, PCCL patients generally require more analgesia, have a longer length of stay, and have the risk of wound infection at the suprapubic access/postoperative catheter site.
- Transurethral and percutaneous treatments can be performed under local anaesthesia in selected patients, with holmium laser lithotripsy using a flexible cystoscope the logical 'next step' if SWL is inappropriate or ineffective.

Evidence base Stone-free rate for different treatments

A systematic review of bladder stone treatment, published in *European Urology* in 2019, assessed 25 studies including 2340 patients with the following conclusions:

- The stone-free rate (SFR) for adults with bladder stones is lower with SWL than TUCL.
- SFRs for TUCL were equivalent for laser and pneumatic stone fragmentation.

- SFRs were the same for TUCL and PCCL but with a shorter procedure duration (approximately a 10-minute saving) and hospital stay (0.8 days).
- SFRs were the same for open cystolithotomy versus TUCL and PCCL, with shorter procedures catheterization time and hospital stay for the endoscopic approaches (but the reviewers commented that this was based on low quality of evidence).
- SFRs were the same for TUCL using a nephroscope or a cystoscope but shorter by a mean difference of nearly 23 minutes with a nephroscope.

A final word from the expert

As stone volumes increase, so does the number of fragments created when treating them. Although SWL may be appropriate for small-volume stones <10 mm (especially if aiming to avoid general/regional anaesthesia), the mainstay of stone treatment is performed as an endourological procedure. This is achieved per urethram in the majority of cases, reserving the percutaneous approach for larger-volume stones (30–40 mm or more), particularly in patients with complex anatomy (lack of urethral access or bladder reconstruction). Open surgery is needed in a small minority of patients, generally because of huge stones of 50–60 mm or more.

Provided the stone size is appropriate, endoscopic treatments have excellent (i.e. close to 100%) stone clearance rates with shorter catheter dwell time and faster convalescence than open surgery. TUCL has less risk and a shorter hospital stay than the percutaneous approach so is the treatment of choice for bladder stones when feasible; the use of a nephroscope via the urethra provides a rapid, safe, and effective means to treat bladder stones with a long-term urethral stricture rate similar to a cystoscopic technique.

The 'index patient', that is, a man with bladder stones secondary to benign prostatic enlargement, can safely have both issues treated at once. Simultaneous holmium laser enucleation of the prostate and holmium laser cystolitholapaxy increases the total operation time, but does not influence the risk of important postoperative complications or treatment outcome. Stones of any size and composition, and prostates of practically any size can be treated endoscopically using the holmium laser. TURP can also be combined with PCCL as a faster alternative to TURP following TUCL in patients with large bladder calculi and large prostates, reducing the fragmentation time for the former and using the suprapubic access site as an outflow channel to improve the vision during the latter.

Adaptations to PCCL include the use of a bladder evacuator to wash out fragments via the Amplatz sheath, or deploying a laparoscopic entrapment sac to retain the stones in close proximity of the nephroscope for treating them. These modifications facilitate the treatment of larger calculi, including those in urinary diversions, to achieve complete stone clearance in a single sitting.

In conclusion, the combination of endourological techniques allows a bespoke approach to manage bladder stones in most situations, and will no doubt continue to extend the threshold for open cystolithotomy, and thereby confirm John Wickham's observation that 'only the largest renal tract stones still require open surgery'.

Further reading

History/overview/general references

DeFoor W, Minevich E, Reddy P, et al. Bladder calculi after augmentation cystoplasty: risk factors and prevention strategies. *J Urol.* 2004;172(5 Pt 1):1964–1966.

Donaldson JF, Ruhayel Y, Skolarikos A, et al. Treatment of bladder stones in adults and children: a systematic review and meta-analysis on behalf of the European Association of Urology Urolithiasis Guideline Panel. *Eur Urol.* 2019;76(3):352–367.

Papatsoris AG, Varkarakis I, Dellis A, Deliveliotis C. Bladder lithiasis: from open surgery to lithotripsy. *Urol Res.* 2006;34(3):163–167.

Philippou P, Moraitis K, Masood J, Junaid I, Buchholz N. The management of bladder lithiasis in the modern era of endourology. *Urology.* 2012;79(5):980–986.

Stav K, Dwyer PL. Urinary bladder stones in women. *Obstet Gynecol Surv.* 2012;67(11):715–725.

Wickham JE. Treatment of urinary tract stones. *BMJ.* 1993;307(6916):1414–1417.

Technique

Bansal A, Kumar M, Sankhwar S, et al. Prospective randomized comparison of three endoscopic modalities used in treatment of bladder stones. *Urologia.* 2016;83(2):87–92.

Breda A, Mossanen M, Leppert J, Harper J, Schulam PG, Churchill B. Percutaneous cystolithotomy for calculi in reconstructed bladders: initial UCLA experience. *J Urol.* 2010;183(5):1989–1993.

Elbahnasy AM, Farhat YA, Aboramadan AR, Taha MR. Percutaneous cystolithotripsy using self-retaining laparoscopic trocar for management of large bladder stones. *J Endourol.* 2010;24(12):2037–2041.

Ener K, Agras K, Aldemir M, Okulu E, Kayigil O. The randomized comparison of two different endoscopic techniques in the management of large bladder stones: transurethral use of nephroscope or cystoscope? *J Endourol.* 2009;23(7):1151–1155.

Eyre KS, Eyre DW, Reynard JM. Morbidity associated with operative management of bladder stones in spinal cord-injured patients. *Spinal Cord.* 2015;53(11):795–799.

Floyd MS Jr, Stubington SR. Mitrofanoff cystolitholapaxy: an innovative method of stone clearance in a hostile abdomen with an inaccessible urethra. *Urol J.* 2015;12(2):2115–2118.

Kara C, Resorlu B, Cicekbilek I, Unsal A. Transurethral cystolithotripsy with holmium laser under local anesthesia in selected patients. *Urology.* 2009;74(5):1000–1003.

Kumar A, Dalela D, Dalela D, Goel A, Paul S, Sankhwar SN. The twin Amplatz sheath method: a modified technique of percutaneous cystolithotripsy for large bladder stones in female patients. *J Surg Tech Case Rep.* 2013;5(2):109–111.

Loeb S, Semins MJ, Matlaga BR. Novel technique for fragment removal after percutaneous management of large-volume neobladder calculi. *Urology.* 2012;80(2):474–476.

Okeke Z, Shabsigh A, Gupta M. Use of Amplatz sheath in male urethra during cystolitholapaxy of large bladder calculi. *Urology.* 2004;64(5):1026–1027.

Paez E, Reay E, Murthy LN, Pickard RS, Thomas DJ. Percutaneous treatment of calculi in reconstructed bladder. *J Endourol.* 2007;21(3):334–336.

Teichman JM, Rogenes VJ, McIver BJ, Harris JM. Holmium:yttrium-aluminum-garnet laser cystolithotripsy of large bladder calculi. *Urology.* 1997;50(1):44–48.

Tugcu V, Polat H, Ozbay B, Gurbuz N, Eren GA, Tasci AI. Percutaneous versus transurethral cystolithotripsy. *J Endourol.* 2009;23(2):237–241.

Wollin TA, Singal RK, Whelan T, Dicecco R, Razvi HA, Denstedt JD. Percutaneous suprapubic cystolithotripsy for treatment of large bladder calculi. *J Endourol.* 1999;13(10):739–744.

Benign prostate hyperplasia and stones

Aron M, Goel R, Gautam G, Seth A, Gupta NP. Percutaneous versus transurethral cystolithotripsy and TURP for large prostates and large vesical calculi: refinement of technique and updated data. *Int Urol Nephrol.* 2007;39(1):173–177.

Bosco PJ, Nieh PT. Extracorporeal shock wave lithotripsy in combination with transurethral surgery for management of large bladder calculi and moderate outlet obstruction. *J Urol.* 1991;145(1):34–36.

Nseyo UO, Rivard DJ, Garlick WB, Bennett AH. Management of bladder stones: should transurethral prostatic resection be performed in combination with cystolitholapaxy? *Urology.* 1987;29(3):265–267.

Romero-Otero J, García González L, García-Gómez B, et al. Analysis of holmium laser enucleation of the prostate in a high-volume center: the impact of concomitant holmium laser cystolitholapaxy. *J Endourol.* 2019;33(7):564–569.

Shah HN, Hegde SS, Shah JN, Mahajan AP, Bansal MB. Simultaneous transurethral cystolithotripsy with holmium laser enucleation of the prostate: a prospective feasibility study and review of literature. *BJU Int.* 2007;99(3):595–600.

Sinik Z, Isen K, Biri H, et al. Combination of pneumatic lithotripsy and transurethral prostatectomy in bladder stones with benign prostatic hyperplasia. *J Endourol.* 1998;12(4):381–384.

Sofer M, Kaver I, Greenstein A, et al. Refinements in treatment of large bladder calculi: simultaneous percutaneous suprapubic and transurethral cystolithotripsy. *Urology.* 2004;64(4):651–654.

Tangpaitoon T, Marien T, Kadihasanoglu M, Miller NL. Does cystolitholapaxy at the time of holmium laser enucleation of the prostate affect outcomes? *Urology.* 2017;99:192–196.

Zhao J, Shi L, Gao Z, Liu Q, Wang K, Zhang P. Minimally invasive surgery for patients with bulky bladder stones and large benign prostatic hyperplasia simultaneously: a novel design. *Urol Int.* 2013;91(1):31–37.

SECTION 3

Upper urinary tract benign disease

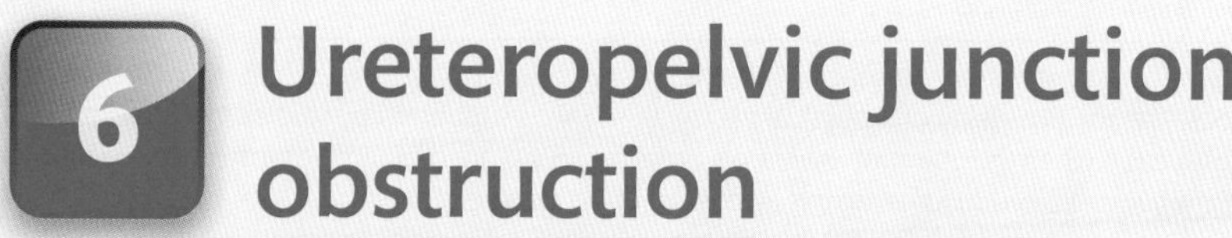

6 Ureteropelvic junction obstruction

Sanjeev Pathak

Expert commentary Neil Oakley

Case history

A 29-year-old male presented to the emergency unit with abdominal pain. He had sudden onset of right loin and abdominal pain. He described the pain as excruciatingly severe, radiating from the loin to groin and was unable to gain comfort. There were no associated lower urinary tract symptoms. He felt nauseous, with no vomiting and no other gastrointestinal symptoms. There was no previous history of kidney stones or urinary tract infections. Interestingly, in the past, he had suffered with intermittent right loin pain exacerbated with alcohol intake. Regarding his general health, there was no previous significant medical or surgical history. He had no known drug allergies or prescription medication. There was a strong family history of kidney stones (maternal and paternal family). He worked as a full-time chef.

On examination, he appeared to be in discomfort. He had mild pyrexia of 37.9°C, pulse rate of 88 beats per minute, blood pressure of 140/75 mmHg, pulse oximetry of 96%, and respiratory rate of 18 breaths per minute. Abdominal examination demonstrated tenderness but no guarding in the right periumbilical region and loin. There were no palpable abdominal masses. Genital examination was unremarkable.

He was given pain relief with per rectal diclofenac (a non-steroidal anti-inflammatory drug). His blood tests revealed a haemoglobin level of 164 g/L (normal range: 131–166 g/L) and white cell count of 14 × 10^9/L (normal range: 3.5–9.5 × 10^9/L); his serum calcium and uric acid levels were normal. Urine dipstick was positive for red and white cells but negative for nitrites. Clinically, the differential diagnoses included right ureteric calculi or pyelonephritis. He underwent a low-dose, non-contrast computed tomography (CT) scan of the abdomen and pelvis. The CT scan was reported as a horseshoe kidney with bilateral, multiple renal calculi but no ureteric calculi, and there was inflammation of the right peri-pelvicalyceal system and hydronephrosis (Figure 6.1). He was transferred to the urology team. Initially, he was treated with intravenous antibiotics and, subsequently, discharged home with an oral course of co-amoxiclav. His urine and blood cultures were negative for bacterial growth.

Learning point Epidemiology of UPJO

- Congenital UPJO: incidence 1 in 2000 live births screened by routine antenatal ultrasound.[6]
- Males are more commonly affected than females (2:1).
- Aetiology:
  - Functional obstruction: results from impaired smooth muscle differentiation in the upper ureter and renal pelvis.

Clinical tip Salient history

Classical symptoms of acute ureteric colic:

- Sudden onset of severe colicky pain.
- Radiation loin to groin.
- Associated fever and elevated white cell count raises possibility of infected, obstructed kidney.

Classical presentation of ureteropelvic junction obstruction (UPJO):

- Onset and exacerbation of pain with alcohol and caffeinated drinks.
- Onset and exacerbation of pain with diuretics.
- Asymptomatic UPJO may result in irreversible 'silent renal loss'.

Learning point
Epidemiology of renal stones

Risk factors for developing stones:

- Sex: three times more likely in men.[1,2]
- Family history of kidney stones: increased risk of 30% in first-degree relative.
- Occupation: increased risk in cooks/chefs.
- Incidence of renal stones in patients with UPJO and horseshoe kidney is 20%.[3,4] Patients with UPJO and concurrent renal calculi carry the same metabolic risk as other stone formers in the general population.[5]

- Mechanical obstruction: presence of aberrant lower pole crossing vessels in up to 50% of cases; does raise the possibility of a physical obstruction. This is supported by studies that show relief of obstruction when the aberrant lower pole crossing vessels are mobilized and 'hitched'—Hallström technique or ligated.[7] However, this area is still under debate.

Learning point Horseshoe kidney

- Horseshoe kidney incidence is 1 in 500 of the general population but the stone incidence is 20–30%.[3,4]
- Aetiology:
  - Failure of the kidneys to ascend, possibly due to failure of regression of caudal blood supply (e.g. persistent accessory iliac vessels).
  - Lower poles fuse together—isthmus.
  - Inferior mesenteric artery—landmark of isthmus.
- Horseshoe kidney is disproportionately associated with an increased incidence of UPJO.
- Associated with Edwards, Turner, and Down syndromes.

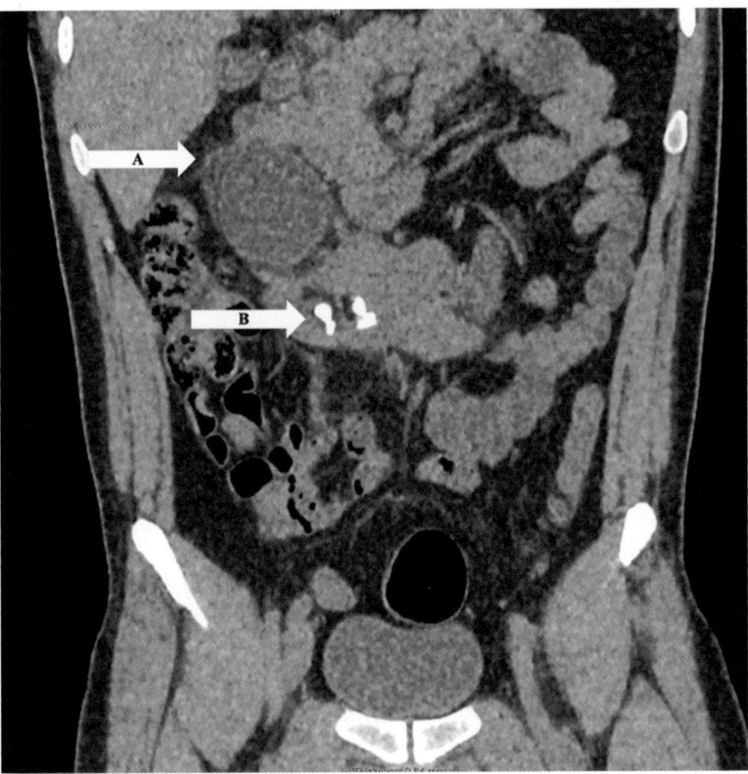

Figure 6.1 Coronal view of a non-contrast CT scan of abdomen and pelvis. This shows right peri-pelvicalyceal inflammation (arrow A) and multiple calculi in the right moiety (arrow B) of a horseshoe kidney.

Evidence base National Institute for Health and Care Excellence 2019 guidelines

Diagnostic imaging: 'offer urgent (within 24 hours of presentation), low-dose non-contrast CT to adults with suspected renal colic. If a woman is pregnant, offer ultrasound instead of CT'.[8]

Pain relief: 'offer a non-steroidal anti-inflammatory drug (NSAID) by any route as first-line treatment for adults, children and young people with suspected renal colic'.[8]

Expert comment Drainage of kidney

For patients with pyonephrosis (i.e. pus in the collecting system due to obstruction), then the old surgical adage of 'if there is pus about, let it out' is as true today as it has ever been. Antibiotics do not penetrate well into an infected collecting system and patients with pyonephrosis are going to be profoundly septic and will need drainage. Many patients, however, even in the presence of obstruction, do not develop pyonephrosis due to upper urinary tract infection and will resolve with conservative measures.

This patient did not have clinical features of infected collection in that his temperature was not swinging, it was not high-grade pyrexia, he was normotensive and only slightly tachycardiac, and, therefore, a trial of fluid and antibiotics was entirely reasonable. If he had not settled, then drainage would have been indicated and whether nephrostomy or stent would depend on local expertise. The nephrostomy has a small risk of significant haemorrhage but guarantees drainage under local anaesthetic whereas a stent involves anaesthesia for a potentially unstable patient and has a higher risk of bacteraemia crisis.

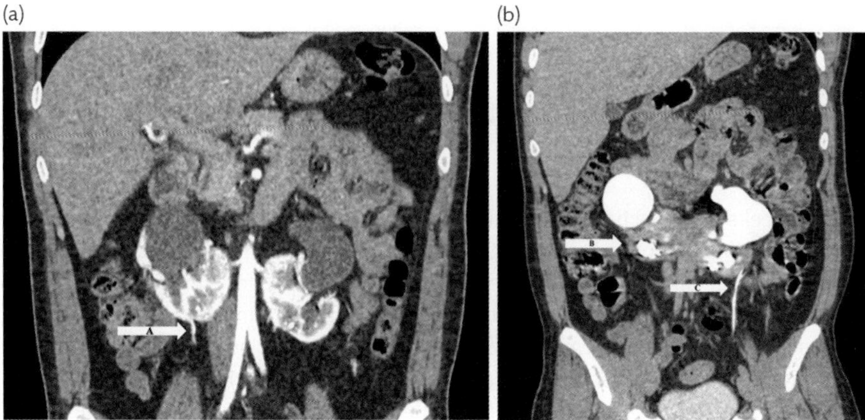

Figure 6.2 Coronal view of a CT urogram. (a) Arterial phase showing an accessory artery entering the right lower moiety of horseshoe kidney arising from right common iliac artery (arrow A). (b) Excretory-phase CT urogram showing absence of contrast in the right ureter in keeping with right ureteropelvic junction obstruction of the horseshoe kidney (arrow B). Contrast is seen in left ureter (arrow C).

The patient underwent a couple of radiological scans, and a technetium-99m mercaptoacetyltriglycine (MAG3) renogram showed 45% function of the right moiety with an obstructed drainage pattern in keeping with UPJO. Unfortunately, following the MAG3 renogram, he developed right loin pain that lasted a few hours but eventually subsided. The CT urogram (arterial phase and excretory phase) confirmed multiple arterial blood vessels supplying the obstructed right moiety (Figure 6.2). Thereafter, his case was discussed at the endourology multidisciplinary team meeting. At the meeting, the stone burden was assessed, and all the calyces were identified by three-dimensional reconstruction images. Potential management options were explored.

Evidence base Radiological tests used as a work-up for UPJO

Anatomical imaging

- Ultrasound scan of renal tract: determines hydronephrosis with assessment of renal parenchyma.
- Non-contrast CT scan of abdomen and pelvis: ureteric calculi.
- Contrast CT scan of abdomen and pelvis: delineates vascular anatomy (e.g. crossing vessels).
- CT urogram/magnetic resonance urogram: level of obstruction.

Functional imaging

- MAG3 renogram: confirms obstruction and relative function. The radiolabelled isotope is injected intravenously, 15 minutes following administration of furosemide (a diuretic). Four types of renogram curves are described[9]:
  - Type 1: normal uptake with prompt washout.
  - Type 2: a rising uptake curve with no response to diuretics, which suggests obstruction.
  - Type 3a: an initially rising curve that falls rapidly in response to diuretics, which suggests non-obstructive dilatation.
  - Type 3b: an initially rising curve that neither falls promptly nor continues to rise (equivocal).
- Whitaker test: largely, a historical test but has a role in equivocal cases of obstruction. This is an invasive, dynamic test that measures the pressure gradient between the renal pelvis and bladder. It

requires a nephrostomy tube and urinary catheter connected to pressure transducers. The patient is prone and diluted contrast media is infused in an antegrade manner at a rate of 10 mL/min.[10]
- Pressure gradient <15 cmH_2O = non-obstructed.
- Pressure gradient between of 15–22 cmH_2O = equivocal.
- Pressure gradient >22 cmH_2O = obstructed.

At 8 weeks post discharge, the patient was reviewed in the outpatient clinic. I explained the diagnosis of congenital right UPJO with bilateral, multiple renal calculi. We discussed all the options available, particularly the rationale for surgery. We agreed to deal with the stone burden in the left moiety once the right moiety had been treated. He underwent an uncomplicated, dismembered right pyeloplasty plus pyelolithotomy plus antegrade JJ stent insertion via a low, right subcostal incision. During the operation, the relevant vascular anatomy to the right moiety was identified and preserved, and the abnormal ureteropelvic junction segment was excised. Using a flexible cystoscope for identification, all renal calculi were removed with a nitinol tipless stone extractor. The Anderson–Hynes pyeloplasty was performed.[11]. The renal pelvis was deliberately not reduced in size. The abdominal drain was removed on day 2, urethral catheter on day 3, and the patient was discharged home on day 4. He underwent a flexible cystoscopy and JJ stent removal at 6 weeks, followed by a MAG3 renogram at 3 and 12 months. The histopathological findings reported were subepithelial fibrosis and mild disarray of the muscularis bundles. He is asymptomatic and has good drainage from the right moiety. Currently, he prefers to be managed conservatively for the stone burden in the left moiety.

Expert comment Why not manage conservatively?

In cases of asymptomatic UPJO, conservative management is feasible because the aim of surgery is to protect renal function and to alleviate symptoms. If the UPJO is incidentally detected, this may indicate a stable chronic pathological entity and intervention has risks of nephrectomy and anastomotic stenosis.

Previous evidence would suggest that the progression of renal loss in UPJO treated conservatively and observed by serial renography may occur in one in ten patients but is unlikely without symptoms. Once a patient has had a symptomatic episode, it is generally accepted that these are likely to recur.

Therefore, indications for intervention include:

- Recurrent pain
- Previous septic episode/pyonephrosis
- Progressive renal loss on renography/morphological features suggesting risk of complication (gross hydronephrosis or stones)
- Lifestyle in which complications are likely, such as young age or contact sports, then surgical correction is mandated.

Interestingly, following his MAG3 renogram, the patient developed right loin pain that lasted a few hours but eventually subsided. This is referred to as Dietl's crisis and is classical of UPJO.[12]

Expert comment Intervention options

Endopyelotomy is a potential treatment for UPJO; however, the success rates are widely variable and are less reliable regarding long-term de-obstruction rates than pyeloplasty. There are morphological factors that would suggest an unfavourable outcome from endopyelotomy such as degree of hydronephrosis, presence of lower pole crossing vessels, and worse ipsilateral split renal function.[13]

In this case, not only are there renal stones which would require an a percutaneous nephrolithotomy but the surgical anatomy (i.e. the horseshoe kidney) would add additional complication to an endopyelotomy. A pyeloplasty remains the gold standard for definitive de-obstruction of UPJO regarding symptom relief and renographic function, and in this case will allow stone clearance during the same procedure.

The options for performing a pyeloplasty in a horseshoe kidney would be open, laparoscopic, or robotic assisted. The benefits of a laparoscopic/robotic approach would be small incisions and less respiratory compromise and fewer long-term wound complications. This has become accepted as the standard approach; however, with a more complex renal anatomy, a higher degree of expertise to access each of the calyces would be extremely challenging laparoscopically. Use of the DaVinci robot with the articulating wrist would allow access to all calyces but would require intraoperative robotic ultrasound to check for stone clearance; again, this would be extremely challenging.

Expert comment Why insert a ureteric stent?

The use of a ureteric stent is to ensure safe drainage of the renal pelvis of the urine across the anastomosis while it heals. Anastomotic leaks are a risk of pyeloplasty (although possibly less in robotic cases with the facilitated suturing), and diverting urine by a ureteric stent reduces these; if they do occur they are usually managed by reinserting a urethral catheter. A nephrostomy also reduces leakage but may not act as a scaffold for the healing anastomosis to remain patent. Pyeloplasty is performed in the paediatric population without ureteric stents without long-term sequalae.[14] In adults, a randomized study has shown no adverse consequences in ureteric stent removal at 1 week over 4 weeks. It might be tempting, therefore, to remove stents early because of symptoms; however, animal studies have revealed that it can take a week for the mucosa to heal following ureteric disruption and up to 4 weeks for the muscularis layer to be histologically healed. Hence the reason why ureteric stents are traditionally kept in for 6 weeks. In the presence of stone disease, a stent is mandatory in case of distal ureteric stone migration.

Expert comment Why leave capacious right renal pelvis?

An aggressive reduction pyeloplasty is likely to give a faster return to a more normal-looking excretion curve on a renogram and possibly reduce sluggish drainage in the long term. It does not, however, improve pain or functional outcomes when compared with a more conservative reduction in renal pelvis size; furthermore, post-pyeloplasty resolution of dilatation and hydronephrosis is uncommon.[15] In addition, the greater the reduction in tissue, the greater the operative difficulty. More dissection is required leading to risk to renal blood supply; more suturing is required: the greater the gap between pelvis and ureter (and hence difficulty in opposing the two), and the greater chance of inadvertently closing a calyx. In the presence of stone disease, however, the possibility of a large redundant pelvis having a sump-like effect to collect stone fragments and facilitate possible future stone formation and the possibility that too large a pelvis may make future flexible ureterorenoscopy technically more difficult.

A final word from the expert

This case highlights the complexity of unilateral UPJO in a relatively young patient with a horseshoe kidney and bilateral renal stones. Therefore, I strongly recommend that this type of case be discussed at the multidisciplinary team meeting. Thorough planning is vital to ensure counselling of the patient with short- and long-term management objectives. Preoperative planning, particularly with three-dimensional CT reconstruction images, will identify accessory vessels such as those arising from iliac vessels, thus avoiding inadvertent injury. Furthermore, this will aid in the identification of stones within calyces. Although minimally invasive (laparoscopic and robot-assisted) pyeloplasty is increasingly the gold standard in adults,[16] this is not the case in horseshoe kidney with UPJO, as demonstrated with small case series reports.[17,18] In this case, given the presence of a significant calyceal stone burden, open surgery was considered the best approach for stone clearance and drainage. However, the future direction is likely to be robot assisted given the increasing experience in robotic surgery, albeit in specialist centres.

Following pyeloplasty, if the drainage from the kidney is normal on renogram at 12 months, patients may be discharged from further follow-up.[19] In this case, postoperative repeat MAG3 renograms at 3 and 12 months showed good drainage. I would recommend long-term follow-up due to:

- Risk of recurrent urinary stone formation.
- Unresolved stone burden in left moiety.
- Risk of stone complications—pain, infections, and stone migration.

Although the patient is reluctant to receive further treatment, I would encourage treatment of the stone burden in the left moiety.

References

1. Soucie JM, Thun MJ, Coates RJ, McClellan W, Austin H. Demographic and geographic variability of kidney stones in the United States. *Kidney Int.* 1994;46(3):893–899.
2. Hiatt RA, Dales LG, Friedman GD, Hunkeler EM. Frequency of urolithiasis in a prepaid medical care program. *Am J Epidemiol.* 1982;115(2):255–265.
3. Janetschek G, Kunzel KH. Percutaneous nephrolithotomy in horseshoe kidneys. Applied anatomy and clinical experience. *Br J Urol.* 1988;62(2):117–122.
4. Cussenot O, Desgrandchamps F, Ollier P, Teillac P, Le Duc A. Anatomical bases of percutaneous surgery for calculi in horseshoe kidney. *Surg Radiol Anat.* 1992;14(3):209–213.
5. Husmann DA, Milliner DS, Segura JW. Ureteropelvic junction obstruction with a simultaneous renal calculus: long-term followup. *J Urol.* 1995;153(5):1399–1402.
6. Woodward M, Frank D. Postnatal management of antenatal hydronephrosis. *BJU Int.* 2002;89(2):149–156.
7. Keeley FX Jr, Bagley DH, Kulp-Hugues D, Gomella LG. Laparoscopic division of crossing vessels at the ureteropelvic junction. *J Endourol.* 1996;10(2):163–168.
8. National Institute for Health and Care Excellence. Renal and ureteric stones: assessment and management. NICE guideline [NG118]. National Institute for Health and Care Excellence. 2019. https://www.nice.org.uk/guidance/ng118
9. O'Reilly PH, Lawson RS, Shields RA, Testa HJ. Idiopathic hydronephrosis—the diuresis renogram: a new non-invasive method of assessing equivocal pelvioureteral junction obstruction. *J Urol.* 1979;121(2):153–155.
10. Whitaker RH. Methods of assessing obstruction in dilated ureters. *Br J Urol.* 1973;45(1):15–22.
11. Anderson JC, Hynes W. Retrocaval ureter; a case diagnosed pre-operatively and treated successfully by a plastic operation. *Br J Urol.* 1949;21(3):209–214.
12. Dietl J. Wandernde nieren and deren einklemmung. *Wien Med Wohenschr.* 1864;14(2):153–161.
13. Samarasekera D, Chew BH. Endopyelotomy still has an important role in the management of ureteropelvic junction obstruction. *Can Urol Assoc J.* 2011;5(2):134–136.
14. Smith KE, Holmes N, Lieb JI, et al. Stented versus nonstented pediatric pyeloplasty: a modern series and review of the literature. *J Urol.* 2002;168(3):1127–1130.
15. Carpenter CP, Tolley E, Tourville E, Sharadin C, Giel DW, Gleason JM. Hydronephrosis after pyeloplasty: 'will it go away?' *Urology.* 2018;121:158–163.

16. Light A, Karthikeyan S, Maruthan S, Elhage O, Danuser H, Dasgupta P. Peri-operative outcomes and complications after laparoscopic vs robot-assisted dismembered pyeloplasty: a systematic review and meta-analysis. *BJU Int.* 2018;122(2):181–194.
17. Potretzke AM, Mohapatra A, Larson JA, Benway BM. Transmesenteric robot-assisted pyeloplasty for ureteropelvic junction obstruction in horseshoe kidney. *Int Braz J Urol.* 2016;42(3):626–627.
18. Spencer CD, Sairam K, Challacombe B, Murphy D, Dasgupta P. Robot-assisted laparoscopic pyeloplasty for the management of pelvi-ureteric junction obstruction in horseshoe kidneys: initial experience. *J Robot Surg.* 2009;3(2):99–102.
19. O'Reilly PH, Brooman PJ, Mak S, et al. The long-term results of Anderson-Hynes pyeloplasty. *BJU Int.* 2001;87(4):287–289.

CASE

7 Oncocytoma

Andrew Deytrikh

Expert commentary Georgina Reall, James Lenton, and Anthony Browning

Case history

A 30-year-old lady is referred by her general practitioner as a 2-week wait to the urology outpatient department having presented with amenorrhoea. A subsequent ultrasound scan (USS) of the abdomen and pelvis, arranged in primary care, demonstrated a large (59 × 59 × 53 mm) solid vascular mass arising from the left kidney.

The patient was otherwise fit and well with no past medical history. There was no family history of renal cancer and her performance status was 0. She was an ex-smoker of 10 pack-years, drank approximately 40 units of alcohol per week, and took the combined oral contraceptive pill.

Her renal function was within normal limits with an estimated glomerular filtration rate (eGFR) of 117 mL/min/1.73 m^2 and a creatinine level of 60 μmol/L. Further imaging in the form of computed tomography (CT) of the chest and abdomen with renal phase was arranged. This revealed a 7.3 cm enhancing lesion arising from the left kidney, with no involvement of the renal vein or associated lymphadenopathy. Of note, a left-sided inferior vena cava (IVC) was described (Figure 7.1). These images were subsequently discussed in the urology cancer multidisciplinary team (MDT) meeting, confirming a double IVC with dominant left side below the level of the renal vein, and with a differential diagnosis which included oncocytoma or renal cell carcinoma (RCC). If the latter were to be true, then this lesion would be radiologically staged as T2aN0M0.

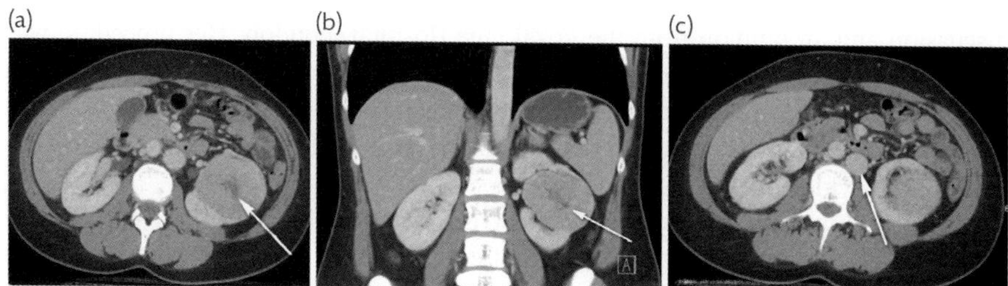

Figure 7.1 CT abdomen and pelvis. (a) Axial and (b) coronal contrast-enhanced CT scans showing a 7.3 cm relatively homogeneously enhancing central renal mass with a large central scar (arrow) consistent with an oncocytoma. (c) Axial CT imaging showing an incidental left-sided IVC, not associated with an oncocytoma but an important observation in order to prevent inadvertent damage at the time of surgery.

Learning point Incidence

The clinical condition and concept of oncocytomas was first described in 1942 by Zippel,[1] and subsequently the first case series was published in 1976.[2] We now know that renal oncocytomas represent between 3% and 7% of all renal tumours,[3,4] making them the commonest benign renal neoplasm. The incidence is higher in men than women with an up to three times male preponderance,[3–5] with a peak incidence of between 40 and 60.[6] Ninety-five per cent of oncocytomas are unilateral.[3] They are formed of epithelial cells with an eosinophilic cytoplasm due to their numerous mitochondria, the basic component of which is known as the 'oncocyte'. It is thought that renal oncocytomas originate from distal renal tubule epithelium, most likely intercalated cells of the collecting duct.[7,8]

Learning point Clinical presentation

Oncocytomas are not entities specific to the kidney. They have been described in a number of organs, namely the salivary and thyroid glands, as well as the adrenals and kidney.[3] The majority of oncocytomas are asymptomatic at presentation and are identified incidentally, more so now and going forward given the use of cross-sectional imaging, but a minority (17–21%) do present with symptoms (haematuria, flank pain, abdominal mass).[3,4] Clinically, renal oncocytosis may occur in a sporadic form without any underlying disease, or may occur in association with other conditions including chronic renal failure, long-term haemodialysis, and Birt–Hogg–Dubé syndrome.[9]

Expert comment Left IVC

The fact that the patient has a dominant left IVC is not in itself a cause for concern, and the operative approach, even with a left-sided renal tumour, does not require an overhaul. Prior to any renal surgery, vascular variants should be noted, and appropriate and proportional consideration given. The benefit of reviewing these images alongside a uroradiologist cannot be overstated, and can prove invaluable. In this particular case, the left gonadal vein was found to drain directly into the IVC, and was preserved at the time of surgery. A prior appreciation of the anatomy will mitigate against any unpleasant surprises.

MDT discussion also explored the role of percutaneous biopsy of this renal lesion; however, this line of investigation was not pursued as the patient preferred definitive operative intervention rather than surveillance for her renal lesion. In this situation, foregoing a percutaneous biopsy is entirely reasonable as it is unlikely to change the upfront management. We will come on to discuss this point further.

The patient was counselled for a left laparoscopic radical nephrectomy, following discussion and an opinion from the Royal Free Hospital, London. Her procedure was uncomplicated; she was discharged on her first postoperative day and was given dalteparin venous thromboembolism prophylaxis for 4 weeks. Histology was reviewed and confirmed the presence of an oncocytoma (Figure 7.2) with clear resection margins and no evidence of malignancy.

Her creatinine level stabilized at 73 μmol/L and her eGFR was 93 mL/min/1.73 m^2 at 2 years postoperatively. The plan going forward was to continue USS surveillance of the right kidney for several years, the exact duration of which was not specified, to ensure no contralateral recurrence.

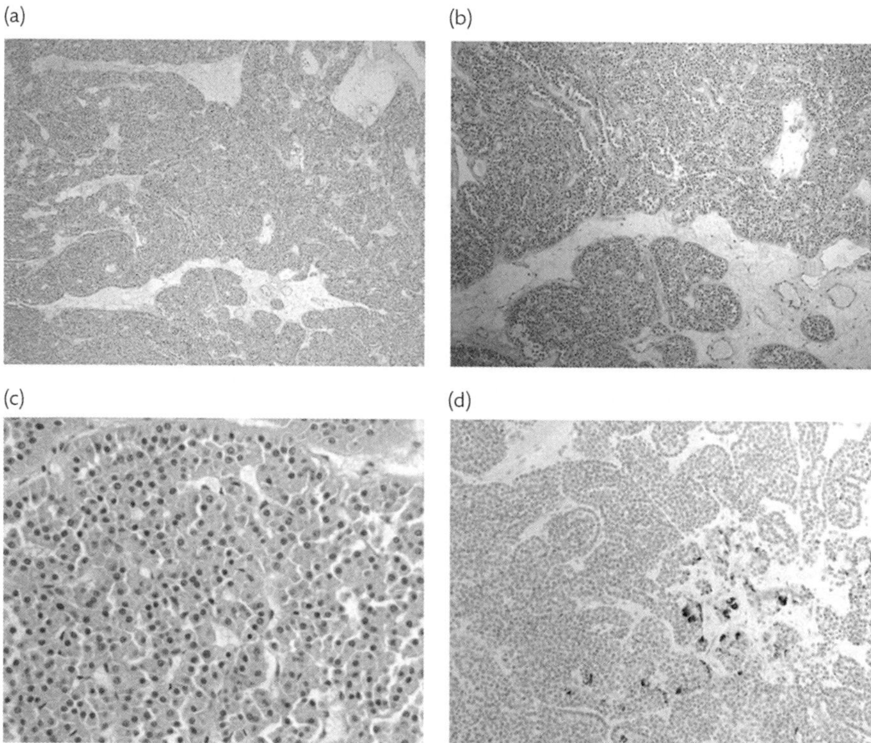

Figure 7.2 Histology slides. (a) A low-power view of a nested oncocytoma with hypocellular myxoid stroma (× 40, haematoxylin and eosin (H&E) stain). (b) A medium-power view showing uniformity of tumour cells (× 100, H&E stain). (c) A high-power view of oncocytes with uniform round nuclei and granular eosinophilic cytoplasm (× 400, H&E stain). (d) CK7 immunohistochemistry showing focal patchy, strong positivity typical in oncocytoma.

Learning point Histopathology

Macroscopically, the typical gross appearance of an oncocytoma is a solid, 5–8 cm, well-circumscribed lesion, often described as mahogany or tan in colour with a central pale scar (usually seen in larger tumours). Microscopically, they have a nested architecture (other patterns, e.g. tubulocystic and trabecular, are also seen) and the cells are described as oncocytic (polygonal with copious granular eosinophilic cytoplasm, central small round nuclei). The background hypocellular stroma is hyalinized or myxoid. Focal degenerative atypia resulting in bizarre nuclear morphology can be present. 'Invasion' or extension into perinephric fat is sometimes seen; however, there should be no necrosis and very few mitoses should be present.

Expert comment Histological and immunohistochemical features

On a well-sampled resection with typical histological and immunohistochemical features, it is reasonable to confidently diagnose oncocytoma. On small core biopsies showing typical morphology, increased confidence in the diagnosis may be gained from radiological and clinical input at MDT meetings. In the absence of this supporting information, a cautious biopsy report of 'oncocytic neoplasm with features compatible with an oncocytoma' might be recommended; if any histological features fall outside of the typical range expected, good communication with the urologist is essential in determining appropriate management for these patients.

Discussion

Surgical resection via partial or radical nephrectomy for oncocytomas is considered curative. When any surgical management strategy is being considered, there are additional patient, disease, and operative factors that all require consideration. So, by the nature of individuals, surgical resection may not be the strategy of choice for everyone. This discussion with the patient will be informed by the diagnostics, and of key concern for oncocytomas, cross-sectional imaging in the form of CT and possible percutaneous biopsy of the lesion are the mainstay.

Diagnostic imaging

CT imaging is the modality of choice for diagnosis, with magnetic resonance imaging (MRI) being reserved for situations where CT is contraindicated. The dilemma and indeed the challenge, is that radiographic features of oncocytomas are similar to that of RCC, making a positive radiological diagnosis particularly difficult. The classical CT description of an oncocytoma would be a well-defined, usually homogeneously enhancing mass, typically with the presence of a central spoke or stellate scar, but this can be mimicked by necrosis in RCC, and is not considered specific or pathognomonic.[10,11] Additionally, RCCs and oncocytomas are both hypervascular lesions that show enhancement and washout as hypoenhancement in the nephrogenic phase, further clouding the waters.[12] The use of standard magnetic resonance imaging has also been assessed for distinguishing oncocytomas from RCCs; however, similar hurdles are encountered with regard to the degree of overlap in radiological features between the two conditions.[13] Specifically, oncocytomas are usually intermediate to high signal on T2-weighted imaging with similar post-contrast findings as CT.[14] A recent study looking at MRI characteristics of oncocytomas verses chromophobe RCCs concluded that the signal intensity following contrast was higher in oncocytomas as well as the relative wash-in of contrast and could be used as a discriminatory marker, though the authors state that further research is required in this area.[15]

Newer techniques may help in the differentiation of oncocytomas from RCCs, although to date none have been incorporated into standard practice. A recent meta-analysis of technetium-99m sestamibi single-photon emission computed tomography/CT concluded that the technique had a high sensitivity and specificity for characterizing benign and low-grade lesions, and while this may improve confidence when recommending active surveillance, the authors did not go as far as suggesting patients could be discharged from imaging follow-up.[16] Work has also recently been forthcoming regarding the role of mass spectrometry imaging to allow discrimination of renal oncocytoma from RCC subtypes. Mass spectrometry imaging has been used to study the metabolic and lipid profiles of various renal tissues including renal oncocytoma, RCC, and normal renal tissue.[17] Of note, the authors reported renal oncocytoma and chromophobe RCC, which present the most significant morphological overlap, were investigated and predictive modelling yielded 100% accuracy in discriminating these tumour subtypes.[17] But again, this has not yet been incorporated into standard practice, and is to date experimental, but shows potential for application to the clinical setting.

Expert comment CT characterization of a renal mass

CT characterization of a renal mass may suggest the diagnosis of on oncocytoma; however, there are currently no features which are diagnostic, with considerable overlap with malignant lesions. A number of methods may in the future provide a more definite diagnosis. Until that point, the management of oncocytomas must assume a malignant risk and incudes resection, biopsy, and surveillance. If surveillance is chosen (either with or without biopsy), then imaging intervals should follow local protocols as for the surveillance of malignant renal lesions. If the mass can be accurately measured using ultrasound, this may be used for follow-up, otherwise patients will require CT or MRI.

Percutaneous biopsy

The role of renal mass biopsy for cases of radiologically suspected oncocytoma has been much debated. The ability to accurately diagnose oncocytoma versus the more sinister RCC negates the unnecessary risk of losing part or all of a renal unit, to treat what is a benign condition. However, the converse is also true. Surveillance based on biopsy results risks delaying treatment of an RCC if the biopsy specimen provides a false negative. A recent systematic review and meta-analysis examined this issue. It found that one in three renal biopsies suggesting oncocytoma were ultimately incorrect when the final histology of nephrectomy specimens was reviewed, and that one in four will actually have RCC.[18] Surgical pathology of suspected oncocytomas revealed chromophobe RCC was the most prevalent variant. The authors concluded that biopsy of a renal mass was found to be unreliable in confidently diagnosing oncocytoma.[18] There is another concern surrounding the role of renal mass biopsy in the accurate diagnosis of oncocytoma. Whether a preoperative renal biopsy provides a representative sample of the mass lesion must be taken into account. The existence of hybrid tumours, a scenario where oncocytomas and RCC coexist, has been described, with an incidence of between 2% and 32%.[19] The differential diagnosis usually includes chromophobe RCC (eosinophilic variant) and clear cell RCC (with granular cytoplasm). If necrosis is present, if there is an increased mitotic rate or atypical mitotic figures are identified, if spindle or clear cells are seen, the diagnosis of oncocytoma should be strongly reconsidered. A panel of immunohistochemistry can be helpful including CK7, vimentin, CD10, RCC, and CD117. The most useful of these is CK7 where the typical pattern of staining in oncocytoma is focal patchy strong positivity. Differentiating malignant eosinophilic renal tumours from benign oncocytomas is fraught with challenges, and often relies on immunohistochemistry, in addition to morphology from the operative specimen, for the most reliable diagnosis.[3,20]

Learning point Surveillance and follow-up

Although oncocytomas are benign in nature, there have been reports of oncocytic cells invading fat[21] and even associated vascular structures, including the renal vein.[22] It is, however, extremely rare that oncocytomas are associated with metastatic spread.[23] For those patients that opt for the non-operative approach, follow-up with some form of surveillance is an important consideration. There are rare reports in the literature of malignant transformation of oncocytomas, and the more common risk of progression to chronic kidney disease.[24]

The natural history of oncocytomas is still poorly understood. There has been limited work to assess this, but the suggestion from one small series was that the natural evolution of an oncocytoma was to increase in size.[25] The authors identified two key markers that they used as indications for surgery. These were the initial tumour volume and the velocity by which this volume increased over time.[25] Despite this, there is certainly no evidence-based consensus as to what a surveillance programme should look like, or what the trigger points used to switch from surveillance to surgical intervention may be.

Expert comment Surveillance

The relative minority of patients who embark on surveillance of their suspected oncocytoma upfront, would reasonably have a biopsy of the lesion from the outset, notable by the absence of an RCC subtype in the specimen. Although no strict evidence base exists, a reasonable surveillance protocol in this cohort may look like a 6-month USS, followed by annual USS imaging. Patient symptoms, size increase of the lesion, and patient choice would act as triggers for intervention.

A final word from the expert

In 2022, the original decision-making difficulties first identified in 1942 with these renal lesions has not diminished, and is perhaps more pronounced as the emergence of incidentalomas with cross-sectional imaging has become established. Adjuncts such as percutaneous biopsy, CT imaging, and immunohistochemistry act as an aid to inform both clinician and patient and therefore guide management strategies. When a plan for surgical treatment has been made, partial nephrectomy should always be considered where feasible. Patients with suspected oncocytomas are often young, and the removal of an entire renal unit should be carefully considered and avoided where possible, given the propensity for development of chronic kidney disease later in life. This carries with it significant cardiovascular risk and associated morbidity and mortality, as a result of treating what is thought to be a benign condition. The extent to which patients are able to proportionately weigh up these longer-term risks associated with nephrectomy against the renal lesion on the CT scan in front of them is unclear. For those individuals who are under surveillance for their suspected oncocytoma, local protocols will dictate the frequency and modality of such follow-up. We know that there is user variability associated with USS imaging, but repeated CT scans add an additional cumulative risk of radiation exposure in what has already been discussed as an often-younger cohort of patients. Urologists will continue to be faced with the diagnostic dilemma of correctly discerning a renal lesion as an oncocytoma with confidence, as opposed to the more sinister RCC. This point represents the cornerstone in the management of this benign condition.

References

1. Zippel L. Zur Kenntinis der Oncocyten. *Virchow Arch Path Anat.* 1942;308:360–382.
2. Klein MJ, Valensi QJ. Proximal tubular adenoma of kidney with so called oncocytic features. A clinicopathologic study of 13 cases of a rarely reported neoplasm. *Cancer.* 1976;38(2):906–914.
3. Perez-Ordonez B, Hamed G, Campbell S, et al. Renal oncocytoma: a clinicopathologic study of 70 cases. *Am J Surg Pathol.* 1997;21(8):871–883.
4. Amin MB, Crotty TB, Tickoo SK, Farrow GM. Renal oncocytoma: a reappraisal of morphologic features with clinicopathologic findings in 80 cases. *Am J Surg Pathol.* 1997;21(1):1–12.
5. Lieber MM. Renal oncocytoma. *Urol Clin North Am.* 1993;20(2):355–359.
6. Ponholzer A, Reiter WJ, Maier U. Organ sparing surgery for giant bilateral renal oncocytoma. *J Urol.* 2002;168(6):2531–2532.
7. Zerban H, Nogueira E, Riedasch G, et al. Renal oncocytoma: origin from the collecting duct. *Virchows Arch B Cell Pathol Incl Mol Pathol.* 1987;52(5):375–387.
8. Nogueira E, Bannasch P. Cellular origin of rat renal oncocytoma. *Lab Invest.* 1988;59(3):337–343.

9. Kuroda N, Tanaka A, Ohe C, et al. Review of renal oncocytosis (multiple oncocytic lesions) with focus on clinical and pathobiological aspects. *Histol Histopathol.* 2012;27(11):1407–1412.
10. Davidson AJ, Hayes WS, Hartman DS, et al. Renal oncocytoma and carcinoma: failure of differentiation with CT. *Radiology.* 1993;186(3):693–696.
11. Hilton S. Imaging of renal cell carcinoma. *Semin Oncol.* 2000;27(2):150–159.
12. Paño B, Macías N, Salvador R, et al. Usefulness of MDCT to differentiate between renal cell carcinoma and oncocytoma: development of a predictive model. *AJR.* 2016;206(4):764–774.
13. Pretorius ES, Siegelman ES, Ramchandani P, et al. Renal neoplasms amenable to partial nephrectomy: MR imaging. *Radiology.* 1999;212(1):28–34.
14. Kay F, Pedrosa I. Imaging of solid renal masses. *Urol Clin North Am.* 201845(3):311–330.
15. Akin I, Altay C, Guler E, et al. Discrimination of oncocytoma and chromophobe renal cell carcinoma using MRI. *Diagn Interv Radiol.* 2019;25(1):5–13.
16. Wilson M, Katlariwala P, Murad MH, et al. Diagnostic accuracy of 99mTc-sestamibi SPECT/CT for detecting renal oncocytomas and other benign renal lesions: a systematic review and meta-analysis. *Abdom Radiol (NY).* 2020;45(8):2532–2541.
17. Zhang J, Li SQ, Lin JQ, et al. Mass spectrometry imaging enables discrimination of renal oncocytoma from renal cell cancer subtypes and normal kidney tissues. *Cancer Res.* 2020;80(4):689–698.
18. Patel HD, Druskin SC, Rowe SP, et al. Surgical histopathology for suspected oncocytoma on renal mass biopsy: a systematic review and meta-analysis. *BJU Int.* 2017;119(5):661–666.
19. Haifler M, Copel L, Sandbank J, et al. Renal oncocytoma—are there sufficient grounds to consider surveillance following prenephrectomy histologic diagnosis. *Urol Oncol.* 2012;30(4):362–368.
20. Gorin MA, Rowe SP, Allaf ME. Oncocytic neoplasm on renal mass biopsy: a diagnostic conundrum. *Oncology.* 2016;30(5):426–435.
21. Williamson SR. Renal oncocytoma with perinephric fat invasion. *Int J Surg Pathol.* 2016;24(7):625–626.
22. Hes O, Michal M, Sima R, et al. Renal oncocytoma with and without intravascular extension into the branches of renal vein have the same morphological, immunohistochemical and genetic features. *Virchows Arch.* 2008;452(3):285–293.
23. Decet CB, Bostwick DG, Blute ML, et al. Renal oncocytoma: multifocality, bilateralism, metachronous tumour development and coexistent renal cell carcinoma. *J Urol.* 1999;162(1):40–42.
24. National Comprehensive Cancer Network. NCCN guideline with NCCN evidence blocks—kidney cancer. Version 3.2019. National Comprehensive Cancer Network. 2019. https://www.nccn.org/guidelines/guidelines-with-evidence-blocks
25. Neuzillet Y, Lechevallier E, Andrew M, et al. Follow-up of renal oncocytoma diagnosed by percutaneous tumor biopsy. *Urology.* 2005;66(6):1181–1185.

SECTION 4
Prostate cancer

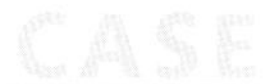

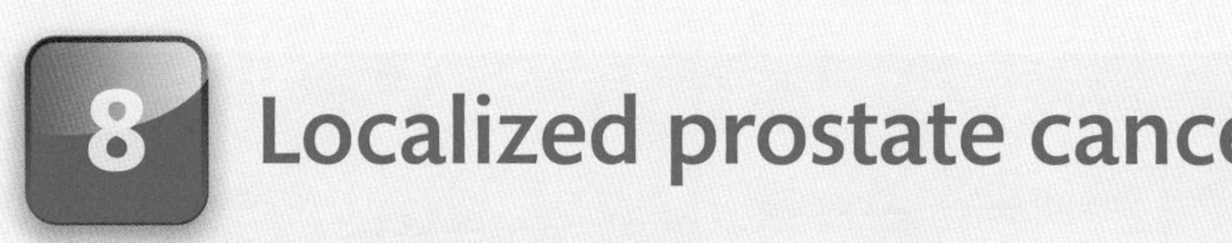

8 Localized prostate cancer

Omer Altan and Alastair Lamb

Expert commentary Freddie C. Hamdy

Case history

A 60-year-old scientist was referred for a urology consultation by his general practitioner on the prostate cancer diagnostic pathway with a persistently elevated serum prostate-specific antigen (PSA) value of 5.35 ng/mL and 7.98 ng/mL on two successive measurements. This was precipitated by a history of haematospermia and symptoms of prostatitis, which settled after antibiotic treatment, but the post-treatment PSA value remained persistently high.

He had a past medical history of type 1 diabetes, arthritis, hypertension, and was taking naproxen, valsartan, statins, and omeprazole. He had no past surgical history. He was otherwise fit and active with moderate to good erectile function. Clinical examination was unremarkable, while digital rectal examination revealed a mildly enlarged benign-feeling prostate with a left-sided firm nodule towards the apex, raising the suspicion of prostate cancer. The patient was counselled about the significance of the raised PSA and suspicious digital rectal examination and the need to investigate him further with a prostate multiparametric magnetic resonance imaging (mpMRI) scan and prostate biopsy.

Clinical tip Initial assessment

- The patient should be made aware early in the diagnostic pathway about the clinical suspicion of prostate cancer.
- The patient needs to be informed about the most common risks of prostate biopsy, whether transrectal ultrasound (TRUS) guided or using the transperineal approach—risks include haematuria, acute urinary retention, and sepsis.[1–3]
- If available, consider offering local anaesthetic transperineal (LATP) biopsy for improved targeting of visible lesions on imaging, particularly in the anterior region of the prostate, improved systematic sampling, and probable reduction in sepsis.[4–7]
- It is important to document whether the patient had a previous history of antibiotic use for urinary tract infections or other conditions which required quinolones (previous TRUS biopsy), as his colonic flora might have become resistant to quinolones which are commonly used for urinary tract infection prophylaxis pre and post TRUS biopsy.
- A voiding cystometry should be performed prior to prostate biopsy to obtain baseline voiding pattern information. This is one of the essential eligibility criteria for brachytherapy if the diagnosis of prostate cancer is confirmed (threshold Qmax 12 mL/s or higher).
- Erectile function prior to biopsy should be documented, which will be useful to plan treatment as necessary, ideally using validated questionnaires (e.g. International Index of Erectile Function).
- Offer pre-biopsy imaging in the form of mpMRI or biparametric MRI of the prostate, with interpretation based on the Prostate Imaging Reporting and Data System (PI-RADS) (or Likert) classification from 1 to 5.[8–10]

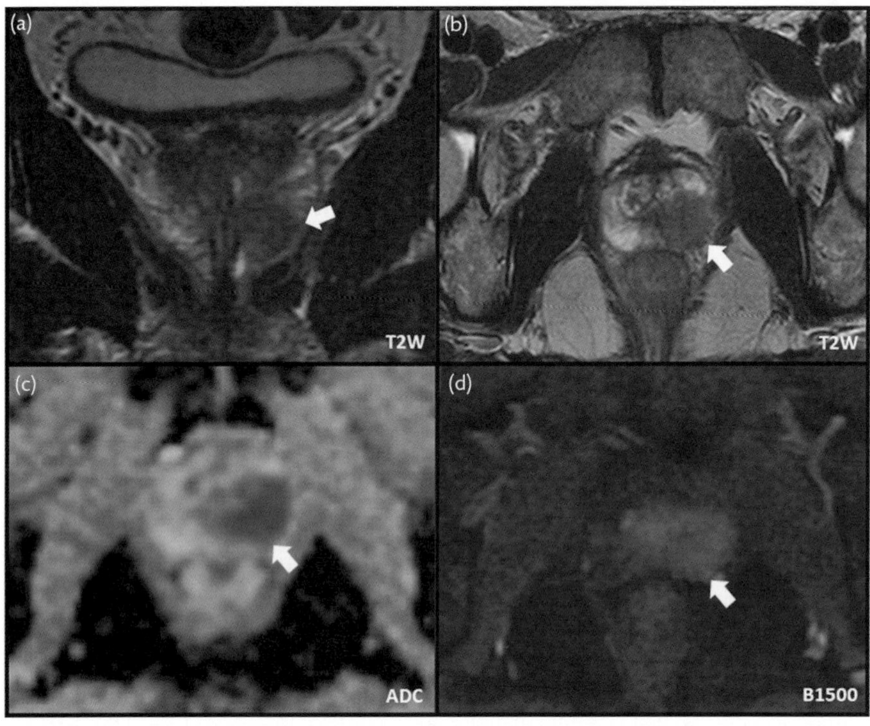

Figure 8.1 Multiparametric magnetic resonance imaging (mpMRI) of the prostate. Coronal and axial T2 weighted (a, b), axial apparent diffusion coefficient (c), and high B-value (d) parameters.

The patient underwent a mpMRI scan of his prostate (Figure 8.1). The prostate volume was 26 cc and there was a 21 mm area of decreased T2 signal within the left peripheral zone posterolaterally, in the mid-portion of the gland, showing restricted diffusion and early enhancement, classified as PI-RADS 5 lesion. There was also broad capsular abutment.

The patient was offered TRUS-guided targeted and systematic biopsies (Table 8.1).

Table 8.1 Biopsy results

	Left	Right
Cores and Gleason Grade Group (GGG)	5 of 5 cores positive for GGG3 (Gleason 4 + 3 = 7)	5 of 5 cores positive for GGG2 (Gleason 3 + 4 = 7)
Tissue involvement	90%	40%
Maximum core length	16 mm (100% of core)	11 mm (60% of core)
Perineural invasion	Yes	No
Extraprostatic extension	No	No
Lymphovascular invasion	No	No

Bilateral adenocarcinoma, maximum Gleason 7 (4 + 3), Grade Group 3.

Learning point PI-RADS

PI-RADS version 2 classification is a scoring system for mpMRI of the prostate which indicates the likelihood of a lesion to represent significant prostate cancer. This is based on the assessment of T2-weighted, diffusion-weighted, and dynamic contrast enhancement imaging. Based on these, a score of 1-5 is given to each lesion. PI-RADS 1–2 lesions are low risk that are unlikely to represent serious disease, PI-RADS 3 lesions are considered equivocal, while PI-RADS 4–5 lesions are considered suspicious and more likely to reveal cancer at the moment of prostate biopsy. The Likert system for scoring is similar but represents a sequential grading of risk from 1 to 5. Interpretation of the mpMRI can be challenging in younger men.[9,10] MRI is a useful tool for local staging and can help preoperative planning should the patient require radical surgery, particularly to determine the appropriateness and risks of neurovascular bundle (NVB) sparing.

An MRI description of 'capsular abutment' can sometimes indicate a higher risk of capsular and extracapsular involvement and locally advanced prostate cancer (T3a disease).[11] If the MRI shows a PI-RADS 1–2 abnormality, the patient can be counselled towards expectant management as the likelihood of finding clinically significant prostate cancer is low, approximately 5–15% regardless of PSA density.[12]

According to the Prostate MRI Imaging Study (PROMIS) trials, up to 27% of patients could avoid prostate biopsies.[13]

If the clinical suspicion of disease outside visible abnormalities is high, then the patient should be offered systematic TRUS or LATP.

Learning point Biopsy approaches

- Transrectal biopsies, although widely available in most units carry the disadvantage of a sepsis rate of up to 5%.[2]
- Performing MRI cognitive or fusion prostate biopsies have a similar diagnostic yield for clinically significant prostate cancer.[19]
- TRUS biopsy has a lower detection rate compared to MRI-targeted biopsies for clinically significant prostate cancer and a higher detection rate for clinically insignificant prostate cancer according to the Prostate Evaluation for Clinically Important Disease: Sampling Using Image Guidance or Not? (PRECISION) trial.[13,14]
- Other studies have shown that when performing MRI-targeted biopsies only, there is a risk for missing clinically significant prostate cancer, concluding that both systematic and targeted biopsies should be performed.[12]

Expert comment Additional systematic biopsies

In the presence of an mpMRI-visible lesion, targeted biopsies should be performed[14] and we would advocate additional systematic biopsies due to the approximately 30% rate of non-target clinically significant prostate cancer detection and to aid planning of radical treatment.[5,15–18] It is sensible, for data auditing purposes, to send these separately for histopathological analysis.

Expert comment LATP

LATP prostate biopsies could be a good alternative to TRUS prostate biopsies. They may have superior diagnostic accuracy but lower risk of urinary sepsis with equivalent patient tolerability.[5] A randomised trial to answer this question (TRANSLATE Trial; NIHR131233) began across several sites in the UK in early 2022.

Given the predominance of Gleason pattern 4 disease, the patient received an MRI of his bone marrow which was negative for metastatic bone disease. The patient's prostate cancer was categorized as high-volume, intermediate-risk disease, cT2cN0M0, with a risk of extracapsular extension on the left side of the prostate, based on radiological and digital rectal examination findings.

The patient was counselled in parallel consultations by the urologist and clinical oncologist (radiation oncologist) and offered different forms of radical treatment as either surgery, in the form of laparoscopic robot-assisted radical prostatectomy (RARP) and extended pelvic lymph node dissection (PLND), or neoadjuvant androgen deprivation therapy followed by external beam radiotherapy.

The patient's choice was to receive a RARP. He expressed a particular preference for bilateral NVB sparing, despite the fact that during the initial surgical consultation he was advised that in view of the findings, the approach recommended would be to receive a RARP with wide excision of the NVB on the left side and a nerve-sparing procedure on the right side, as well as bilateral PLND. The clinical challenge was the suspicion of locally advanced disease (T3a on the left side), which would pose a significant risk of positive surgical margins (PSMs) should a nerve-sparing procedure be considered.

Clinical tip MRI and preoperative planning

In addition to clinical staging, the MRI scan can be helpful with the preoperative planning of radical prostatectomy in defining extent of the disease, suspicion of extracapsular extension, and prediction of risk of urinary leakage.

The case was discussed extensively at the RARP planning meeting, and the consensus was to offer a RARP with bilateral nerve sparing and intraoperative frozen sections of the prostatic edge corresponding to the left and right NVB respectively. The membranous urethral length (MUL) measured 18 mm—an important consideration as the tumour was close to the apex, and there is emerging evidence of the relevance of the urethral length in regaining early continence after surgery.[24,25]

Evidence base ProtecT and patient-reported outcomes

It is critical to counsel patients regarding the evidence of treatment effectiveness of conventional therapies in localized prostate cancer. The Prostate Testing for Cancer and Treatment (ProtecT) trial has shown that surgery or external beam radiation with neoadjuvant androgen deprivation are equally effective in reducing the risk of disease progression and metastasis at an average of 10 years following diagnosis.[20,21]

The side effect profiles, however, are different, as shown by the ProtecT trial's patient-reported outcomes, and the patient needs to measure the trade-off between treatments and potential side effects in order to make an informed decision, assisted by his treating clinician.[22,23]

Expert comment MUL

A preoperative MUL of <6 mm can leave men permanently incontinent. A MUL <10 mm often leads to delayed recovery of continence. A longer MUL >16 mm measured on the coronal T2-weighted MRI slices likely results in a high rate of recovery in urinary continence following radical prostatectomy.[24]

The patient underwent a RARP with bilateral PLND and with a bilateral NVB-sparing technique. The prostate specimen was sliced at the level of the lateral margins (Figure 8.2), adjacent to the NVB, and sent for frozen section analysis. Foci of adenocarcinoma (Gleason Grade Group 2) were detected 0.8 mm away from the margin, which was clear. Both NVBs were thus preserved, and bilateral extended PLND was performed.

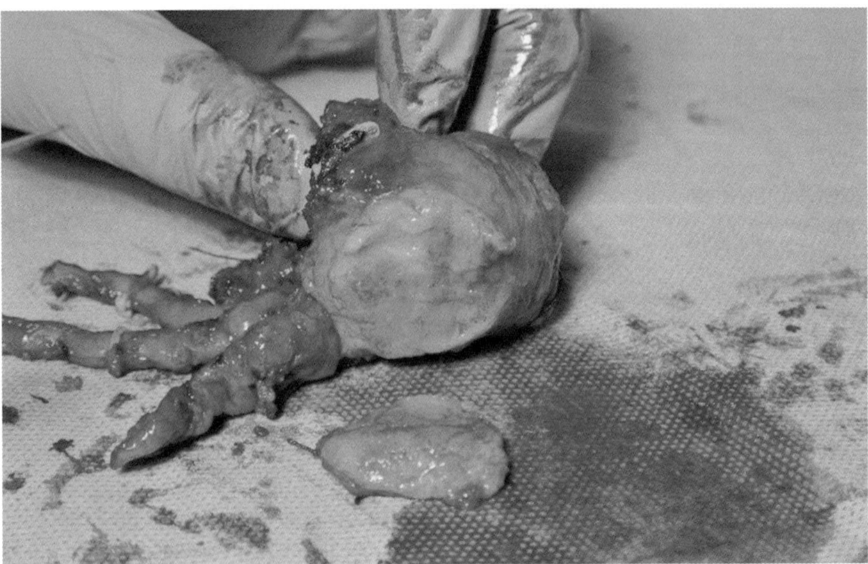

Figure 8.2 Prostate specimen after removal through Alexa™ camera port with angled sagittal section taken to provide frozen sections from circumferential margins.
Modified from NeuroSAFE technique.[26]

Evidence base NeuroSAFE

The NeuroSAFE protocol for radical prostatectomy has been developed in an attempt to:

- Improve functional outcome by preserving the NVBs when appropriate and in the absence of detectable cancer cells at the sample margin by frozen section histopathological examination
- Reduce the incidence of PSM by undertaking wide excision of the NVBs if cancer cells are present at frozen section of the margins. The technique is currently the subject of a randomized controlled trial to provide evidence of its effectiveness.[26,27]

The patient made an uneventful postoperative recovery and was discharged home with a urethral catheter the following day. His catheter was removed after 7 days. At 6 weeks, he regained full continence without the use of a pad, and was achieving moderate spontaneous erection. His postoperative PSA level was <0.01 ng/mL.

The final pathology report confirmed bilateral Gleason score 7 (4 + 3), Grade Group 3, pT3b pN0 prostate cancer. All margins were clear of prostate cancer cell infiltration.

The discrepancy between the initial staging cT2 and final pathology pT3b justified the initial planning for RARP, bilateral PLN, and using the modified NeuroSAFE protocol.

A final word from the expert

Given the high rate of postoperative upstaging of clinically localized (cT2) to extracapsular locally advanced prostate cancer (pT3) disease, consideration should be given to mpMRI appearances in addition to other clinical parameters in planning radical treatment for these patients. Novel and emerging imaging techniques such as prostate-specific membrane antigen positron emission tomography–CT scans need to be evaluated further in an attempt to improve the staging of prostate cancer preoperatively, to detect extraprostatic and local invasion of prostate cancer cells before administration of radical surgery. While in this particular case a NeuroSAFE-like protocol was followed in order to minimize the risk of a PSM while preserving the NVBs, the technique is used routinely only in a limited number of centres worldwide, due to resource implications and the additional time needed for the frozen section biopsies, with close engagement from expert histopathologists. The technique is the subject of a randomized controlled trial led by colleagues in London, UK.[27–28]

Precision surgery for prostate cancer is reaching new dimensions. Prostate-specific membrane antigen fluorescence conjugated tracers and radioligand guidance are being developed in order to visualize cancer cells intraoperatively in real time, improve detection of lymph node disease and extraprostatic cancer cells, reduce PSM at surgery and unfavourable pathological outcomes, and achieve complete disease excision, while improving functional outcomes by preservation of NVBs where appropriate. As these new technologies develop further and continue to be evaluated, careful counselling and managing the patient and his partner's expectations are critical to the patient's experience and satisfaction, as well as oncological outcomes throughout his treatment journey.

References

1. Rosario DJ, Lane JA, Metcalfe C, et al. Short term outcomes of prostate biopsy in men tested for cancer by prostate specific antigen: prospective evaluation within ProtecT study. *BMJ*. 2012;344:d7894.

2. Batura, D, Gopal Rao G. The national burden of infections after prostate biopsy in England and Wales: a wake-up call for better prevention—authors' response. *J Antimicrob Chemother.* 2013;68(10):2419–2420.
3. Loeb S, Vellekoop A, Ahmed HU, et al. Systematic review of complications of prostate biopsy. *Eur Urol.* 2013;64(6):876–892.
4. Lopez JF, Campbell A, Omer A, et al. Local anaesthetic transperineal (LATP) prostate biopsy using a probe-mounted transperineal access system: a multicentre prospective outcome analysis. *BJU Int.* 2021;128(3):311–318.
5. Omer A, Lamb AD. Optimizing prostate biopsy techniques. *Curr Opin Urol.* 2019;29(6):578–586.
6. Stefanova V, Buckley R, Flax S, et al. Transperineal prostate biopsies using local anesthesia: experience with 1,287 patients. prostate cancer detection rate, complications and patient tolerability. *J Urol.* 2019;201(6):1121–1126.
7. Marra G, Zhuang J, Beltrami M et al. Transperineal freehand multiparametric MRI fusion targeted biopsies under local anaesthesia for prostate cancer diagnosis: a multicentre prospective study of 1014 cases. *BJU Int.* 2021 Jan;127(1):122–130. doi:10.1111/bju.15121. Epub 2020 Aug 2.
8. Sathianathen NJ, Omer A, Harriss E, et al. Negative predictive value of multiparametric magnetic resonance imaging in the detection of clinically significant prostate cancer in the prostate imaging reporting and data system era: a systematic review and meta-analysis. *Eur Urol.* 2020;78(3):402–414.
9. Turkbey B, Rosenkrantz AB, Haider MA, et al. Prostate Imaging Reporting and Data System Version 2.1: 2019 Update of Prostate Imaging Reporting and Data System Version 2. *Eur Urol.* 2019;76(3):340–351.
10. Schieda N, Quon JS, Lim C, et al. Evaluation of the European Society of Urogenital Radiology (ESUR) PI-RADS scoring system for assessment of extra-prostatic extension in prostatic carcinoma. *Eur J Radiol.* 2015;84(10):1843–1848.
11. de Rooij M, Hamoen EH, Witjes JA, Barentsz JO, Rovers MM. Accuracy of magnetic resonance imaging for local staging of prostate cancer: a diagnostic meta-analysis. *Eur Urol.* 2016;70(2):233–245.
12. Bryant RJ, Hobbs CP, Eyre KS, et al. Comparison of prostate biopsy with or without prebiopsy multiparametric magnetic resonance imaging for prostate cancer detection: an observational cohort study. *J Urol.* 2019;201(3):510–519.
13. Ahmed HU, El-Shater Bosaily A, Brown LC, et al. Diagnostic accuracy of multi-parametric MRI and TRUS biopsy in prostate cancer (PROMIS): a paired validating confirmatory study. *Lancet.* 2017;389(10071):815–822.
14. Kasivisvanathan V, Rannikko AS, Borghi M, et al. MRI-targeted or standard biopsy for prostate-cancer diagnosis. *N Engl J Med.* 2018;378(19):1767–1777.
15. Neale A, Stroman L, Kum F, et al. Targeted and systematic cognitive freehand guided transperineal biopsy—is there still a role for systematic biopsy? *BJU Int.* 2020;126(2):280–285.
16. Dell'Oglio P, Stabile A, Soligo M, et al. There is no way to avoid systematic prostate biopsies in addition to multiparametric magnetic resonance imaging targeted biopsies. *Eur Urol Oncol.* 2020;3(1):112–118.
17. Drost FH, Osses D, Nieboer D, et al. Prostate magnetic resonance imaging, with or without magnetic resonance imaging-targeted biopsy, and systematic biopsy for detecting prostate cancer: a Cochrane systematic review and meta-analysis. *Eur Urol.* 2020;77(1):78–94.
18. Drost FH, Osses DF, Nieboer D, et al. Prostate MRI, with or without MRI-targeted biopsy, and systematic biopsy for detecting prostate cancer. *Cochrane Database Syst Rev.* 2019;4:CD012663.
19. Wegelin O, van Melick HHE, Hooft L, et al. Comparing three different techniques for magnetic resonance imaging-targeted prostate biopsies: a systematic review of in-bore versus magnetic resonance imaging-transrectal ultrasound fusion versus cognitive registration. Is there a preferred technique? *Eur Urol.* 2017;71(4):517–531.

20. Hamdy FC. The Prostate Testing for Cancer and Treatment (ProtecT) study: what have we learnt? *BJU Int.* 2016;118(6):843.
21. Johnston TJ, Shaw GL, Lamb AD, et al. Mortality among men with advanced prostate cancer excluded from the ProtecT trial. *Eur Urol.* 2017;71(3):381–388.
22. Donovan JL, Hamdy FC, Lane JA, et al. Patient-reported outcomes after monitoring, surgery, or radiotherapy for prostate cancer. *N Engl J Med.* 2016;375(15):1425–1437.
23. Lane A, Metcalfe C, Young GJ, et al. Patient-reported outcomes in the ProtecT randomized trial of clinically localized prostate cancer treatments: study design, and baseline urinary, bowel and sexual function and quality of life. *BJU Int.* 2016;118(6):869–879.
24. Kim LHC, Patel A, Kinsella N, Sharabiani MTA, Ap Dafydd D, Cahill D. Association between preoperative magnetic resonance imaging-based urethral parameters and continence recovery following robot-assisted radical prostatectomy. *Eur Urol Focus.* 2020;6(5):1013–1020.
25. Mungovan SF, Sandhu JS, Akin O, Smart NA, Graham PL, Patel MI. Preoperative membranous urethral length measurement and continence recovery following radical prostatectomy: a systematic review and meta-analysis. *Eur Urol.* 2017;71(3):368–378.
26. Beyer B, Schlomm T, Tennstedt P, et al. A feasible and time-efficient adaptation of NeuroSAFE for da Vinci robot-assisted radical prostatectomy. *Eur Urol.* 2014;66(1):138–144.
27. Shaw GL, Rajan P, Sooriakumaran P, et al. The NeuroSAFE PROOF study (an RCT to evaluate the use of frozen section technology to improve oncological and functional outcomes in robotic radical prostatectomy). *Eur J Surg Oncol.* 2017;43(11):2213.
28. Dinneen E, Haider A, Grierson J, et al. NeuroSAFE frozen section during robot-assisted radical prostatectomy (RARP): peri-operative and histopathological outcomes from the NeuroSAFE PROOF feasibility randomised controlled trial. *BJU Int.* 2020;127:676–686. doi:10.1111/bju.15256

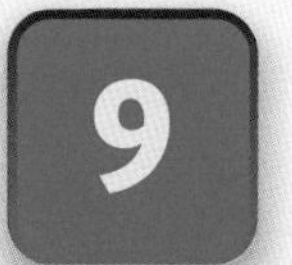

Oligometastatic prostate cancer

Francesco Claps, Fabio Traunero, Nicola Pavan, and Prasanna Sooriakumaran

Expert commentary Prasanna Sooriakumaran

Case history

A 68-year-old man was found with a prostate-specific antigen (PSA) level of 41 ng/mL on routine evaluation. Digital rectal examination revealed an enlarged, multinodular prostate gland. His past medical history was unremarkable.

Laboratory data showed the following: haemoglobin level 13.4 g/dL, haematocrit 42%, white blood cell count 8100/mm^3, normal differential, platelets 230,000/mm^3, creatinine 1.0 mg/dL, and normal alkaline phosphatase and liver function tests. A chest X-ray was negative, but bone scanning and abdominal computed tomography scanning identified a single bone metastasis in the left iliac spine. The patient had a diagnosis of oligometastatic prostate cancer (PCa). After a multidisciplinary consultation, the patient was selected as eligible for the Testing Radical Prostatectomy in Men with Oligometastatic Prostate Cancer that has Spread to the Bone (TRoMbone) trial and he was randomized to the surgical arm.

As per the clinical protocol, before surgery the patient received 9 months of androgen deprivation therapy (ADT) and six cycles of neoadjuvant chemotherapy with docetaxel. No evidence of severe toxicity was reported. His PSA level before surgery was <0.01 ng/mL.

He underwent robot-assisted radical prostatectomy with lymph node dissection. The total operative time was 250 minutes, with 210 minutes of console time. The final pathology report revealed a prostatic adenocarcinoma with a Gleason score of 7 (4 + 3) with established capsular involvement. Negative surgical margins (R0) were achieved. In addition, one of 12 lymph nodes removed was positive for disease. During the surgical procedure no complications were reported, and the patient remained complication free in the postoperative period. The catheter was removed on postoperative day 14. At routine follow-up to 6 months, his PSA level remained stable, and the patient became continent at 3 months (less than one pad per day).

Diagnosis: pT3b, N1, M1a (single iliac bone metastasis), R0, Gleason score 7 (4 + 3) adenocarcinoma of the prostate.

Expert comment Characterizing newly diagnosed metastatic PCa

With the spread in testing of PSA in men older than 50 years, there has been an increase in the number of men diagnosed with clinically non-metastatic PCa. Nevertheless, 10–20% of all newly diagnosed PCa is in men with metastatic disease.[1] There remains debate as to the best treatment for men with advanced PCa.

Moreover, increasing developments of non-invasive local and systemic staging allow an accurate characterization of patients newly diagnosed with metastatic prostate cancer (mPCa).[2] As a consequence, it is widely accepted that there is a need to quantify the burden of disease, introducing the concepts of 'low-volume' and 'high-volume' disease in the metastatic setting.

Learning point Definition of metastatic disease

Using criteria that take into account the number and location of the lesions, several definitions of metastatic load have been proposed.[3,4] In particular, the new state of oligometastatic disease is defined as the *development of three or fewer non-castrate lesions outside of the primary tumour*.[1,5] This 'oligometastatic' state is thought to represent a transitory state between high-risk localized/locally advanced disease and widely disseminated metastatic cancer.

Expert comment Reasons to locally treat oligometastatic disease

There are several postulated reasons to locally treat oligometastatic disease. First of all, treatment of metastases alongside the primary tumour could produce a benefit in long-term survival or cure.[6,7] In addition, treatment of oligometastatic cancer can help in controlling disease-related morbidity and reducing the risk of tumour spread.[1]

In particular, in PCa, Parker et al.[8] investigated the role of radiotherapy to the primary tumour for newly diagnosed mPCa. The results of this randomized controlled phase III trial demonstrated that prostate radiotherapy improves overall survival for men with oligometastatic PCa.

Cytoreductive or radical surgery, radiotherapy, or combined therapies have been shown to improve survival in other metastatic diseases as well. Radical surgery in metastatic glioblastoma,[9] colorectal cancer,[10] and renal cell carcinoma[11] have been associated with improved survival outcomes. Hence, it is not that surprising that local therapy to the primary tumour in oligometastatic PCa may have merit.

Expert comment Postulated approach in the treatment of oligometastatic PCa

Historically, men with high-risk localized PCa have been managed most commonly with radiotherapy, ADT, or both, while surgery has been discouraged in this setting, due to concerns about side effects and inadequate disease control.[12] Nevertheless, retrospective studies report encouraging results for surgery over radiotherapy with the advantage of avoiding ADT in many patients. However, no randomized data are currently available to evaluate surgery versus radiotherapy plus ADT in terms of survival outcomes and/or toxicity (predominantly genitourinary toxicity and sexual dysfunction for surgery, and predominantly gastrointestinal toxicity for radiotherapy), but the ongoing randomized Scandinavian Prostate Cancer Group (SPCG)-15 trial will provide us with valuable information on this matter in the future.[13] Until then, it appears sensible to offer both treatments with equipoise. Hence, if radiotherapy improves survival in oligometastatic PCa, and surgery improves survival in metastatic disease in other tumour types, it would be worth interrogating the role of surgery in oligometastatic PCa.

One postulated approach in the treatment of oligometastatic PCa is a multimodal approach:

1. Local therapy of the primary tumour (radiotherapy or surgery).
2. Metastasis-directed therapy.
3. Systemic therapy.

It must be said that patients with good performance status and limited or no comorbidity may be more commonly considered for surgery, highlighting a bias of choice compared to patients undergoing radiotherapy. Preoperative ADT can also affect surgical outcomes with worse functional outcomes and an increased risk of complications in these patients.[14]

Evidence base Multimodal treatment of high-risk or locally advanced PCa

Although too soon to make recommendations, the use of neoadjuvant chemotherapy in association with surgery is currently being tested as part of the multimodal treatment of high-risk or locally advanced PCa.[15] Future analysis and longer follow-up of these trials will provide valuable information. Currently, the European Association of Urology PCa guidelines recommend radical prostatectomy with extended pelvic lymph node dissection (ePLND) in a multimodal approach (with possible postoperative radiotherapy and ADT), or external beam radiation therapy at a dose of 76–78 Gy, or external beam radiation therapy with brachytherapy boost with long-term ADT in men with life expectancies of >10 years.[16] The STAMPEDE trial confirmed the value of radical therapy (hazard ratio 0.48; 95% confidence interval 0.29–0.79) in a non-randomized comparison.[17]

In the case we describe, the standard of care was ADT plus chemotherapy with docetaxel. We investigated whether robotic prostatectomy plus pelvic lymphadenectomy was technically feasible and safe after systemic therapy had commenced, in this situation. This would help inform the question of whether surgery could be considered as an alternative to radiotherapy as local therapy for men presenting with oligometastatic PCa. Other investigators are examining similar questions.

Learning point European Association of Urology guidelines for radical treatment of locally advanced disease

Recommendations	Strength rating
Radical prostatectomy (RP)	
Offer RP to highly selected patients with locally advanced PCa as part of multimodal therapy	Strong
ePLND	
Perform an ePLND in locally advanced PCa	Strong
Radiotherapeutic treatments	
In patients with locally advanced PCa, offer radiotherapy in combination with long-term ADT	Strong
Offer long-term ADT for at least 2 years	Weak

Clinical tip Technical points associated with radical prostatectomy

Features of high-volume, bulky local disease in men with oligometastatic cancer, combined with its biological aggressiveness, can make the radical prostatectomy challenging. Here are some technical points:

- Periprostatic fat is commonly more adherent to the capsule and surrounding tissue.
- Performing a bladder-sparing technique is not always possible. It is better to avoid positive surgical margins and make a wide dissection.
- Performing the posterior dissection is difficult with poor planes between Denonvilliers' fascia and the prostate and the rectum; extreme care is required to avoid a rectal injury.
- Dissection of the endopelvic fascia and the pelvic lymphadenectomy can be challenging as the tissues can be adherent to surrounding structures.
- Nerve sparing is not recommended as patients have bulky disease and planes are adherent.

Evidence base Surgery in Metastatic Carcinoma of Prostate (SIMCAP) trial

Preliminary results of this multi-institutional international phase II–III study that aims to assess the efficacy of cytoreductive radical prostatectomy in men with newly diagnosed mPCa was published by Yuh et al. in a phase I safety trial setting.[18] Eligible men had biopsy-proven PCa and evidence of lymph node or bone metastasis by conventional imaging, or biopsy. The initial study cohort was composed of 32 patients with a mean age of 64 years. In 37.5% of cases neoadjuvant treatment (ADT in combination or not with chemotherapy) was reported. As primary endpoint, the overall complication rate was 31.25%. Of note, major complications defined as >3 points according to the Clavien–Dindo classification occurred in two (6.25%) patients. Mean blood loss was 267.7 mL (range 50–950 mL). Positive surgical margins occurred in 65.6% of patients, pT3b in 62.5%. As secondary endpoints, at median follow-up of 214 days, a PSA nadir <0.2 ng/mL under ADT was reported in 19 (67.9%) patients.

Evidence base Local treatment of Metastatic Prostate Cancer (LoMP) trial

This multicentric prospective study evaluated the role of cytoreductive radical prostatectomy with extended pelvic lymphadenectomy versus standard of care in patients newly diagnosed with mPCa.[19] Inclusion criteria were multidisciplinary oncological consultation, histologically confirmed PCa, and the presence of at least one metastatic lesion (cM1) after staging with abdominopelvic computed tomography and bone scan. CHAARTED definitions were used to define the disease volume. Forty-six patients were recruited: 17 (37%) underwent surgery and were significantly younger, had lower initial PSA levels, and less high-volume disease compared to their counterparts. In this group of patients, no intraoperative complications were reported. After 3 months, 70.6% of patients treated with surgery versus 44.8% patients treated with standard of care were continent and had no local symptoms.

Expert comment Safety and feasibility of surgical approach

In this unusual clinical case scenario, we operated on a patient with oligometastatic PCa who had undergone best systemic therapy with ADT and chemotherapy. If surgery of the primary tumour is a well-established concept in the treatment of several metastatic malignancies including ovarian tumours, various gastrointestinal tumours, and renal cell carcinoma, there is growing evidence that local control of disease may be useful also in mPCa. Furthermore, STAMPEDE arm H assessed the efficacy of radiotherapy to the primary tumour in M1 disease[8]; thus, cytoreductive radical prostatectomy (CRP) has recently garnered research interest. To date, considering the improvements in minimally invasive surgery, CRP feasibility is becoming more widely accepted. Starting from a multi-institutional retrospective experience including 106 men with M1a and M1b PCa who underwent CRP, an overall complication rate of 20.8% was reported. The most common complications were need of blood transfusion (14.2%), symptomatic lymphocele (8.5%), and anastomotic leak (6.6%) but no significant differences were found considering the burden of disease (M1a vs M1b). In addition, cancer-specific survival at 2 years of follow-up was 88.7%.[20]

With a prospective design, Poelaert et al.[19] compared two groups: group A, a carefully selected cohort of 17 asymptomatic men with mPCa who received ADT plus CRP, and group B, 29 men with mPCa who received standard of care. The robotic approach was performed in 94.1% of cases and only seven minor complications were reported at 90 days after surgery.

Using prospective data, Steuber et al.[21] compared 43 patients with low-volume mPCa who underwent CRP with 40 patients who received standard of care. Of note, the cohort who received CRP experienced a significant lower number of locoregional complications (7 vs 35, $p < 0.01$). No significant oncological benefit, in terms of overall and castration resistant-free survival, was reported.[21] The lack of further locoregional complications represents a relevant CRP goal. The escalation due to the increasing number of drugs available as well as advances in targeted therapy of specific somatic mutations have expanded the overall survival of these patients. Thus, the treatment of local progression-related symptoms such as haematuria, ureteric obstruction, urge incontinence, and obstructive voiding represents a clinical scenario that need to be faced.

Yuh et al. sought out to demonstrate feasibility and assess safety in a cohort of patients with mPCa in an international multi-institutional setting. Regarding 90-day complication rates, a total of ten events were reported: according to the Clavien–Dindo system eight minor and two major, including one death in which a patient developed rapid progressive disease.[18]

Phase II and III studies are warranted to determine efficacy and to confirm these results but these preliminary data suggest that the complication rates are similar to those of radical prostatectomy in clinically localized PCa.

A final word from the expert

The future is getting brighter for men with mPCa. More and more systemic agents are being proven to improve survival, and local therapy has a proven efficacy in oligometastatic disease. This case illustrates that surgery to remove the primary tumour might be a viable alternative to radiotherapy for these men, to further increase the therapeutic options available to them. The TRoMbone study[22] is the first randomized controlled trial examining the safety and feasibility of randomization to systemic therapy plus radical prostatectomy in synchronous oligometastatic PCa. Inclusion criteria were the following:

- Male aged 18–74 years.
- Diagnosed with synchronous oligometastatic PCa (one to three skeletal lesions on bone-specific imaging, no visceral metastases).
- Locally resectable tumour (clinical stage cT1–T3).
- Eastern Cooperative Oncology Group (ECOG) performance status 0–1.

The initial protocol randomized these patients to radical prostatectomy and ePLND within 3 months of starting standard care versus standard care alone. After the introduction of docetaxel as first-line therapy in hormone-sensitive patients, the protocol was then amended to follow systemic therapy for up to 12 months before surgery. Among the 176 patients screened, 71 were eligible and 51 (71.8%) were randomized including 25 to radical prostatectomy. Of note, all surgeries were conducted with robotic assistance, and results are awaited.

References

1. Stevens DJ, Sooriakumaran P. Oligometastatic prostate cancer. *Curr Treat Options Oncol.* 2016;17(12):62.
2. Corfield J, Perera M, Bolton D, Lawrentschuk N. 68Ga-prostate specific membrane antigen (PSMA) positron emission tomography (PET) for primary staging of high-risk prostate cancer: a systematic review. *World J Urol.* 2018;36(4):519–527.
3. Sweeney CJ, Chen YH, Carducci M, et al. Chemohormonal therapy in metastatic hormone-sensitive prostate cancer. *N Engl J Med.* 2015;373(8):737–746.
4. Fizazi K, Tran NP, Fein L, et al. Abiraterone plus prednisone in metastatic, castration-sensitive prostate cancer. *N Engl J Med.* 2017;377(4):352–360.
5. Ost P, Bossi A, Decaestecker K, et al. Metastasis-directed therapy of regional and distant recurrences after curative treatment of prostate cancer: a systematic review of the literature. *Eur Urol.* 2015;67(5):852–863.
6. Weichselbaum RR, Hellman S. Oligometastases revisited. *Nat Rev Clin Oncol.* 2011;8(6):378–382.
7. MacDermed DM, Weichselbaum RR, Salama JK. A rationale for the targeted treatment of oligometastases with radiotherapy. *J Surg Oncol.* 2008;98(3):202–206.
8. Parker CC, James ND, Brawley CD, et al. Radiotherapy to the primary tumour for newly diagnosed, metastatic prostate cancer (STAMPEDE): a randomised controlled phase 3 trial. *Lancet.* 2018;392(10162):2353–2366.
9. Nitta T, Sato K. Prognostic implications of the extent of surgical resection in patients with intracranial malignant gliomas. *Cancer.* 1995;75(11):2727–2731.
10. Temple LKF, Hsieh L, Wong WD, Saltz L, Schrag D. Use of surgery among elderly patients with stage IV colorectal cancer. *J Clin Oncol.* 2004;22(17):3475–3484.
11. Mickisch GHJ, Garin A, Van Poppel H, De Prijck L, Sylvester R. Radical nephrectomy plus interferon-alfa-based immunotherapy compared with interferon alfa alone in metastatic renal-cell carcinoma: a randomised trial. *Lancet.* 2001;358(9286):966–970.
12. Stewart SB, Boorjian SA. Radical prostatectomy in high-risk and locally advanced prostate cancer: Mayo Clinic perspective. *Urol Oncol.* 2015;33(5):235–244.
13. Stranne J, Brasso K, Brennhovd B, et al. SPCG-15: a prospective randomized study comparing primary radical prostatectomy and primary radiotherapy plus androgen deprivation therapy for locally advanced prostate cancer. *Scand J Urol.* 2018;52(5–6):313–320.
14. De Groote R, Nathan A, De Bleser E, et al. Techniques and outcomes of salvage robot-assisted radical prostatectomy (sRARP). *Eur Urol.* 2020;78(6):885–892.
15. Eastham JA, Heller G, Halabi S, et al. CALGB 90203 (Alliance): radical prostatectomy (RP) with or without neoadjuvant chemohormonal therapy (CHT) in men with clinically localized, high-risk prostate cancer (CLHRPC). *J Clin Oncol.* 2019;37(15 Suppl):5079–5079.
16. Mottet N, Cornford P, van den Bergh RCN, et al. EAU–EANM–ESTRO–ESUR–SIOG guidelines on prostate cancer 2019. European Association of Urology. 2019. https://uroweb.org/guideline/prostate-cancer/
17. James ND, Spears MR, Clarke NW, et al. Impact of node status and radiotherapy on failure-free survival in patients with newly-diagnosed non-metastatic prostate cancer: data from > 690 patients in the control arm of the STAMPEDE Trial. *Int J Radiat Oncol.* 2014;90(1):S13.
18. Yuh BE, Kwon YS, Shinder BM, et al. Results of phase 1 study on cytoreductive radical prostatectomy in men with newly diagnosed metastatic prostate cancer. *Prostate Int.* 2019;7(3):102–107.
19. Poelaert F, Verbaeys C, Rappe B, et al. Cytoreductive prostatectomy for metastatic prostate cancer: first lessons learned from the multicentric prospective Local Treatment of Metastatic Prostate Cancer (LoMP) trial. *Urology.* 2017;106(5):146–152.

20. Sooriakumaran P, Karnes J, Stief C, et al. A multi-institutional analysis of perioperative outcomes in 106 men who underwent radical prostatectomy for distant metastatic prostate cancer at presentation. *Eur Urol.* 2016;69(5):788–794.
21. Steuber T, Berg KD, Røder MA, et al. Does cytoreductive prostatectomy really have an impact on prognosis in prostate cancer patients with low-volume bone metastasis? Results from a prospective case-control study. *Eur Urol Focus.* 2017;3(6):646–649.
22. Sooriakumaran P. Testing radical prostatectomy in men with prostate cancer and oligometastases to the bone: a randomized controlled feasibility trial. *BJU Int.* 2017;120(5):E8–E20.

CASE

Newly diagnosed metastatic prostate cancer

Adnan Ali and Noel W. Clarke

Expert commentary Noel W. Clarke

Case history

A previously fit 69-year-old man developed non-specific musculoskeletal aches and pains. His general practitioner measured the prostate-specific antigen (PSA) level which was raised to 1200 ng/mL, triggering a referral for further investigation. Prostate biopsies showed a Gleason score 7 (4 + 3) adenocarcinoma with tertiary pattern 5. Bone and computed tomography (CT) scans demonstrated widespread metastatic disease without visceral involvement. Relevant past history included a pneumothorax 40 years previously but nothing else relevant.

Following discussion, the multidisciplinary team recommended treatment included life-long androgen deprivation therapy (ADT), with anti-androgen 'flare' protection and docetaxel. The patient was counselled regarding treatment and was commenced on a gonadotropin-releasing hormone (GnRH) agonist combined with six 3-weekly cycles of docetaxel (75mg/m^2) with prednisolone 10 mg daily. Full blood counts, bilirubin, alanine aminotransferase, aspartate aminotransferase, and alkaline phosphatase values were obtained prior to each treatment cycle. The patient had no serious chemotherapy-related side effects and went on to complete six cycles of therapy. Grade 1 treatment-related toxicities included fatigue, skin/nail changes, and dysgeusia. On completion of chemotherapy, prednisolone was reduced progressively and stopped. One month after the sixth docetaxel cycle, all grade 1 toxicities (fatigue, dysgeusia, fatigue, cold feet) resolved. However, he still had nail changes, hot flushes, and impotence. None were especially bothersome.

Learning point First-line treatment options for newly diagnosed metastatic prostate cancer

ADT remains the primary therapy in untreated metastatic prostate cancer, which depends on androgens for its sustained growth. Androgen suppression is achieved either by surgical or medical castration (testosterone levels <50 ng/mL). Bilateral orchiectomy is highly effective but has largely been replaced by 'medical castration' using either luteinizing hormone-releasing hormone (i.e. GnRH) agonists or antagonists. GnRH agonists are used most commonly and are delivered as depot injections 1-, 2-, 3-, 6-, or 12-monthly. GnRH antagonists are administered by monthly subcutaneous injection. Oral anti-androgens can be used as an alternative, often with reduced androgen-linked side effects but they are less effective in overt metastatic disease. Their use in modern practice is mainly to prevent disease flare at the outset of treatment.

Until recently, ADT monotherapy was the first-line management option for newly diagnosed M1 prostate cancer. However, since 2015, large phase III trials have evaluated ADT combined with other treatments.[1-16] Currently, three different ADT combination treatments are known to improve survival:

- Docetaxel.
- Novel anti-androgenics (abiraterone, enzalutamide, apalutamide).
- Prostate radiotherapy in patients with low metastatic burden.

Currently, the choice among these treatments largely depends on patient comorbidity and preference, metastatic burden, and availability of treatment. Although some patients in the currently reported trials received triple combination therapy, the data are currently immature to recommend such combinations.

Evidence base Clinical trials showing survival benefit in M1 hormone-naïve prostate cancer: docetaxel and abiraterone

Over the last decade, various phase III randomized trials have evaluated the addition of different treatment combinations with standard ADT in M1 hormone-naïve prostate cancer (mHNPC). All systemic treatments (docetaxel, abiraterone, enzalutamide, apalutamide) are first-line options regardless of metastatic burden. Prostate radiotherapy is also recommended for patients with low metastatic burden (defined as patients with only M1a disease or fewer than four bone metastases and no visceral disease on standard imaging).

Docetaxel

Three trials, GETUG-15, CHAARTED, and STAMPEDE arm C, have evaluated the combination of ADT + docetaxel over ADT alone. A meta-analysis of these trials confirmed the improvement in overall survival with the addition of docetaxel to ADT (hazard ratio (HR) 0.77; 95% confidence interval (CI) 0.68–0.87).[14] A subgroup analysis in the CHAARTED study showed more pronounced benefit in patients with high-metastatic burden (HR 0.63; 95% CI 0.50–0.79).[12] However, no such difference in survival based on metastatic burden (interaction p = 0.827) was observed in the long-term follow-up data for M1 patients in the STAMPEDE comparison.[8] Addition of docetaxel to ADT is a recommended option for all fit M1 patients regardless of metastatic burden.

Abiraterone

Two trials, LATITUDE and STAMPEDE arm G, have evaluated the combination of ADT + 1000 mg abiraterone with 5 mg prednisolone/prednisone daily. LATITUDE randomized 1199 patients with high-risk mHNPC, with risk defined as the presence of at least two of the following: Gleason score ≥8, at least three bone metastases, or presence of visceral metastases.[10] The addition of abiraterone to ADT showed significantly improved overall survival (HR 0.66; 95% CI 0.56–0.78). A similar benefit in survival was observed in the STAMPEDE trial for M1 patients (HR 0.63; 95% CI 0.52–0.76).[9] A post hoc analysis demonstrated this survival benefit regardless of high or low metastatic burden (p-interaction = 0.77) and risk (p-interaction = 0.39).[7]

Evidence base Clinical trials showing survival benefit in mHNPC: anti-androgens

Enzalutamide

Two trials, ENZAMET and ARCHES, have evaluated the combination of ADT + enzalutamide. ENZAMET randomized 1125 men with mHNPC to either ADT + non-steroidal anti-androgen (bicalutamide, nilutamide, or flutamide) versus ADT + enzalutamide. Enzalutamide showed significant improvement in overall survival (HR 0.67; 95% CI 0.52–0.86).[11] At interim analysis, the ARCHES trial's primary endpoint of improved radiographic progression-free survival was improved significantly with ADT + enzalutamide (HR 0.39; 95% CI 0.30–0.50).[16]

Apalutamide

The combination of apalutamide with ADT has been evaluated in the phase III TITAN trial where 525 patients were assigned to receive ADT + apalutamide and 527 to ADT + placebo. The addition of apalutamide to ADT improved overall survival (HR 0.67; 95% CI 0.51–0.89) with no significant differences according to disease volume.[15]

Darolutamide

A further randomized trial of the third 'anti-androgenic amide', darolutamide, is currently being evaluated in combination with ADT in mHNPC (ARASENS trial). Results are awaited.

Evidence base Prostate radiotherapy in mHNPC

The HORRAD and STAMPEDE trials have evaluated ADT ± prostate radiotherapy in this setting. HORRAD randomized 446 patients to receive ADT or ADT + radiotherapy. Improved overall survival was suggested in a subgroup of 160 patients with one to five bone metastases (HR 0.68; 95% CI 0.42–1.10).[6] STAMPEDE arm H randomized 2061 men to ADT ± radiotherapy. In a prespecified subgroup analysis by metastatic burden, prostate radiotherapy improved survival in patients with low metastatic burden (HR 0.68; 95% CI 0.52–0.90).[5] Further exploratory analysis has refined the definition of low metastatic burden, which predicts survival benefit with ADT + prostate radiotherapy as only non-regional lymph node metastasis (M1a) or fewer than four bone metastases without any visceral disease.[4]

Expert comment Continuous versus intermittent ADT

A number of trials have evaluated intermittent versus continuous ADT in mHNPC. None have shown a clear survival benefit with continuous over intermittent ADT but there is a constant trend towards improved overall survival with continuous ADT, although intermittent ADT may favour better quality of life.

All recent trials showing survival benefit when combining ADT with other treatments have used continuous ADT.

Clinical tip Flare phenomenon

If GnRH agonists are used, there is a transient increase in luteinizing hormone which can cause a surge in testosterone after the first injection. This may induce worsening of disease if there is an impending spinal cord compression or urinary tract obstruction. Therefore, an anti-androgen should be added for 1 week prior to GnRH analogue administration and for 2 weeks thereafter to decrease the incidence of any such unfavourable clinical effects. This is especially important in patients with symptomatic and/or high-volume disease. Orchidectomy and GnRH antagonists do not cause flare. In patients with impending spinal cord compression or urinary obstruction, one of these two therapies should be used instead of GnRH agonists.

Expert comment Timing of ADT

In mHNPC, immediate treatment with ADT is required in all patients unless there is a specific contraindication such as serious comorbidity/frailty with anticipated short life expectancy. In the majority of cases, combination treatment either with docetaxel-based chemotherapy or novel anti-androgenics should be the standard of care. This will improve life expectancy and delay the onset of serious complications.

Learning point Common adverse effects of ADT

Use of ADT has adverse effects which affect quality of life. Additionally, it increases fat mass, decreases lean body mass, increases fasting plasma insulin levels, decreases insulin sensitivity, and increases serum levels of cholesterol and triglycerides. This metabolic dysregulation heightens the risk of cardiovascular morbidity and metabolic syndrome. Patients should be appropriately screened and counselled about these side effects prior to treatment. Common side effects include the following:

- Cardiovascular and metabolic complications: screening and intervention to prevent and treat diabetes, dyslipidaemia, and cardiovascular diseases are recommended in patients starting long-term ADT.
- Sexual dysfunction: this is common in men receiving ADT. Most men who are potent prior to ADT have decreased libido and erectile dysfunction after treatment. Management is non-specific and centres around pretreatment counselling of patients and partners.
- Hot flushes: most men receiving ADT report vasomotor symptoms that manifest as hot flushes. These are associated with sweating, sleep disturbances, and, sometimes, nausea. Effective management can be difficult. Treatment approaches include use of serotonin reuptake inhibitors (e.g. venlafaxine or sertraline) and alternative hormonal treatment (e.g. low-dose megestrol acetate or cyproterone acetate at low dose).
- Fatigue/anaemia: fatigue is a common side effect. Regular exercise is recommended and may help. Low-grade anaemia secondary to marrow suppression is also associated with ADT. This may be contributory.
- Osteoporosis and osteopenia: see ' Learning point' box for management of bone health.
- Other side effects: these include thinning of body hair and decrease in penile and testicular size.

Learning point Management of bone health during ADT

ADT reduces bone and muscle mass. This increases the risk of osteoporotic fractures. Bone loss, measured by bone mineral density (BMD) can be assessed by dual-energy X-ray absorptiometry (DXA) or predicted using Fracture Risk Assessment Tool (FRAX)® scoring. BMD decreases with ADT by 2–3%/year, and declines steadily thereafter long. -term, accompanied by reducing muscle mass. This treatment-related sarcopenia increases the risk of falls. Therefore, preventive management for osteoporosis is recommended in all patients starting long-term ADT which include:

- Use of systemic bone protection with bisphosphonates or RANK ligand inhibition (denosumab)
- Lifestyle changes, particularly weight-bearing and aerobic exercise, smoking cessation, and reduced alcohol consumption
- Calcium 1000–1200 mg daily from food and supplements
- Vitamin D_3 400–1000 IU daily.

Estimated fracture risk assessed by the FRAX® algorithm guides use of anti-fracture therapies. For men ≥50 years old with low BMD (T-score −1.0 to −2.5, osteopenia) at the femoral neck, hip, or lumbar spine by DXA and a 10-year probability of either hip fracture ≥3% or major osteoporotic fracture ≥20%:

- Denosumab or bisphosphonate is recommended to increase BMD.
- A DXA scan after 1 year of ADT is recommended.

Clinical tip Use of bone protective agents

Bone protective agents such as denosumab and zoledronic acid at low dose have only a minimal risk of significant complications. Before starting patients on such agents, serum calcium should be measured and monitored periodically during treatment. Hypocalcaemia if identified should be corrected before starting treatment. During treatment, unless hypercalcaemic, daily calcium (≥500 mg) and vitamin D (≥400 IU equivalent) is recommended in all patients. It is important to recognize that the bone-protective dose of these agents is much lower than that used in the late stages of progressive castration-resistant disease.

Clinical tip Monitoring progression

Serial evaluation of serum PSA every 3–6 months during treatment is the mainstay of monitoring disease progression but alkaline phosphatase is also important, particularly in low-PSA secretors. The need for radiographic evaluation (bone scan or CT/magnetic resonance imaging (MRI)) is based on changes in PSA and/or development of new symptoms. Treatment should not be stopped based on PSA progression alone. At least two of the three criteria (PSA progression, radiographic progression, or clinical deterioration) should be fulfilled.

Nineteen months after his last docetaxel cycle, the patient's PSA level started increasing and he reported new low back pain. An updated bone scan showed no clear evidence of progression but he was started on 50 mg of bicalutamide. His PSA stabilized at 6 ng/mL and the back pain improved. However, after 2 months the PSA rose to 10 ng/mL. At this point bicalutamide was stopped and further options were discussed with the patient. After a wash out period of 6 weeks, enzalutamide 160 mg daily was commenced. The patient was followed regularly, remaining asymptomatic, but the PSA level increased slowly from 12 to 19 ng/mL over a 6-month period. A CT scan showed stable disease but a further bone scan showed multifocal areas of activity, particularly extensive in the spine at T12 and L2. The increase in PSA level continued, reaching 38 ng/mL within 4 months. At this time-point the patient had two episodes of lower abdominal and back pain radiating down both legs, managed by codeine-based analgesia. Updated CT and bone scans failed to show evidence of further progression. The enzalutamide dose was therefore continued. Two months later, the patient was admitted complaining of lumbar back pain radiating to the groins and testicles. Urgent imaging showed no evidence of spinal cord compression and a single 8 Gy fraction of radiotherapy to T12–L4 was administered. Enzalutamide was stopped at this point and patient started on dexamethasone 0.5 mg. This induced a short-lived decrease in PSA level and stilboestrol 1 mg once daily was added along with aspirin 75 mg to reduce the risk of thrombosis.

Given the extensive nature of the patient's bone metastases, but his good condition overall, further treatment options were discussed. The patient agreed to proceed with six cycles of 4-weekly radium-223. Haematological indices were checked and seen to be stable before each of six cycles administered. Following completion, the patient continued on dexamethasone and stilboestrol. Right-sided pelvic pain developed 3 months later, requiring local radiotherapy with a single 8 Gy fraction. Dexamethasone and stilboestrol were continued and the patient reported he was well overall with his main complaint being tiredness. His electrolyte and haemoglobin levels were checked to assess for upper tract obstruction and the need for blood transfusion. Haemoglobin was maintained at 9.4 g/dL. Over the coming weeks his overall condition deteriorated, with complaints of pain in various places requiring opiate-based analgesia. His disease followed a relentless course thereafter requiring palliative support and ultimately hospice care. He died nearly 7 years after his initial diagnosis.

Clinical tip Role of imaging and evaluation of metastatic burden

Staging and evaluation of metastatic burden is currently recommended based on conventional imaging, that is, a technitium-99m methylene diphosphonate bone scan and cross-sectional imaging based on CT/MRI. Metastatic burden is prognostic for systemic treatments and predictive of survival benefit from prostate radiotherapy.

Learning point Treatment options for metastatic castration-resistant prostate cancer

The majority of men with metastatic prostate cancer will eventually show evidence of disease progression following primary ADT-based therapy. This is usually manifest as an increase in serum PSA, development of new or progression of existing metastases or development of symptoms. These also include lower urinary tract and bone-marrow related problems. Such men, with castrate levels of serum testosterone (<50 ng/dL) are considered to have metastatic castration-resistant prostate cancer (mCRPC). Treatment options at progression which have been shown to improve survival include chemotherapy, novel ADT, systemic radionuclides, and, more recently, DNA repair inhibition[17–26]:

- Chemotherapy: docetaxel, cabazitaxel.
- Novel ADT: abiraterone, enzalutamide.
- Systemic radionuclides: radium-223.
- DNA repair inhibition: olaparib.

The choice of treatment depends on prior systemic therapies, the site/extent of disease involvement, presence of symptoms, and evidence of somatic/germline mutations in homologous recombination repair (HRR) genes. Whenever possible, these patients should be included in clinical trials.

Learning point Management of bone metastasis complications

Bone metastases are the most common site of metastasis in prostate cancer and often lead to skeletal complications. These, referred to as skeletal-related events (SREs), include pathological fracture, the need for radiotherapy or surgery to bone, and spinal cord compression. The overarching treatment goals are to improve survival, relieve pain, improve mobility, and prevent or delay such complications arising:

- Systemic treatment with docetaxel, abiraterone, enzalutamide, radium-223, or zoledronic acid all reduce SREs and remain central to prevention and management of these complications.
- Even with the best available treatment, pain is a common symptom which is managed as required using established analgesics.
- Isolated painful bony metastases can be managed effectively with a single fraction of 8 Gy. The onset of pain relief varies from a few days to 4 weeks.
- Surgery, including vertebroplasty/kyphoplasty, is usually reserved for patients who have pathological fractures or spinal cord compression.

Clinical tip Spinal cord compression

Patients should be educated to recognize the warning signs of spinal cord compression. Once suspected, high-dose corticosteroids should be given immediately and spinal MRI performed urgently. Neurosurgery or orthopaedic surgery should be consulted straight away for discussion regarding decompression followed by external beam radiotherapy. If surgery is not appropriate, external beam radiotherapy ± secondary systemic therapy is preferred.

Evidence base Third-line treatment options following docetaxel and abiraterone/enzalutamide in mCRPC

The CARD trial evaluated the safety and efficacy of chemotherapy with cabazitaxel in mCRPC following prior treatment with docetaxel and progression within 12 months compared to abiraterone or enzalutamide.[23] At median follow-up of 9.2 months, third-line cabazitaxel improved survival over novel ADT (HR 0.64; 95% CI 0.46–0.89; $p = 0.008$). The median overall survival was 13.6 months with cabazitaxel and 11 months with standard therapy. Grade 3 or higher adverse events occurred in 56.3% of patients receiving cabazitaxel and in 52% of those receiving a novel androgen.

Evidence base Radium-223 in mCRPC

The phase III randomized, double-blind, placebo-controlled ALSYMPCA trial evaluated radium-223, an alpha emitter, which selectively targets bone metastases. Men who had received, were not eligible to receive, or declined docetaxel were randomized in a 2:1 ratio to receive six injections of radium-223 at 50 kBq per kilogram at 4-week intervals. Radium-223 improved overall survival significantly (median 14.9 vs 11.3 months; HR 0.70; 95% CI 0.58–0.83; $p < 0.001$).[22]

Another trial, ERA-223, showed that in mCRPC patients with bone metastasis the addition of radium-223 to abiraterone did not improve symptomatic skeletal event-free survival and was associated with an increased frequency of osteoporotic bone fractures compared with placebo. Use of this drug combination is not recommended without bone protection with bisphosphonates. Following ERA-223, the European Medicines Agency restricted its use only after docetaxel and at least one AR targeted agent had been used and failed.[19]

Evidence base Olaparib in mCRPC

Defects in genes involved in HRR directly or indirectly confer sensitivity to poly (adenosine diphosphate-ribose) polymerase (PARP) inhibitors such as olaparib. The PROfound trial randomized men with mCRPC progressing on anti-androgenics who had alteration in any of 15 prespecified DDR genes to receive olaparib versus an alternative ADT. Tumour testing was conducted centrally using archival or recent biopsy tissue from primary or metastatic sites. In 245 patients with at least one alteration in *BRCA1*, *BRCA2*, or *ATM*, olaparib improved radiological progression-free survival (HR 0.34; 95% CI 0.25–0.47) and overall survival (HR 0.64; 95% CI 0.43–0.97).[24] Olaparib can be considered after new hormonal agents for patients with mCRPC with alteration in *BRCA1* or *BRCA2*.

Future directions Ongoing trials, molecular biomarkers, and next-generation imaging

Currently, a number of ongoing trials are evaluating local (surgery and radiotherapy), systemic, and metastasis-directed therapy alone or in combination. These trials are likely to report in future years. Additionally, molecular biomarkers are being evaluated to identify predictive indicators which can then be used to select patients for specific treatment. Next-generation imaging such as whole-body MRI and prostate-specific membrane antigen radionuclide scans are being evaluated: these may improve staging and stratification of novel treatments by detecting occult metastasis.

Expert comment DNA damage and repair genes

Defects in DNA damage repair (known as DDR or HRR defects) can be familial (germ line) or tumour derived (somatic). A significant proportion of men with metastatic prostate cancer harbour these genetic aberrations. Such genes, including *BRCA2*, which are involved in HRR are potential predictors of response to PARP inhibitors. Men with a family history of prostate cancer and with other cancer syndromes arising from HRR mutations should be considered for genetic testing and counselling. A large phase III trial (PROpel) is currently evaluating the efficacy, safety, and tolerability of olaparib versus placebo when given with abiraterone to mCRPC patients following first-line ADT failure.

Discussion

With a number of different trials reporting survival benefit, the choice of first-line treatment currently depends on patient preference and fitness, drug availability, side effects, and metastatic burden. A key decision requires the evaluation of metastatic burden based on conventional imaging (bone scan and CT/MRI). Prostate radiotherapy in M1 patients can be considered when the metastatic burden is low, defined as the

Table 10.1 Key adverse events of systemic agents used in metastatic prostate cancer

Agent	Key adverse effects
Abiraterone	Hypokalaemia, hypertension, hyperglycaemia, oedema
Cabazitaxel	Diarrhoea, haematuria, peripheral neuropathy, alopecia, myelosuppression
Docetaxel	Alopecia, neuropathy, fluid retention, myelosuppression, febrile neutropenia
Enzalutamide	Musculoskeletal pain, fatigue, hot flushes, hypertension
Radium-223	Nausea, vomiting, diarrhoea, myelosuppression
Olaparib	Anaemia, nausea, fatigue (including asthenia), decreased appetite, diarrhoea, vomiting, thrombocytopenia, cough

presence of non-regional lymph node metastasis or fewer than four bone metastases and no visceral metastasis[1–6] on standard imaging. Systemic treatment with docetaxel, abiraterone, apalutamide, and enzalutamide have shown to improve survival when added to ADT regardless of metastatic burden.[7–16]

The patient reviewed here presented with extensive bone metastases. For such patients with high metastatic burden, the long-term follow-up data from the STAMPEDE docetaxel comparison show a median survival of approximately 3 years, with one in three men surviving beyond 5 years (5-year survival 34%). It is therefore important to recognize that prolonging life is not the only goal of management. Consideration of overall quality of life and the avoidance of serious cancer-related complications are paramount. This requires multidisciplinary care with input from uro-oncologists and palliative care teams working jointly.

Over a 7-year period following his diagnosis, this man went on to receive docetaxel, enzalutamide, and radium-223. All these treatments have side effects (Table 10.1) and patients need counselling about these prior to treatment initiation in addition to mitigation of their effects where possible while they are on treatment.[17–26] Bone is the commonest site of metastasis and patients often require management of pain and complications arising therefrom. In patients with extensive symptomatic bone metastases without visceral disease, radium-223 can improve survival, reduce symptomatic SREs, and reduce bone pain. Zoledronic acid also reduces SREs including long bone fracture and cord compression but its use should not be for > 24 months as osteonecrosis of the jaw then becomes more common. Painful bone metastases will require palliative measures, including single 8 Gy fraction radiotherapy, opioid-based analgesics, and, where necessary, orthopaedic fixation and urgent spinal surgery for cord compression. Blood transfusion and relief of upper urinary tract obstruction is also a regular requirement.

A final word from the expert

Sixteen per cent of patients presenting with prostate cancer have metastases when first seen and they constitute 40% of the deaths arising from this disease. Combination therapy with ADT and chemotherapy or novel anti-androgenics is the standard of care, with radiotherapy to the primary site when disease burden is low. This new approach, based on data derived from large-scale trials, has improved treatment options for patients in recent years and combination therapies, stratified for risk, have increased life expectancy and quality of life for many. However, in most, the disease will ultimately progress, requiring a coordinated and subspecialized approach to treatment, treatment sequencing, and the management of the treatment-related side effects. In managing these patients, clinicians must be familiar with modern treatment options and the best way to sequence/direct therapy using the continually evolving data as they emerge. Clinicians must also remember that optimal management of metastatic prostate cancer is multidisciplinary, involving various clinical groups, but always with the patient at the centre.

References

1. European Association of Urology. Guidelines: prostate cancer. European Association of Urology. 2019. https://uroweb.org/guideline/prostate-cancer/
2. National Comprehensive Cancer Network. Clinical practice guidelines in oncology—prostate cancer. Version 2.2019. National Comprehensive Cancer Network. 2019. https://www.nccn.org/professionals/physician_gls/pdf/prostate.pdf
3. European Society for Medical Oncology. Treatment recommendations for cancer of the prostate. European Society for Medical Oncology. 2019. https://www.esmo.org/Guidelines/Genitourinary-Cancers/Cancer-of-the-Prostate/eUpdate-Treatment-Recommendations
4. Ali SA, Hoyle A, James ND, et al. Benefit of prostate radiotherapy for patients with lymph node only or < 4 bone metastasis and no visceral metastases: exploratory analyses of metastatic site and number in the STAMPEDE 'M1|RT comparison'. *Ann Oncol.* 2019;30(Suppl 5):v325–v355.
5. Parker CC, James ND, Brawley CD, et al. Radiotherapy to the primary tumour for newly diagnosed, metastatic prostate cancer (STAMPEDE): a randomised controlled phase 3 trial. *Lancet.* 2018;392(10162):2353–2366.
6. Boeve LMS, Hulshof M, Vis AN, et al. Effect on survival of androgen deprivation therapy alone compared to androgen deprivation therapy combined with concurrent radiation therapy to the prostate in patients with primary bone metastatic prostate cancer in a prospective randomised clinical trial: data from the HORRAD trial. *Eur Urol.* 2019;75(3):410–418.
7. Hoyle AP, Ali A, James ND, et al. Abiraterone in 'high-' and 'low-risk' metastatic hormone-sensitive prostate cancer. *Eur Urol.* 2019;76(6):719–728.
8. Clarke NW, Ali A, Ingleby FC, et al. Addition of docetaxel to hormonal therapy in low- and high-burden metastatic hormone sensitive prostate cancer: long-term survival results from the STAMPEDE trial. *Ann Oncol.* 2019;30(12):1992–2003.
9. James ND, de Bono JS, Spears MR, et al. Abiraterone for prostate cancer not previously treated with hormone therapy. *N Engl J Med.* 2017;377(4):338–351.
10. Fizazi K, Tran N, Fein L, et al. Abiraterone acetate plus prednisone in patients with newly diagnosed high-risk metastatic castration-sensitive prostate cancer (LATITUDE): final overall survival analysis of a randomised, double-blind, phase 3 trial. *Lancet Oncol.* 2019;20(5):686–700.
11. Davis ID, Martin AJ, Stockler MR, Begbie S, Chi KN, Chowdhury S, et al. Enzalutamide with standard first-line therapy in metastatic prostate cancer. *N Engl J Med.* 2019;381(2):121–131.
12. Kyriakopoulos CE, Chen YH, Carducci MA, et al. Chemohormonal therapy in metastatic hormone-sensitive prostate cancer: long-term survival analysis of the randomized phase III E3805 CHAARTED Trial. *J Clin Oncol.* 2018;36(11):1080–1087.
13. Sweeney CJ, Chen YH, Carducci M, et al. Chemohormonal therapy in metastatic hormone-sensitive prostate cancer. *N Engl J Med.* 2015;373(8):737–746.
14. Vale CL, Burdett S, Rydzewska LHM, et al. Addition of docetaxel or bisphosphonates to standard of care in men with localised or metastatic, hormone-sensitive prostate cancer: a systematic review and meta-analyses of aggregate data. *Lancet Oncol.* 2016;17(2):243–256.

15. Chi KN, Agarwal N, Bjartell A, et al. Apalutamide for metastatic, castration-sensitive prostate cancer. *N Engl J Med.* 2019;381(1):13–24.
16. Armstrong AJ, Szmulewitz RZ, Petrylak DP, et al. ARCHES: a randomized, phase III study of androgen deprivation therapy with enzalutamide or placebo in men with metastatic hormone-sensitive prostate cancer. *J Clin Oncol.* 2019;37(32):2974–2986.
17. Ryan CJ, Smith MR, de Bono JS, et al. Abiraterone in metastatic prostate cancer without previous chemotherapy. *N Engl J Med.* 2013;368(2):138–148.
18. de Bono JS, Logothetis CJ, Molina A, et al. Abiraterone and increased survival in metastatic prostate cancer. *N Engl J Med.* 2011;364(21):1995–2005.
19. Smith M, Parker C, Saad F, et al. Addition of radium-223 to abiraterone acetate and prednisone or prednisolone in patients with castration-resistant prostate cancer and bone metastases (ERA 223): a randomised, double-blind, placebo-controlled, phase 3 trial. *Lancet Oncol.* 2019;20(3):408–419.
20. Beer T, Armstrong A, Rathkopf D, et al. Enzalutamide in metastatic prostate cancer before chemotherapy. *N Engl J Med.* 2014;371(5):424–433.
21. Scher H, Fizazi K, Saad F, et al. Increased survival with enzalutamide in prostate cancer after chemotherapy. *N Engl J Med.* 2012;367(13):1187–1197.
22. Parker C, Nilsson S, Heinrich D, et al. Alpha emitter radium-223 and survival in metastatic prostate cancer. *N Engl J Med.* 2013;369(3):213–223.
23. de Wit R, de Bono J, Sternberg C, et al. Cabazitaxel versus abiraterone or enzalutamide in metastatic prostate cancer. *N Engl J Med.* 2019;381(26):2506–2518.
24. de Bono J, Mateo J, Fizazi K, et al. Olaparib for metastatic castration-resistant prostate cancer. *N Engl J Med.* 2020;382(22):2091–2102.
25. Oudard S, Fizazi K, Sengeløv L, et al. Cabazitaxel versus docetaxel as first-line therapy for patients with metastatic castration-resistant prostate cancer: a randomized phase III trial—FIRSTANA. *J Clin Oncol.* 2017;35(28):3189–3197.
26. de Bono J, Oudard S, Ozguroglu M, et al. Prednisone plus cabazitaxel or mitoxantrone for metastatic castration-resistant prostate cancer progressing after docetaxel treatment: a randomised open-label trial. *Lancet.* 2010;376(9747):1147–1154.

SECTION 5

Bladder cancer

CASE

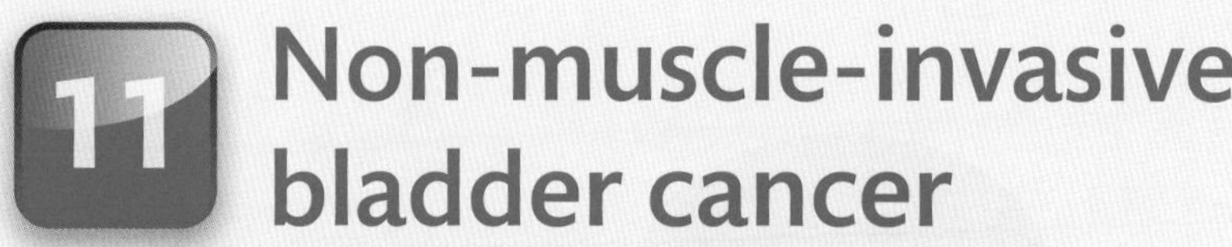

11 Non-muscle-invasive bladder cancer

Samantha Conroy

Expert commentary Aidan P. Noon

Case history

An 82-year-old gentleman was referred to the urology department for further investigations and management of an isolated episode of visible haematuria and dysuria; no evidence of urinary tract infection had been identified.

His past medical history included aortic stenosis with mild left ventricular systolic dysfunction, hypertension, atrial fibrillation (for which he was anticoagulated), and type 2 diabetes mellitus. He was an ex-smoker (with a 50 pack-year history), but had no occupational risk factors for bladder cancer (BC). He lived alone with once-daily carers due to limited mobility from his heart failure.

His assessment included clinical history and examination, upper tract computed tomography (CT) urogram, and flexible cystoscopy. He was haemodynamically stable and passing clear urine, with prior blood testing confirming a haemoglobin level of 106 g/L and a serum creatinine level of 128 µmol/L.

Flexible cystoscopy identified a 2.5 cm papillary tumour on the posterior wall of the bladder, which looked suspicious for high-grade disease. He did not have a biopsy at the time of flexible cystoscopy due to his anticoagulation. The CT urogram revealed no evidence of synchronous upper tract disease or ureteric obstruction.

Due to this gentleman's performance status (Eastern Co-operative Oncology Group performance status 3), frailty, and comorbidities, he underwent a full anaesthetic assessment prior to surgical resection and was deemed high risk for surgery. A multidisciplinary decision was made to proceed in the first instance with a flexible cystoscopy and tissue biopsy (after managing his anticoagulation).

Histology from the flexible cystoscopy revealed a high-grade G3pTa urothelial cell carcinoma (UCC), which confirmed the diagnosis of high-risk UCC; however, formal transurethral resection of the bladder tumour (TURBT) was required to assess the depth of invasion. A joint decision was made to proceed with urgent TURBT, under spinal anaesthetic, to guide future management options.

TURBT confirmed a 3.5 cm G3pT1 solitary lesion with no evidence of muscle invasion or carcinoma *in situ* (CIS). Figure 11.1 describes the multidisciplinary team (MDT) approach used to make combined clinician–patient decisions in the next stages of his care.

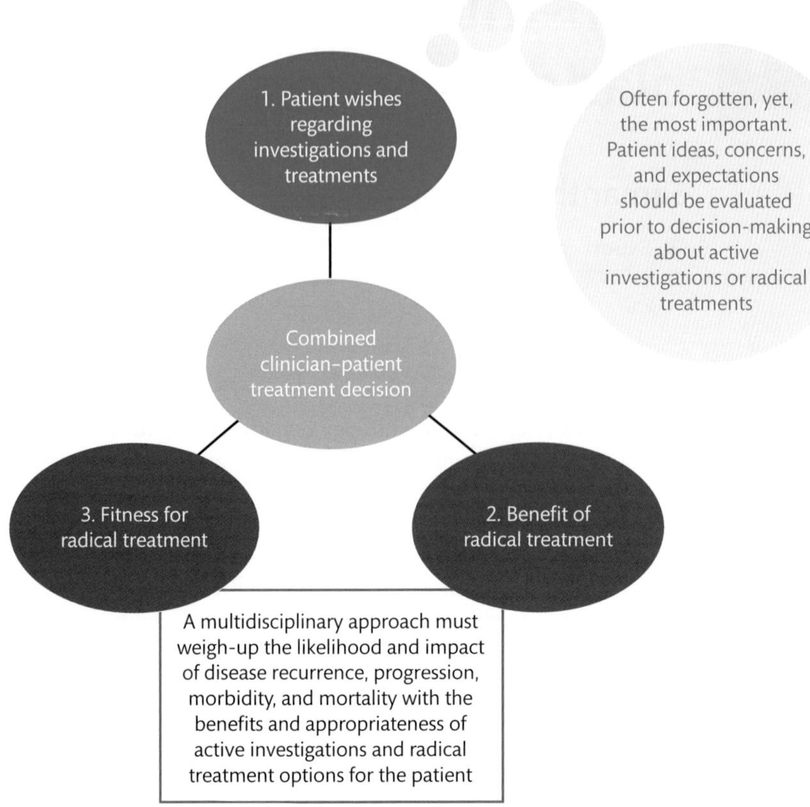

Figure 11.1 Considerations prior to active investigation and/or radical therapies in NMIBC.

Learning point Background and management

BC is the tenth most common cancer in the UK[1] with approximately 10,000 newly diagnosed cases per year.[2] The majority of patients present with non-muscle-invasive tumours,[3] also known as non-muscle-invasive bladder cancer (NMIBC), which, histologically, is confined to either the urothelium or the subepithelial connective tissues, but not invading the detrusor muscle.[4]

The primary treatment modality for NMIBC is transurethral resection. However, due to heterogeneous rates of recurrence and progression, adjuvant intravesical therapy or surgery is often required.[5]

A difficulty faced by many urologists occurs when first-line treatment options fail. Synthesizing a patient-centred treatment plan in this cohort, particularly in those who are not fit for surgery, can be extremely difficult.

Evidence base Treatment patterns, morbidity, and mortality in the elderly

A large population-based study evaluated all newly diagnosed BC cases. Cancer-specific and other-cause mortality rates at 5 years were equal (19% and 19%, respectively). This suggests that elderly patients diagnosed with BC are just as likely to die of other causes as they are from their cancer.[6]

Learning point Classification of NMIBC

Recurrence and progression rates in NMIBC are heterogeneous, ranging from 15% to 78% and 0.2% to 45% within 5 years of diagnosis, respectively (Figure 11.2).[7] Therefore, NMIBC is categorized into three distinct groups: low-, intermediate-, and high-risk disease. When risk stratifying a patient, urologists must consider tumour size, grade, multiplicity, recurrence, depth of invasion, concurrent CIS, and histopathological variants.[8] This risk stratification is essential in predicting recurrence and progression, which aid patient-centred management decisions.

Table 11.1 One-year and 5-year predicted recurrence and progression risks based on the patient's flexible cystoscopy and TURBT findings

EORTC risk calculator	Flexible cystoscopy staging (2.5 cm, G3pTa)	TURBT staging (3.5 cm, G3pT1)
1-year recurrence	24%	38%
1-year progression	1%	5%
5-year recurrence	46%	62%
5-year progression	6%	17%

Using the European Organisation for Research and Treatment of Cancer (EORTC) NMIBC risk stratification calculator, Table 11.1 depicts the change in recurrence and progression risk when a patient is histologically upstaged from pTa to pT1 disease in NMIBC. Hence, highlighting the need for accurate and timely staging.

The patient was reviewed in a specialist BC clinic. A joint decision was made not to attempt re-resection of his tumour given his frailty and comorbidities. As he was not fit for radical cystoprostatectomy (RC), he was offered intravesical bacillus Calmette–Guérin (BCG).

Learning point Recommended management of high-risk NMIBC

High-risk NMIBC can be further subdivided into either *high-risk* or *highest-risk* disease. Highest-risk NMIBC displays the following clinical and/or histological characteristics[9]:

- pT1 tumour with evidence of lymphovascular invasion.
- Multiple, large, or recurrent high-grade G2/G3pT1 tumours.
- All high-grade G2/G3pT1 tumours with concurrent CIS.
- CIS in the prostatic urethra.
- Some histological variants of UCC.

For patients with highest-risk disease, RC is the recommended first-line treatment option. However, due to the increasing comorbidity and polypharmacy that parallels an ageing population, alternative approaches to RC are becoming more widely accepted. Intravesical BCG is an acceptable alternative in such circumstances, but in a climate of BCG manufacturing shortages[10] and high volume of BCG failures, it is essential to identify more alternative and successful adjuvant therapies.

Learning point BCG regimen and efficacy

BCG is a live attenuated vaccine that has been used as an intravesical agent to treat BC for many years. Intravesical BCG's mechanism of action on BC cells is not yet fully understood, although it is thought to activate acquired and innate immune responses, facilitating the recognition and destruction of BC cells. The optimal intravesical schedule for BCG should include induction, followed by 1–3 years of maintenance. An example of a 3-year schedule[9] is shown here:

- Induction: 6 × weekly instillations of BCG.
- Maintenance: 3 × weekly instillations given at 3, 6, 12, 18, 24, 30, and 36 months.
- Regular check cystoscopies throughout.

Intravesical BCG is effective as an adjuvant immunotherapeutic agent, where meta-analysis data have confirmed reductions in the risk of recurrence and progression in NMIBC compared to controls.[11] Its effect is superior to other chemotherapeutic agents, such as ambient mitomycin C (MMC), for high-risk NMIBC and CIS; however, the true benefit is usually only seen in those who complete both induction and maintenance treatment.[11] Unfortunately, it is estimated that only one-third of patients will complete the full 3-year induction and maintenance schedule,[12] due to side effects, toxicity, and failure.

Learning point BCG side effects, complications, and contraindications

Due to BCG's mechanism of action, patients usually develop inflammatory side effects that manifest in the form of lower urinary tract symptoms (dysuria, frequency, urgency, and haematuria) and urinary tract infections. These symptoms can occasionally be severe, relentless, and intolerable for patients.

The most clinically significant complication to be aware of is localized or systemic granulomatous infection. Patients typically present with high fever, confusion, and clinical signs of sepsis. BCG sepsis—a rare and potentially life-threatening condition—requires prompt identification, resuscitation, and involvement of the infectious diseases team, who often initiate lengthy antitubercular therapy with or without supportive steroids in the acute phase.[13]

Absolute contraindications to intravesical BCG treatment include:

- Immunocompromised patients or those on immunosuppressive medication
- Symptomatic urinary tract infection; or, patients with a breach of the urothelium, suggested by having had a recent TURBT (within the last 14 days)
- Recent catheter-related trauma, or visible haematuria.

Note: a relative contraindication to intravesical BCG therapy is complete incontinence, which reduces intravesical dwelling time and, therefore, efficacy of treatment.

Learning point Classifying BCG failures

BCG failures can be subclassified as one of the following[9]:

1. Muscle-invasive tumour detected during follow-up period.
2. BCG-refractory tumour:
   - High-grade non-muscle-invasive tumour identified at 3-month endoscopic check—further BCG therapy is linked with increased risk of progression.
   - CIS present at 3- and 6-month checks—additional BCG can achieve complete response in >50%.
   - New high-grade tumour identified during BCG treatment (note: low-grade tumours not considered BCG failure).

After completing BCG induction, a flexible check cystoscopy was performed to avoid the anaesthetic risk associated with rigid cystoscopy. A new, concerning patchy erythematous area was identified and biopsied, as the patient had been pre-warned about stopping anticoagulation.

Histology confirmed a high-grade G3pTa UCC and a re-staging CT scan showed no evidence of muscle-invasive or metastatic disease. The patient, therefore, had BCG-refractory disease. Because he was asymptomatic, and unfit for RC, he was offered the following management strategies:

- Intravesical hyperthermic MMC.
- Active surveillance (AS).

Future directions The role of AS in NMIBC

AS is not currently recommended in high-risk NMIBC, but is currently being evaluated in a non-inferiority phase III randomized controlled trial in Japan[14] as an alternative strategy to intravesical BCG after complete TURBT resection (pT0 on re-resection). For low-risk NMIBC, AS has been advocated as a potential strategy in a well-defined, compliant population with low-risk, low-volume, pTa disease.[15] AS aims to reduce the morbidity of repeated surgical procedures and/or adjuvant treatments.

Expert comment Watchful waiting in high-risk NMIBC in patients unfit for RC

Watchful waiting is another relatively novel concept in NMIBC. When managing unfit or frail patients, an MDT decision should be made (Figure 11.1), with active patient involvement about the need for and benefit of repeated investigations and treatments.

When managing low-volume, asymptomatic disease, in patients with a short life expectancy or significant comorbidity, clinicians must consider the benefits and risks of TURBT to identify progression to muscle-invasive disease. If the patient is unsuitable for or unwilling to undergo radical treatment (surgery or chemoradiotherapy), watchful waiting seems a reasonable management strategy for those failing first-line bladder-preserving therapies.

Learning point Alternative chemotherapy agents 1: standard MMC therapy

Mechanism of action

- Cytotoxic.
- Alkylates DNA.

Recommendation

Adjuvant therapy in those with intermediate-risk disease.

Comparison with BCG

A large meta-analysis has shown[16]:

- Higher risk of recurrence in MMC (but lower recurrence rates when compared to induction-only BCG patients)
- No observed significant differences in progression or survival.

Dosing schedule

Induction and maintenance phases (no definitive recommended schedule):

- Induction phase: 6–8 weekly instillations (60–120-minute duration).
- Maintenance phase: 3 weekly instillations.
- The need for ongoing maintenance therapy is dictated by tolerability and response (can be repeated to a maximum duration of 1 year).

Adverse effects

- Dysuria, frequency, haematuria, urinary tract infection, allergic skin rash, urethral stricture (2–50%).
- Severe allergic reaction, bladder fibrosis (<1%).

Clinical tip Alternative treatment strategies for unfit patients in the context of BCG failure

There has been growing motivation among urologists to identify more novel therapies and/or devices that can provide a feasible and efficacious alternative to intravesical BCG therapy in those unfit for RC. Current alternatives include use of intravesical chemotherapy, device-assisted therapy, alternative immunotherapies, and conservative management with either AS or watchful waiting.

Learning point Alternative chemotherapy agents 2: epirubicin (and other anthracyclines such as doxorubicin)

Mechanism of action

- Anthracycline.
- Inhibits DNA replication, transcription, and repair.

Recommendation

Not currently recommended in isolation over MMC or BCG.

Comparison with BCG

- Inferior disease-specific survival and higher progression, when used in isolation.
- In combination with BCG, has shown promising effects on disease recurrence and progression (without significantly increasing toxicity).[17]

Dosing schedule

Similar schedule to intravesical MMC.

Adverse effects

Similar to MMC.

Learning point Alternative chemotherapy agents 3: gemcitabine

Mechanism of action

- Cytotoxic.
- Antimetabolite (impairs DNA synthesis).

Recommendation

- Traditionally used systemically for locally advanced or metastatic BC (in combination with cisplatin or carboplatin).
- Ongoing research into its intravesical use, although early data are promising.

Comparison with BCG

A recent meta-analysis, comparing five randomized controlled trials with follow-up of 1–4 years, highlighted no significant difference between intravesical BCG and gemcitabine for risk of recurrence or progression.[18]

Dosing schedule

- No definitive schedule defined. Similar to MMC.
- Once-weekly instillations for 6–8 weeks.
- Maintenance therapy proposed as a once-monthly dose for up to 1 year.

Adverse effects

- Similar to MMC.
- Significantly lower incidence of haematuria and dysuria than BCG.[18]

Learning point Alternative chemotherapy agents 4: device-assisted thermochemotherapy with MMC

Mechanism of action

Thermochemotherapy is thought to increase urothelial permeability to allow for greater depth of drug delivery. It can be delivered via:

- SYNERGIO device: electromagnetic radiation is transmitted via a catheter to produce homogeneous heating of the bladder tissues, along with concomitant instillation of MMC
- COMBAT BRS device: external dry aluminium conduction system that recirculates the MMC solution at a given temperature.

Comparison with BCG

Early research has suggested:

- Better recurrence-free survival for high-grade disease and equivocal response rates for CIS, when compared to patients who have only undergone 1 year of BCG therapy.[19]
- More data are required for to compare outcomes with maintenance BCG.

Dosing schedule

Similar to standard MMC.

Adverse effects

- Similar to standard MMC.
- Significantly higher rates of frequency, haematuria, and bladder spasm.[20]

Learning point Combination immunotherapy: durvalumab and BCG therapy (POTOMAC study)

Mechanism of action

- Durvalumab is an immunoglobulin G1 monoclonal antibody that targets and binds to the programmed death-ligand 1 (PD-L1) and programmed cell death-1 (PD-1) receptors.
- Binding of these receptors is thought to initiate pathways that activate antitumour immune responses.
- BCG mechanism has been explained earlier in the case.
- *Note*: systemic durvalumab has shown promising overall survival results for metastatic urothelial carcinoma in those who have previously progressed despite first-line therapy.[21]

Dosing schedule

To be confirmed after the results of the POTOMAC trial.[22]

Adverse effects

- Adverse effects of BCG have been described earlier in the case.
- Systemic durvalumab may cause the following general and immune-mediated side effects:
  - General: fatigue, musculoskeletal pain, nausea, constipation, and acute kidney injury.
  - Immune mediated: pneumonitis, hepatitis, colitis, endocrinopathies, dermatitis and immunocompromise.

Evidence base POTOMAC trial

The POTOMAC trial is a phase III randomized, open-label, multicentre, global study of durvalumab and BCG administered as combination therapy versus BCG alone in high-risk, BCG-naïve NMIBC patients.[22]

It is currently recruiting to compare combined and standard immunotherapy:

- BCG induction and maintenance + durvalumab versus
- BCG induction + durvalumab versus
- BCG induction and maintenance.

The trial aims to recruit almost 1000 patients worldwide, with the primary outcome being disease-free survival. Secondary outcomes will assess side effects, tolerability, health-related quality of life, disease progression, and overall survival.

Learning point Alternative immunotherapy

An example is interferon alpha (IFNα) therapy.[23]

Mechanism of action

IFNα has been shown to increase T-cell and natural killer recognition of tumour cells by control/manipulation of antigen presentation and dendritic maturation.

Recommendation

Phase III trial data are required prior to widespread use.

Comparison with BCG

A recent phase II randomized controlled trial, evaluating IFNα with a surfactant-enhanced recombinant adenovirus vector rAd–IFNα/Syn3, has shown promising efficacy in BCG-refractory disease, with 35% of patients being recurrence free at 12 months.[23]

Dosing schedule

- Dose not yet confirmed.
- Proposed schedule: one 60-minute instillation, repeated at 4, 7, and 10 months if confirmed as disease free on cystoscopy.

Adverse effects

- Limited available data; however, usually well tolerated.
- Urgency, dysuria, haematuria, nocturia, and pollakiuria (often transient and self-limiting).

Between the choice of AS and hyperthermic MMC, the patient chose active treatment. He completed induction hyperthermic MMC, which was well tolerated, but cystoscopic assessment showed minimal change in the patchy, erythematous area (graded G3pTa). He was initiated on a maintenance cycle of hyperthermic MMC; however, during his second instillation he developed a palmar rash and opted out of further treatment.

Expert comment
Checkpoint inhibitors

Advances in our understanding of UCC and the complex molecular pathways by which it evades antitumour responses have played an important role in developing targeted immunotherapies. In particular, the binding and inhibition of PD-L1 and PD-1 checkpoint molecules.

These novel immunotherapies are a very promising treatment modality for high-risk NMIBC patients. Investigation of their use both in isolation and in conjunction with existing therapies will play a vital role for targeted BC therapy in the future.

Subsequently, a joint patient–clinician decision was made to keep the patient under clinic review; however, there would be no surveillance cystoscopies unless he became symptomatic.

A final word from the expert

NMIBC is a challenging condition to manage. The nature of this disease means it is expensive to manage and burdensome for the patient. For fit patients, with normal life expectancy, the emphasis must obviously be to prevent disease progression. However, for patients who are unfit, with reduced life expectancy, a personalized approach must be adopted that strikes a balance between the risks of diagnosis and/or treatment and potential symptoms. Increasingly, newer treatments are being used or being evaluated in clinical trials which will hopefully lead to further management options for both the fittest and the frailest of patients.

References

1. Antoni S, Ferlay J, Soerjomataram I, Znaor A, Jemal A, Bray F. Bladder cancer incidence and mortality: a global overview and recent trends. *Eur Urol.* 2017;71(1):96–108.
2. Cancer Research UK. Bladder cancer statistics. Cancer Research UK. n.d. https://www.cancerresearchuk.org/health-professional/cancer-statistics/statistics-by-cancer-type/bladder-cancer
3. Cumberbatch MGK, Jubber I, Black PC, et al. Epidemiology of bladder cancer: a systematic review and contemporary update of risk factors in 2018. *Eur Urol.* 2018;74(6):784–795.
4. Brierley J, Gospodarowicz MK, Wittekind C, eds. *TNM Classification of Malignant Tumours*. 8th ed. Chichester: Wiley-Blackwell; 2017.
5. Au JLS, Jang SH, Wientjes MG. Clinical aspects of drug delivery to tumors. *J Control Release.* 2002;78(1–3):81–95.
6. Noon AP, Albertsen PC, Thomas F, Rosario DJ, Catto JWF. Competing mortality in patients diagnosed with bladder cancer: evidence of undertreatment in the elderly and female patients. *Br J Cancer.* 2013;108(7):1534–1540.
7. Sylvester RJ, van der Meijden APM, Oosterlinck W, et al. Predicting recurrence and progression in individual patients with stage Ta T1 bladder cancer using EORTC risk tables: a combined analysis of 2596 patients from seven EORTC trials. *Eur Urol.* 2006;49(3):466–477.
8. National Institute for Health and Care Excellence. Bladder cancer: risk classification in non-muscle-invasive bladder cancer. National Institute for Health and Care Excellence. 2015. https://www.nice.org.uk/guidance/ng2/resources/nmibc-risk-classification-table-pdf-3779101
9. Compérat E, Gontero P, Mostafid AH, et al. EAU guidelines on non-muscle-invasive bladder cancer (TaT1 and CIS). European Association of Urology. 2017. https://uroweb.org/wp-content/uploads/EAU-Guidelines-on-Non-muscle-Invasive-Bladder-Cancer-2020.pdf
10. Mostafid AH, Palou Redorta J, Sylvester R, Witjes JA. Therapeutic options in high-risk non-muscle-invasive bladder cancer during the current worldwide shortage of bacille Calmette-Guérin. *Eur Urol.* 2015;67(3):359–360.
11. Sylvester RJ, van der Meijden APM, Lamm DL. Intravesical bacillus Calmette-Guerin reduces the risk of progression in patients with superficial bladder cancer: a meta-analysis of the published results of randomized clinical trials. *J Urol.* 2002;168(5):1964–1970.
12. Liu CY, Chuang CK, Chang YH, et al. Maintenance bacillus Calmette–Guérin therapy prolongs recurrence-free survival in non-muscle-invasive bladder cancer: a real-world experience. *Urol Sci.* 2015;26(2):96–100.
13. Koya MP, Simon MA, Soloway MS. Complications of intravesical therapy for urothelial cancer of the bladder. *J Urol.* 2006;175(6):2004–2010.

14. Kunieda F, Kitamura H, Niwakawa M, et al. Watchful waiting versus intravesical BCG therapy for high-grade pT1 bladder cancer with pT0 histology after second transurethral resection: Japan Clinical Oncology Group Study JCOG1019. *Jpn J Clin Oncol.* 2012;42(11):1094–1098.
15. Hernández V, Llorente C, de la Peña E, Pérez-Fernández E, Guijarro A, Sola I. Long-term oncological outcomes of an active surveillance program in recurrent low grade Ta bladder cancer. *Urol Oncol.* 2016;34(4):165.e19–165.e23.
16. Malmström PU, Sylvester RJ, Crawford DE, et al. An individual patient data meta-analysis of the long-term outcome of randomised studies comparing intravesical mitomycin C versus bacillus Calmette-Guérin for non-muscle-invasive bladder cancer. *Eur Urol.* 2009;56(2):247–256.
17. Houghton BB, Chalasani V, Hayne D, et al. Intravesical chemotherapy plus bacille Calmette-Guérin in non-muscle invasive bladder cancer: a systematic review with meta-analysis. *BJU Int.* 2013;111(6):977–983.
18. Ye Z, Chen J, Hong Y, Xin W, Yang S, Rao Y. The efficacy and safety of intravesical gemcitabine vs Bacille Calmette-Guérin for adjuvant treatment of non-muscle invasive bladder cancer: a meta-analysis. *Onco Targets Ther.* 2018;11:4641–4649.
19. Sadée C, Kashdan E. A model of thermotherapy treatment for bladder cancer. *Math Biosci Eng.* 2016;13(6):1169–1183.
20. Tan WS, Palou J, Kelly J. Safety and tolerability analysis of hyperthermic intravesical mitomycin to mitomycin alone in HIVEC I and HIVEC II: an interim analysis of 307 patients. *Eur Urol Suppl.* 2017;16(3):e1150–e1151.
21. Powles T, O'Donnell PH, Massard C, et al. Efficacy and safety of durvalumab in locally advanced or metastatic urothelial carcinoma: updated results from a phase 1/2 open-label study. *JAMA Oncol.* 2017;3(9):e172411.
22. De Santis M, Abdrashitov R, Hegele A, et al. A phase III, randomized, open-label, multicenter, global study of durvalumab and bacillus Calmette-Guérin (BCG) versus BCG alone in high-risk, BCG-naïve non-muscle-invasive bladder cancer (NMIBC) patients (POTOMAC). *J Clin Oncol.* 2019;37(7 Suppl):TPS500–TPS500.
23. Shore ND, Boorjian SA, Canter DJ, et al. Intravesical rAd–IFNα/Syn3 for patients with high-grade, bacillus Calmette-Guerin-refractory or relapsed non-muscle-invasive bladder cancer: a phase II randomized study. *J Clin Oncol.* 2017;35(30):3410–3416.

CASE

12 Muscle-invasive bladder cancer

Samantha Conroy

Expert commentary James W.F. Catto

Case history

A 71-year-old gentleman, with a solitary right kidney, was reviewed in a haematuria clinic after being referred by his general practitioner with persistent, asymptomatic, non-visible haematuria. His medical history included well-controlled hypertension and hypercholesterolaemia, for which he was taking amlodipine and simvastatin, respectively. He was a non-smoker and was independent with his daily activities.

On clinical assessment, he was asymptomatic and haemodynamically stable. He underwent the following investigations:

- Urine dipstick analysis, confirming the presence of non-visible haematuria.
- Baseline blood tests, showing a haemoglobin level of 121 g/L, a creatinine concentration of 79 μmol/L, an estimated glomerular filtration rate of 89 mL/min/1.73 m^2, and creatinine clearance of 100 mL/min.
- Flexible cystoscopy, which identified a large posterior wall bladder tumour, close to the right ureteric orifice.
- Computed tomography (CT) intravenous urography, which confirmed a posterior bladder mass, but showed no evidence of ureteric obstruction or synchronous upper tract malignancy.

The working diagnosis was explained to the patient and he was scheduled for an urgent transurethral resection of his bladder tumour (TURBT).

Rigid cystoscopy confirmed a solitary, 4 cm, solid tumour on the right posterior wall of the bladder. It was close to, but not invading, the right ureteric orifice. The tumour was resected down to and including detrusor muscle, taking care to avoid the ureteric orifice.

The histological and radiological findings were discussed at the uro-oncology multidisciplinary team meeting, which confirmed a solitary G3pT2 infiltrating bladder tumour with associated carcinoma *in situ* (CIS). CT imaging of the thorax, abdomen, and pelvis identified one 7.8 mm in diameter right-sided, internal iliac lymph node (LN), which was felt to be at intermediate risk of being a metastasis. No other locoregional lymphadenopathy or distant metastases were identified.

The outcome of the multidisciplinary team meeting was to proceed with radical cystoprostatectomy (RC), with extended lymphadenectomy, and to arrange an oncological assessment for neoadjuvant chemotherapy (NAC).

Learning point Epidemiology

In 2018, there were 549,393 new cases of bladder cancer (BC) diagnosed worldwide. Over 75% of these patients were male, making it the sixth most frequently diagnosed cancer, in men, worldwide.[1] Most BCs are non-muscle-invasive bladder cancer (NMIBC) tumours confined to the urothelium or subepithelial tissues. Persons presenting with muscle-invasive bladder cancer (MIBC: approximately, 25% of new cases) or developing invasive cancers after prior NMIBC, need radical treatment to achieve cure. Despite using radical treatment, around half of patients with MIBC die from this cancer.[2]

Learning point Aetiology

In order to determine significant personal, environmental, and socioeconomic risk factors for BC, clinicians should obtain a focused history. Known risk factors for BC include[3]:

- Smoking:
  - Greater relative risk for current versus ex-smokers[4]
- Occupational carcinogens:
  - Industries such as aluminium, dye, rubber, coal-tar, dry cleaning, hairdressing, printing, and textiles[5]
- Dietary factors and obesity:
  - Increases with body mass index
- Increasing age:
  - Median age 73 years at diagnosis
- Male sex
- Past medical history of:
  - Radiotherapy, diabetes mellitus, schistosomiasis, pioglitazone, and cyclophosphamide use (conversely, non-steroidal anti-inflammatory drugs and phenobarbital reduce risk)
- Family history of BC
- Socioeconomic status:
  - Increased risk in industrialized areas.

Expert comment Diagnosis and staging of BC

Typically, patients with suspected BC are referred to urology services because of non-visible haematuria or visible haematuria in the presence or absence of associated risk factors. They will undergo a number of investigations including urine cytology, flexible cystoscopy, and urinary tract imaging (ultrasonography or CT) to identify synchronous upper tract tumours. If a bladder tumour is identified, the patient will require a formal TURBT to establish a histological diagnosis and to differentiate between non-muscle-invasive and muscle-invasive disease. MIBC is characterized by a bladder tumour showing evidence of invasion into the detrusor muscle, histologically defined as invasion of the muscularis propria (pT2). In conjunction to histological diagnosis, patients must be evaluated for locoregional or distant metastases.

The tumour, node, metastasis (TNM) system is recommended for staging of BC[6]:

- *Tumour*: Tx—unable to assess tumour; T0 no evidence of tumour; Ta—non-invasive papillary carcinoma; T1—invasion of the lamina propria; T2—invasion of the muscularis propria (2a—inner 50%; 2b—outer 50%); T3—invasion of the perivesical tissue (3a—microscopic invasion; 3b macroscopic invasion); T4—invasion of surrounding organs/structures (T4a—invasion of the prostate, seminal vesicles, uterus, or vagina; T4b—invasion of the pelvic or abdominal wall).
- *Node*: Nx—unable to assess LN status; N0—no regional LN metastases; N1—single LN metastasis in true pelvis; N2—multiple LN metastases in true pelvis; N3—common iliac LN metastases.
- *Metastasis*: M0—no distant metastases; M1—metastases present (M1a—LN metastases outside of the pelvis; M1b—metastases present in other organs or parts of the body).

Around 33–55% of patients found with pT1 (NMIBC) disease on initial TURBT, have persistent disease on re-resection and up to 25% are upstaged to pT2 disease (MIBC)[7] These figures highlight the need for accurate and timely staging.

Clinical tip Pathology subtypes

Histological classification of BC plays an important role in determining future management. Around 90% of all BCs are urothelial cell carcinomas (UCCs), thus, only a small proportion of BCs are non-urothelial histological subtypes; these include squamous, adenocarcinoma, small cell, sarcoma, and melanoma. The outcomes and systemic regimens for non-urothelial BCs differ and so care should be adapted accordingly.

Almost all MIBCs are high-grade UCCs. Therefore, histological and/or radiological stage have greater prognostic value than grade. However, some morphological subtypes of UCCs behave differently to pure UCCs in terms of treatment response and prognosis; these variants include micropapillary, small cell (neuroendocrine), lymphoepithelioma, nested, plasmacytoid, and those with squamous components, and should be considered when making decisions about patient care.

Expert comment Current challenges in BC pathological staging

The under-staging of MIBC is a particular concern for patient care. This most commonly arises when at TURBT a cancer is staged as NMIBC (and invasive components are not apparent). To clarify the diagnosis, a re-resection TURBT, ideally within 6 weeks of the initial resection, is advocated for patients with high risk of upstaging (e.g. high-grade NMIBC, stage T1, lack of detrusor muscle in TURBT specimen, CIS).[9] Disease that progresses from NMIBC to MIBC has a worse cancer-specific survival than for cancers that present as *de novo* MIBC.[10]

This raises two important questions;

1. Are we staging high-risk NMIBC appropriately—or should pT1 disease be subclassified?
2. Do we need to treat high-risk NMIBC more aggressively in the first instance?

Future directions Genetic subclassification

Advances in our molecular understanding of BC has also allowed genetic subclassification of tumours into luminal, luminal papillary, luminal unstable, stromal rich, basal/squamous, and neuroendocrine like.[8] In the future, these molecular characteristics may aid clinical decision-making and play a role in targeted therapy.

Evidence base BRAVO randomized controlled trial

Radical cystectomy against intravesical BCG immunotherapy for high-risk non-muscle-invasive bladder cancer (BRAVO) was a multicentre, parallel-group, randomized controlled feasibility study to evaluate acceptability and feasibility of a phase III randomized controlled trial comparing maintenance BCG with radical cystectomy for high-risk NMIBC.[11,12] Recruitment to the study was challenging, attributable to multiple factors including patient preference, lack of clinician equipoise, and logistical difficulties. The study highlighted the challenges in managing this cohort of patients: around 10% of all new high-risk NMIBCs harboured lethal disease, and thus may benefit from primary RC; but a significant proportion successfully underwent bladder-preserving therapy while maintaining pre-diagnosis quality of life. Hence, clinicians must use risk-adapted and patient-centred strategies.[11]

Future directions Subcategorization of pT1 tumours

Predicting the progression and response of pT1 tumours (currently classified as high-risk NMIBC) is challenging, hence, a second TURBT within 6 weeks of the original resection is recommended.[13]

More recently, the American Joint Committee on Cancer have recommended sub-classification of pT1 disease into those that have minor or extensive invasion of the lamina propria, however, do not yet have a validated method of doing so.[14] Future subcategorization of pT1 disease may provide a more effective risk stratification system for those with 'borderline' muscle-invasive disease.

Clinical tip Accurate histological staging of BC

Accurate histological staging is essential and clinicians must be aware of how surgical technique impacts on tissue analysis.

- Surgical factors that may interfere with analysis include cautery or thermal damage to tissues and tangential tissue segmentation, making it difficult to orientate.[14]
- Therefore, 'en bloc' resection of small tumours and fractional resection of larger tumours is recommended.
- Detrusor muscle should always be obtained for analysis, and where possible, sent as a separate sample to the tumour.

Shortly after the multidisciplinary team meeting, the patient was reviewed by a uro-oncologist with the view to starting NAC as soon as possible, as to not delay RC. As part of the assessment, repeat baseline blood tests were requested. His repeat urea and electrolyte results showed a significant rise in creatinine concentration (104 μmol/L from 79 μmol/L) with an associated reduction in his estimated glomerular filtration rate (65 mL/min/1.73 m^2 from 89 mL/min/1.73 m^2) and creatinine clearance (73 mL/min from 100 mL/min).

In the context of the patient's solitary kidney and the proximity of the resected infiltrating tumour to the right UO, the clinicians were concerned about potential malignant ureteric obstruction. He was fully assessed for evidence of pre-renal and renal causes of his acute kidney injury, but none were identified. Post-renal obstruction, therefore, was the most likely cause.

Clinically, he was euvolaemic, systemically well, and had no signs or symptoms of coexisting urinary tract infection. An urgent, non-contrast CT scan was performed, showing mild to moderate right-sided hydroureteronephrosis, traceable down to the right vesicoureteric junction.

Having confirmed the ureteric obstruction, a joint decision was made to site a percutaneous nephrostomy (PCN), with the goal of facilitating temporary urinary diversion and preserving renal function to facilitate NAC.

Expert comment Options for acute urinary diversion

Two methods commonly used for acute urinary diversion are ureteric stents and PCN. The modality of diversion is dependent on the aetiology, urgency, technical expertise required for diversion and bladder function/capacity, as well as patient choice. Although there is no consensus between stenting and PCN in BC, PCN is preferred in the neoadjuvant setting because it offers more definitive urinary drainage and lower rates of tumour seeding to the upper tracts.[15]

Temporizing PCN provides an option for preserving renal function in the neoadjuvant setting to optimize patients prior to NAC and RC. PCN may be regarded as a potential infective focus during chemotherapy, but this is counter-balanced by assisting in the resolution of urinary stasis and associated urinary tract sepsis, as well as contributing towards improving renal function, minimizing the delay to definitive surgery.

Within 72 hours of PCN insertion, the patient's estimated glomerular filtration rate had increased to baseline. He was re-reviewed by the oncology team, who were now happy for him to proceed with NAC. He completed four cycles of systemic cisplatin and gemcitabine without significant side effects or complications.

The patient's definitive treatment was open RC with ileal conduit formation and extended lymphadenectomy. The procedure was uneventful, with no immediate anaesthetic or surgical complications. A total of 465 mL of blood was lost intraoperatively. Because he had a very good postoperative urine output via the ileal conduit, and now had ureteroileal anastomotic stents (placed intraoperatively), the right PCN was removed on table at the end of surgery.

Learning point Neoadjuvant chemotherapy

The prognosis of patients with MIBC undergoing RC remains poor.[2] NAC has been shown to improve 5-year survival rates by around 5%[13,16] and so is recommended for platinum-eligible patients with T2–T4a cN0M0 disease. Table 12.1 describes the potential benefits and risks of NAC in MIBC.

Cisplatin-based combination chemotherapy is the optimal NAC regimen in MIBC. Cisplatin can be combined with either gemcitabine or with methotrexate, vinblastine, and doxorubicin (Adriamycin®) (MVAC). Gemcitabine is more commonly used, as comparative trials suggest gemcitabine is less toxic and has similar efficacy to MVAC.[17] Carboplatin may be used as an alternative in patients with contraindications to cisplatin.

- Cisplatin mechanism of action:
  - Alkylating agent.
  - Interferes with DNA replication and repair.
- Action recommendation:
  - Cisplatin-based NAC should be offered to those with MIBC who have no evidence of locoregional or distant metastases.
- Contraindications:
  - Eastern Cooperative Oncology Group (ECOG) score ≥2.
  - Poor renal function (creatinine clearance <60 mL/min).
  - Evidence of heart failure (≥ class III New York Heart Association heart failure).
  - Evidence of neuropathy (≥ grade 2).
  - Hearing impairment (≥ grade 2).
- Adverse effects[18]:
  - Common: nephrotoxicity, ototoxicity, bone marrow suppression, nausea/vomiting, diarrhoea, fatigue.
  - Uncommon: neurotoxicity, allergic reactions, cardiac arrhythmias.

Table 12.1 Advantages and disadvantages of NAC in patients with MIBC

Advantages of NAC	Disadvantages of NAC
Better compliance and tolerated pre-cystectomy than after	Potentially delays definitive treatment for those with tumours that are not chemosensitive
Treatment for metastatic disease at low volume. Metastases are the cause of death in most MIBC patients	Potential to over-treat those who have not been staged by conventional TURBT and imaging
Can identify in vivo sensitivity of tumour to NAC	Side effect profile
Clear evidence that it does not increase surgical morbidity	

Clinical tip Management of MIBC

Radical treatment (RC or radiotherapy) is the main curative treatment for MIBC. The choice between surgery or radiotherapy reflects disease factors (stage, hydronephrosis, presence of CIS), patient factors (fitness, comorbidities), bladder function (capacity and compliance), and patient preference. Optimal factors for bladder-sparing radiotherapy are unclear but may include low-volume or unifocal disease (and clearance at TURBT), good bladder capacity, lack of CIS, and a good response to NAC. Most RCs are performed with a curative intent. However, in certain cases palliative cystectomy may be performed for symptomatic relief.

The timing of RC is important. Studies have shown that delaying RC for >90 days may significantly impact survival, particularly in those with pT2 disease.[19] Therefore, patients ideally should be optimized for surgery within this time frame, to avoid unnecessary disease progression which may affect prognosis and survival (Figure 12.1).

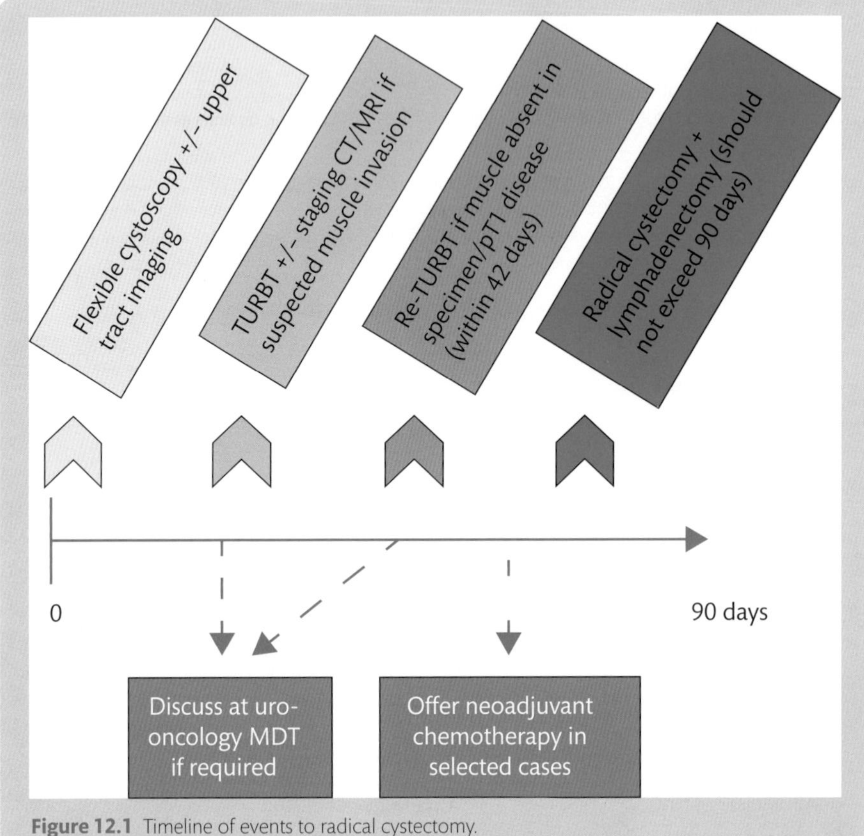

Figure 12.1 Timeline of events to radical cystectomy.

Expert comment Lymphadenectomy during RC

Many authorities advocate pelvic lymph node dissection (LND) at the time of RC. LND has a role in staging the cancer and may have a therapeutic benefit. However, the procedure lengthens the duration of surgery and can slow patient recovery (lymphatic fluid may prolong ileus and may require drainage). Conventionally, pelvic LND includes removal of LNs up to the ureteric crossing of the common iliac vessels (namely the internal iliac, presacral, obturator, and external iliac nodes). More extensive LND approaches are practised, with extended lymphadenectomy including LNs up to the aortic bifurcation and super-extended lymphadenectomy including LNs up to the inferior mesenteric artery. The optimal extent of LND required in MIBC is debatable.

LND staging

Preoperative imaging (CT or MRI) should identify enlarged LNs with a diameter of >8 mm in the pelvis and 10 mm in the abdomen, which in the context of a known pelvic malignancy, should be treated as suspicious for malignant deposits.[13] However, not all malignant LNs are enlarged and, conversely, some enlarged LNs are inflamed. As such, lymphadenectomy clarifies the stage and this can be used to stratify the need for adjuvant treatment and predict recurrence.

LND therapy

The therapeutic benefit from lymphadenectomy is unclear. Proponents report patients with nodal metastasis who are cured from MIBC and non-randomized data suggesting better outcomes with lymphadenectomy.[20,21] However, there are no randomized data comparing LND to no LND, and recent comparisons of limited versus extended LND show no difference in survival.[21,22]

Therefore, when deciding on the need for and extent of lymphadenectomy, one should consider the likely disease burden, patient fitness, and technical implications for the surgical procedure.

Evidence base Extended versus limited lymphadenectomy for MIBC

A prospective, phase III, multicentre trial evaluated extended LND versus limited LND in patients undergoing RC for high-risk NMIBC and MIBC.[22] A total of 401 patients were randomized with the primary endpoint being recurrence-free survival and secondary endpoints including cancer-specific and overall survival. This trial showed no statistically significant benefit of extended over limited LND for the primary or secondary endpoints described. However, it did suggest that 11% of patients would have had metastatic LNs left behind had they undergone limited rather than extended LND. Extended LND may therefore play a role in a selected cohort with more aggressive and radiologically node-negative disease (pT2–4N0).

Learning point Urinary diversion during RC

The main routes of urinary diversion are:

1. Incontinent: ileal conduit or ureterocutaneostomy
2. Continent: orthotopic neobladder (ileal or ileal/caecal) or continent cutaneous diversion
3. Rectosigmoid: such as a Mainz or Mansoura pouch.

The choice of urinary diversion includes patient, oncological, and surgical factors.

Patient factors

- Patient fitness (ileal conduit is faster and less complicated).
- Comorbidities (various neobladder exclusions such as renal impairment, Crohn's disease, etc.).
- Life expectancy (neobladders are better with longer recovery).
- Insight and engagement, pre-existing benign urethral disease, or incontinence.

Oncological factors

- Evidence of UCC at a surgical margin.
- Coexisting urethral tumours or N2–3 disease (all of which exclude an orthotopic reconstruction).

Surgical/institutional factors

- Centre volume, surgeon experience, and surgeon preference.

Postoperatively, the patient was initiated on the Enhanced Recovery After Surgery (ERAS; see 'Learning point' box on postoperative care) protocol, and made good progress with pain control, mobilization, oral intake, and stoma care on the ward. His postoperative blood investigations were unremarkable. He was discharged 5 days after his surgery with 28 days of low-molecular-weight heparin and continued to make a good recovery in the community.

Expert comment Palliative cystectomy in locally advanced BC

Although the primary aim of RC is for curative intent, this is not its sole purpose. Palliative cystectomy and urinary diversion may be offered on a case-by-case basis (e.g. symptomatic tumour, upper tract obstruction, low metastatic burden, high performance status), to patients with symptomatic disease, without alternative options.

Learning point Postoperative care

The aim of postoperative care is to enable patients to reach complete recovery, as soon as possible, to their preoperative state. A multidisciplinary approach should be used to determine the most suitable location for postoperative recovery on a case-by-case basis, which in some, may require higher level care in the initial stages.

More recently, there has been a push to improve perioperative and postoperative outcomes from RC. ERAS protocols have been implemented to good effect in many non-urological specialities for major surgery; the principles of ERAS are as follows[23]:

1. Appropriate preoperative assessment, optimization, caloric loading with avoidance of bowel preparation, and prolonged fasting.
2. Perioperative standardized anaesthetic protocols.
3. Early postoperative oral feeding, mobilization, and drain/catheter removal where appropriate.

Specific adaptations of ERAS protocols for RC are described in Table 12.2.[24] In a recent, single-centre randomized controlled trial, patients who underwent RC followed by ERAS (when compared to controls) had the following benefits[23]:

Table 12.2 ERAS® components for RC used at a high-volume single centre

Domain	Item	Elements
Clinic	Preoperative counselling and education	Advice about maintaining activity levels, dietary and alcohol advice, details of admission and recovery, written material detailing postoperative recovery plan
	Prehabilitation exercise	Walking for 1 hour per day
	Preoperative medical optimization	Optimization of comorbidities, smoking cessation advice, plan social aspects of discharge
	Correction of anaemia	Oral iron supplements or intravenous iron
Prior to admission	Bowel preparation	Omitted. Normal diet until preoperative fasting
	Self-administered thromboprophylaxis	LMWH injection 12 hours prior to surgery administered at home
	Preoperative carbohydrate loading	Preoperative carbohydrate loading (careful use in diabetic patients)
Admission	Preoperative oral intake	Clear fluid until 2 hours preoperatively, solid food until 6 hours preoperatively
	Pre-anaesthesia medication	Avoidance of long-acting sedatives
Anaesthesia	Standard anaesthetic protocol	
	Antimicrobial prophylaxis	24 hours intravenous Augmentin®
	Skin preparation	Two-stage preparation: spray alcoholic 2% chlorhexidine gluconate and paint aqueous 10% povidone-iodine
	Thromboembolic prophylaxis	Thromboembolic compression stockings, 28 days of pharmacological prophylaxis with LMWH starting day before surgery, intraoperative pneumatic compression stockings
	Regional analgesia	Epidural anaesthesia omitted, rectus sheath catheters (0.125% bupivacaine) for first 48 hours
	Perioperative fluid management	Avoid overhydration (<1 L crystalloid until bladder removed). Vasopressors to maintain arterial hypotension
	Nasogastric intubation	No nasogastric tube or it is removed at the end of surgery
	Preventing intraoperative hypothermia	Use of a warming blanket
Surgery	Minimally invasive approach	Mini-open cystectomy incision or robotic approaches
	Resection site drainage	Consider omitting pelvic drain
	Urinary drainage	Ureteral stents or transurethral neobladder catheter should be used. Stents removed as an outpatient or catheter removed after cystogram for neobladder patients
	Wound closure	2/0 polydioxanone suture (Ethicon®) to rectus sheath. 3/0 subcuticular Monocryl® (poliglecaprone) suture (Ethicon®) to skin
Postoperative	Postoperative diet	Chewing gum to start at 4 hours after surgery, oral fluids to start evening of surgery—30 mL/hour of clear non-fizzy fluids. Resume diet when passing flatus, mobile, and pain controlled
	Prevention of postoperative nausea and vomiting	Antiemetics as needed, early resumption of oral fluids
	Postoperative analgesia	Rectus sheath catheters, patient-controlled opiates, intravenous paracetamol/acetaminophen 1 g four times daily until diet resumed
	Early mobilization	6 hours out of bed on postoperative day (POD) 1, walk 10 m on POD 1, 50 m on POD 2, >100 m on POD 3+
	Audit	Audit compliance. Understand problems. Keep resource within team

- Significant improvement in physical and emotional functioning scores after surgery between days 3 and 7 and on discharge.
- Significant reduction in wound healing problems, deep vein thrombosis, and postoperative fever.
- Significantly lower demand for postoperative analgesia.
- Increased oral intake postoperatively (as early as day 3).

A final word from the expert

RC with lymphadenectomy remains the best chance of cure in those with muscle-invasive disease. The preparation for curative treatment is twofold; firstly, providing the patient with an accurate diagnosis at the earliest opportunity. Once the diagnosis of MIBC has been made, the patient can be adequately counselled about the best possible modalities of treatment—whether this be radical curative approaches or palliative treatments. This will almost certainly involve a multidisciplinary approach and, in the majority of patients, RC should be considered.

Secondly, if the patient opts for RC, they must be adequately prepared for the procedure. Not only should this involve the provision of NAC, to improve oncological outcomes in those who are eligible, but also surgical optimization with a thorough preoperative assessment. RC with lymphadenectomy is a huge physiological undertaking, so consideration of extent of disease, age, comorbidities, medication, preoperative function, and nutritional status will aid the decision about whether radical treatment is feasible and appropriate.

Occasionally, ensuring that a patient is optimized for surgery may involve delaying RC, as performing major surgery in a suboptimized patient may lead to poorer outcomes. In the case described, protecting, and optimizing renal function was imperative; neoadjuvant insertion of a PCN both ensured that the solitary right kidney was protected from malignant ureteric obstruction, and also facilitated the delivery of NAC that would have otherwise been inappropriate with declining renal function.

Therefore, thorough optimization and meticulous preparation of patients prior to RC not only facilitates the delivery of multimodal therapy to improve oncological outcomes, but helps to limit the associated morbidity from RC.

References

1. Bray F, Ferlay J, Soerjomataram I, Siegel RL, Torre LA, Jemal A. Global cancer statistics 2018: GLOBOCAN estimates of incidence and mortality worldwide for 36 cancers in 185 countries. *CA Cancer J Clin.* 2018;68(6):394–424.
2. Noon AP, Albertsen PC, Thomas F, Rosario DJ, Catto JWF. Competing mortality in patients diagnosed with bladder cancer: evidence of undertreatment in the elderly and female patients. *Br J Cancer.* 2013;108(7):1534–1540.
3. Cumberbatch MGK, Jubber I, Black PC, et al. Epidemiology of bladder cancer: a systematic review and contemporary update of risk factors in 2018. *Eur Urol.* 2018;74(6):784–795.
4. Cumberbatch MG, Rota M, Catto JWF, La Vecchia C. The role of tobacco smoke in bladder and kidney carcinogenesis: a comparison of exposures and meta-analysis of incidence and mortality risks. *Eur Urol.* 2016;70(3):458–466.
5. Cumberbatch MGK, Cox A, Teare D, Catto JWF. Contemporary occupational carcinogen exposure and bladder cancer. *JAMA Oncol.* 2015;1(9):1282–1290.
6. Eble JN, Sauter G, Epstein JI, Sesterhenn IA. *Pathology and Genetics of Tumours of the Urinary System and Male Genital Organs*. Lyon: International Agency for Research on Cancer; 2004.

7. Compérat E, Gontero P, Mostafid AH, et al. EAU guidelines on non-muscle-invasive bladder cancer (TaT1 and CIS). European Association of Urology. 2017. https://uroweb.org/wp-content/uploads/EAU-Guidelines-on-Non-muscle-Invasive-Bladder-Cancer-2020.pdf
8. Kamoun A, de Reyniès A, Allory Y, et al. A consensus molecular classification of muscle-invasive bladder cancer. *Eur Urol.* 2020;77(4):420–433.
9. Gordon PC, Thomas F, Noon AP, Rosario DJ, Catto JWF. Long-term outcomes from re-resection for high-risk non–muscle-invasive bladder cancer: a potential to rationalize Use. *Eur Urol Focus.* 2019;5(4):650–657.
10. Van Den Bosch S, Witjes JA. Long-term cancer-specific survival in patients with high-risk, non-muscle-invasive bladder cancer and tumour progression: a systematic review. *Eur Urol.* 2011;60(3):493–500.
11. Catto JWF, Gordon K, Collinson M, et al. Radical cystectomy against intravesical BCG for high-risk high-grade nonmuscle invasive bladder cancer: results from the randomized controlled BRAVO-feasibility study. *J Clin Oncol.* 2021;39(3):202–214.
12. Oughton JB, Poad H, Twiddy M, et al. Radical cystectomy (bladder removal) against intravesical BCG immunotherapy for high-risk non-muscle invasive bladder cancer (BRAVO): a protocol for a randomised controlled feasibility study. *BMJ Open.* 2017;7(8):e017913.
13. Witjes JA, Compérat E, Cowan NC, et al. EAU guidelines on muscle-invasive and metastatic bladder cancer. European Association of Urology. 2016. https://uroweb.org/wp-content/uploads/EAU-Guidelines-Muscle-invasive-and-Metastatic-Bladder-Cancer-Guidelines-2016.pdf
14. Magers MJ, Lopez-Beltran A, Montironi R, et al. Staging of bladder cancer. *Histopathology.* 2019;74(1):112–134.
15. Kiss B, Furrer MA, Wuethrich PY, Burkhard FC, Thalmann GN, Roth B. Stenting prior to cystectomy is an independent risk factor for upper urinary tract recurrence. *J Urol.* 2017;198(6):1263–1268.
16. International Collaboration of Trialists; Medical Research Council Advanced Bladder Cancer Working Party (now the National Cancer Research Institute Bladder Cancer Clinical Studies Group); European Organisation for Research and Treatment of Cancer Genito-Urinary Tract Cancer Group; et al. International phase III trial assessing neoadjuvant cisplatin, methotrexate, and vinblastine chemotherapy for muscle-invasive bladder cancer: long-term results of the BA06 30894 trial. *J Clin Oncol.* 2011;29(16):2171–2177.
17. von der Maase H, Sengelov L, Roberts JT, et al. Long-term survival results of a randomized trial comparing gemcitabine plus cisplatin, with methotrexate, vinblastine, doxorubicin, plus cisplatin in patients with bladder cancer. *J Clin Oncol.* 2005;23(21):4602–4608.
18. Astolfi L, Ghiselli S, Guaran V, et al. Correlation of adverse effects of cisplatin administration in patients affected by solid tumours: a retrospective evaluation. *Oncol Rep.* 2013;29(4):1285–1292.
19. Nielsen ME, Palapattu GS, Karakiewicz PI, et al. A delay in radical cystectomy of >3 months is not associated with a worse clinical outcome. *BJU Int.* 2007;100(5):1015–1020.
20. Bruins HM, Veskimae E, Hernandez V, et al. The impact of the extent of lymphadenectomy on oncologic outcomes in patients undergoing radical cystectomy for bladder cancer: a systematic review. *Eur Urol.* 2014;66(6):1065–1077.
21. Karl A, Carroll PR, Gschwend JE, et al. The impact of lymphadenectomy and lymph node metastasis on the outcomes of radical cystectomy for bladder cancer. *Eur Urol.* 2009;55(4):826–835.
22. Gschwend JE, Heck MM, Lehmann J, et al. Extended versus limited lymph node dissection in bladder cancer patients undergoing radical cystectomy: survival results from a prospective, randomized trial. *Eur Urol.* 2019;75(4):604–611.
23. Karl A, Buchner A, Becker A, et al. A new concept for early recovery after surgery for patients undergoing radical cystectomy for bladder cancer: results of a prospective randomized study. *J Urol.* 2014;191(2):335–340.
24. Pang KH, Groves R, Venugopal S, Noon AP, Catto JWF. Prospective implementation of enhanced recovery after surgery protocols to radical cystectomy. *Eur Urol.* 2018;73(3):363–371.

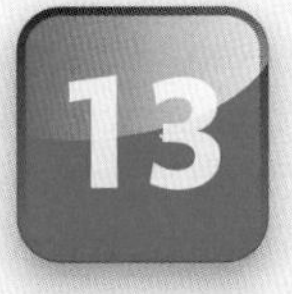

Progression of high-grade non-muscle-invasive bladder cancer

Naomi L. Neal

Expert commentary Richard J. Bryant and Andrew Protheroe

Case history

A 73-year-old gentleman was referred urgently to the urology department following an episode of painless visible haematuria, without any other lower urinary tract symptoms. He had a background history of hypertension, cardiomyopathy, type 2 diabetes, and a previous ventricular fibrillation cardiac arrest with subsequent insertion of a pacemaker. Clinical examination was unremarkable, and flexible cystoscopy revealed a 2–3 cm papillary bladder tumour on the left side of the bladder lateral to the ureteric orifice. A computed tomography (CT) urogram revealed a left-sided bladder tumour but was otherwise unremarkable, with normal upper urinary tracts (Figure 13.1).

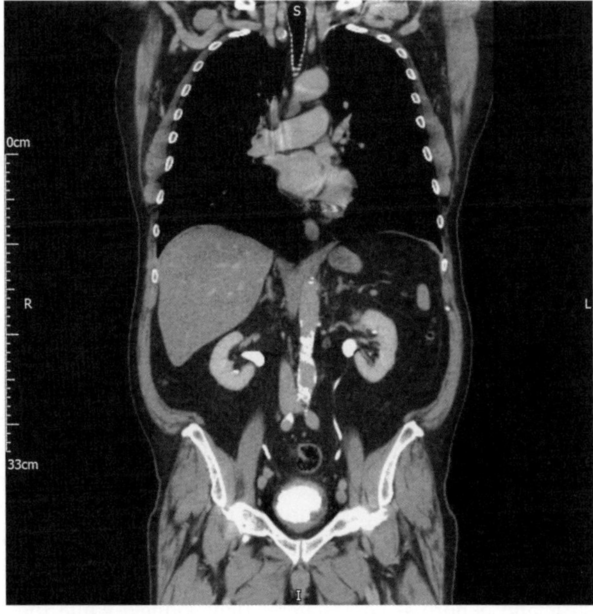

Figure 13.1 The initial CT urogram demonstrates a left-sided bladder filling defect and normal upper urinary tracts, with no lymphadenopathy.

A transurethral resection of bladder tumour (TURBT) was undertaken. This confirmed the presence of a 2–3 cm papillary lesion lateral to the left ureteric orifice, with no macroscopic solid component. The remainder of the bladder appeared normal on cystoscopic inspection. A complete resection of the lesion was undertaken, followed by a single instillation of postoperative mitomycin C. Histological examination of the surgical specimen confirmed the presence of G3pT1 transitional cell carcinoma (TCC); however, there was no muscularis propria in the specimen, and therefore a re-resection TURBT was performed 6 weeks later. The re-resection of the previous bladder tumour site, which did visibly detect overt tumour at cystoscopy, again revealed G3pT1 TCC of the bladder upon histological examination of the specimen; however, the muscularis propria was free of tumour. At outpatient clinic follow-up, the treatment options were discussed with the patient, with these comprising bladder conservation therapy using intravesical bacillus Calmette–Guérin (BCG) instillation therapy, or radical cystectomy (RC) and ileal conduit urinary diversion. The patient elected to receive a bladder preservation approach strategy using BCG.

Clinical tip Re-resection TURBT

Re-resection TURBT is advised within 2–6 weeks if there is an incomplete primary tumour resection, or if there is no muscularis propria in the surgical specimen (unless there is a Ta low-grade cancer or primary carcinoma *in situ* (CIS)), or in cases of T1 tumours. The re-resection specimen may contain residual cancer in around a third of primary Ta, and half of all T1, cases.[1] Twenty-five to forty-five per cent of initial high-grade non-muscle-invasive bladder cancer (HGNMIBC) cases are upstaged to muscle-invasive bladder cancer (MIBC) at early re-resection. Early re-resection of initial HGNMIBC is associated with an increased recurrence-free survival, and improved outcomes (recurrence-free survival, progression-free survival, and overall survival) after BCG treatment.[2]

Learning point Early RC versus bladder preservation therapy with BCG

Patients with HGNMIC can be offered bladder preservation therapy with BCG, or RC. Aggressive treatment is required due to the high risk of disease progression, which occurs in 30% of T1G3 and 80% of HGNMIBC cases with concomitant CIS.

Patients who experience HGNMIBC disease progression to MIBC following bladder preservation therapy have a worse prognosis than those who initially present with MIBC.[3] RC is recommended over BCG for the highest risk category patients, including those with HGNIMBC T1 tumours with concurrent CIS, multiple or large or recurrent T1 high-grade tumours, and some forms of variant histology of urothelial carcinoma.

Expert comment
Treatment discussions

Treatment discussions should include a balance of the risk of progression to MIBC and death (50% and 30%, respectively, by 15 years after BCG treatment) versus the side effects of RC.

The patient commenced induction BCG; however, at this stage a worldwide shortage of BCG became apparent, and this resulted in the patient receiving an incomplete full induction course. A subsequent check cystoscopy under general anaesthetic revealed an apparent solid lesion on the left side wall of the bladder, resulting in the left ureteric orifice being non-visible during cystoscopic inspection, while the remainder of the bladder including the right ureteric orifice was unremarkable. The recurrent bladder tumour was re-resected, with subsequent histology confirming recurrent G3pT1 urothelial carcinoma with concomitant CIS, with uninvolved muscularis propria. A repeat CT urogram at that stage revealed a left hydronephrosis and hydroureter to the vesicoureteric junction (Figure 13.2), and a normal contralateral right kidney, while the renal function remained normal. The option of a RC and ileal conduit formation was considered at this stage; however, given the patient's high risk for radical surgery owing to his cardiac

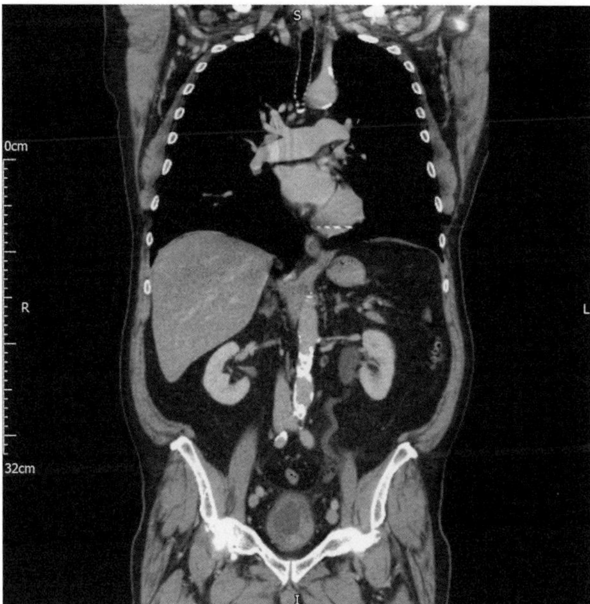

Figure 13.2 A follow-up CT urogram revealed a left hydronephrosis and hydroureter to the vesicoureteric junction.

comorbidity, a further re-do TURBT was performed, and on this occasion the relatively small amount of residual disease on the left side wall of the bladder was resected macroscopically clear, including the scar tissue around the left ureteric orifice, which resulted in drainage of the left ureter. Subsequent histology revealed T1 TCC of the bladder along with chronic inflammation, and the patient elected to receive a full course of induction BCG given that this was now available following resolution of the worldwide shortage.

Learning point Morbidity of RC, and outcomes for RC following BCG failure

RC includes the surgical removal of the bladder, distal ureters, and lymph nodes, together with the prostate and seminal vesicles in men, and adjacent vagina and uterus in women. The morbidity for this surgery is between 30% and 60%, with many of the risks being associated with the urinary diversion, including stoma complications, ureteroileal strictures, metabolic disturbances, and subsequent urinary stone formation.[4] Other risks include paralytic ileus, anastomotic leak, venous thromboembolism, myocardial infarction, pulmonary complications, cerebrovascular events, and wound dehiscence or hernia development. The mortality after RC is approximately 5%.

The presence of CIS, tumour size >3 cm, and multiple tumours at diagnosis are predictors of pathological upstaging to T3/4 and/or N+ disease after RC following BCG failure.[5] Patients with recognized progression prior to RC have a shorter time to cancer death compared to those upstaged on RC histology. It is possible that younger patients benefit from upfront RC rather than bladder-preserving BCG treatment.

Three subsequent check cystoscopies over the next year revealed various erythematous areas in the bladder; these were each confirmed to be benign with chronic inflammation on histological examination of biopsy specimens, and the patient continued on maintenance BCG instillation therapy. A surveillance CT scan revealed the improvement of the previous hydronephrosis and hydroureter, and the patient's renal function remained normal. A further subsequent check cystoscopy under general anaesthetic showed no apparent

Expert comment
Approaches to RC

Clinical trials comparing open and minimally invasive approaches (including robotic cystectomy in the Intracorporeal Robot Assisted Radical Cystectomy (iROC) trial) are ongoing, but currently appear to show no significant difference other than perhaps a small reduction in blood transfusion rates and length of hospital stay.[6] Even in the modern era with great surgical advances and techniques, RC remains a morbid operation.

active intravesical disease; however, the left ureteric orifice was re-resected as this had appeared to have re-stenosed, the subsequent histology from this procedure confirming the presence of inflammation only, with no active TCC of the bladder on histology.

Learning point Outcomes for BCG intravesical therapy

Fifteen-year follow-up studies of patients receiving BCG for NMIBC show progression in around 50%. Around 30% of patients die from disease progression, and only 27% survive with an intact bladder. Around 25% of patients develop upper urinary tract cancer.

The Spanish Oncology Group (CUETO) has identified risk factors for disease recurrence, including being female, having had a previous recurrence, multiplicity of tumours, and presence of CIS.[7] Predictors of progression include age, previous recurrence, high-grade disease, T1 stage, and recurrent disease at the first check cystoscopy at 3 months.

The patient underwent a further surveillance CT scan, which revealed the presence of a 16 mm apparent tumour nodule in the region of the left vesicoureteric junction, which was not visible intravesically at cystoscopy, and enlarged pelvic lymph nodes (Figure 13.3) and an enlarged aortocaval lymph node, suspicious for metastatic disease recurrence based on radiological criteria. The patient was reviewed in the medical oncology clinic, and was informed of the concern regarding possible metastatic TCC recurrence. The options of upfront chemotherapy in the form of gemcitabine and carboplatin, or surveillance, were discussed, and the patient elected to receive a period of surveillance in the first instance, as he was asymptomatic. His radiological imaging remained stable at the next surveillance CT scan; however, a few months later a check flexible cystoscopy under local anaesthetic revealed tumour recurrence at the bladder base along with an area of erythema over the left lateral wall of the bladder.

Expert comment Metastatic TCC of the bladder

The concern with the patient at this point is that he now has metastatic disease, albeit with a limited burden of lymph nodal disease, despite the histology still demonstrating HGNMIBC. It is appropriate in this situation to offer systemic chemotherapy, if the multidisciplinary team were in agreement that this was in keeping with radiographic development of metastatic disease, given the known risk that this may occur with HGNMIBC.

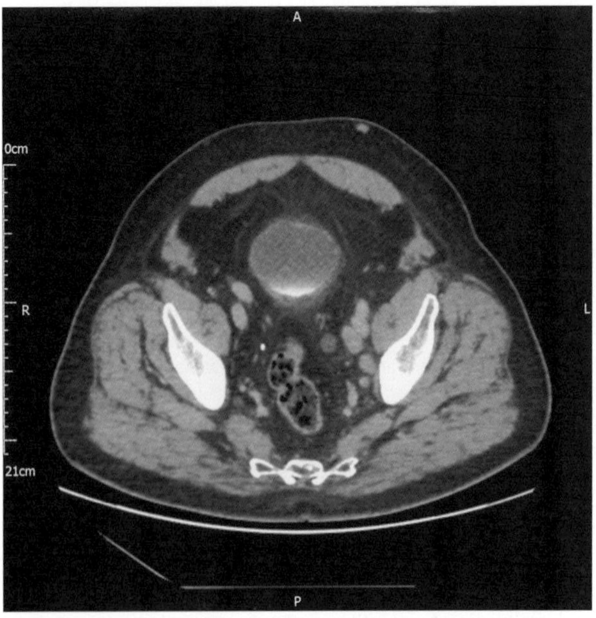

Figure 13.3 A surveillance CT scan revealed the presence of enlarged pelvic lymph nodes.

Learning point Chemotherapy and immunotherapy for metastatic TCC of the bladder

The standard first-line chemotherapy combination for metastatic BC is gemcitabine and cisplatin,[8] which has an overall response rate of approximately 50%, and a median survival of around 14 months. MVAC (methotrexate, vinblastine, Adriamycin® (doxorubicin), and cisplatin) would be an acceptable alternative first-line chemotherapy regimen.[9,10] The response rate to a cisplatin-based combination has been reported to be between 36% and 71%.[11] The preference for treating BC patients is always to give a cisplatin-based combination of chemotherapeutic agents, as this has demonstrated better outcomes.[11–13] Criteria to determine cisplatin ineligibility have been developed and published.[14] If the toxicity of cisplatin is a concern then a combination of gemcitabine and carboplatin could be offered, although this has a lower response rate (28–56%)[11] and poorer overall survival.

If patients are ineligible to receive cisplatin, immunotherapy in the form of a checkpoint inhibitor can now be offered. This is based on two phase II studies investigating atezolizumab (from the IMvigor 210 study group) or pembrolizumab (from the KEYNOTE-052 study group).[15,16] The KEYNOTE-052 study, investigating 'upfront' single-agent pembrolizumab, demonstrated a 24% overall response following the use of this agent.[16] However, the European Medicines Agency has restricted the use of pembrolizumab for untreated urothelial carcinoma, such that it should now only be used in adults with high levels of programmed death-ligand 1 (PD-L1) expression in their tumours. This recommendation is based on unpublished findings in the KEYNOTE-361 and IMvigor-130 studies, where decreased survival in individuals with tumours with low PD-L1 expression was demonstrated in patients receiving pembrolizumab, compared with those who received cisplatin or carboplatin-based chemotherapy.

A further TURBT was therefore performed, where an anterior bladder neck tumour was resected, and histology of this specimen revealed recurrent G3pT1 TCC. The scarred left ureteric orifice was re-resected in order to 'uncap' the left ureter, and a retrograde ureterogram was performed which showed no ureteric tumour, and a left-sided ureteric stent was inserted in order to maintain drainage of the left upper urinary tract and maintain normal renal function ahead of further treatment. Unfortunately, the patient subsequently developed intractable stent symptoms, and so the stent was removed at a check flexible cystoscopy 4 months later.

Due to concerns regarding cardiac comorbidity and the presence of limited lymph nodal metastatic disease, the patient was still not a candidate for RC at this point, and further cross-sectional imaging in the form of a repeat CT scan revealed the presence of enlarging pelvic and retroperitoneal lymph nodes (Figure 13.4) suggestive of progressive metastatic TCC. The management options at this point comprised either chemotherapy, or bladder and pelvis radiotherapy, with the option of possible subsequent chemotherapy. A further staging CT scan confirmed progression of the para-aortic and left iliac lymphadenopathy, and in light of this, the preferred management option was chemotherapy, with possible consolidation radiotherapy if the patient was suitable for this in due course.

The patient commenced first-line chemotherapy in the form of gemcitabine and carboplatin, and this was well tolerated, with a subsequent CT scan showing a good response to chemotherapy. His condition remained under active review with serial cross-sectional imaging. Future options, should imaging reveal further lymph node metastatic progression, could include possible immunotherapy, or second-line chemotherapy.

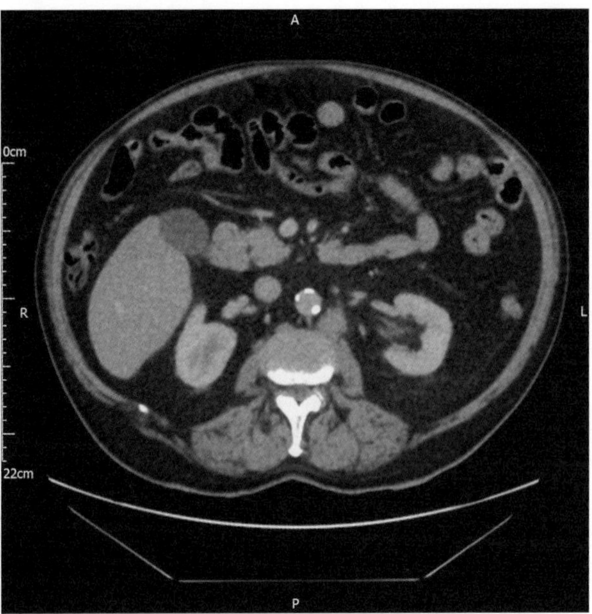

Figure 13.4 A repeat CT scan revealed the presence of enlarging pelvic and retroperitoneal lymph nodes, suggestive of progressive metastatic urothelial carcinoma.

Learning point Second-line chemotherapy options

Up until recently, the treatment options for patients with metastatic TCC were limited, with chemotherapy being the only available systemic treatment. Invariably, when patients developed disease recurrence following first-line chemotherapy for metastatic disease, that disease was aggressive, with rapid progression and only limited options for further treatment.

Second-line chemotherapy was usually offered to those patients who were fit enough to receive it. A number of chemotherapy drugs have single-agent activity, but the US Food and Drug Administration has approved none of these in the second-line setting. In Europe, single-agent vinflunine is approved following a study that demonstrated a 2.6-month survival advantage over best supportive care in patients fit enough to receive chemotherapy.[17] However, taxanes are probably the most commonly used second-line chemotherapy single agents. Paclitaxel and docetaxel are associated with a modest overall risk reduction of 10–30% and an overall survival improvement of 6–9 months.[18–20]

Future directions New combinations of immunotherapy

After a prolonged period of time where there were limited available options for patients with metastatic BC, suddenly and excitingly the doors are now being opened for new and improved therapies. Multiple new potential combinations of immunotherapy and other targeted agents are being investigated in clinical studies, with the potential to improve patient treatment outcomes in the future.

Evidence base Immunotherapy

Immunotherapy with checkpoint inhibitor agents has become available and is now licensed for metastatic urothelial cancer, and this has increased the treatment options for patients. Checkpoint inhibitors, which either block programmed cell death-1 (PD-1) or PD-L1, are now licensed and available as treatment options for patients with metastatic BC. Initial reports of the use of these agents suggested encouraging activity and safety.[21] This led to the acquisition of phase III data, in particular from the KEYNOTE-45 study,[22] which compared pembrolizumab (a PD-1 inhibitor) to standard-dose chemotherapy (investigator's choice of paclitaxel, docetaxel, or vinflunine). This study demonstrated a significantly longer survival (3 months) with pembrolizumab, and a higher response rate (21.1% vs 11.4% in the whole group). As a result, immunotherapy is now licensed and funded as a second-line treatment option following post-chemotherapy disease recurrence. Several immune checkpoint inhibitors are now licensed for advanced urothelial cancer, including pembrolizumab and nivolumab (PD-1 inhibitors), and atezolizumab, avelumab, and durvalumab (PD-L1 inhibitors).

A final word from the expert

Bladder cancer is a malignancy that is moderately sensitive to chemotherapy treatment options, and this has therefore been the mainstay of systemic therapy until very recently. The historical chemotherapy regimens used have been MVAC; cisplatin, methotrexate, and vinblastine; and a combination of gemcitabine and cisplatin. Over the last 20 years, combined gemcitabine and cisplatin has emerged to be the preferred global first-line chemotherapy combination, in view of better toxicity and equivalent response rates and overall survival compared to MVAC. Gemcitabine and cisplatin response rates are around 50%, with an approximately 14-month median survival in this population of patients. Metastatic BC is a particularly aggressive form of malignancy, and a significant proportion of patients are not eligible to receive cisplatin due to their comorbidities and poor performance status, particularly in the form of concomitant renal function impairment. It is estimated that up to around 50% of these patients are not eligible for cisplatin treatment. Where necessary, cisplatin has traditionally been substituted with carboplatin in this group of patients; however, carboplatin has slightly lower outcomes in terms of response rates and overall survival compared against cisplatin.

The treatment options for patients with subsequent disease relapse following initial chemotherapy have been very limited, in part because of the aggressive nature of the disease, and further because of the poor fitness of many patients. There has also been a general lack of good evidence that further chemotherapy is beneficial in this disease relapse situation. Vinflunine is licensed as a second-line chemotherapy treatment option; however, there have been concerns regarding the design of clinical trials using this agent. Taxanes, particularly single-agent paclitaxel, have also been used globally as second-line chemotherapy agents.

The treatment landscape for patients with BC has recently changed significantly with the development of immune checkpoint inhibitor drugs. Indeed, PD-1 and PDL-1 inhibitors have been licensed. These agents are now funded and available mainly as second-line treatments in the metastatic disease setting, although they can be used 'upfront' for patients who are ineligible for cisplatin, though only if their tumour expresses PD-1.

References

1. Grimm MO, Steinhoff C, Simon X, Spiegelhalder P, Ackermann R, Vogeli TA. Effect of routine repeat transurethral resection for superficial bladder cancer: a long-term observational study. *J Urol.* 2003;170(2 Pt 1):433–437.
2. Sfakianos JP, Kim PH, Hakimi AA, Herr HW. The effect of restaging transurethral resection on recurrence and progression rates in patients with nonmuscle invasive bladder cancer treated with intravesical bacillus Calmette-Guérin. *J Urol.* 2014;191(2):341–345.
3. Moschini M, Sharma V, Dell'oglio P, et al. Comparing long-term outcomes of primary and progressive carcinoma invading bladder muscle after radical cystectomy. *BJU Int.* 2016;117(4):604–610.
4. Shabsigh A, Korets R, Vora KC, et al. Defining early morbidity of radical cystectomy for patients with bladder cancer using a standardized reporting methodology. *Eur Urol.* 2009;55(1):164–176.
5. Soria F, Pisano F, Gontero P, et al. Predictors of oncological outcomes in T1G3 patients treated with BCG who undergo radical cystectomy. *World J Urol.* 2018;36(11):1775–1781.
6. Catto JWF, Khetrapal P, Ambler G, et al. Robot-assisted radical cystectomy with intracorporeal urinary diversion versus open radical cystectomy (iROC): protocol for a randomised controlled trial with internal feasibility study. *BMJ Open.* 2018;8(8):e020500.
7. Fernandez-Gomez J, Solsona E, Unda M, et al. Prognostic factors in patients with non-muscle-invasive bladder cancer treated with bacillus Calmette-Guérin: multivariate analysis of data from four randomized CUETO trials. *Eur Urol.* 2008;53(5):992–1001.

8. von der Maase H, Hansen SW, Roberts JT, et al. Gemcitabine and cisplatin versus methotrexate, vinblastine, doxorubicin, and cisplatin in advanced or metastatic bladder cancer: results of a large, randomized, multinational, multicenter, phase III study. *J Clin Oncol.* 2000;18(17):3068–3077.
9. Loehrer PJ, Einhorn LH, Elson PJ, et al. A randomized comparison of cisplatin alone or in combination with methotrexate, vinblastine, and doxorubicin in patients with metastatic urothelial carcinoma: a cooperative group study. *J Clin Oncol.* 1992;10(7):1066–1073.
10. Logothetis CJ, Dexeus FH, Finn L, et al. A prospective randomized trial comparing MVAC and CISCA chemotherapy for patients with metastatic urothelial tumors. *J Clin Oncol.* 1990;8(6):1050–1055.
11. Galsky MD, Chen GJ, Oh WK, et al. Comparative effectiveness of cisplatin-based and carboplatin-based chemotherapy for treatment of advanced urothelial carcinoma. *Ann Oncol.* 2012;23(2):406–410.
12. Dreicer R, Manola J, Roth BJ, et al. Phase III trial of methotrexate, vinblastine, doxorubicin, and cisplatin versus carboplatin and paclitaxel in patients with advanced carcinoma of the urothelium. *Cancer.* 2004;100(8):1639–1645.
13. Dogliotti L, Cartenì G, Siena S, et al. Gemcitabine plus cisplatin versus gemcitabine plus carboplatin as first-line chemotherapy in advanced transitional cell carcinoma of the urothelium: results of a randomized phase 2 trial. *Eur Urol.* 2007;52(1):134–141.
14. Galsky MD, Hahn NM, Rosenberg J, et al. A consensus definition of patients with metastatic urothelial carcinoma who are unfit for cisplatin-based chemotherapy. *Lancet Oncol.* 2011;12(3):211–214.
15. Balar AV, Galsky MD, Rosenberg JE, et al. Atezolizumab as first-line treatment in cisplatin-ineligible patients with locally advanced and metastatic urothelial carcinoma: a single-arm, multicentre, phase 2 trial. *Lancet.* 2017;389(10064):67–76.
16. Balar AV, Castellano D, O'Donnell PH, et al. First-line pembrolizumab in cisplatin-ineligible patients with locally advanced and unresectable or metastatic urothelial cancer (KEYNOTE-052): a multicentre, single-arm, phase 2 study. *Lancet Oncol.* 2017;18(11):1483–1492.
17. Bellmunt J, Théodore C, Demkov T, et al. Phase III trial of vinflunine plus best supportive care compared with best supportive care alone after a platinum-containing regimen in patients with advanced transitional cell carcinoma of the urothelial tract. *J Clin Oncol.* 2009;27(27):4454–4461.
18. McCaffrey JA, Hilton S, Mazumdar M, et al. Phase II trial of docetaxel in patients with advanced or metastatic transitional-cell carcinoma. *J Clin Oncol.* 1997;15(5):1853–1857.
19. Vaughn DJ, Broome CM, Hussain M, Gutheil JC, Markowitz AB. Phase II trial of weekly paclitaxel in patients with previously treated advanced urothelial cancer. *J Clin Oncol.* 2002;20(4):937–940.
20. Jones RJ, Hussain SA, Protheroe AS, et al. Randomized phase II study investigating pazopanib versus weekly paclitaxel in relapsed or progressive urothelial cancer. *J Clin Oncol.* 2017;35(16):1770–1777.
21. Powles T, Eder JP, Fine GD, et al. MPDL3280A (anti-PD-L1) treatment leads to clinical activity in metastatic bladder cancer. *Nature.* 2014;515(7528):558–562.
22. Bellmunt J, de Wit R, Vaughn DJ, et al. Pembrolizumab as second-line therapy for advanced urothelial carcinoma. *N Engl J Med.* 2017;376(11):1015–1026.

SECTION 6

Upper urinary tract cancer

Localized renal cancer with inferior vena cava tumour thrombus

Tobias Klatte, Antony C.P. Riddick, and Grant D. Stewart

Expert commentary Jose A. Karam

Case history

A 61-year-old patient is referred by his general practitioner with a 4-week history of intermittent right loin pain. He does not report haematuria or systemic symptoms. His current World Health Organization performance status is 0. Except for a right inguinal hernia repair 20 years ago, he has not had any previous surgeries. He is not on any regular medications but takes paracetamol when he has pain. The clinical examination is unremarkable. Routine blood tests and the urine dipstick are normal. He undergoes an ultrasound study, which shows a large right renal tumour. The subsequent computed tomography (CT) scan of the chest, abdomen, and pelvis confirms a large, heterogeneous, enhancing right renal mass with a tumour thrombus extending into the infrahepatic inferior vena cava (IVC, Mayo level II) (Figure 14.1).[1] There is no evidence of metastatic disease in the chest, abdomen, or pelvis. The clinical stage is T3bN0M0.

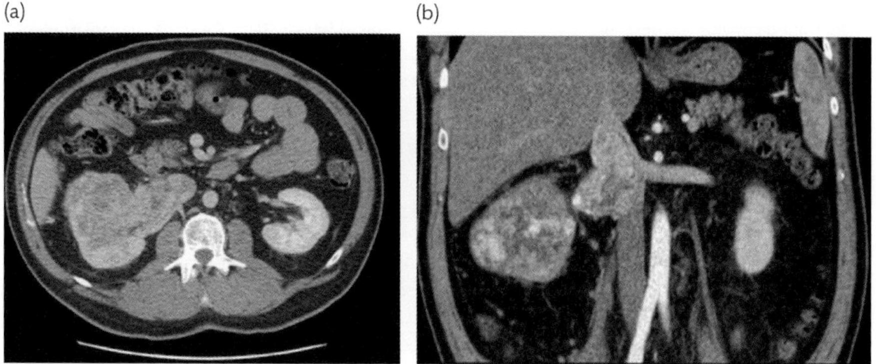

Figure 14.1 Contrast-enhanced CT scan demonstrating heterogeneous right renal tumour with extension into the infrahepatic IVC. (a) Axial; (b) coronal.
Reproduced with permission.[1]

Learning point Diagnostic imaging

CT scans of the chest, abdomen, and pelvis are usually performed initially and subsequently supplemented by magnetic resonance imaging (MRI) scans at many centres (Figure 14.2). Data established decades ago[2] suggested that MRI scans may be superior to CT in delineating the cephalad extent of the venous tumour thrombus (VTT) and may be able to distinguish a bland thrombus (non-enhancing, benign) from a tumour thrombus (enhancing, malignant). However, more recent studies suggest that there are no clinically meaningful differences between MRI and contemporary CT technology[3–5] and that a CT scan alone may be sufficient.[6] It cannot be overemphasized that up-to-date imaging must be obtained within 7–10 days of the scheduled date for optimal surgical planning. This imaging strategy excludes rapid tumour progression that would change management.

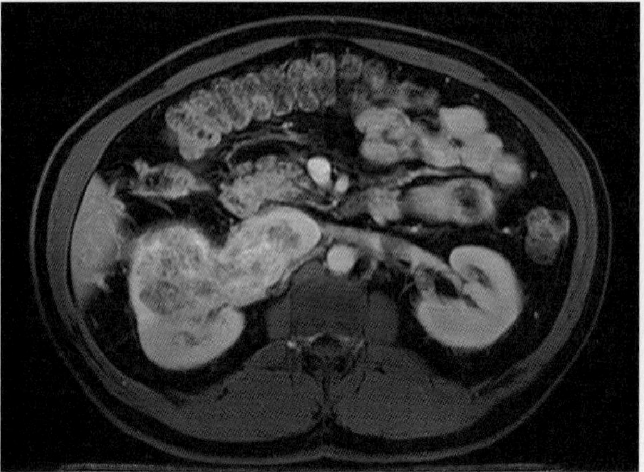

Figure 14.2 Axial water LAVA-Flex (GE Medical) gradient echo MRI demonstrating right renal tumour extending and distending the renal vein and IVC.
Reproduced with permission.[1]

Learning point Vascular anatomy on imaging

In surgical candidates, several additional vascular features warrant attention while reviewing the scan. Arterial anatomy is crucial, as early arterial control is desired; this lowers blood loss and leads to thrombus 'shrinkage' by decreasing venous back pressure. In right-sided cases, arterial control can be achieved by identifying the renal artery in the inter-aorto-caval space if there are no bulky lymph nodes. The anatomy of lumbar veins should be studied, as ligation is essential to achieve a bloodless field during cavotomy. The gonadal vein and adrenal vein are often prominent as they may provide a collateral circulation for the kidney with an obstructed renal vein.

Expert comment Cavotomy and haemostasis

Ligation of the right gonadal vein and the right adrenal vein, in addition to the lumbar veins, is crucial for excellent haemostasis during cavotomy.

Learning point Anteroposterior diameter of the IVC

An important feature is the anteroposterior diameter of the IVC at the level of the renal vein ostium. An increasing diameter is associated with an increased risk of IVC wall invasion,[7] which generally necessitates IVC resection and possibly reconstruction to achieve negative resection margins. An anteroposterior diameter of ≥24 mm (odds ratio (OR) 4.4), right-sided tumour location (OR 3.3), and radiographic complete occlusion of the IVC at the renal vein ostium (OR 4.9) are all significant predictors of the need for IVC resection and should be assessed.[8]

Learning point Venacavography

Invasive venacavography is reserved for surgical candidates in whom both contrast CT and MRI are contraindicated, or if findings are equivocal. Transabdominal ultrasound may be used as an adjunct modality in select cases, but requires highly trained personnel and is often indeterminate.[9] Finally, initial (i.e. preoperative) transoesophageal echocardiography is highly accurate for staging of VTT, but does not provide additional information to CT/MRI.[10] Rather, it is used as a baseline investigation for cardiac anatomy and function. Intraoperative continuous echocardiography can assist both surgeons and anaesthetists during the operation, as it provides real-time imaging during surgery while monitoring cardiovascular and fluid status.[11]

Learning point Clinical, surgical, and pathological staging

Clinical staging of localized renal cell carcinoma (RCC) is based on imaging and physical examination. The most commonly used clinical classification system is the tumour, node, and metastasis (TNM) system, which is supplemented by a surgical VTT classification (Table 14.1).

Based on imaging, the tumour is classified clinically according to TNM. The eighth edition of the TNM classification was implemented for all new cancer diagnoses from 1 January 2018. For tumours with IVC-VTT, the primary clinical tumour (cT) stage is always T3b, T3c, or T4. Pathological tumour (pT) stage needs to be guided by the operating surgeon as the pathologist will not be able to discern between pT3b and pT3c based on the appearance of the tumour thrombus.

Clinical N stage refers to regional retroperitoneal lymph nodes and is based on the short-axis diameter on cross-sectional imaging. The short-axis diameter is the longest perpendicular diameter to the longest (i.e. long-axis) lymph node diameter.[12] The historical cut-off for retroperitoneal nodes is ≥10 mm,[12] although this remains controversial. The risk of positive lymph nodes is 20% in nodes ≥7 mm, 29% in nodes ≥10 mm, 47% in nodes ≥15 mm, and 66% in nodes ≥20 mm.[13] Adding additional imaging parameters to multivariable models does not improve the net benefit over measurement of the short-axis diameter alone.[13] Finally, M stage refers to distant or non-regional lymph node metastases and is assessed clinically. pM1 can be assigned in rare circumstances in which a metastatic deposit is sent for pathology, that is, after surgical removal (most commonly an ipsilateral adrenal metastasis) or biopsy of a metastasis.[14]

A variety of surgical VTT classifications have been published, all of which are directly related to surgical management. The authors use the Mayo classification according to Neves and Zincke,[15] which is shown in Table 14.1.

Table 14.1 Clinical and surgical classification of VTT

Classification	Class	Description
TNM[14]	T3b	Tumour grossly extends into IVC below diaphragm
	T3c	Tumour grossly extends into IVC above diaphragm or invades wall of the vena cava
	T4	Tumour invades beyond Gerota's fascia (including contiguous extension into ipsilateral adrenal gland)
Mayo classification[15]	I	Tumour extends into IVC <2 cm from renal vein ostium
	II	Tumour extends into IVC >2 cm from renal vein ostium but under the major hepatic veins
	III	Tumour extends into IVC at or above major hepatic veins
	IV	Tumour extends into IVC above diaphragm

Source data from: Brierley JD, Gospodarowicz MK, Wittekind C. Union for International Cancer Control (UICC) *TNM Classification of Malignant Tumours*. 8th ed. Chichester, West Sussex, UK: Wiley Blackwell; 2017 and Neves RJ, Zincke H. Surgical treatment of renal cancer with vena cava extension. *Br J Urol*. 1987 May;59(5):390–395.

Expert comment Correct staging

One way to facilitate the correct staging is by having the urological surgeon include the tumour thrombus level with the specimen details sent to pathology.

The scans were reviewed in the multidisciplinary team (MDT) meeting. This confirmed the presence of probable right renal cancer with extension into the IVC well below the major hepatic veins, equalling a VTT level of II according to the Mayo classification. There were no features suggestive of IVC wall involvement. A single right renal artery was present. There was no intra-abdominal lymphadenopathy. The MDT panel discussed presurgical systemic therapy (as part of a clinical trial) versus immediate surgery and recommended offering immediate surgical resection. The patient was brought back to clinic and the outcome of the MDT meeting was discussed. The patient agreed to undergo surgery. He was thoroughly consented to understand the indication, complications, and all possible outcomes of the disease and procedure.

Expert comment Planning for VTT surgery

Aim to schedule surgery as soon as possible, ideally within 2 weeks, to avoid tumour extension or embolization. We generally use prophylactic doses of anticoagulation between presentation to clinic and time of surgery. However, there are no prospective data to support the use of therapeutic anticoagulation in patients with IVC thrombus prior to surgery, in the absence of bland tumour thrombus, deep vein thrombosis, or pulmonary embolism. Presurgical IVC filter placement cranial to the IVC tumour thrombus should not be performed. Similarly, presurgical renal artery embolization is generally not needed. The only clinical scenario when we perform renal artery embolization is in patients who present with Budd-Chiari syndrome. In these patients, we reassess for surgical candidacy around 2 months after renal artery embolization, to check if Budd-Chiari syndrome has resolved. For tumour thrombus level III or higher, the surgery will ideally take place in a thoracic/cardiac operating room, in the presence of a cardiac anaesthesiologist, a thoracic/cardiac surgeon (in addition to a urological surgeon), transoesophageal echocardiography machine, and cardiac pump on standby.

Learning point Presurgical systemic therapy

Downstaging of locally advanced or initially unresectable primary RCC is the aim of presurgical systemic approaches with tyrosine kinase inhibitors (TKIs) and often discussed as a potential option in MDT meetings. At present, there are no published case series with immune checkpoint inhibitors alone or in combination with TKIs. Several retrospective case series evaluated the impact of targeted therapy in patients with VTT. For this case, we performed a quantitative data synthesis of eight retrospective case series with a total of 109 patients using standard random effects models (Publication cut-off: 4 January 2019) (Figure 14.3). Four studies focused on mixed groups of targeted therapies,[16–19] two on sunitinib,[20,21] one on axitinib,[22] and one on pazopanib.[23] The median number of treatment cycles was two. Overall, 65.1% of patients (95% confidence interval (CI) 47.9–79.1) showed a measurable decrease in VTT height with a mean reduction of 2.0 cm (95% CI 1.8–2.5), while 19.4% (95% CI 12.5–28.8) showed an increase in VTT height. The VTT level decreased in 22.6% (95% CI 14.9–32.9), remained stable in 73.6% (95% CI 64.1–81.4), and increased in 7.2% (95% CI 3.4–14.3). (*Note*: these proportions are derived from separate random effects models and therefore do not add up to 100%.) Results were most favourable for sunitinib and axitinib.[16,18,22]

There is only one ongoing prospective trial in this setting. NAXIVA (Neoadjuvant study of AXItinib for reducing extent of venous tumour thrombus in clear cell renal cell cancer with Venous invAsion; NCT0349481) is a single-arm phase II feasibility trial of neoadjuvant axitinib on 20 patients with clear cell RCC and VTT. The primary endpoint is change in VTT level.

In summary, the effect of targeted therapies on tumour thrombi is variable although it may alter surgical management in select patients. Current guidelines do not recommend presurgical systemic therapy outside of clinical trials.

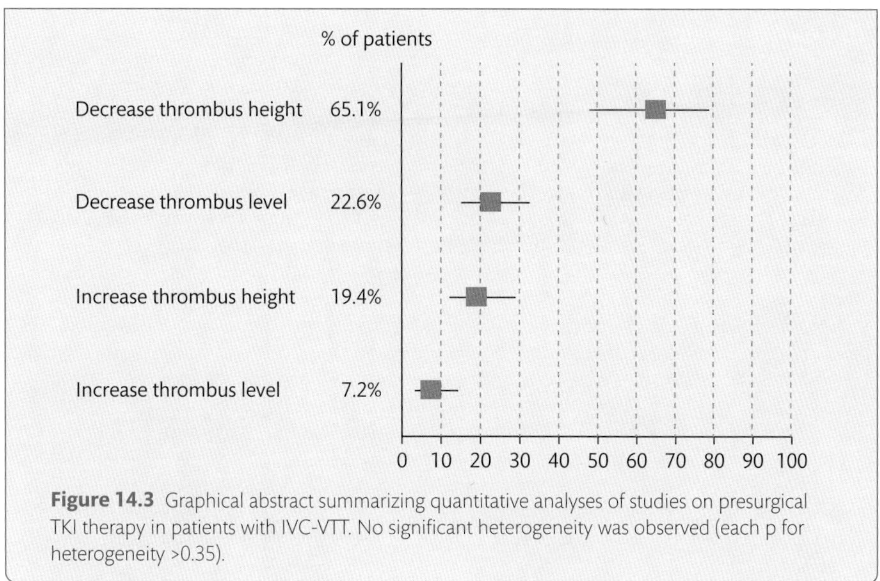

Figure 14.3 Graphical abstract summarizing quantitative analyses of studies on presurgical TKI therapy in patients with IVC-VTT. No significant heterogeneity was observed (each p for heterogeneity >0.35).

The patient was placed in the supine position. Antibiotic prophylaxis with 160 mg of gentamicin was given. Laparotomy was performed using a rooftop incision. A Thompson retractor was placed. The right hemicolon and hepatic flexure were mobilized off Gerota's fascia. The small bowel was mobilized and the duodenum Kocherized. Hepatic ligaments and adhesions between the lower margin of the liver and Gerota's fascia were then divided. The supra- and infrarenal vena cava and the left renal vein were then fully exposed, and slings were passed around these structures (Figure 14.4a). The renal artery was identified in the inter-aortocaval groove and divided between polyglactin 1 ties. Lumbar veins were divided between polyglactin 4-0 ties. The kidney was then fully mobilized. Intraoperative ultrasound was applied, confirming infrahepatic tumour thrombus. A tourniquet was applied around the proximal and distal cava and the left renal vein. An elliptic incision was made around the right renal vein ostium and extended 4 cm cephalad using Potts scissors. The right kidney, right renal vein, and the IVC thrombus were then removed en bloc (Figure 14.4b,c). The lumen of the cava was irrigated using heparinized saline and subsequently closed with a running Prolene® 4-0 suture. The tourniquets were released and no bleeding encountered. The wound was closed in 2 layers using running polydioxanone 1. The intraoperative blood loss was 400 mL, and the operating time was 210 minutes.

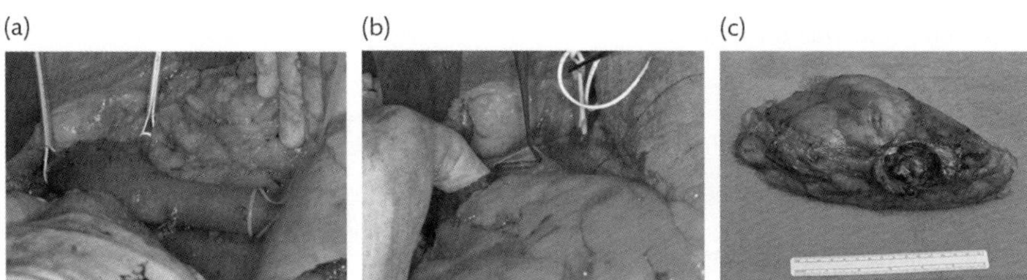

Figure 14.4 Intraoperative images. (a) Control of the infrarenal and suprarenal vena cava and left renal vein with slings, which will be used as tourniquet. All lumbar veins have been divided at this stage. (b) After cavotomy, the tumour thrombus is removed. (c) The renal tumour was excised in continuity with the thrombus. Reproduced with permission.[1]

Expert comment Approach to VTT surgery

- We usually provide venous thromboembolism prophylaxis prior to surgery using heparin.
- A midline incision is my preferred approach, it provides quick entry and closure, as well as excellent access to the retroperitoneum, especially when coupled with a Thompson retractor. In rare cases where more cranial extension is needed, the skin can be opened for another 5 cm and the xiphoid process can be resected, which allows for even more retraction and exposure.
- It is important to control and divide all short hepatic veins for level II thrombi in order to allow full mobilization of the IVC as cranial as possible caudal to the major hepatic veins.
- I fully mobilize the IVC after the right renal artery has been controlled. This can be achieved early in the surgery after identifying the left renal vein, cleaning the preaortic nodes, lifting the left renal vein anteriorly with a vein retractor, then finding the right renal artery posterior to the left renal vein, which is the safest location for control in IVC thrombectomy surgeries. After the right renal artery is controlled and divided, the IVC is isolated cranially and caudally, and so is the left renal vein, with vessel loops or umbilical tapes placed loosely placed around these structures.
- We generally leave the kidney *in situ* without any mobilization in order to minimize the risk of tumour thrombus embolization, which could occur during handling of the kidney.
- For cranial IVC control, we generally use a clamp instead of a tourniquet as sometimes we need to resect more IVC wall cranially that planned for/expected, and this would be more stable compared to a tourniquet which could become loose if the IVC is opened too close to it. This can be used for caudal IVC control as well.
- I generally use a 15-blade to perform the cavotomy as it is less likely to violate the tumour thrombus when opening the IVC wall, given the blade's convex shape (in contradistinction to an 11-blade, for example).
- It is helpful to have in the surgical set reverse Potts scissors in addition to regular Potts scissors to allow for more versatility in the resection of IVC wall. It is very important to resect the renal vein ostium. A bovine pericardium patch should be available on standby in these types of surgeries in case the IVC wall is resected more than expected preoperatively.
- It is helpful to have a No. 1 Penfield dissector available for this surgery, as it is a very useful tool to dissect an adherent thrombus away from IVC wall.
- My preference for caval closure is to use two separate Prolene® sutures, one starting from each corner of the cavotomy and then tied together. Some additional manoeuvres that can be used is to put the table in Trendelenburg position and opening the clamps temporarily prior to tying the Prolene® sutures in order to minimize the risk of embolism. If already in use, transoesophageal echocardiography can be used to check the heart for air when this is done.

Pathology showed a clear cell RCC with invasion of the perirenal fat, renal sinus fat, and the collecting system. As the thrombus extended into the infra-diaphragmatic cava but not the caval wall, the final T classification was 3b. The maximum size of the primary tumour was 9 cm. There were areas of coagulative tumour necrosis. Tumour cell nucleoli were eosinophilic and clearly visible at 100 × magnification. There was no sarcomatoid or rhabdoid dedifferentiation. The final International Society of Urological Pathology (ISUP) grade was 3. The tumour did not reach the perirenal resection margin. There were ten negative lymph nodes. The final stage was T3bN0M0, and the Leibovich score was 6 ('high risk').

Learning point Risk stratification

An accurate prediction of the individual probability of recurrence based on multivariable prognostic models is essential to counsel patients, individualize surveillance, and select patients for adjuvant clinical trials. The Leibovich prognostic score[24] and the University of California Integrated Staging System (UISS)[25] are the most commonly used postoperative prognostic models and can be assigned from routine clinicopathological data (Table 14.2).[26] The Leibovich score does include patients with N+ disease, while UISS treats those as metastatic. While the Leibovich score was developed for clear cell RCC, UISS includes all RCC subtypes.

Table 14.2 The Leibovich score and UISS for postoperative risk stratification of clinically localized renal cell carcinoma

Name	Feature		Points
Leibovich Score (T1–4N any M0)	T classification	T1a	0
		T1b	2
		T2	3
		T3 or T4	4
	N classification	pNx or pN0	0
		pN+	2
	Tumour size	<10 cm	0
		≥10 cm	1
	Nuclear grade	G1 or G2	0
		G3	1
		G4	3
	Tumour necrosis	Absent	0
		Present	1
	Stratification based on total points	0–2	Low risk
		3–5	Intermediate risk
		6–11	High risk
UISS (T1–4N0M0)	T1, grade 1–2, ECOG PS 0		Low risk
	T1, grade 1–2, ECOG PS ≥1		Intermediate risk
	T1, grade 3–4, any ECOG PS		Intermediate risk
	T2, any grade, any ECOG PS		Intermediate risk
	T3, grade 1, any ECOG PS		Intermediate risk
	T3, grade 2–4, ECOG PS 0		Intermediate risk
	T3, grade 2–4, ECOG PS ≥1		High risk
	T4, any grade, any ECOG PS		High risk

ECOG, Eastern Cooperative Oncology Group; PS, performance status.
Adapted from reference[26].

The postoperative course was uneventful and the patient was discharged home on postoperative day 5. He completed a 28-day course of subcutaneous low-molecular-weight heparin injections. Following release of the pathology report, the case was re-discussed at the MDT meeting. The panel recommended 'high-risk follow-up' and offered participation in an adjuvant clinical trial. The patient was counselled that the risk of disease recurrence is approximately 50%.

Learning point Surveillance and adjuvant therapy

At present, postoperative surveillance remains the standard of care for patients with completely resected non-metastatic RCC. There is little evidence in this field and therefore little agreement among professional bodies regarding the optimal surveillance regimen. The authors of this case follow the EAU schedule (Table 14.3).[27]

Adjuvant trials are typically superiority placebo-controlled clinical phase III trials, which are initiated following successful drug testing in the metastatic setting. There have been numerous investigations over the past decades on a range of interventions, including radiotherapy, hormone therapy, cytokines, and vaccines. Many of these trials were underpowered and, with the exception of one vaccine trial,[28] none produced convincing data of benefit. Several trials investigating the use of TKIs and mammalian target of rapamycin inhibitors are now published or currently in follow-up (Table 14.4).[29–32] Only one trial (S-TRAC[29]) showed an improvement in disease-free survival (of 1.2-year delay in progression for 1 year of sunitinib therapy), adjuvant therapy with TKI is therefore not recommended by the European Association of Urology guidelines panel.[27] Recently, adjuvant pembrolizumab at a dose of 200 mg once every 3 weeks for up to 17 cycles (approximately 1 year) improved disease-free survival

Table 14.3 Surveillance schedule proposed by the European Association of Urology

Risk profile	Surveillance schedule				
	6 months	1 year	2 years	3 years	>3 years
Low	Ultrasound	CT	Ultrasound	CT	CT once every 2 years; counsel about recurrence risk of ~10%
Intermediate/high	CT	CT	CT	CT	CT once every 2 years

Table 14.4 Overview of adjuvant trials with TKIs and mTOR inhibitors

Trial and identifier	Arms	N	Subtype	Outcome
ASSURE NCT00326898	Sunitinib vs sorafenib vs placebo for 1 year	1943	Clear cell or non-clear cell	No improvement in disease-free or overall survival[29]
ATLAS NCT01599754	Axitinib vs placebo for 3 years	724	Clear cell	No improvement in disease-free survival[30]
PROTECT NCT01235962	Pazopanib vs placebo for 1 year	1500	Clear cell	No improvement in disease-free survival[31]
S-TRAC NCT00375674	Sunitinib vs placebo for 1 year	615	Clear cell	Improvement in disease-free survival, no improvement in overall survival[32]
EVEREST NCT01120249	Everolimus vs placebo for 1 year	1545	Clear cell or non-clear cell	In follow-up, results not available yet
SORCE NCT00492258	Sorafenib vs placebo for 1–3 years	1656	Clear cell or non-clear cell	In follow-up, results not available yet

mTOR, mechanistic target of rapamycin.

in patients with high-risk clear cell renal cell carcinoma compared to placebo.[33] Final overall survival data are not available yet. The Renal Cell Carcinoma European Association of Urology guidelines panel issued a weak recommendation for the adjuvant use of pembrolizumab.[34] It is worth noting that several other adjuvant immune-oncological trials are currently recruiting patients. Ongoing trials involve nivolumab (PROSPER RCC), atezolizumab (IMMotion010), nivolumab plus ipilimumab (CheckMate 914), and durvalumab/durvalumab plus tremelimumab (RAMPART). Many of these agents and combinations showed impressive clinical activity in metastatic RCC.

A final word from the expert

IVC tumour thrombectomy is still a tremendous operation with potential for mortality and morbidity. Urological surgeon experience is paramount to the success of this operation. Appropriate preoperative evaluation (clinical, radiographic, anaesthetic, and cardiac) and a MDT approach are also crucial to achieve optimal outcomes. While this surgery is being done with robotic assistance more frequently, the standard of care is still open surgery, which allows handling of vascular and cardiac emergencies in an expeditious manner. It is ideal to concentrate the performance of IVC tumour thrombectomies to a few urologists in each department in order to optimize their experience and minimize intraoperative and postoperative complications, and to achieve complete resection of all tumour. Since most of these patients (if they present without metastatic disease) are at high risk of recurrence, they should be offered adjuvant therapy (where approved), and an adjuvant clinical trial (where available). Alternatively, careful surveillance should be performed.

References

1. Sut M, Riddick ACP. Management of renal cell carcinoma with vena cava involvement. BJUI Knowledge. 26 April 2017. https://www.bjuiknowledge.org/modules/management-renal-cell-carcinoma-vena-cava-involvement/
2. Goldfarb DA, Novick AC, Lorig R, et al. Magnetic resonance imaging for assessment of vena caval tumor thrombi: a comparative study with venacavography and computerized tomography scanning. *J Urol.* 1990;144(5):1100–1114.
3. Hallscheidt PJ, Fink C, Haferkamp A, et al. Preoperative staging of renal cell carcinoma with inferior vena cava thrombus using multidetector CT and MRI: prospective study with histopathological correlation. *J Comput Assist Tomogr.* 2005;29(1):64–68.
4. Lawrentschuk N, Gani J, Riordan R, Esler S, Bolton DM. Multidetector computed tomography vs magnetic resonance imaging for defining the upper limit of tumour thrombus in renal cell carcinoma: a study and review. *BJU Int.* 2005;96(3):291–295.
5. Guo H, Song Y, Na Y. Value of abdominal ultrasound scan, CT and MRI for diagnosing inferior vena cava tumour thrombus in renal cell carcinoma. *Chin Med J (Engl).* 2009;122(19):2299–2302.
6. Guzzo TJ, Pierorazio PM, Schaeffer EM, Fishman EK, Allaf ME. The accuracy of multidetector computerized tomography for evaluating tumor thrombus in patients with renal cell carcinoma. *J Urol.* 2009;181(2):486–491.
7. Zini L, Destrieux-Garnier L, Leroy X, et al. Renal vein ostium wall invasion of renal cell carcinoma with an inferior vena cava tumor thrombus: prediction by renal and vena caval vein diameters and prognostic significance. *J Urol.* 2008;179(2):450–454.
8. Psutka SP, Boorjian SA, Thompson RH, et al. Clinical and radiographic predictors of the need for inferior vena cava resection during nephrectomy for patients with renal cell carcinoma and caval tumour thrombus. *BJU Int.* 2015;116(3):388–396.
9. Kallman DA, King BF, Hattery RR, et al. Renal vein and inferior vena cava tumor thrombus in renal cell carcinoma: CT, US, MRI and venacavography. *J Comput Assist Tomogr.* 1992;16(2):240–247.
10. Glazer A, Novick AC. Preoperative transesophageal echocardiography for assessment of vena caval tumor thrombi: a comparative study with venacavography and magnetic resonance imaging. *Urology.* 1997;49(1):32–34.
11. Calderone CE, Tuck BC, Gray SH, Porter KK, Rais-Bahrami S. The role of transesophageal echocardiography in the management of renal cell carcinoma with venous tumor thrombus. *Echocardiogr Mt Kisco N.* 2018;35(12):2047–2055.
12. Ganeshalingam S, Koh DM. Nodal staging. *Cancer Imaging.* 2009;9(1):104–111.
13. Gershman B, Takahashi N, Moreira DM, et al. Radiographic size of retroperitoneal lymph nodes predicts pathological nodal involvement for patients with renal cell carcinoma: development of a risk prediction model. *BJU Int.* 2016;118(5):742–749.
14. Brierley JD, Gospodarowicz MK, Wittekind C. *TNM Classification of Malignant Tumours.* 8th ed. Chichester: Wiley Blackwell; 2017.
15. Neves RJ, Zincke H. Surgical treatment of renal cancer with vena cava extension. *Br J Urol.* 1987;59(5):390–395.
16. Cost NG, Delacroix SE, Sleeper JP, et al. The impact of targeted molecular therapies on the level of renal cell carcinoma vena caval tumor thrombus. *Eur Urol.* 2011;59(6):912–918.
17. Bigot P, Fardoun T, Bernhard JC, et al. Neoadjuvant targeted molecular therapies in patients undergoing nephrectomy and inferior vena cava thrombectomy: is it useful? *World J Urol.* 2014;32(1):109–114.

18. Peng C, Gu L, Wang L, et al. Role of presurgical targeted molecular therapy in renal cell carcinoma with an inferior vena cava tumor thrombus. *Onco Targets Ther.* 2018;11:1997–2005.
19. Fukuda H, Kondo T, Takagi T, Iizuka J, Nagashima Y, Tanabe K. Limited benefit of targeted molecular therapy for inferior vena cava thrombus associated with renal cell carcinoma. *Int J Clin Oncol.* 2017;22(4):767–773.
20. Ujike T, Uemura M, Kawashima A, et al. Clinical and histopathological effects of presurgical treatment with sunitinib for renal cell carcinoma with inferior vena cava tumor thrombus at a single institution. *Anticancer Drugs.* 2016;27(10):1038–1043.
21. Horn T, Thalgott MK, Maurer T, et al. Presurgical treatment with sunitinib for renal cell carcinoma with a level III/IV vena cava tumour thrombus. *Anticancer Res.* 2012;32(5):1729–1735.
22. Tanaka Y, Hatakeyama S, Hosogoe S, et al. Presurgical axitinib therapy increases fibrotic reactions within tumor thrombus in renal cell carcinoma with thrombus extending to the inferior vena cava. *Int J Clin Oncol.* 2018;23(1):134–141.
23. Terakawa T, Hussein AA, Bando Y, et al. Presurgical pazopanib for renal cell carcinoma with inferior vena caval thrombus: a single-institution study. *Anticancer Drugs.* 2018;29(6):565–571.
24. Leibovich BC, Blute ML, Cheville JC, et al. Prediction of progression after radical nephrectomy for patients with clear cell renal cell carcinoma: a stratification tool for prospective clinical trials. *Cancer.* 2003;97(7):1663–1671.
25. Zisman A, Pantuck AJ, Wieder J, et al. Risk group assessment and clinical outcome algorithm to predict the natural history of patients with surgically resected renal cell carcinoma. *J Clin Oncol.* 2002;20(23):4559–4566.
26. Klatte T, Rossi SH, Stewart GD. Prognostic factors and prognostic models for renal cell carcinoma: a literature review. *World J Urol.* 2018;36(12):1943–1952.
27. Ljungberg B, Albiges L, Abu-Ghanem Y, et al. European Association of Urology guidelines on renal cell carcinoma: the 2019 update. *Eur Urol.* 2019;75(5):799–810.
28. Jocham D, Richter A, Hoffmann L, et al. Adjuvant autologous renal tumour cell vaccine and risk of tumour progression in patients with renal-cell carcinoma after radical nephrectomy: phase III, randomised controlled trial. *Lancet.* 2004;363(9409):594–599.
29. Haas NB, Manola J, Uzzo RG, et al. Adjuvant sunitinib or sorafenib for high-risk, non-metastatic renal-cell carcinoma (ECOG-ACRIN E2805): a double-blind, placebo-controlled, randomised, phase 3 trial. *Lancet.* 2016;387(10032):2008–2016.
30. Gross-Goupil M, Kwon TG, Eto M, et al. Axitinib versus placebo as an adjuvant treatment of renal cell carcinoma: results from the phase III, randomized ATLAS trial. *Ann Oncol.* 2018;29(12):2371–2378.
31. Motzer RJ, Haas NB, Donskov F, et al. Randomized phase III trial of adjuvant pazopanib versus placebo after nephrectomy in patients with localized or locally advanced renal cell carcinoma. *J Clin Oncol.* 2017;35(35):3916–3923.
32. Ravaud A, Motzer RJ, Pandha HS, et al. Adjuvant sunitinib in high-risk renal-cell carcinoma after nephrectomy. *N Engl J Med.* 2016;375(23):2246–2254.
33. Chouieiri et al. Adjuvant Pembrolizumab after Nephrectomy in Renal-Cell Carcinoma. *N Engl J Med.* 2021;385(8):683–694.
34. Bedke et al. Updated European Association of Urology Guidelines on the Use of Adjuvant Pembrolizumab for Renal Cell Carcinoma. *Eur Urol.* 2021;81(2):134–137.

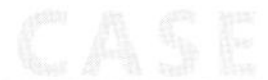

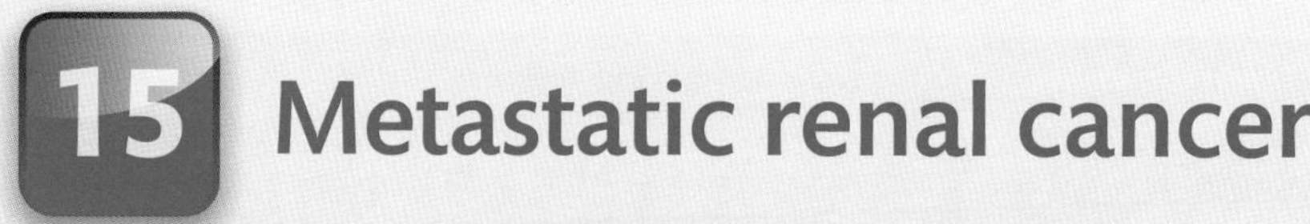

15 Metastatic renal cancer

Joana B. Neves and Maxine G. B. Tran

Expert commentary Axel Bex

Case history

A 43-year-old previously fit male presented with intermittent abdominal discomfort for the previous 2 years, with symptomatic worsening in the previous months. He had no family history of kidney cancer, tuberous sclerosis, or epilepsy. On examination, a palpable abdominal mass was felt. On cross-sectional imaging of chest, abdomen, and pelvis, a large tumour was found in the right kidney, measuring 24 cm in the largest axis (Figure 15.1). There was no clinical evidence of invasion of the renal vein or adjacent structures, or of macroscopic metastatic disease. A right open radical nephrectomy was planned.

Clinical tip Signs and symptoms of renal masses

The classical triad of visible haematuria, flank pain, and a palpable abdominal mass associated with renal tumours is most frequently seen with large tumours. These signs can also be present independently. On physical examination, a varicocele in males can indicate renal vein invasion. Constitutional symptoms can be present. Less frequently, a renal tumour can be found in the investigation of paraneoplastic syndromes such as secondary polycythaemia or hyper-reninemia. Otherwise, the majority of renal tumours are small, localized, and clinically silent.[1]

Learning point The role of surgery in large renal masses

For patients diagnosed with large renal tumours that are suspected renal cell carcinoma (RCC) and appear to be localized (cM0), the standardized curative approach is radical nephrectomy. Whenever possible, minimally invasive (laparoscopy and robot-assisted surgery) surgical approaches tend to be preferred due to observational evidence pointing towards reduced length of hospital stay, reduced blood loss, lower analgesic use, and faster postoperative recovery.[2]

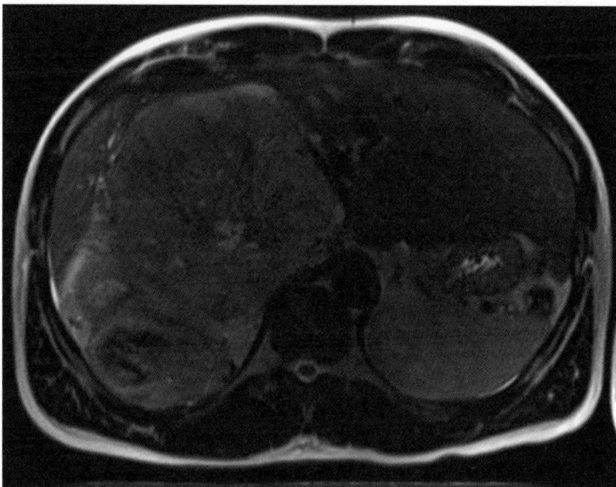

Figure 15.1 Magnetic resonance axial image at diagnosis depicting the large renal mass abutting the liver (T2-weighted sequence).

Expert comment Minimally invasive and open approaches

Although there is no tumour size threshold to advise between minimally invasive and open approaches, minimally invasive surgery for large tumours (>10 cm) is likely to be technically more challenging due to space limitations and will require a large incision for tumour removal, thus a traditional open approach can be more appropriate.

Intraoperatively, the decision to also perform ipsilateral adrenalectomy and lymphadenectomy was done for the presented case. Surgery was complicated by intraoperative injury to liver segments V and VIII, which were superficial and managed conservatively. There was no evidence of capsular breach or tumour spillage intraoperatively (Figure 15.2).

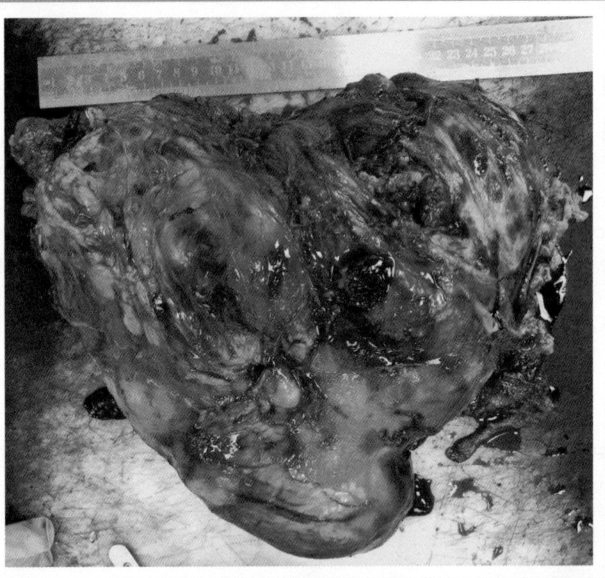

Figure 15.2 Surgical specimen.

Evidence base Lymph node dissection for non-urothelial renal tumours

A randomized controlled trial and systematic review question the impact on oncological outcomes of lymph node dissection at the time of nephrectomy.[3,4] Thus, the trade-off between potential surgical complications from performing lymphadenectomy and oncological benefit for cases where no clinical suspicious nodes are found, does not seem warranted.

However, when clinical suspicion of node-positive disease on cross-sectional imaging or intraoperatively is present, consideration should be given to performing the additional procedure as there are observational data suggesting an increased cancer-specific survival when more than ten nodes are removed and node-positive disease is confirmed.[5]

Evidence base Adrenalectomy for non-urothelial renal tumours

Traditionally, ipsilateral adrenalectomy was an integral component of radical nephrectomy. Adrenal involvement by disease is rare and no beneficial oncological impact has been documented from performing adrenalectomy.[6] Currently, the adrenal is preserved unless there is clinical suspicion of involvement (either preoperatively on staging imaging or intraoperatively).

Evidence base Adjuvant therapies for non-urothelial renal tumours

The ASSURE,[7] PROTECT,[8] SORCE,[9] and S-TRAC[10] randomized controlled trials have addressed the issue of adjuvant therapy for RCC, showing no survival benefit of additional systemic treatment with tyrosine kinase inhibitors after surgery for intermediate or high-risk cases.

To date, in Europe no adjuvant therapies have been approved for RCC or other kidney tumours. In the US, based on disease-free survival data for high-risk patients on S-TRAC, sunitinib (a tyrosine kinase inhibitor with anti-vascular endothelial growth factor activity) has been approved by the Food and Drug Administration as adjuvant therapy.

A diagnosis of epithelioid angiomyolipoma (AML) was histologically confirmed after analysis of the surgical specimen. The tumour replaced almost all of the kidney; it was macroscopically a multinodular brownish mass with extensive necrotic areas and an ill-defined border. Maximal diameter of the tumour was 240 mm and it weighed 2980 g. Microscopically, it exhibited a classical triphasic structure composed of smooth muscle, adipose tissue, and blood vessels, intermingled with areas of polygonal epithelioid cells with mild atypia and of bizarre multinucleated epithelioid giant cells. Mitotic figures, including atypical forms, were present, as was coagulative necrosis. The tumour had little recognizable fat. On immunohistochemical analysis, the tumour was positive for Melan A, HMB45, smooth muscle actin (SMA), and vimentin. There was weak positivity for CD117, e-cadherin, and AMRC. PAX8, CAIX, RCC, CK7 were negative. Excision was deemed complete but the tumour was found to be invading the hilar and perinephric adipose tissue, as well as the renal vein. Fourteen nodes were retrieved (one hilar, 12 paracaval, and one mesenteric), all free of disease. No adrenal metastasis was found.

Expert comment Histological considerations

Most adult kidney tumours are of epithelial origin, with the most common subtype being clear cell (cc) RCC. The other 14 subtypes of RCC according to the last 2016 World Health Organization (WHO) pathology classification,[11] are collectively termed non-clear cell RCC. In addition, there are also other types of kidney tumours, usually rare, that have mesenchymal origin or mixed epithelial and mesenchymal origins.

Most available evidence on disease management for patients with renal tumours derives largely from data in the context of RCC or, more frequently, ccRCC. This poses additional complexities when deciding the management of renal tumours of mesenchymal origin and consideration of referral to a tertiary specialist centre should be given.

Learning point Characteristics of epithelioid AMLs

Renal AMLs are lesions composed of varied proportions of classical smooth muscle cells, mature adipocytes (fat cells), pericytes (also known as perivascular epithelioid cells), and thick-walled, irregular, blood vessels. They represent one of the most frequent benign kidney masses, and the most frequent renal benign lesion of mesenchymal origin. Atypical AMLs have been described, including oncocytoma-like AMLs and epithelioid AMLs.

Epithelioid AMLs are rare, are described as a separate entity to AMLs since the 2004 WHO pathology classification,[12] and have a morphology that can resemble high-grade RCC or RCC with sarcomatoid differentiation. Microscopically, the predominance of epithelioid cells (cells of neural crest origin, thought to be the precursor cell also in classical AMLs), the low-fat cell content, and cytologic atypia are the main features distinguishing epithelioid AMLs from classical AMLs.

Tumours thought to originate from perivascular epithelioid cells (PECs), such as classical and epithelioid AMLs belong to the PEComa family.[13-16]

Microscopic features

- Predominant epithelioid cells with spindle cell morphology, clear or eosinophilic cytoplasm, with large nuclei and prominent eosinophilic nucleoli (according to the 2016 WHO pathology classification, the diagnostic criteria for epithelioid AML include >80% of the tumour to be composed of these cells[11]).[13–16]
- Epithelioid cells are admixed with lymphocytes and sit close to thick-walled blood vessels (perivascular).
- Multinucleate, pleomorphic enlarged ganglion-like cells.
- Low adipose cell content.

Typical immunoreactivity

- Positive for melanocytic markers such as HMB-45, HMB-50, Melan-A, microphthalmia transcription factor; variable positivity for mesenchymal markers such as SMA.[13–15]
- Negative for epithelial markers such as cytokeratins and epithelial membrane antigen.

Expert comment Radiological appearances of AML

Radiologically, the presence of epithelioid AML can be suspected when fat-containing lesions suggestive of AMLs have a large solid component. However, this feature is not pathognomonic. Frequently, the fat content in epithelioid AMLs can be low enough not to be distinguishable on cross-sectional imaging. Likewise, they can also be radiologically indistinguishable from classical AMLs.[14,17,18]

Given the understanding of the potential malignant behaviour of epithelioid AMLs, as well as the presence of poor prognostic features, the patient was offered postoperative surveillance. This was accomplished with a first scan at 6 months and another at 12 months, with a plan to continue yearly surveillance for 5 years postoperatively.

One year after surgery, the finding of an ill-defined heterogeneous lesion arising in the right nephrectomy bed abutting the right portal vein and encasing the inferior vena cava, left renal vein, and common hepatic artery was documented. There were also large nodal deposits lying against the psoas muscle measuring at least 6 cm and multiple liver hypodensities with peripheral arterial enhancement seen at the caudate lobe and segments IV, V, VI, and VII, consistent with metastatic deposits (Figure 15.3). The chest was clear.

Evidence base Features associated with potential malignant behaviour in epithelioid AMLs

- Most of the tumour composed of epithelioid cells (published thresholds vary between >70% and >95%).[20,22]
- Presence of coagulative necrosis.[20–23]
- Perinephric fat invasion.[20,23]
- Renal vein invasion.[20,22]
- More than two mitotic figures per ten high-power fields.[21]
- Atypical mitotic activity.[21]
- Large size (published thresholds vary between >7 cm or >9 cm).[20,22,23]
- Confirmed tuberous sclerosis (TS) syndrome or presence of concomitant classical AML.[20]

Learning point Malignant behaviour of epithelioid AMLs

Epithelioid AMLs can display malignant behaviour and metastasize in up to a third of cases, shortening life expectancy.[13,19–23] Metastasis occurs most frequently to the liver, lungs, and to regional lymph nodes. The same clonal genetic profile between primary and metastatic lesions has been documented in a case report.[24]

(a)

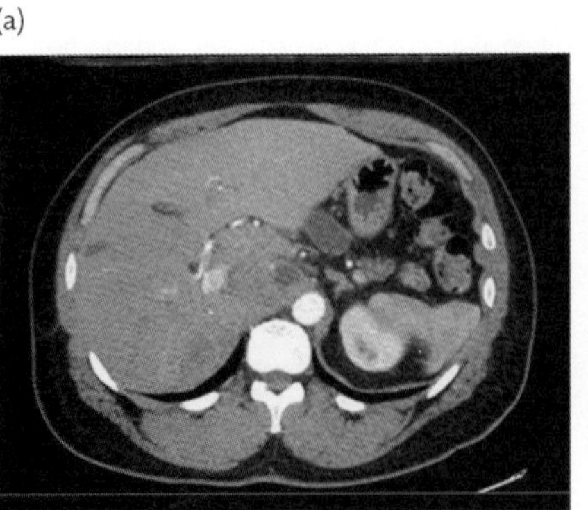

(b)

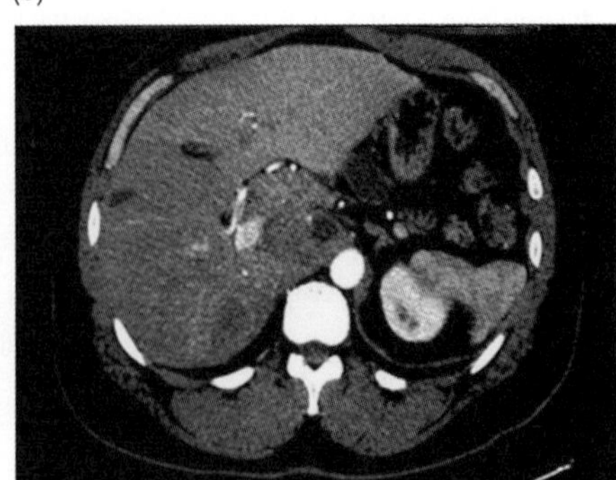

Figure 15.3 Computed tomography axial images at the time of regional and metastatic (liver) disease recurrence. Arterial phase, (a) abdomen window; (b) liver window.

Evidence base Genetic hallmarks of epithelioid AMLs

Classical AMLs can be associated with TS syndrome, an autosomal dominant disease associated with mutations of the *TSC1* and *TSC2* genes and consequent perturbation of the mammalian target of rapamycin (mTOR) signalling pathway. Likewise, epithelioid AMLs can be sporadic in up to three quarter of cases.[13,15,20] Similar to sporadic classical AMLs, sporadic epithelioid AMLs are also commonly associated with mutations in the *TSC* genes[25,26] and activation of the mTORC1 pathway can be documented using immunohistochemistry.[26,27]

Genetically, silencing of TP53 is a distinguishing feature between classical and epithelioid AMLs, attesting to the potential malignant transformation seen in these atypical cases.[13,28,29]

Biopsy-proven liver metastases were diagnosed. Due to the high metastatic burden, local management of metastasis with surgery or radiotherapy was not appropriate. The patient's care was transferred to the oncology team, with a view to starting systemic therapy.

Expert comment Biopsy of metastatic lesions

Biopsy of suspected kidney cancer-associated metastatic lesions, especially in the context of disease of low metastatic potential, can be useful in guiding disease management and ascertain the need for further treatment.

Expert comment Prognostic features

Radical nephrectomy for large renal tumours can be a challenging procedure and in the presented case there was intraoperative liver injury (segments V and VIII). Despite tumour resection margins being reported as clear, and no intraoperative spillage of tumour, renal bed recurrence, liver metastasis (caudate lobe and segments IV, V, VI, and VII), as well as lymph node metastasis developed during the first 12 months following surgery.

Poor prognostic features on histology (presence of mitotic figures, which were atypical, coagulative necrosis, and perinephric adipose tissue and renal vein invasion) point towards aggressive disease biology, and progression of disease to the liver and lymph nodes is frequently found in metastatic epithelioid AMLs.[20]

Evidence base Systemic therapy for kidney cancer

Until recently, the management of advanced kidney cancer has been disappointing. Primary renal malignancies were recognized as radio- and chemoresistant entities. A breakthrough arose 40 years ago, with the realization that immune modulation using intravenous interleukin-2, despite its high-risk side effect profile, was useful in this arena.[30] Insights into the biology of von Hippel–Lindau syndrome led to the recognition of the role of hypoxia-inducible factor pathway activation as a driver event in ccRCC, and to the approval of antiangiogenic drugs in 2006, the first of which was sunitinib.[31] Shortly after, the mTOR pathway inhibitors temsirolimus and everolimus arrived on the scene.[32]

Currently, the development of a new form of immune modulation via checkpoint inhibition, has once again changed the management of metastatic RCC and these drugs are now the first-line option for intermediate- and high-risk cases.[33]

Currently, no phase III trials have been reported for metastatic kidney tumours that are not ccRCC.[34] Again, this exposes the current difficulties in managing rarer metastatic kidney tumours.

Evidence base Systemic therapy for malignant epithelioid AMLs

A recent multicentre observational retrospective study evaluated the oncological outcomes of four systemic therapy regimens (anthracycline based, gemcitabine based, vascular endothelial growth factor inhibitor, and mTOR inhibitors) in 53 patients with locally advanced or metastatic PEComas, 11 of whom had epithelioid AMLs.[35] The best response rate and progression-free survival were achieved with mTOR inhibition (76.9% and 9 months respectively). Sarcoma chemotherapy regimens had the lowest responses. Dramatic tumour responses of metastatic epithelioid AMLs to mTOR inhibitors[25,26,36,37] have also been reported previously.

Evidence base Local management of recurrent and metastatic lesions of renal primary lesions

There is observational evidence pointing towards an oncological benefit of excising isolated local RCC recurrences.[38] Likewise, for RCC cases with low metastatic burden amenable to metastasectomy of all deposits, observational data indicate improved oncological outcomes and delay of start of systemic therapy.[39]

Discussion

The initial management of a clinically localised large renal tumour is mainly surgical. It is clear for malignant cases that postoperative follow-up with imaging is required to detect early or late metastatic spread. However, follow-up guidelines are less defined for cases such as epithelioid AMLs, which are not definitely classified as malignant. In the case presented, the previous knowledge that these lesions have potential malignant behaviour, the size of the primary, and the presence of poor prognostic features indicated the need for postoperative surveillance. Indeed, the patient developed local and distant recurrence which was not amenable to surgical management and systemic therapies had to be considered.

The paucity of studies dedicated to histological subtypes other than ccRCC and the consequent lack of high-level evidence introduce many uncertainties to the management of patients with rare kidney tumour subtypes. Surgical management should be the standard management option in non-metastatic disease and can also be considered in locally recurrent or metastatic disease amenable to complete disease clearance. The systemic therapies approved for ccRCC have often been untested in rarer subtypes. In the case of epithelioid AMLs, there is a plausible biological rationale and real-world evidence that treatment with mTOR inhibitors may improve oncological outcomes for patients with metastatic disease.

A final word from the expert

In recent years, tremendous advances have been made on the morphologic reclassification of renal tumours, as well as the understanding of renal tumour genomics. The number of tumour subtypes seems to be increasing but research is still very much focused on ccRCC. Due to this, the 'one-size-fits-all' approach is still being used for the management of rarer cancer subtypes, which may have distinct natural histories and molecular drivers. The conversation and research on renal tumours need to be broadened. The clinical and scientific community needs to establish international collaborations to drive the discovery of molecular drivers and the development of tailored approaches for rare renal tumour subtypes.

References

1. Lee CT, Katz J, Fearn PA, Russo P. Mode of presentation of renal cell carcinoma provides prognostic information. *Urol Oncol.* 2002;7(4):135–140.
2. MacLennan S, Imamura M, Lapitan MC, et al. Systematic review of oncological outcomes following surgical management of localised renal cancer. *Eur Urol.* 2012;61(5):972–993.
3. Blom JH, van Poppel H, Marechal JM, et al. Radical nephrectomy with and without lymph-node dissection: final results of European Organization for Research and Treatment of Cancer (EORTC) randomized phase 3 trial 30881. *Eur Urol.* 2009;55(1):28–34.

4. Bhindi B, Wallis CJD, Boorjian SA, et al. The role of lymph node dissection in the management of renal cell carcinoma: a systematic review and meta-analysis. *BJU Int.* 2018;121(5):684–698.
5. Whitson JM, Harris CR, Reese AC, Meng MV. Lymphadenectomy improves survival of patients with renal cell carcinoma and nodal metastases. *J Urol.* 2011;185(5):1615–1620.
6. Weight CJ, Mulders PF, Pantuck AJ, Thompson RH. The role of adrenalectomy in renal cancer. *Eur Urol Focus.* 2016;1(3):251–257.
7. Haas NB, Manola J, Uzzo RG, et al. Adjuvant sunitinib or sorafenib for high-risk, non-metastatic renal-cell carcinoma (ECOG-ACRIN E2805): a double-blind, placebo-controlled, randomised, phase 3 trial. *Lancet.* 2016;387(10032):2008–2016.
8. Motzer RJ, Haas NB, Donskov F, et al. Randomized phase III trial of adjuvant pazopanib versus placebo after nephrectomy in patients with localized or locally advanced renal cell carcinoma. *J Clin Oncol.* 2017;35(35):3916–3923.
9. Eisen TQG, Frangou E, Smith B, et al. LBA56Primary efficacy analysis results from the SORCE trial (RE05): adjuvant sorafenib for renal cell carcinoma at intermediate or high risk of relapse: an international, randomised double-blind phase III trial led by the MRC CTU at UCL. *Ann Oncol.* 2019;30:v891–v892.
10. Ravaud A, Motzer RJ, Pandha HS, et al. Adjuvant sunitinib in high-risk renal-cell carcinoma after nephrectomy. *N Engl J Med.* 2016;375(23):2246–2254.
11. Moch H, Humphrey PA, Ulbright TM, Reuter VE, eds. *WHO Classification of Tumours of the Urinary System and Male Genital Organs.* 4th ed. Lyon: IARC Press; 2016.
12. Eble JN, Sauter G, Epstein JI, Sesterhenn IA, eds. *Classification of Tumours: Pathology and Genetics of Tumours of the Urinary System and Male Genital Organs.* Lyon: IARC Press; 2004.
13. Mete O, van der Kwast TH. Epithelioid angiomyolipoma: a morphologically distinct variant that mimics a variety of intra-abdominal neoplasms. *Arch Pathol Lab Med.* 2011;135(5):665–670.
14. Cui L, Zhang JG, Hu XY, et al. CT imaging and histopathological features of renal epithelioid angiomyolipomas. *Clin Radiol.* 2012;67(12):e77–e82.
15. Aydin H, Magi-Galluzzi C, Lane BR, et al. Renal angiomyolipoma: clinicopathologic study of 194 cases with emphasis on the epithelioid histology and tuberous sclerosis association. *Am J Surg Pathol.* 2009;33(2):289–297.
16. He W, Cheville JC, Sadow PM, et al. Epithelioid angiomyolipoma of the kidney: pathological features and clinical outcome in a series of consecutively resected tumors. *Mod Pathol.* 2013;26(10):1355–1364.
17. Liu Y, Qu F, Cheng R, Ye Z. CT-imaging features of renal epithelioid angiomyolipoma. *World J Surg Oncol.* 2015;13:280.
18. Hassan M, El-Hefnawy AS, Elshal AM, Mosbah A, El-Baz M, Shaaban A. Renal epithelioid angiomyolipoma: a rare variant with unusual behavior. *Int Urol Nephrol.* 2014;46(2):317–322.
19. Ribalta T, Lloreta J, Munne A, Serrano S, Cardesa A. Malignant pigmented clear cell epithelioid tumor of the kidney: clear cell ('sugar') tumor versus malignant melanoma. *Hum Pathol.* 2000;31(4):516–519.
20. Nese N, Martignoni G, Fletcher CD, et al. Pure epithelioid PEComas (so-called epithelioid angiomyolipoma) of the kidney: a clinicopathologic study of 41 cases: detailed assessment of morphology and risk stratification. *Am J Surg Pathol.* 2011;35(2):161–176.
21. Brimo F, Robinson B, Guo C, Zhou M, Latour M, Epstein JI. Renal epithelioid angiomyolipoma with atypia: a series of 40 cases with emphasis on clinicopathologic prognostic indicators of malignancy. *Am J Surg Pathol.* 2010;34(5):715–722.
22. Lei JH, Liu LR, Wei Q, et al. A four-year follow-up study of renal epithelioid angiomyolipoma: a multi-center experience and literature review. *Sci Rep.* 2015;5:10030.
23. Zheng S, Bi XG, Song QK, et al. A suggestion for pathological grossing and reporting based on prognostic indicators of malignancies from a pooled analysis of renal epithelioid angiomyolipoma. *Int Urol Nephrol.* 2015;47(10):1643–1651.

24. Martignoni G, Pea M, Rigaud G, et al. Renal angiomyolipoma with epithelioid sarcomatous transformation and metastases: demonstration of the same genetic defects in the primary and metastatic lesions. *Am J Surg Pathol.* 2000;24(6):889–894.
25. Espinosa M, Roldan-Romero JM, Duran I, et al. Advanced sporadic renal epithelioid angiomyolipoma: case report of an extraordinary response to sirolimus linked to TSC2 mutation. *BMC Cancer.* 2018;18(1):561.
26. Wagner AJ, Malinowska-Kolodziej I, Morgan JA, et al. Clinical activity of mTOR inhibition with sirolimus in malignant perivascular epithelioid cell tumors: targeting the pathogenic activation of mTORC1 in tumors. *J Clin Oncol.* 2010;28(5):835–840.
27. Kenerson H, Folpe AL, Takayama TK, Yeung RS. Activation of the mTOR pathway in sporadic angiomyolipomas and other perivascular epithelioid cell neoplasms. *Hum Pathol.* 2007;38(9):1361–1371.
28. Kawaguchi K, Oda Y, Nakanishi K, et al. Malignant transformation of renal angiomyolipoma: a case report. *Am J Surg Pathol.* 2002;26(4):523–529.
29. Li W, Guo L, Bi X, Ma J, Zheng S. Immunohistochemistry of p53 and Ki-67 and p53 mutation analysis in renal epithelioid angiomyolipoma. *Int J Clin Exp Pathol.* 2015;8(8):9446–9451.
30. Bukowski RM. Natural history and therapy of metastatic renal cell carcinoma: the role of interleukin-2. *Cancer.* 1997;80(7):1198–1220.
31. Rock EP, Goodman V, Jiang JX, et al. Food and Drug Administration drug approval summary: sunitinib malate for the treatment of gastrointestinal stromal tumor and advanced renal cell carcinoma. *Oncologist.* 2007;12(1):107–113.
32. Voss MH, Molina AM, Motzer RJ. mTOR inhibitors in advanced renal cell carcinoma. *Hematol Oncol Clin North Am.* 2011;25(4):835–852.
33. Ljungberg B, Albiges L, Abu-Ghanem Y, et al. European Association of Urology guidelines on renal cell carcinoma: the 2019 update. *Eur Urol.* 2019;75(5):799–810.
34. Giles RH, Choueiri TK, Heng DY, et al. Recommendations for the management of rare kidney cancers. *Eur Urol.* 2017;72(6):974–983.
35. Sanfilippo R, Jones RL, Blay JY, et al. Role of chemotherapy, VEGFR inhibitors, and mTOR inhibitors in advanced perivascular epithelioid cell tumors (PEComas). *Clin Cancer Res.* 2019;25(17):5295–5300.
36. Kohno J, Matsui Y, Yamasaki T, et al. Role of mammalian target of rapamycin inhibitor in the treatment of metastatic epithelioid angiomyolipoma: a case report. *Int J Urol.* 2013;20(9):938–941.
37. Shitara K, Yatabe Y, Mizota A, Sano T, Nimura Y, Muro K. Dramatic tumor response to everolimus for malignant epithelioid angiomyolipoma. *Jpn J Clin Oncol.* 2011;41(6):814–816.
38. Margulis V, McDonald M, Tamboli P, Swanson DA, Wood CG. Predictors of oncological outcome after resection of locally recurrent renal cell carcinoma. *J Urol.* 2009;181(5):2044–2051.
39. Dabestani S, Marconi L, Hofmann F, et al. Local treatments for metastases of renal cell carcinoma: a systematic review. *Lancet Oncol.* 2014;15(12):e549–e561.

CASE

16 Upper urinary tract urothelial carcinoma

Richard Nobrega

Expert commentary Mark Sullivan

Case history

A 74-year-old gentleman presents to his district general hospital as a 2-week wait with visible haematuria. His flexible cystoscopy was normal, and his renal function revealed an estimated glomerular filtration rate of 49 mL/min with a serum creatinine of 126 μmol/L. A computed tomography urogram (CTU) revealed bilateral ureteric filling defects: a right ureteric lesion at L4/L5 and left ureteric lesion at L3/L4 with a long stricture distally. His right kidney was hydronephrotic (Figure 16.1).

Subsequent cystoscopy was undertaken under general anaesthesia demonstrating a normal bladder. Retrograde study on the right showed dense ureteric filling defects and an impassable right ureter with both rigid and flexible ureteroscopy. A left retrograde study confirmed the computed tomography (CT) findings of a distal ureteric stricture with more proximal filling defects. Cytology was aspirated and the left ureter was subsequently perforated on attempting rigid ureteroscopy; biopsy was unsuccessful and a JJ stent left in situ. Cytology showed atypical cells only. The patient was then referred to our tertiary centre upper tract MDT for further management given the high index of suspicion for bilateral upper tract urothelial carcinomas (UTUC). The right side was thought likely to be a high-grade invasive tumour while on the left, possibly superficial disease proximal to a long benign distal ureteric stricture.

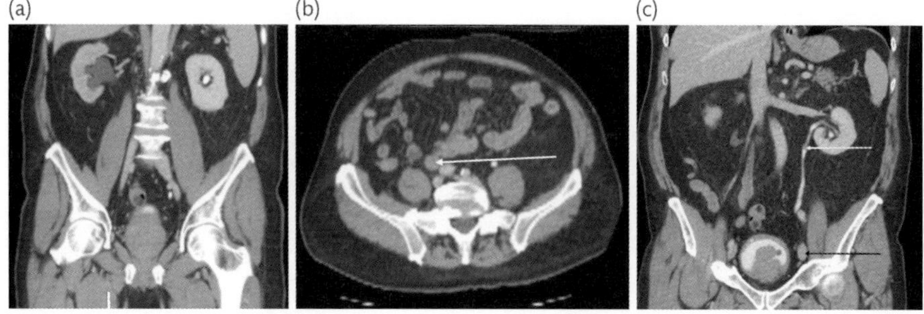

Figure 16.1 (a) CTU of case study patient with bilateral UTUC showing dilated right kidney. (b) Blue arrow shows irregular, thickened distal right ureter radiologically suspicious for high-grade disease. (c) A dilated distal left ureter just above the stricture indicated by the green arrow and filling defects within the left proximal and mid ureter shown by the blue arrow also suspicious for TCC.

Learning point Incidence, clinical presentation, and diagnosis of UTUC

UTUCs are malignant lesions that arise from the lining of the proximal urinary tract from the renal pelvis to the distal ureter. Non-urothelial cancers are rare at <5%. The incidence of UTUC is slowly rising but it remains a rare tumour when compared with bladder cancers, which are ten times more common.[1,2]

The European Association of Urology (EAU) guidelines suggest that 60% of upper tract tumours are invasive at diagnosis compared with 15–25% of bladder tumours.[3,4] This compares with bladder cancer where approximately 30% are invasive at diagnosis.[5] UTUC is twice as common in men compared with women and peak incidence in patients aged 70–90 years.[6]

The most common presentation of UTUC is painless visible or non-visible haematuria. In 17% of cases it is associated with a synchronous bladder tumour.[7] Recurrence in the bladder occurs in 24–47% of UTUC patients[8–10] compared with 2–6% recurrence in the contralateral upper tract.[11–13] CTU is the gold-standard investigation for UTUC, and as per Figures 16.2 and 16.3 shown from current EAU guidance, it forms part of the pre-intervention risk stratification and management algorithm.[14] The European Society of Urogenital Radiology (ESUR) also advocates CTU.[15] Positive urine cytology is highly suggestive of UTUC in the presence of a normal cystoscopy although it has a high specificity and low sensitivity with a high false-negative rate in low-grade tumours.[16]

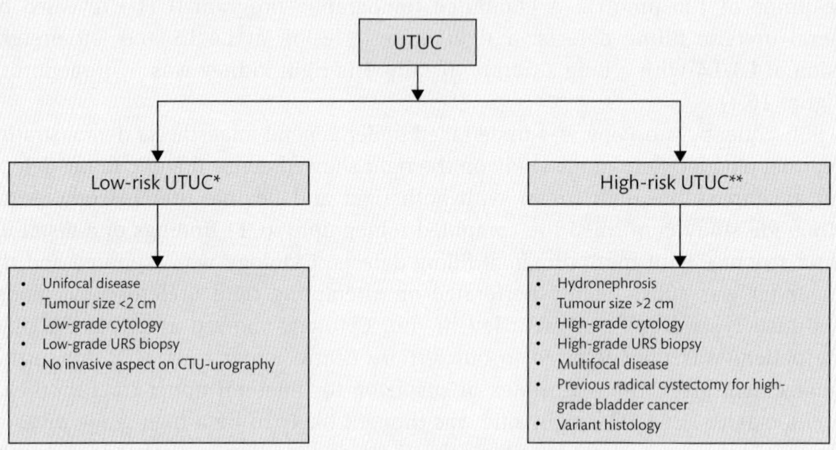

CTU = computed tomography urography; URS = ureteroscopy; UTUC = upper urinary tract urothelial carcinoma.
**All these factors need to be present.*
***Any of these factors need to be present.*

Figure 16.2 Pre-intervention risk stratification of UTUC.
Adapted from EAU 2020 UTUC guidelines with permission (www.uroweb.org/guideline).

Learning point Pre-intervention risk stratification and management of UTUC

The EAU guidelines on UTUC stratify UTUC into low risk and high risk based on a variety of pre-intervention features including tumour size, cytology, ureteric biopsy, CTU, and previous radical cystectomy for bladder cancer (Figure 16.2). The subsequent management of UTUC is based on this risk stratification, with high-risk disease being managed with radical nephroureterectomy (RNU) with or without template lymphadenectomy (Figure 16.3).

Expert comment The need for rigid/flexible ureteroscopy?

If you have convincing CTU findings for invasive transitional cell carcinoma (TCC) as in this case and your retrograde study confirms this, obtaining positive cytology is more valuable than pursuing with a difficult ureteroscopy and causing a perforation and having to leave a stent without taking any biopsies. Stents tend to cause periureteric inflammation and can make nephroureterectomy more difficult. There is also a theoretical risk of tumour seeding on perforation.

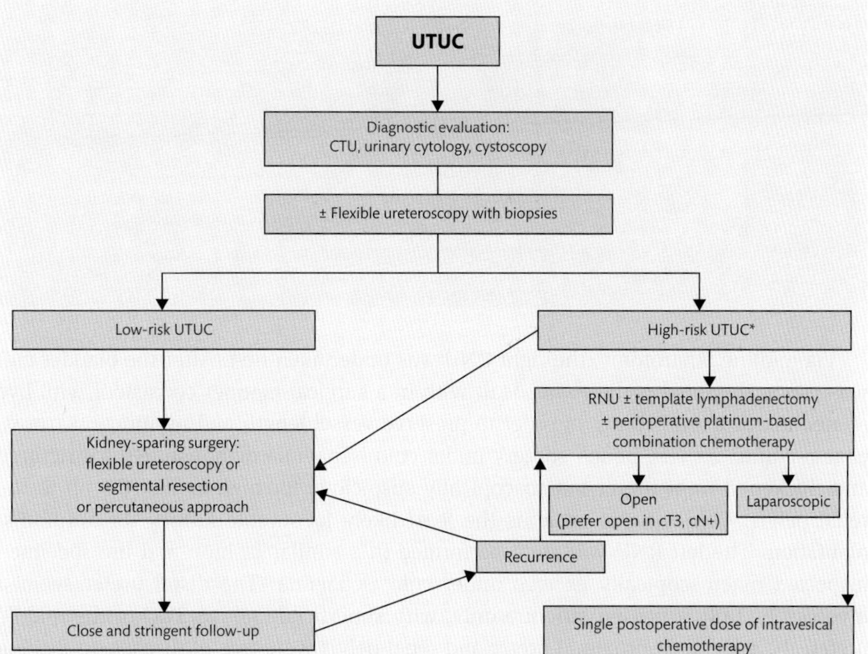

Figure 16.3 Proposed flowchart for the management of UTUC.
Adapted from EAU 2020 UTUC guidelines with permission (www.uroweb.org/guideline)

Evidence base Ureteroscopy before RNU and dissemination

Does ureteroscopy before RNU cause dissemination? A meta-analysis of eight studies (N = 3975) showed a cancer-specific survival hazard ratio of 0.76 (95% confidence interval 0.59–0.99; p = 0.04) (in favour of ureteroscopy). Overall survival, recurrence-free survival, and metastasis-free survival were all equivalent.[17]

The patient is otherwise fit with a history of hypertension and benign prostate enlargement. His regular medications are codeine, finasteride, lactulose, and amlodipine. Unfortunately, preoperatively the patient developed shortness of breath and a CT pulmonary angiogram showed a pulmonary embolus necessitating anticoagulation with treatment dose low-molecular-weight heparin (dalteparin). After further preoperative assessment and echocardiography he was deemed fit for surgery and bridged perioperatively as per local haematology advice.

This patient with suspected bilateral UTUC was discussed at our tertiary multidisciplinary team meeting and a decision made for Open bilateral nephroureterectomies via midline laparotomy and *ex vivo* bench surgery under cold ischaemia for both kidneys with the intent of autotransplantation of the more favourable kidney with renal pelvis free of TCC and viable ureter for bladder reimplantation.

Expert comment Management of bilateral high-grade UTUC

UTUC is rare in itself, with bilateral high-grade disease even more so. Given the paucity of published management on these cases with most evidence being low level, there is no established treatment protocol. Midline laparotomy and bilateral nephroureterectomies is a viable option in a patient with high-grade, invasive bilateral disease involving the renal pelvis and proximal ureters. Other options would be to consider nephroureterectomy on the side of high-grade/invasive disease and either renal autotransplantation, ileal interposition or if feasible a Boari flap if on the contralateral side, the renal pelvis with or without the upper ureter is free of invasive tumour. With a distal invasive ureteric tumour, a distal ureterectomy and reimplantation can be considered.

Expert comment Nephron-sparing surgery in bilateral UTUC

The challenge in this situation is for patients to recognise that with nephron-sparing surgery, there may be an increased risk of recurrence in the remaining renal unit(s), but they may accept this, if it is the only options of maintaining adequate renal function and stay off dialysis. One also should consider at this point the ease of endoscopic access to the remaining renal unit for surveillance and/or endoscopic ablation of recurrences. If there was high-grade disease on one side, and the contralateral ureter had low-grade disease only, an endoscopic approach could be taken with the low-grade disease initially and RNU on the contralateral side. Close 3-monthly endoscopic surveillance with or without laser ablation would be the mainstay of treatment to the remaining kidney and ureter containing low-grade disease.

Via midline laparotomy, the right RNU was undertaken first. After the bladder cuff was taken, the renal pedicle was dealt with in a surgical manner consistent with live related donor nephrectomy in order to preserve vessel length and minimize warm ischaemic time. *Ex vivo* bench surgery under cold ischaemia demonstrated a strictured and thickened right ureter macroscopically suspicious for high-grade TCC up to the renal pelvis. This was set aside as the least likely favourable kidney for autotransplantation. The left RNU was then performed in a similar fashion and the specimen inspected macroscopically *ex vivo* under cold ischaemia. The distal ureter seemed involved by only a benign stricture only, with superficial-looking TCC in the middle ureter; the very most proximal ureter and renal pelvis were free of disease on flexible renoscopy and were thus separated from the ureteric TCC under cold ischaemia. The vessels were prepared as for renal transplantation. Renal autotransplantation was performed in the right iliac fossa in an ordinary extraperitoneal fashion with single renal artery and vein anastomosed to the external iliac vessels and direct ureterovesical reimplantation performed.

Clinical tip Technical elements of autotransplantation

The kidney should only be devascularized once it and the entire ureter have been dissected free, irrespective of the method of excision at the bladder end, in so doing keeping warm ischaemia to a minimal. Once out, the kidney is perfused with transplant medium (e.g. Soltran) and put on ice. Bench surgery starts with sharp dissection of the fat off the kidney to expose the pedicle and collecting system. The ureter is inspected macroscopically and a flexible ureterorenoscope used to identify tumour burden. In the case of bilateral disease, this can help identify the kidney best preserved for autotransplantation. The ureter is excised as far proximally as is required and a final flexible ureterorenoscopy performed to check all macroscopic disease has been removed. The bench surgery can usually be performed in 30–45 minutes, not that dissimilar to standard bench surgery times for preparing a donor nephrectomy.

Evidence base Autotransplantation

Renal autotransplantation is a rare, safe, and effective surgical procedure for the treatment of complex urological conditions. It was first reported by J.D. Hardy in 1963 when he repaired a high ureteric injury following aortic surgery by reimplanting the repaired kidney into the ipsilateral iliac fossa.[18]

The longest follow-up on patients with renal autotransplants was reported by Holmäng and Johansson in 2005.[19] Their study was conducted on 23 patients with urothelial carcinoma in the upper urinary tract, operated with resection and autotransplantation then followed for 7–20 years. Nine of these patients had either bilateral UTUC or disease in a single kidney. Of these nine, two survived without needing dialysis or having recurrences for 127 and 238 months, respectively. Three patients required haemodialysis 0–3 times weekly for 27, 85, and 108 months, respectively. Three patients with low-grade disease developed invasive recurrences in the autotransplanted kidney after 16, 27, and 90 months, respectively, and later died from the disease. One patient died in an accident after 14 months.

Expert comment Autotransplantation

Renal pelvic resection, ureterectomy, and renal autotransplantation with direct pyelo- or ureterocystostomy implies increased radicality and safety in the conservative treatment of patients with urothelial tumours of the upper urinary tract. The technique also simplifies follow-up. If a recurrence is diagnosed, it can often be treated by the transurethral route. The procedure should be considered as an alternative in the treatment of patients with bilateral tumours of the ureter and/or renal pelvis and in patients with a ureteric and/or pelvic tumour within a solitary kidney.[20] It should be noted that both Pettersson's and Holmäng's groups only advocate autotransplantation in the context of UTUC in a solitary kidney or bilateral disease.[21] This is due to the significant surgical morbidity and mortality of an autotransplant and the risk of recurrence in the preserved renal unit when compared to a RNU in a patient who has a normal contralateral kidney.

The patient in this case study had their catheter removed after a cystogram at 14 days (Figure 16.4). Rigid cystoscopy at 8 weeks allowed removal of JJ stent from the renovesical anastomosis. Inspection of the bladder at this time and biopsy of the transplant ureteric orifice and flexible renoscopy of the autotransplant was normal. Final histology showed:

- Right: G3T1 TCC + carcinoma *in situ*, clear margins
- Left: low-grade TCC mid ureter, no carcinoma *in situ*, clear margins.

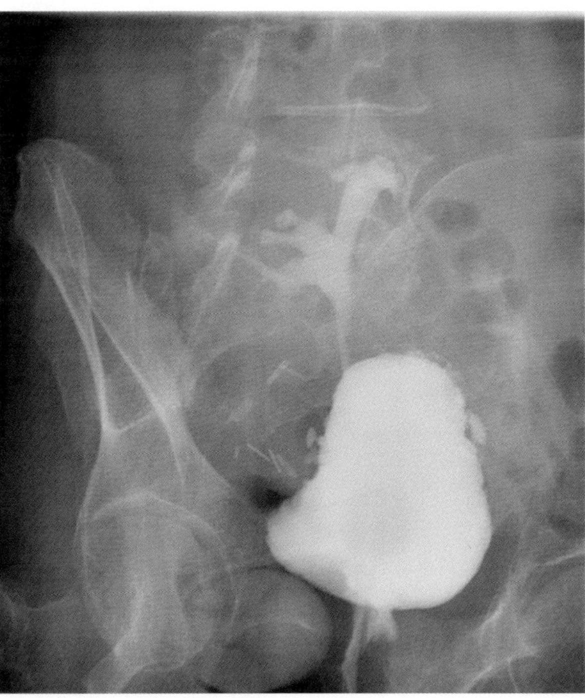

Figure 16.4 Cystogram post bilateral RNU and renal autotransplantation. Check cystogram 2 weeks post bilateral RNU and autotransplant demonstrating no leak and non-dilated well-opacified pelvicalyceal system of autotransplanted kidney. Metal clips are at the site of the vascular anastomosis with the external iliac vessels.

Clinical tip Post-RNU mitomycin C

All patients should receive a single course of intravesical 40 mg mitomycin C post RNU. Logistically, the best way to give this is for the patient to come back to a specialist nurse clinic or urology triage the day of their postoperative cystogram (day 10–14), at which point mitomycin C can be given if there is no leak. The evidence for this is laid out in the ODMIT-C trial.[22]

Evidence base Benign disease following RNU

In a Korean series in 2014 in which 244 patients underwent RNU without biopsy over 6 years, seven patients had (2.9%) benign disease (five in the ureter, two in the renal pelvis).[23]

Learning point Five-year disease-specific survival rates by tumour stage in UTUC

The UTUC 5-year disease-specific survival rates stratified by tumour stage range from 100% in pTa/carcinoma *in situ* to <5% in pT4 disease (Table 16.1).[24]

There are subtle differences in managing UTUC between the EAU guidelines and what is practised in the UK. Moon et al.[25] summarized what we practice in the UK and made a comparison with the EAU guidelines (Table 16.2).

Table 16.1 Disease-specific 5-year survival rates by tumour stage in UTUC

Stage	Disease-specific 5-year survival rates by tumour stage (%)
pTa/CIS	100
pT1	91.7
pT2	72.6
pT3	40.5
pT4	<5.0

CIS, carcinoma *in situ*.
Adapted from Craig et al. Prognostic factors, recurrence, and survival in transitional cell carcinoma of the upper urinary tract: a 30-year experience in 252 patients. *Urology*, Volume 52, Issue 4, 594–601.

Table 16.2 A comparison of the major differences between the EAU guidance and UK practice

EAU	UK practice
Low risk UUT-TCC should be offered kidney-sparing surgery	In the presence of a normal contralateral kidney NU remains the current standard of care for the majority cases of UUT-UC
Invasive or large tumours are a contraindication to laparoscopic NU	Laparoscopic NU is the most common surgical option for UUT-UC and significant numbers of patients will have invasive disease
Lymphadenectomy is recommended for invasive UUT-UC	Lymph node dissection is not performed routinely
Neoadjuvant chemotherapy is optional	Neoadjuvant chemotherapy is not offered
Annual CT-IVU for all stages of disease	Annual CT for high-risk tumours only (pT1 and above)
Routine use of urine cytology in follow-up	Urine cytology is not offered as routine follow-up

CT, computed tomography; CT-IVU, computed tomography intravenous urography; NU, nephroureterectomy; UUT-TCC, upper urinary tract transitional cell carcinoma.
Adapted from Moon et al. Urothelial carcinomas of the upper urinary tract – how does UK practice compare with European guidelines: is there a difference? *Journal of Clinical Urology* 2018;11(2):139–143.

A final word from the expert

Bilateral simultaneous nephroureterectomy and nephroureterectomy of a single kidney as radical treatment for high-grade urothelial carcinoma of the upper tract is relatively rare. However, surgical techniques to deal with the oncological burden while avoiding the rendering of a patient anephric should be considered. With an ageing population and patients rightly valuing quality of life, bearing in mind the potential burden of dialysis on our patients is important. It should be noted that to be listed for a renal transplant in the UK, patients have to be cancer-free for 5 years. Given that 50% of patients with UTUC will have a bladder recurrence, once patients are anephric it is likely they may never receive a transplant as they will at some point have a *de novo* bladder cancer while on surveillance and thus be removed from, or never reach, the transplant waiting list. This case demonstrates that careful multidisciplinary team planning and joint working with our nephrology and transplant colleagues can allow us to offer and perform nephron-sparing surgery under cold ischaemia in selected cases of UTUC bilaterally or in a solitary kidney in patients who would otherwise become anephric and require renal replacement therapy. Autotransplantation for upper tract TCC from our institution has followed five patients from 2004 to 2019, with a mean 3-year follow-up and shows a cancer-specific survival of 100%: 100% of patients are recurrence-free and 100% of patients are dialysis free. These patients are highly selected, require a very careful informed discussion of recurrence risk, and need meticulous intensive follow-up utilizing cytology, CTU, and ureteroscopy.

References

1. National Cancer Intelligence Network. *Bladder Cancer Incidence, Mortality and Survival Rates in the United Kingdom*. London: Public Health England; 2013.
2. National Cancer Intelligence Network. *Renal Pelvis and Ureter Cancer Incidence, Mortality and Survival Rates in the United Kingdom*. London: Public Health England; 2013.
3. Babjuk M, Oosterlinck W, Sylvester R, et al. EAU guide- lines on non-muscle-invasive urothelial carcinoma of the bladder, the 2011 update. *Eur Urol*. 2011;59(6):997–1008.
4. Margulis V, Shariat SF, Matin SF, et al. Outcomes of radical nephroureterectomy: a series from the Upper Tract Urothelial Carcinoma Collaboration. *Cancer*. 2009;115(6):1224–1233.
5. Stewart GD, Bariol SV, Grigor KM, et al. A comparison of the pathology of transitional cell carcinoma of the bladder and upper urinary tract. *BJU Int*. 2005;95(6):791–793.
6. Siegel RL, Miller KD, Jemal A. Cancer statistics, 2017. *CA Cancer J Clin*. 2017;66(1):7–33.
7. Cosentino M, Palou J, Gaya JM, et al. Upper urinary tract urothelial cell carcinoma: location as a predictive factor for concomitant bladder carcinoma. *World J Urol*. 2013;31(1):141–145.
8. Xylinas E, Rink M, Margulis V, et al. Multifocal carcinoma in situ of the upper tract is associated with high risk of bladder cancer recurrence. *Eur Urol* 2012;61(5):1069–1070.
9. Zigeuner RE, Hutterer G, Chromecki T, et al. Bladder tumour development after urothelial carcinoma of the upper urinary tract is related to primary tumour location. *BJU Int*. 2006;98(6):1181–1186.
10. Novara G, De Marco V, Dalpiaz O, et al. Independent predictors of metachronous bladder transitional cell carcinoma (UC) after nephroureterectomy for UC of the upper urinary tract. *BJU Int*. 2008;101(11):1368–1374.
11. Li WM, Shen JT, Li CC, et al. Oncologic outcomes following three different approaches to the distal ureter and bladder cuff in nephroureterectomy for primary upper urinary tract urothelial carcinoma. *Eur Urol*. 2010;57(6):963–969.
12. Mazeman E. Tumours of the upper urinary tract calyces, renal pelvis and ureter. *Eur Urol*. 1976;2(3):120–126.
13. Novara G, De Marco V, Dalpiaz O, et al. Independent predictors of contra-lateral metachronous upper urinary tract transitional cell carcinoma after nephroureterectomy: multi-institutional dataset from three European centers. *Int J Urol*. 2009;16(2):187–191.
14. Rouprêt M, Babjuk M, Böhle A, et al. *Urothelial Carcinomas of the Upper Urinary Tract*. Arnham: European Association of Urology; 2015.
15. Van Der Molen AJ, Cowan NC, Mueller-Lisse UG, Nolte-Ernsting CC, Takahashi S, Cohan RH. CT urography: definition, indications and techniques: a guideline for clinical practice. *Eur Radiol*. 2008;18(1):4–17.

16. Messer J, Shariat SF, Brien JC, et al. Urinary cytology has a poor performance for predicting invasive or high-grade upper-tract urothelial carcinoma. *BJU Int*. 2011;108(5):701–705.
17. Guo RQ, Hong P, Xiong GY, et al. Impact of ureteroscopy before radical nephroureterectomy for upper tract urothelial carcinomas on oncological outcomes: a meta-analysis. *BJUI*. 2018;121(2):184–193.
18. Dean RH, Meacham PW, Weaver FA. Ex vivo renal artery reconstructions: indications and techniques. *J Vasc Surg*. 1986;4(6):546–552.
19. Holmäng S, Johansson SL. Tumours of the ureter and renal pelvis treated with resection and renal autotransplantation: a study with up to 20 years of follow-up. *BJU Int*. 2005;95(9):1201–1205.
20. Pettersson S, Brynger H, Henriksson C, Johansson SL, Nilson AE, Ranch T. Treatment of urothelial tumors of the upper urinary tract by nephroureterectomy, renal autotransplantation, and pyelocystostomy. *Cancer*. 1984;54(3):379–386.
21. Pettersson S, Brynger H, Johansson S, Nilson AE. Extracorporeal surgery and autotransplantation for carcinoma of the pelvis and ureter. *Scand J Urol Nephrol*. 1979;13(1):89–93.
22. O'Brien T, Ray E, Singh R, et al. Prevention of bladder tumours after nephroureterectomy for primary upper urinary tract urothelial carcinoma: a prospective, multicentre, randomised clinical trial of a single postoperative intravesical dose of mitomycin C (the ODMIT-C trial). *Eur Urol*. 2011;60(4):703–710.
23. Hong K, Kwon T, You D, et al. Incidence of benign results after laparoscopic radical nephroureterectomy. *J Soc Laparoendosc Surg*. 2014;18(4):e2014.00335.
24. Hall MC, Womack S, Sagalowsky AI, Carmody T, Erickstad MD, Roehrborn CG. Prognostic factors, recurrence, and survival in transitional cell carcinoma of the upper urinary tract: a 30-year experience in 252 patients. *Urology*. 1998;52(4):594–601.
25. Moon A, Frew J, Johnson MI. Urothelial carcinomas of the upper urinary tract – how does UK practice compare with European guidelines: is there a difference? *J Clin Urol*. 2018;11(2):139–143.

SECTION 7

Penile cancer

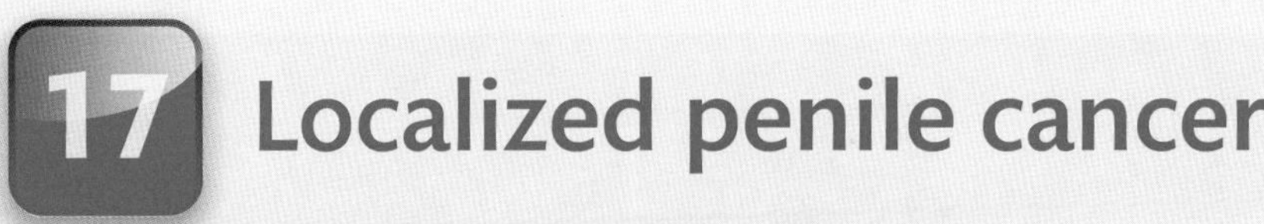

17 Localized penile cancer

Ian Eardley

Expert commentary Ian Eardley

Case history

A 58-year-old married man presented with a 3-month history of a painful ulcerating lesion on his glans penis. He had initially consulted with his general practitioner who had treated him with topical antifungal cream. When this failed to provide any benefit, a urological opinion was sought. The man was otherwise well and he took no regular medication. On examination he was circumcised and there was a peri-meatal ulcer of the glans penis with a palpable firm mass within the glans penis approximately 1 cm in diameter (Figure 17.1). There was no palpable inguinal lymphadenopathy. A staging penile magnetic resonance imaging (MRI) scan confirmed a small tumour that was invading the corpus spongiosum of the glans penis but that did not invade the corpora cavernosa (Figure 17.2). There was no evidence of inguinal lymphadenopathy on the MRI scan. An incisional penile biopsy, performed under local anaesthesia confirmed a G3 squamous cell carcinoma (SCC).

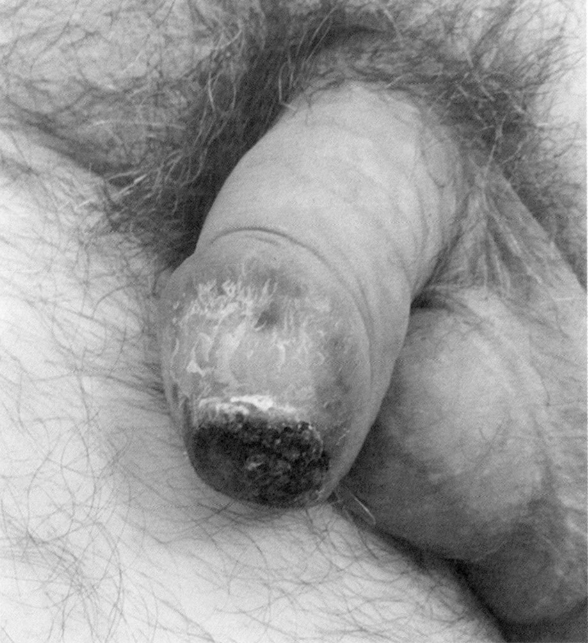

Figure 17.1 Squamous cell carcinoma of the penis. There is an ulcerating lesion in the peri-meatal region. A small firm mass was palpable within the glans penis.

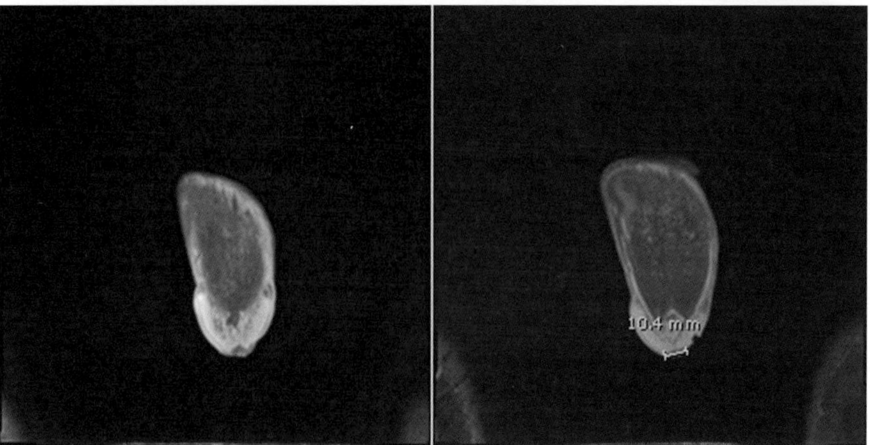

Figure 17.2 MRI scan of the penis. The MRI shows a plaque of tumour in the peri-meatal region of the glans penis approximately 10.4 mm in diameter.

Learning point Epidemiology and aetiology of penile cancer

Penile cancer is uncommon in the Western world, where it accounts for <1% of male cancers. However, there is substantial variation in incidence internationally, such that penile cancer can account for up to 10% of male cancers in parts of Africa, South Asia, and South America.[1]

The incidence increases with age and risk factors include human papillomavirus (HPV) infection, lichen sclerosis, phimosis, and smoking.[2,3]

Circumcision early in life is protective. As such, penile cancer is rarely seen in those cultures that practise circumcision in the neonatal period or in childhood.[2]

HPV-related tumours account for around half of the clinical cases seen in the UK and are associated particularly with warty carcinomas and with basaloid carcinomas. The commonest HPV subtypes are types 16 and 18.[3-5]

There are a number of premalignant penile lesions. Penile intraepithelial neoplasia (PeIN), which usually presents as a red patch on the glans or in prepuce will progress to carcinoma in up to a third of cases. In contrast, although lichen sclerosis and Bowenoid papulosis can progress to invasive cancer, they do so infrequently. Other conditions that can progress to invasive cancer include giant condyloma (Buschke–Löwenstein tumour), Bowen's disease, and Paget's disease.

Clinical tip Staging of penile cancer

Clinical staging of primary penile cancer is based primarily upon clinical examination. The most important clinical features to identify are whether there is a phimosis and whether the tumour clinically involves the corpus spongiosum and/or the corpus cavernosum. The most commonly used imaging modalities are ultrasound[6] and MRI, with the latter having good sensitivity and specificity for differentiating invasion of corpus spongiosum from invasion of corpus cavernosum.[7] MRI is usually performed following an artificially induced erection.

The procedure for identifying lymph node involvement depends upon whether there is evidence of lymphadenopathy on clinical examination of the groins. If there are no palpable nodes in either groin then dynamic sentinel node biopsy is the preferred staging technique (see later 'Learning point' box on sentinel node biopsy). If there are palpable nodes, an abdominal pelvic computed tomography (CT) scan will determine the extent of the nodal involvement in the groins and the pelvis while an 18-fluorodeoxyglucose (FDG) positron emission tomography/CT scan can demonstrate metastatic disease.[8]

The tumour, node, and metastasis (TNM) staging of penile cancer (Table 17.1) was updated in 2016 (published in 2017).[9,10] Although there were a number of changes, the most notable was a redefinition of T2 and T3 tumours, with the former reflecting invasion of the corpus spongiosum and the latter reflecting invasion of the corpus cavernosum.

Table 17.1 TNM penile cancer staging, 2016

Primary tumour	
Tx	Primary tumour cannot be assessed
T0	No evidence of primary tumour
Tis	Carcinoma *in situ*
Ta	Non-invasive verrucous carcinoma
T1a	Tumour invades subepithelial connective tissue No lymphovascular invasion and not poorly differentiated
T1b	Tumour invades subepithelial connective tissue Either lymphovascular invasion or poorly differentiated
T2	Tumour invades corpus spongiosum with or without urethral invasion
T3	Tumour invades corpus cavernosum with or without urethral invasion
T4	Tumour invades other adjacent structures
Regional lymph nodes	
pNx	Regional lymph nodes cannot be assessed
pN0	No regional nodal metastasis
pN1	One *or* two unilateral inguinal lymph node metastases
pN2	More than two unilateral nodal metastasis *or* bilateral inguinal nodal metastasis
pN3	Pelvic nodal metastasis *or* extracapsular spread of any nodal metastasis
Distant metastases	
M0	No distant metastasis
M1	Distant metastasis
Histopathological grading	
Gx	Grade of differentiation cannot be assessed
G1	Well differentiated
G2	Moderately differentiated
G3	Poorly differentiated
G4	Undifferentiated

Following multidisciplinary team review, the patient was counselled regarding treatment options. He wished to maintain as much penile length as possible and wished, if possible, to remain sexually active. Accordingly, he chose to undergo glansectomy with split-skin grafting of the corpora cavernosa rather than partial penectomy. Surgery was undertaken successfully without significant complications. A split-skin graft was taken from the thigh and fixed to the corporal tips with a tie-over dressing (Figure 17.3). The dressing remained in place, in conjunction with an indwelling catheter for 1 week.

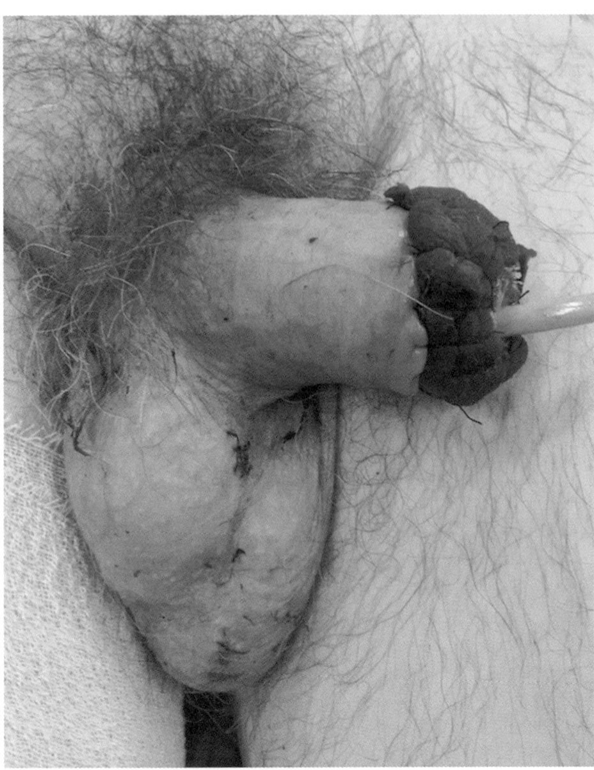

Figure 17.3 Post-glansectomy image. Tie-over dressing (soaked in povidone-iodine) following glansectomy and skin graft with urethral catheter. Both dressing and catheter remain *in situ* for about 7 days.

Expert comment Rationale for conservative surgery in localized penile cancer

Until the early years of this century, the traditional view was that a clear margin of at least 2 cm was required to achieve a cure for men with penile cancer. In recent years, it has become clear that conservative surgery is both effective and safe in the treatment of localized penile cancer, with a number of recent studies confirming that conservative surgery can achieve safe outcomes with resection margins of only a few millimetres. Local recurrence rates of 5–10% are typically reported following conservative surgery.[11–13]

Accordingly, circumcision can effectively treat tumours affecting the prepuce while tumours that are confined to the glans penis (Ta, T1, and T2 tumours) can be treated by glansectomy with skin grafting of the corporal tips. For patients with small superficial Ta tumours, perhaps associated with penile intraepithelial neoplasia, glans resurfacing is an option.

More radical surgery is required for more proximal tumours. For tumours invading the corpora cavernosa a partial penectomy will usually suffice. For more proximal tumours a total penectomy may be necessary in order to achieve complete tumour resection, combined with a perineal urethrostomy.

In some cases, where the extent of the tumour within the corpora cavernosa is unclear, perioperative frozen section can be a useful adjunct.

Clinical tip Glansectomy and glans resurfacing technique and outcomes

Glansectomy takes advantage of the plane between the corpora cavernosa and the glans penis. Using a circumcising incision, it is possible to enter this plane, and to remove the glans penis from the corporal tips with division of the urethra ventrally. Following spatulation of the urethra the corporal tips can receive a split-skin graft, usually taken from the thigh. The graft is quilted in place, and fixed with a tie-over dressing that stays in place for around 7 days. Urinary drainage is achieved using an indwelling catheter that remains *in situ* until the glans dressing has been removed. Such surgery can be performed either as a day case or with overnight stay.

More proximally invading tumours can still benefit from reconstruction providing that the tumour is confined to the tips of the corporate cavernosa. Excision of the corporal tips in continuity with the glans can be followed by primary repair of the corpora with skin grafting over the top.

Glans resurfacing involves removal of the skin from the glans penis, usually undertaken in conjunction with a circumcision. A split skin graft can be used to cover the spongiosal tissue. Spatulation of the meatus is necessary and the postoperative care is as described for glansectomy.

Expert comment Conservative surgery

The primary purpose of conservative surgery is to maintain penile length and penile function. Although the functional outcomes of conservative surgery are relatively poorly documented, what literature is available suggests that the outcomes are good. The cosmetic appearances are reasonable, and a significant number of men are able to retain sexual function, although there is inevitably some loss of sensation. Urinary function is retained with full continence, although urinary spraying is common, such that some men need to sit down in order to pass urine while others use disposable funnels to hold over the phallus when standing to pass urine, thereby directing the urinary stream.

Histology showed a T2G3 SCC, basaloid type, with negative surgical margins. The tumour extended to 7 mm from the resection margin.

Learning point Histological types of penile cancer

Penile cancer is almost always a SCC. There are multiple different histological subtypes of penile cancer. The commonest is the so-called common or usual type of SCC, which accounts for around 50% of cases. Less common types include warty carcinoma (around 10%), verrucous carcinoma (around 5%), and papillary carcinoma (around 10%), which all tend to have a good prognosis.

Both basaloid (around 5%) and sarcomatoid (around 2%) types have a poor prognosis.

There are multiple rare variants including pseudohyperplastic carcinoma, carcinoma cuniculatum, pseudoglandular carcinoma, adenosquamous carcinoma, and clear cell carcinoma.

Subsequently, the patient underwent a CT scan of the abdomen and pelvis that showed no evidence of inguinal nodal disease. He then underwent sentinel lymph node biopsy to assess the inguinal nodes. Surgery was performed under general anaesthesia as a day case with a single node being obtained from each groin.

Learning point Rationale for lymph node assessment

Penile cancer spreads primarily via the lymphatic system in a stepwise and sequential fashion. From the midline, penile tumour spread will occur to the inguinal nodes (in both groins) before spreading further (via the femoral canal) to the pelvic nodes and then on to the para-aortic notes. It is extremely unusual for tumour to 'skip" past one set of nodes to a higher set of lymph nodes. Blood-borne metastasis is also extremely unusual and typically only occurs in late-stage disease.

For patients such as this man, with impalpable inguinal nodes, a number of approaches can be considered. The likelihood of nodal spread is largely dictated by the stage and grade of the primary tumour. Overall, around 20–25% of men with clinically impalpable disease will have micro-metastatic disease with the greatest risk being in those with poorly differentiated (G3) or invasive (T2 or greater) disease. Most guidelines have identified these criteria as representing patients with high-risk disease.

For patients with a low risk of disease (T1 or less, G1 tumours), most guidelines suggest surveillance combining clinical examination and radiological surveillance.

For patients with high-risk disease (T2 or greater and/or G3 tumours), a number of approaches have been advocated. Some advocate bilateral inguinal lymphadenectomy in all high-risk cases (so-called prophylactic inguinal lymphadenectomy), while others support clinical and radiological surveillance. The difficulty with surveillance is that current imaging techniques cannot consistently identify disease in lymph nodes <1 cm in diameter. The difficulty with prophylactic lymphadenectomy is the morbidity associated with that operation.

For these reasons, a 'middle way' using sentinel node biopsy has become generally accepted as the most appropriate approach for staging impalpable inguinal nodal disease, although there are no prospective randomized control trials confirming either safety or efficacy.

Learning point Sentinel node biopsy

Sentinel lymph node biopsy relies upon the concept that lymphatic spread occurs in a sequential, stepwise manner. Using this hypothesis, penile tumours spread from the midline via the lymphatic channels to a 'sentinel' node in each groin. Isolation and examination of this node allows prediction of whether the rest of the nodes in that groin (or basin) are at risk.

To localize the sentinel node, an intradermal injection of colloid particles labelled with technetium-99m is made in the penis to facilitate imaging of the sentinel node on a lymphoscintigram. A few hours later, under general anaesthetic, a further injection of patent blue dye is made into the penis, which complements the radioactive colloid injection. Using a Geiger counter, it is possible to explore both groins to identify radioactive blue sentinel notes. Typically, one or two nodes are found in each groin.

If the sentinel node shows no evidence of tumour, then it is assumed that there is no tumour spread in that groin and no further treatment is required. If the sentinel node does show evidence of tumour, then full inguinal lymphadenectomy is undertaken at a separate operation.

The results of sentinel lymph node biopsy suggest a false-negative rate of 5–10%.[14] The morbidity of sentinel lymph node biopsy is low with occasional wound infections and occasional small lymphoceles.

On the right side, histology of the lymph node showed SCC within the node (no extracapsular spread) while the left side showed no tumour. As a consequence, the patient subsequently underwent a right inguinal lymphadenectomy from which he made a recovery complicated by wound infection and persistent lymphatic drainage with temporary lymphocele formation. There was no additional tumour in the resected lymph nodes. No further adjuvant treatment was necessary.

Learning point Inguinal lymphadenectomy

Inguinal lymphadenectomy is a morbid surgical procedure that involves removing all the superficial inguinal and deep inguinal lymph nodes that lie within the femoral triangle. The surgical margins are the inguinal ligament proximally, the adductor muscles medially, the sartorius muscle laterally, and the crossover of the sartorius muscle and the adductor longus muscle distally. In most cases such as this, a modified surgical approach can be taken with preservation of the long saphenous vein.[15]

Despite preservation of the saphenous vein, there is considerable morbidity with wound infection, lymphoedema, and lymphocele formation all being common. Less frequently, complete wound breakdown can occur. Significant complications occur in 30% or more of patients.[15]

While the lymphoedema is often temporary, in around 5–10% of men it can be persistent. In men who receive adjuvant radiotherapy, the lymphoedema is typically permanent and severe and in patients who need to undergo bilateral lymphadenectomy, the oedema can affect the scrotum and penis.

Indeed, in patients who have undergone a partial penectomy followed by bilateral lymphadenectomy, the penile stump can occasionally end up buried within the lymphoedematous scrotum.

Lymphoedema is best managed by massage and compression stockings and, if it affects the scrotum, by the use of supportive cycling shorts. Surgical treatment is rarely effective. Patients with lymphoedema are potentially prone to subcutaneous streptococcal infections.

Persistent lymphatic drainage and lymphocele is a common complication that is best treated in the early stages by use of a perioperative surgical drain. Following drain removal, intermittent aspiration of the lymphocele, perhaps twice a week, will ultimately lead to resolution, although this may take several weeks.

In patients with extensive nodal disease (pN2) or with extracapsular spread,[16] adjuvant radiotherapy can be used, although there are no randomized trial data to confirm efficacy.[17] While some advocate prophylactic pelvic node resection in such cases, again, there are no trial data to confirm benefit.

Following treatment, the patient remained under follow-up for 5 years, with regular clinical examination and CT scanning. There was no clinical or radiological evidence of recurrence during that time and he was then discharged. Functionally, he was able to stand when passing urine with occasional spraying of urine. Erectile function was maintained despite the glansectomy although there was loss of sensation as a consequence of the skin grafting and accordingly, while he was able to achieve sexual intercourse with penetration, he did have difficulty in achieving an orgasm.

Expert comment Minimally invasive approaches to lymphadenectomy

One approach to reducing the morbidity of lymphadenectomy is to perform the procedure endoscopically either using a laparoscope or even using robotic-assisted techniques.[18] By minimizing the size of the skin incision, the reported complications appear to be much less frequent.[19]

Expert comment Follow-up and prognosis

The outcome of treatment for men with penile cancer is generally good. The overall cancer-specific 5-year survival rate is around 70–80% in most modern series. Adverse prognostic features include tumour histological type, tumour stage, and tumour grade but overall the most important adverse prognostic feature is the presence of nodal disease at presentation.

Local or regional nodal recurrence typically occurs within 2 years of the primary treatment. Accordingly, most centres pursue an intensive (3–4-monthly) follow-up regimen for the first 2 years with regular clinical examination and regular imaging. Follow-up continues for at least another 3 years, albeit with a less intensive regimen (6–12-monthly).[14]

Local recurrence can occur with organ-sparing surgery, and when it does so, is treated by more aggressive surgical excision of the recurrent tumour. Regional recurrence is often less amenable to treatment, but if identified early can be treated by radical surgery with or without adjuvant radiotherapy or chemotherapy.

A final word from the expert

Penile cancer is rare in the Western world and it may be that it becomes even less common in the future with the advent of population immunization programmes against HPV. Modern management entails initial primary local surgical treatment of the primary tumour with subsequent nodal staging and treatment as appropriate.

It is now clear that the primary surgery can be conservative with surgical margins of only a few millimetres being acceptable. This provides for better functional outcomes. In patients without palpable nodal disease in the groin, sentinel node biopsy has become the mainstay of nodal staging with relatively low false-negative rates. This has reduced the need for radical lymphadenectomy with all its associated morbidity. At present, there is no place for adjuvant therapy in patients with localized penile cancer.

The outlook for most men with penile cancer is good, with long-term survival being the norm. Men with inguinal disease at presentation have a less good prognosis and current research is focused on identifying the role of adjuvant therapy.

References

1. Mira S, Chaturvedi A, Misra NC. Penile carcinoma: a challenge for the developing world. *Lancet Oncol.* 2004;5(4):240–247.
2. Maden C, Sherman KJ, Beckmann AM, et al. History of circumcision, medical conditions, and sexual activity and risk of penile cancer. *J Natl Cancer Inst.* 1993;85(1):19–24.
3. Chaux A, Netto GJ, Rodríguez IM, et al. Epidemiologic profile, sexual history, pathologic features, and human papillomavirus status of 103 patients with penile carcinoma. *World J Urol.* 2013;31(4):861–867.
4. Lebelo RL, Boulet G, Nkosi CM, Bida MN, Bogers JP, Mphahlele MJ. Diversity of HPV types in cancerous and pre-cancerous penile lesions of South African men: implications for future HPV vaccination strategies. *J Med Virol.* 2014;86(2):257–265.
5. Muñoz N, Castellsagué X, Berrington de González A, Gissmann L. Chapter 1: HPV in the etiology of human cancer. *Vaccine.* 2006;24(Suppl 3):S3/1–S3/10.
6. Bozzini G, Provenzano M, Romero Otero J, et al. Role of penile Doppler US in the preoperative assessment of penile squamous cell carcinoma patients: results from a large prospective multicenter European study. *Urology.* 2016;90:131–135.
7. Hanchanale V, Yeo L, Subedi N, et al. The accuracy of magnetic resonance imaging (MRI) in predicting the invasion of the tunica albuginea and the urethra during the primary staging of penile cancer. *BJU Int.* 2016;117(3):439–443.
8. Schlenker B, Scher B, Tiling R, et al. Detection of inguinal lymph node involvement in penile squamous cell carcinoma by 18F-fluorodeoxyglucose PET/CT: a prospective single-center study. *Urol Oncol.* 2012;30(1):55–59.
9. Leijte JA, Gallee M, Antonini N, Horenblas S. Evaluation of current TNM classification of penile carcinoma. *J Urol.* 2008;180(3):933–938.
10. Brierley J, Gospodarowicz MK, Wittekind C, eds. *TNM Classification of Malignant Tumours.* 8th ed. Chichester: Wiley-Blackwell; 2017.
11. Shabbir M, Muneer A, Kalsi J, et al. Glans resurfacing for the treatment of carcinoma in situ of the penis: surgical technique and outcomes. *Eur Urol.* 2011;59(1):142–147.
12. Philippou P, Shabbir M, Malone P, et al. Conservative surgery for squamous cell carcinoma of the penis: resection margins and long-term oncological control. *J Urol.* 2012;188(3):803–808.
13. Li J, Zhu Y, Zhang SL, et al. Organ-sparing surgery for penile cancer: complications and outcomes. *Urology.* 2011;78(5):1121–1124.
14. Leijte JA, Kirrander P, Antonini N, Windahl T, Horenblas S. Recurrence patterns of squamous cell carcinoma of the penis: recommendations for follow-up based on a two-centre analysis of 700 patients. *Eur Urol.* 2008;54(1):161–168.
15. Yao K, Tu H, Li YH, et al. Modified technique of radical inguinal lymphadenectomy for penile carcinoma: morbidity and outcome. *J Urol.* 2010;184(2):546–552.
16. Graafland NM, van Boven HH, van Werkhoven E, Moonen LM, Horenblas S. Prognostic significance of extranodal extension in patients with pathological node positive penile carcinoma. *J Urol.* 2010;184(4):1347–1353.
17. Franks KN, Kancherla K, Sethugavalar B, Whelan P, Eardley I, Kiltie AE. Radiotherapy for node positive penile cancer: experience of the Leeds teaching hospitals. *J Urol.* 2011;186(2):524–529.

18. Tobias-Machado M, Tavares A, Ornellas AA, Molina WR, Juliano RV, Wroclawski ER. Video endoscopic inguinal lymphadenectomy: a new minimally invasive procedure for radical management of inguinal nodes in patients with penile squamous cell carcinoma. *J Urol.* 2007;177(3):953–957.
19. Kumar V, Sethia KK. Prospective study comparing video-endoscopic radical inguinal lymph node dissection (VEILND) with open radical ILND (OILND) for penile cancer over an 8-year period. *BJU Int.* 2017;119(4):530–534.

CASE

Advanced and metastatic penile cancer

Hussain Alnajjar

Expert commentary Asif Muneer

Case history

A 69-year-old male presents to hospital with a 6-month history of a progressive phimosis, bleeding, and pain from the distal penis. The phimosis has been present for several years. There are no other previous comorbidities and he is a non-smoker. On clinical examination, he was found to have a palpable penile mass affecting the distal penis and which is extending proximally towards the proximal penile shaft. He had bilateral impalpable inguinal lymph nodes. His imaging studies include an ultrasound scan of the groins and computed tomography scan of the chest, abdomen, and pelvis which were unremarkable. He also underwent penile magnetic resonance imaging (MRI) with alprostadil (Caverject®) which showed that the tumour was invading into the tips of the distal corpora with multiple skip lesions more proximally.

The patient was introduced to a specialist cancer nurse specialist and a biopsy of the lesion was arranged. Subsequently, the penile biopsy and imaging were reviewed at a penile cancer multidisciplinary meeting which confirmed that the lesion was a squamous cell carcinoma with a basaloid subtype. The imaging studies showed no evidence of metastatic disease. The ultrasound of the groins did not detect any morphologically abnormal lymph nodes.

The patient underwent a radical penectomy and perineal urethrostomy and bilateral dynamic sentinel node biopsy.

Learning point Penile-sparing surgery

- Distal penile tumours which involve the glans penis or distal corporal tips have previously been managed by performing a partial penectomy. Penile-preserving surgery is now used where possible which maintains penile length with better cosmetic, functional outcomes and without the detrimental emasculating effects of partial or radical penectomy.
- Austoni et al. described the anatomical distinction between the corpora cavernosa and corpus spongiosum and proposed glansectomy as a penile-preserving surgical option for patients with invasive penile cancer confined to the glans.[3]
- Approximately 80% of all cases of invasive penile carcinoma are potentially amenable to penile-sparing surgery.
- The extent of tumour extension is determined on preoperative MRI with intracavernosal prostaglandin injection used to induce an erection.[4]

Learning point Risk factors

- Risk factors for penile cancer include the following:
  - Phimosis, chronic inflammation, lichen sclerosus, smoking, psoralen and ultraviolet light A phototherapy, human papillomavirus infection,[1] low socioeconomic status, and multiple sexual partners.
- Any suspicious penile lesion should be biopsied. Even in clinically obvious cases, histological confirmation is mandatory before the primary surgical treatment.[2]

The histopathology report confirmed an exophytic grade 3 squamous cell carcinoma, stage pT3 of basaloid subtype arising from the glans, corona, and inner foreskin and infiltrates extensively into the lamina propria, spongiosus, tunica, and distal cavernous erectile tissue with focal obstruction of the distal urethra. There were several skip lesions throughout the corpus cavernosum. There was widespread lymphovascular invasion and focal perineural invasion. The tumour extended to the left corporal margin. The urethral, right corporal, and peripheral skin limits were all free of tumour by > 5 mm. The right sentinel lymph node biopsy detected metastatic disease in one of two lymph nodes excised with the presence of extracapsular spread. The left sentinel lymph node was free of metastatic disease. The patient subsequently underwent a right radical inguinal lymphadenectomy. A further eight right inguinal lymph nodes were removed with metastatic disease present in three of them.

Following surgery, he underwent a further restaging computed tomography scan of the chest, abdomen, and pelvis which revealed multiple new metastatic pulmonary lesions.

Discussion

Penile-preserving surgery

The surgical management of penile cancer is largely directed by the grade and stage of the primary tumour and the extent of involvement of the glans, corpus cavernosum, and penile skin. Advanced disease involving a significant portion of the corpus cavernosum is still best managed by conventional radical surgery. However, in cases where lesions are confined to the glans or just extend into the distal corpus cavernosum, the requirement for radical surgery is no longer a requirement and has resulted in a paradigm shift in surgical practice.

Evidence base Penile-preserving surgery and surgical margins

Previously, clearance margins following surgery required at least 2 cm to be tumour free. However, a number of studies have challenged this hypothesis. Agrawal et al. examined 64 partial and total penectomy specimens to determine the microscopic extension of the primary tumour beyond the macroscopic tumour margin.[5] They reported that 81% did not spread beyond the macroscopic tumour margin and of those that did; only 25% extended more than 5 mm from the margin. They concluded that a 10 mm clearance was adequate for grade 1 and 2 lesions, and 15 mm for grade 3 tumours.[5] A further study reported on 51 cases who underwent penile-sparing surgery and concluded that despite 90% of patients having a margin <20 mm (48% of which were <10 mm), only three (6%) patients had positive margins and only two (4%) developed local recurrence within an average follow-up of 26 months.[6] A follow-up study reviewed 179 patients with invasive penile cancer treated with organ-sparing surgery. Local, regional, and distant metastatic recurrence developed in 16 (8.9%), 19 (10.6%), and nine patients (5.0%). The overall 5-year local recurrence-free rate was 86.3% (95% confidence interval 82.6–90.4). They established that penile-conserving surgery is oncologically safe and a surgical excision margin of <5 mm is adequate.[7] By establishing the effect of reducing the surgical clearance margin on the incidence of local tumour recurrence, these studies have led to the increasing use of penile-preserving procedures in the management of invasive penile carcinoma.

Expert comment Penile-preserving surgery

- Penile-preserving surgery is oncologically safe and a surgical excision margin of <5 mm is adequate.
- Higher local recurrence rates are associated with lesions which have lymphovascular invasion, and are a higher tumour stage and grade.
- It is important to note that most recurrences after penile-preserving surgery are surgically salvageable and local recurrence does not impact on long-term cancer-specific mortality rates.
- Dynamic sentinel lymph node biopsy now offers a less morbid technique to remove inguinal lymph nodes from patients with clinically impalpable inguinal nodes.

Locally advanced penile tumours

Patients presenting with penile lesions located on the glans penis with a palpable invasion into the distal tunica albuginea and corpus cavernosum can undergo a partial penectomy procedure. The preoperative evaluation using MRI to assess the extent of the tumour can aid in the management of these patients as it can demonstrate tumour involvement of the glans penis extending into the distal corporal tips, in which case a glansectomy and distal corporectomy will still preserve the penile length. However, if the tumour shows a more significant proximal extension, then a conventional partial penectomy is performed.

Radical or total penectomy is usually reserved for cases where extensive tumour involvement of the penile shaft necessitates complete excision of the penis and crura. Once more, preoperative MRI is useful in order to demonstrate the proximal extension of the tumour as there may be skip lesions extending proximally. Hence, adequate tumour margins can only be obtained by performing a total penectomy. The surgical dissection does not have to extend to include the crural attachment with the pubic bone unless there is extensive tumour involvement of the proximal crura whereby a radical penectomy is required. If possible, the preservation of the crura aids future reconstruction using phalloplasty procedures as they provide support for the proximal ends of the penile prostheses used during reconstructive surgery. However, in some advanced cases of penile cancer, the tumour extends proximally to involve the crura and pubic bones. In these patients, a conventional radical penectomy is required which involves detaching the crura from the pubic bone. Patients with extensive sarcomas of the penis or recurrent disease in the penile stump may also require a radical penectomy. Rarely, metastatic disease from the genitourinary system presents with multiple nodular lesions within the corpus cavernosum and again MRI is useful for diagnostic evaluation in these situations.

Clinical tip Intraoperative frozen section

An intraoperative frozen section at the time of the primary surgery may help to confirm clear surgical resection margins and hence avoid further revision surgery. However, a 2018 study by Danakas et al. showed that performing frozen section during penectomy does not appear to have any significant impact on the final surgical margin status or the long-term oncological outcomes. Nonetheless, they reported that routine frozen section can be beneficial in select cases.[8]

Locally advanced penile cancer with regional metastasis

At first clinical presentation, it has been shown that 28–64% of men with penile cancer will have clinically palpable inguinal lymph nodes, with the quoted risk of metastatic disease being 47–85% in such individuals (the remainder are due to inflammatory or infective cause). The probability of pelvic nodal metastases is 22–56% if inguinal lymph nodes are involved.[11–13] The presence of inguinal lymph node metastases is the single-most important prognostic indicator in penile cancer. Additional important prognostic factors are the number of positive lymph nodes, the presence of extracapsular spread, and the presence of pelvic node involvement.[14] Micrometastatic disease will occur in about 25% of cases at presentation, where the inguinal lymph nodes are clinically impalpable (cN0), with predictive prognostic factors being tumour stage, grade, and lymphovascular invasion.

Learning point Outcomes of partial and radical penectomies

- The techniques of partial penectomy and radical penectomy have been employed since the first century as it was found that excision of the penile tumour using these techniques results in adequate disease control.
- Patients undergoing these procedures have a low recurrence rate. The local recurrence rate following a partial penectomy is 0–8%.[9,10]
- In terms of functional outcomes, these procedures are deemed drastic with a significant psychological impact related to de-masculinization.

Advanced metastatic inguinal node disease

As originally described by Cabanas, the step-wise metastatic involvement of lymph nodes in patients with penile cancer begins at the level of the inguinal lymph nodes.[15] In advanced disease, the lymph nodes may develop into large palpable lesions which may infiltrate into the overlying skin or become fixed to the underlying fascia or muscle. Unsurprisingly, these large masses are associated with extracapsular extension of tumour and therefore require excision of overlying skin and subcutaneous tissue in order to achieve local control. With metastatic lymph nodes deep to the skin, primary closure of the defect may still be possible by mobilization of the superior and inferior skin flaps. However, larger defects following resection of bulky inguinal metastatic nodes associated with skin ulceration often requires the use of pedicled skin flaps (e.g. vertical rectus abdominis muscle or tensor fascia lata flaps) in order to cover the resulting large defect. Bulky ulcerating inguinal N3 disease can be managed by palliative resection of the tumour and overlying skin followed by coverage of the defect using a pedicled skin flap.[16] This allows palliation with better symptom control such as pain, mobility, and sepsis and reduces the risk of fatal vascular invasion due to malignant infiltration. When circumstances demand a large area of inguinal soft tissue sacrifice, primary closure may be obtained by using scrotal skin[17] or an abdominal wall advancement flap.[18]

Expert comment
Management of fixed nodal mass

The options for patients with penile tumours and a fixed nodal mass are limited. Current chemotherapeutic regimens show a promising yet limited response in the neoadjuvant setting. These patients often present with a poor performance status and are unlikely to tolerate the side effects of chemotherapy. Surgical resection with reconstruction may offer both symptom control and a chance of cure in the absence of distant metastasis.

The role of neoadjuvant and adjuvant chemotherapy/radiotherapy in advanced and metastatic disease

There is a paucity of data related to preoperative chemoradiation regimens in penile cancer prior to surgery in cases of advanced disease. As a result, clear guidelines are not available and a case-by-case approach is currently used to manage these challenging cases. It is clear that treatment of the primary lesion with radiotherapy is not recommended due to the high local recurrence rates and complications. Neoadjuvant radiotherapy does not appear to improve the overall survival according to limited data and may also lead to a delay in surgery in cases which have a limited window of opportunity before vascular or skin infiltration. However, it is often used in other squamous cell carcinoma sites such as head and neck cancers and has led to the development of a multinational trial called InPACT (International Penile Advanced Cancer Trial) to investigate the role of neoadjuvant radiotherapy in penile cancer.

Learning point Metastatic lymph nodes and radiotherapy

Metastatic lymph nodes which have extensively progressed through the skin and present as ulcerating lesions can be managed using external beam radiotherapy to the inguinal regions. Ravi et al.[19] studied 41 patients (66 groins) who were treated with palliative radiotherapy to the inguinal regions for fixed inguinal lymph nodes. They reported that 56% of the patients attained a relief in symptoms. However, the 5-year disease-free survival was only 1%. Additionally, 33 patients were treated with neoadjuvant radiotherapy (40 Gy) over a 4-week period. The incidence of extranodal disease was only 8% with a further 3% suffering recurrence in the groins. This indicates that preoperative radiotherapy can improve local disease control in cases with extensive disease. Although, radiotherapy relieved painful bony metastases, it was deemed ineffective for pelvic node metastases.

Small retrospective case series have shown some advantage in preoperative chemotherapy prior to undergoing surgery. Shammas et al.[20] reported a 28% response using a combination of cisplatin and 5-fluorouracil (FU). Ahmed et al.[21] investigated single-agent use of methotrexate, cisplatin, or bleomycin. They reported overall response rates in 39 with 1.5%, 25%, and 21% for methotrexate, cisplatin, and bleomycin, respectively. Bleomycin and methotrexate showed treatment-related deaths of 7% and 12%, respectively.

In a Southwest Oncology Group Study (SWOG) study, 26 patients were administered single-agent cisplatin at a dose of 50 mg/m^2 (days 1 and 8 of 28-day cycle).[22] The overall response rate obtained in the SWOG study was 15%, with no treatment-related deaths. The aforementioned two studies led to the prospect of combined chemotherapeutic agents in advanced penile cancer. In 1999, a phase II prospective study utilizing bleomycin, methotrexate, and cisplatin was reported.[23] In this study, 45 patients were recruited, of whom 40 were evaluable. The overall response rate was 32.5%, with five treatment-related deaths (12.5%). The median overall survival in this group was 28 weeks. However, the study was discontinued due to the high toxicity rates.

In another study where a combination of paclitaxel, ifosfamide, and cisplatin (TIP) was utilized, 20 patients were evaluated, with an overall response rate of 55% and median overall survivals of 11 months.[24] Therefore, cisplatin or paclitaxel-based combinations seem to provide a good overall response rate with much less toxicity. The TPF study, one of the first national, multicentre, phase II chemotherapy trials in the UK, used docetaxel, cisplatin, and 5-FU. The primary endpoint in this study was response rates in all patients recruited with metastatic or locally advanced disease. Docetaxel, cisplatin, and 5-FU did not reach the predetermined threshold for further research and caused significant toxicity leading to a premature study discontinuation.[25]

The Netherlands Cancer Institute has reported a series of 19 retrospective cases of unresectable penile cancer which were treated with varying regimens, including single-agent bleomycin and cisplatin, and 5-FU, but no Taxol®-based regimen.[26] Overall, 12 patients responded (63%) with two complete and ten partial responses. Of the 12 responders, nine underwent further surgery and eight of these showed no evidence of disease at a median follow-up of 20.4 months. All three patients who did not respond to chemotherapy died within 8 months. The chemotherapy-related deaths were mainly in those patients receiving bleomycin. Pizzocaro et al. undertook a prospective study using paclitaxel, cisplatin, and 5-FU. Of the six patients treated, four patients had a complete response of whom three underwent consolidative surgery with a good outcome.[27] Pagliaro et al. from MD Anderson[24] studied a total of 30 patients with stage N2 or N3 disease who underwent neoadjuvant treatment using paclitaxel, ifosfamide, and cisplatin. Fifty per cent had an objective response with a total of 22 patients (73%) undergoing surgery following chemotherapy. After a median follow-up of 34 months, 9 (30%) patients remained free of recurrence. To date, cisplatin-based chemotherapy has been shown to have a role in the management of patients with advanced penile cancer with reasonable patient responses and furthermore, it may allow advanced disease with skin and muscle involvement deemed irresectable to become resectable. However, there is currently no accepted optimum regimen and further multicentre trials are required to novel targeted therapies.

Evidence base Postoperative radiotherapy for positive lymph nodes

- There is limited evidence in favour of postoperative radiotherapy for prophylaxis in node-positive penile cancer, and its use is controversial although it is offered on a case-by-case basis.
- While a few case series have proposed a survival benefit, particularly in pN3 disease, the data are from extremely small case series. Larger series and/or prospective multicentre studies are needed before its use can receive an evidence-based recommendation.

A final word from the expert

Penile cancer is a rare genital malignancy and advances in surgical techniques and research related to the disease have primarily been aided by the centralization of services in centres throughout Europe. In the UK, this was driven by the Improving Outcomes Guidance which proposed 12 national centres would manage penile cancer. Not only has this allowed a cohort of urological surgeons to become experts in managing the primary tumour using penile-preserving surgical techniques, it has also ensured that dynamic sentinel lymph node biopsy is now the standard of care for patients with clinically impalpable inguinal lymph nodes which has reduced the morbidity associated with open inguinal lymphadenectomy.

Epidemiological studies have also demonstrated that over a 30-year period, the 5-year cancer-specific mortality has remained relatively unchanged.[1] This is largely due to the unresponsiveness of patients with advanced or metastatic disease to the currently available chemotherapy regimens and despite a number of studies which have used multiple agents, advanced disease is relatively chemoresistant.

Research relating to rare disease is often hampered by the lack of funding opportunities, low number of patients available for recruitment, and limited resources such as tissue biorepositories. With the increasing centralization of services, there has now been progress mainly related to whole-exome sequencing and methylation studies which will help to identify key therapeutic targets.

The establishment of international groups such as the International Rare Cancers Initiative and the eUROGEN workstream as part of the European Reference Network has also aided in developing collaborative trials to help recruit patients with advanced disease.

Future research will aim to develop targeted treatment options and investigate the role of immunotherapy focusing on the programmed cell death-1 (PD-1)/programmed death-ligand 1 (PD-L1) immune checkpoint inhibitors.

References

1. Arya M, Li R, Pegler K, et al. Long-term trends in incidence, survival and mortality of primary penile cancer in England. *Cancer Causes Control.* 2013;24(12):2169–2176.
2. Compérat E, Minhas S, Necchi A, et al. Penile cancer. European Association of Urology. 2020. https://uroweb.org/guideline/penile-cancer/
3. Austoni E, Fenice O, Kartalas Goumas Y, Colombo F, Mantovani F, Pisani E. [New trends in the surgical treatment of penile carcinoma.] *Arch Ital Urol Androl.* 1996;68(3):163–168.
4. Kayes O, Minhas S, Allen C, Hare C, Freeman A, Ralph D. The role of magnetic resonance imaging in the local staging of penile cancer. *Eur Urol.* 2007;51(5):1313–1318.
5. Agrawal A, Pai D, Ananthakrishnan N, Smile SR, Ratnakar C. The histological extent of the local spread of carcinoma of the penis and its therapeutic implications. *BJU Int.* 2000;85(3):299–301.
6. Minhas S, Kayes O, Hegarty P, Kumar P, Freeman A, Ralph D. What surgical resection margins are required to achieve oncological control in men with primary penile cancer? *BJU Int.* 2005;96(7):1040–1043.
7. Philippou P, Shabbir M, Malone P, et al. Conservative surgery for squamous cell carcinoma of the penis: resection margins and long-term oncological control. *J Urol.* 2012;188(3):803–808.
8. Danakas AM, Bsirini C, Miyamoto H. The impact of routine frozen section assessment during penectomy on surgical margin status and long-term oncologic outcomes. *Pathol Oncol Res.* 2018;24(4):947–950.
9. Horenblas S, van Tinteren H, Delemarre JF, et al. Squamous cell carcinoma of the penis. II. Treatment of the primary tumour. *J Urol.* 1992;147(6):1533–1538.
10. McDougal WS, Kirchner Jr FK, Edwards RH, et al. Treatment of carcinoma of the penis: the case for primary lymphadenectomy. *J Urol.* 1986;136(1):38–41.
11. Hakenberg OW, Wirth MP. Issues in the treatment of penile carcinoma. A short review. *Urol Int.* 1999;62(4):229–233.
12. Pizzocaro G, Piva L, Bandieramonte G, Tana S. Up-to-date management of carcinoma of the penis. *Eur Urol.* 1997;32(1):5–15.
13. Leijte JA, Kirrander P, Antonini N, Windahl T, Horenblas S. Recurrence patterns of squamous cell carcinoma of the penis: recommendations for follow-up based on a two-centre analysis of 700 patients. *Eur Urol.* 2008;54(1):161–168.

14. Ficarra V, Akduman B, Bouchot O, Palou J, Tobias-Machado M. Prognostic factors in penile cancer. *Urology.* 2010;76(2 Suppl 1):S66–S73.
15. Cabanas RM. An approach for the treatment of penile carcinoma. *Cancer.* 1977;39(2):456–466.
16. Alnajjar HM, MacAskill F, Christodoulidou M, et al. Long-term outcomes for penile cancer patients presenting with advanced N3 disease requiring a myocutaneous flap reconstruction or primary closure- a retrospective single centre study. *Transl Androl Urol.* 2019;8(Suppl 1):S13–S21.
17. Skinner DG. Management of extensive, localized neoplasms of lower abdominal wall. Pubectomy and scrotal skin transfer technique. *Urology.* 1974;3(1)34–37.
18. Tabatabaei S, McDougal WS. Primary skin closure of large groin defects after inguinal lymphadenectomy for penile cancer using an abdominal cutaneous advancement flap. *J Urol.* 2003;169(1):118–120.
19. Ravi R, Chaturvedi HK, Sastry DV. Role of radiation therapy in the treatment of carcinoma of the penis. *Br J Urol.* 1994;74(5):646–651.
20. Shammas FV, Ous S, Fossa SD. Cisplatin and 5-fluorouracil in advanced cancer of the penis. *J Urol.* 1992;147(3):630–632.
21. Ahmed T, Sklaroff R, Yagoda A. Sequential trials of methotrexate, cisplatin and bleomycin for penile cancer. *J Urol.* 1984;132(3):465–468.
22. Gagliano RG, Blumenstein BA, Crawford ED, et al. Cis-diamminedichloroplatinum in the treatment of advanced epidermoid carcinoma of the penis: a Southwest Oncology Group Study. *J Urol.* 1989;141(1):66–67.
23. Haas GP, Blumenstein BA, Gagliano RG, et al. Cisplatin, methotrexate and bleomycin for the treatment of carcinoma of the penis: a Southwest Oncology Group Study. *J Urol.* 1999;161(6):1823–1825.
24. Pagliaro LC, Williams DL, Daliani D, et al. Neoadjuvant paclitaxel, ifosfamide, and cisplatin chemotherapy for metastatic penile cancer: a phase II study. *J Clin Oncol.* 2010;28(24):3851–3857.
25. Nicholson S, Hall E, Harland SJ, et al. Phase II trial of docetaxel, cisplatin and 5FU chemotherapy in locally advanced and metastatic penis cancer (CRUK/09/001). *Br J Cancer.* 2013;109(10):2554–2559.
26. Leijte JA, Kerst JM, Bais E, et al. Neoadjuvant chemotherapy in advanced penile carcinoma. *Eur Urol.* 2007;52(2):488–494.
27. Pizzocaro G, Nicolai N, Milani A. Taxanes in combination with cisplatin and fluorouracil for advanced penile cancer: preliminary results. *Eur Urol.* 2009;55(3):546–551.

SECTION 8

Testicular cancer

CASE

19 Growing teratoma syndrome in testis cancer

Jennifer Clark, Thomas A. Lee, and Vijay A.C. Ramani

Expert commentary Vijay A.C. Ramani

Case history

A fit and well 24-year-old man presented with a right-sided testicular mass and back pain of approximately 6 months' duration. He was working as a plasterer, was unmarried with no children, and living with his mother. He smoked 15–20 cigarettes per day and denied drinking alcohol. At the time of presentation, he had palpable abdominal and supraclavicular lymph node masses. Tumour markers were considerably elevated with an alpha-fetoprotein (AFP) level of 996 ng/mL and a beta human chorionic gonadotropin (β-hCG) level of 6620 ng/mL. He had an obviously abnormal-feeling right testis and testicular ultrasound confirmed a heterogeneous mass suspicious for malignancy.

He was advised of the likely diagnosis of testicular cancer and, following adequate counselling and sperm banking, he underwent a right radical inguinal orchidectomy. Radical orchidectomy was performed via an inguinal approach and the spermatic cord transected at the internal ring. Insertion of testicular prosthesis was discussed with him preoperatively but he opted against this.

Learning point Epidemiology and aetiology

Epidemiology

Primary testicular cancer accounts for around 1% of all male cancers and 5% of all urological cancers and is the commonest solid organ cancer in men aged between 20 and 45 years. Non-seminomatous germ-cell tumours (NSGCTs) are commoner between the ages of 20 and 35 years, whereas seminoma is more common between the ages of 35 and 45 years. Incidence has been increasing in Western societies and is currently around 3–10/100,000 per year. Mortality is low (0.3/100,000) and has fallen significantly since the introduction of platinum-based chemotherapy in 1975.

Aetiology

- **Age**: rare <15 and >60 years (yolk sac tumour and lymphoma more common respectively for these groups).
- **Race**: white Caucasians at highest risk (white males in US 3 × as likely as black males to develop testicular cancer).

- **Cryptorchidism**: 5–10% of patients with testicular cancer have history of cryptorchidism; 3 × risk and 6 × risk of testicular cancer in men who underwent orchidopexy before or after 13 years of age respectively.
- **Germ cell neoplasia insitu (GCNIS)**: 50% will develop invasive germ cell testicular cancer within 5 years.
- **Hereditary**: 4 × increased risk over population if father diagnosed with testicular cancer, 8 × increased risk if brother diagnosed.
- **HIV**: increased risk of seminoma.
- **Previous testicular cancer**: 1–2% of testicular cancers are bilateral. 12 × increased risk of metachronous testicular cancer.

Compiled from EAU guidelines on testis cancer 2019.[1]

Clinical tip Pretreatment fertility assessment should be offered

All patients of reproductive age should be offered a pretreatment fertility assessment including testosterone, luteinizing hormone, and follicle-stimulating hormone levels plus semen analysis and cryopreservation.[2] All centres should have a fast-track arrangement for semen cryopreservation to avoid any delay in management. In cases where the patient has life-threatening complications of metastatic disease, there may not be time for this before commencing urgent chemotherapy.

Histological examination confirmed the presence of a 35 mm postpubertal type cystic teratoma with the presence of germ cell neoplasia *in situ* (GCNIS) (Figure 19.1). There was no lymphovascular invasion and the rete testis, epididymis, and spermatic cord were free of tumour. He was staged at pT1NxMx (see 'Learning point' box on TNM staging)—teratoma postpubertal type.

Expert comment Preoperative essentials

Serum tumour markers

This allows baseline reading and monitoring after orchidectomy and throughout systemic therapy. AFP and β-hCG must decrease according to their half-lives (5–7 days and 2–3 days, respectively) in the absence of metastatic or contralateral disease. Persistence or rise of serum tumour markers

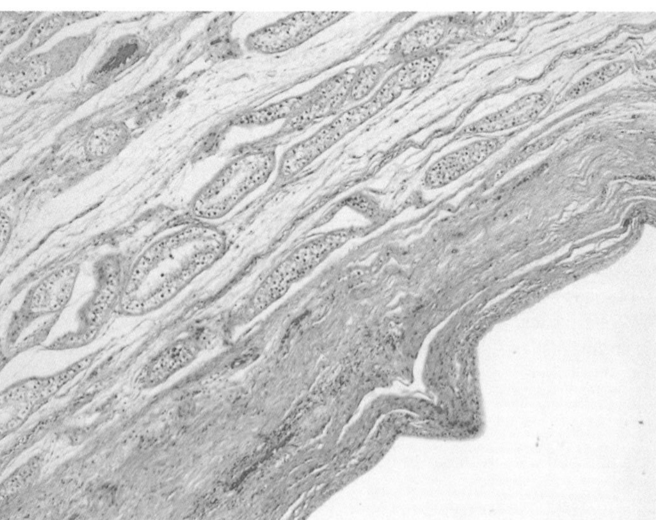

Figure 19.1 Histology from orchidectomy specimen demonstrating GCNIS within tubules and the cystic lining of the teratoma.

after orchidectomy indicates the presence of micro- or macro-metastatic disease. Lactate dehydrogenase (LDH) is not a specific marker but may indicate the extent of tumour burden in metastatic disease.

Sperm banking

All centres should have a fast-track service for sperm banking, which should be done before orchidectomy wherever possible. A small percentage (4%) of patients can be azoospermic[3] after orchidectomy, although some reports indicate this could be higher. This allows fertility planning in azoospermic patients and arrangements for onco-testicular sperm extraction (onco-TESE) at an appropriate centre.

Testicular prosthesis

Insertion of a testicular prosthesis should be offered to patients and it can be inserted at the time of orchidectomy without increased risk of infectious complication.[4] Clinical factors such as extreme size of primary tumour and condition of scrotum, significant metastatic disease requiring urgent chemotherapy, and poorly controlled diabetes may contraindicate primary insertion of a prosthesis.

Contralateral testis biopsy

The risk of contralateral GCNIS is 5%. High-risk groups should be offered contralateral testis biopsy and centres should have specialist multidisciplinary team (SMDT) consensus with oncologists for the management of GCNIS. Age <40 years and testis atrophy (<12 mL) increases the risk of GCNIS to 18%[5] and these patients should be targeted for contralateral testis biopsy.

The patient underwent a staging computed tomography (CT) scan with contrast of the thorax, abdomen, and pelvis showing a bulky conglomerate retroperitoneal nodal mass, which displaced the inferior vena cava (IVC) and completely encased the aorta measuring 14.7 × 8.3 cm. He had no suspicious pulmonary nodules and no bone lesions but did have thrombus in the left internal jugular and subclavian veins (Figure 19.2).

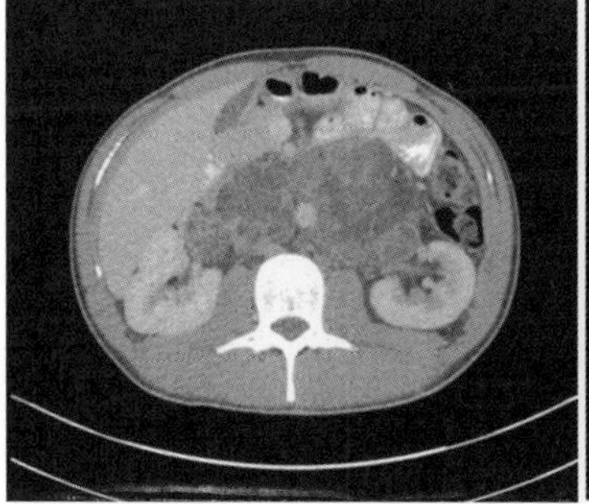
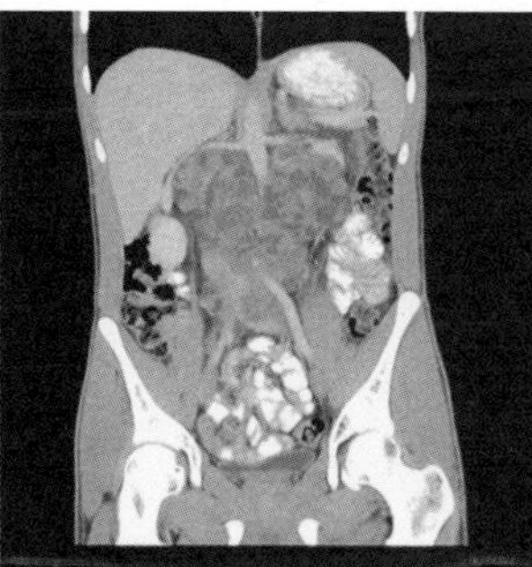
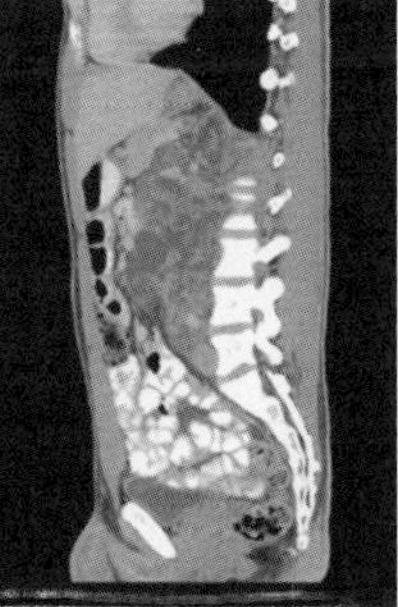

Figure 19.2 Initial CT findings of retroperitoneal nodal mass encasing major vessels.

Learning point TNM staging of testis cancer

See Table 19.1.

Table 19.1 Tumour, lymph node, and metastases (TNM) staging system

T–primary tumour		N–regional lymph nodes		M–distant metastasis	
Tx	Primary tumour not assessed	**Nx**	Regional nodes not assessed	**Mx**	Distant metastasis not assessed
T0	No evidence of primary tumour	**N0**	No evidence of regional node metastasis	**M0**	No evidence of distant metastasis
Tis	Intratubular germ cell neoplasia (ITGCN)	**N1**	Metastasis of 5 or fewer lymph nodes (none >2 cm in maximum diameter)	**M1a**	Metastasis to non-regional lymph nodes or lungs
T1	Limited to testis/ epididymis *without* lymphovascular invasion (LVI), no involvement of tunica vaginalis	**N2**	Lymph node metastasis of between 2 and 5 cm maximum diameter **or** Metastasis of >5 lymph nodes (none >5 cm in maximum diameter)	**M1b**	Distant metastasis other than to non-regional lymph nodes or lungs
T2	Limited to testis/ epididymis *with* LVI *or* involvement of tunica vaginalis	**N3**	Lymph node metastasis of >5 cm maximum diameter		
T3	Invasion of spermatic cord *with/without* LVI				
T4	Invasion of scrotum *with/without* LVI				

Adaptation of TNM staging from EAU guidelines (2020).[1]

Learning point Classification of teratomas (2016)

It is important to note that teratomas are classified based on whether or not they originated from GCNIS.[7]

Germ cell tumours derived from GCNIS

- Teratoma postpubertal type.
- Teratoma with somatic-type malignancy.

Germ cell tumours unrelated to GCNIS

- Teratoma prepubertal type:
  - Dermoid cyst.
  - Epidermoid cyst.
  - Well-differentiated neuroendocrine tumour (monodermal teratoma).
- Mixed teratoma and yolk sac tumour prepubertal type.

Learning point World Health Organization 2016 histopathological classification of germ cell tumours

See Table 19.2.

Table 19.2 World Health Organization 2016 histopathological classification of germ cell tumours

GCNIS derived	Non-GCNIS derived
Seminoma	Spermatocytic tumour
Embryonal carcinoma	Yolk sac tumour (prepubertal)
Yolk sac tumour:	Teratoma (prepubertal)
–Sarcomatoid yolk sac tumour	
Trophoblastic:	
–Choriocarcinoma	
–Other trophoblastic tumours	
Teratoma (postpubertal)	

Adaptation of Williamson SR et al.[6]

Expert comment Postpubertal and prepubertal teratomas

One of the main modifications of the 2016 World Health Organization classification of testis tumours is the clarification of the origin of postpubertal and prepubertal teratoma from GCNIS.[6]

It is important to remember that postpubertal teratomas are associated with GCNIS and have a significant potential to develop metastasis containing both teratomatous and non-teratomatous germ cell elements. This case presented is an illustration of this and the vast majority of adult teratomas should be managed as malignant germ cell tumours. Management of postpubertal teratomas based on the presence or absence of mature or immature elements has no prognostic value as even the 'mature teratoma' in the postpubertal setting has its origins in GCNIS.

Prepubertal teratomas, on the other hand, are characterized by more organized structure, lack of cytological atypia or GCNIS, or impaired spermatogenesis and have not been reported to metastasize. In rare cases, a prepubertal teratoma can be diagnosed in postpubertal testis based on documented histopathological features.[8]

Post orchidectomy, the patient's AFP level peaked at 3077 ng/mL with an β-hCG concentration of just over 18,000 and an LDH level of 440 IU/L. His case was discussed in the regional germ cell multidisciplinary team (MDT) meeting and the final staging was confirmed as pT1N3M0 S2. For prognostic and treatment purposes, this placed him in the intermediate-risk group (S2).

Learning point Serum tumour markers

See Table 19.3.

Table 19.3 Serum tumour markers staging system

S—serum tumour markers					
Sx	Serum markers not assessed				
S0	Normal serum markers				
	LDH (U/l)		**β-hCG (mIU/mL)**		**AFP (ng/mL)**
S1	<1.5 × normal	**and**	<5000	**and**	<1000
S2	1.5–10 × normal	**or**	5000–50,000	**or**	1000–10,000
S3	>10 × normal	**or**	>50,000	**or**	>10,000

Adaptation of TNM staging from EAU guidelines (2020).[1]

Evidence base Prognostic-based system for metastatic germ cell cancer

See Table 19.4.

Table 19.4 Prognostic-based staging system for metastatic germ cell cancers

Good prognosis group	
NSGCT (56% of cases)	**Seminoma (90% of cases)**
• 5-year progression-free survival (PFS) 89% • 5-year overall survival (OS) 92% All of the following: • Testis/retroperitoneal primary • No non-pulmonary visceral metastases • AFP < 1000 ng/mL • hCG < 5000 mIU/mL • LDH <1.5 × normal	• 5-year PFS 82% • 5-year OS 86% All of the following: • Any primary site • No non-pulmonary visceral metastases • Normal AFP • Any level of hCG • Any level of LDH

(continued)

Table 19.4 Continued

Intermediate prognosis group	
NSGCT (28% of cases) • 5-year PFS 75% • 5-year OS 80% Any of the following: • Testis/retroperitoneal primary • No non-pulmonary visceral metastases • AFP 1000–10,000 ng/mL • hCG 5000–50,000 mIU/mL • LDH 1.5–10 × normal	**Seminoma (10% of cases)** • 5-year PFS 67% • 5-year OS 72% All of the following: • Any primary site • Non-pulmonary visceral metastases • Normal AFP • Any hCG • Any LDH
Poor prognosis group	
NSCGT (16% of cases) • 5-year PFS 41% • 5-year OS 48% Any of the following: • Mediastinal primary • Non-pulmonary visceral metastases • AFP > 10,000 ng/mL • hCG > 50,000 mIU/mL • LDH > 10 × normal	**Seminoma** No patients classified as poor prognosis

Adapted from International Germ Cell Cancer Collaborative Group (IGCCCG).[9]

After discussion in the MDT, a plan was made for treatment with four cycles of 5-day bleomycin, etoposide, and cisplatin (BEP) under the care of the medical oncology team. Pretreatment, he underwent audiology and pulmonary function tests alongside full blood work. He was admitted to a dedicated young person's oncology unit for the treatment and had a peripherally inserted central catheter line inserted. Apart from side effects of nausea and fatigue, the patient tolerated chemotherapy well.

Evidence base Evidence for BEP in metastatic NSGCT

Standard treatment of metastatic NSGCT with three to four cycles of BEP chemotherapy depends on the histology of the primary tumour and the prognostic subgroup as defined by the International Germ Cell Cancer Collaborative Group.

De Wit et al., as part of the EORTC Genitourinary Tract Cancer Cooperative Group, reported a randomized study comparing four cycles of etoposide, ifosfamide, cisplatin (VIP) to four cycles of BEP in patients with intermediate-prognosis NSGCT.[10] There were no differences in relapse rate, disease-free rate, and overall survival rate. The VIP regimen was more toxic with regard to bone marrow function with no improved effectiveness.

Clinical tip Pre-chemotherapy testing

- **Audiological studies**: cisplatin ototoxicity can result in high-frequency hearing loss.
- **Pulmonary function tests**: bleomycin can cause potentially life-threatening pulmonary interstitial fibrosis in up to 10% of patients.
- **Renal function tests**: cisplatin can lead to nephrotoxicity so pre- and post-chemotherapy renal function testing as well as hydration during treatment is imperative.
- **Liver function tests**: etoposide can cause elevation in alanine transaminase levels, in particular when used in conjunction with an alkylating agent such as cisplatin, and liver function should be monitored.
- **Cardiac function**: cisplatin has been reported as a risk for arrhythmia and myocarditis. In older patients or those at risk, echocardiography may be recommended.

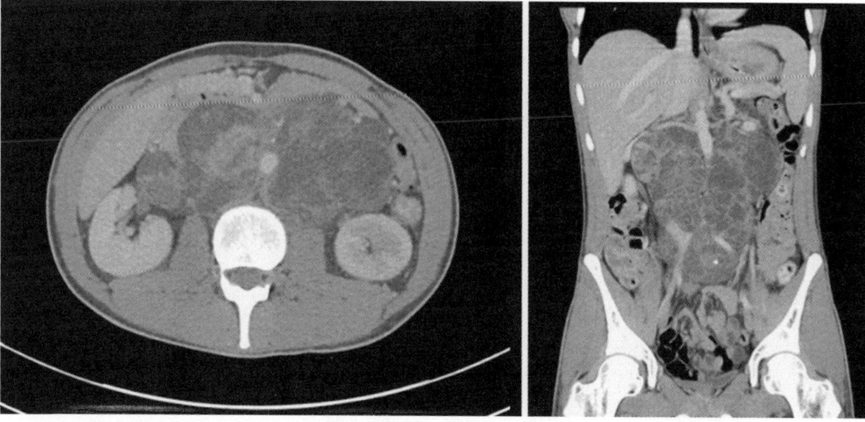

Figure 19.3 CT scan demonstrating progression in size of tumour mass and cystic components.

Unfortunately, shortly following completion of chemotherapy, despite normalization of his tumour markers, the patient was admitted with ongoing back pain, nausea, vomiting, and suspected small bowel obstruction. His nutritional status was poor and he described significant weight loss. He was managed with a nasogastric tube, intravenous fluids, and total parenteral nutrition.

A further CT of the abdomen and pelvis with contrast was performed (Figure 19.3) which showed progression of the bulky mixed density retroperitoneal lymphadenopathy to 16.6 × 8.3 cm, causing obstruction of the third and fourth parts of the duodenum. There was also progressive thrombus within the left brachiocephalic vein.

The patient's case was re-discussed at the germ cell MDT and he was listed for laparotomy and bilateral template retroperitoneal lymph node dissection (RPLND).

Clinical tip Indications for post-chemotherapy RPLND

NSCGT

- Any residual mass >1 cm diameter and normalized serum tumour markers.
- Any residual mass <1 cm diameter and plateauing serum tumour makers.
- Residual mass <1 cm diameter and mature teratoma in primary orchidectomy specimen.
- Residual mass with negative or plateauing markers after salvage chemotherapy.
- Desperation RPLND for patients with chemoresistant masses which are completely resectable.

Seminoma

- Patients with residual mass >3 cm should undergo fluorodeoxyglucose (FDG) positron emission tomography (PET) (risk of viable cancer 12–30%):
  - PET negative → surveillance.
  - PET positive → SMDT discussion regarding radiotherapy/further chemotherapy/surgery.

Compiled from ESMO Consensus Conference 2018.[11]

Expert comment Surgical decision-making in the MDT

Decisions in the testis MDT regarding surgery should be based on (1) indications, (2) timing, and (3) procedure (TIP).

Indications

NSGCT: patients with a post-chemotherapy (usually BEP) residual mass >1 cm and normal or plateauing tumour markers should undergo RPLND. The indications are summarized in the earlier 'Clinical tip' box. The final histology following RPLND shows viable cancer or mature teratoma in up to 10% and 50% of patients, respectively. Approximately 40% of patients have fibrotic or necrotic tissue in the final specimen and currently there are no tests to identify these patients. Particular attention should be paid to those patients with postpubertal 'mature' teratoma in the orchidectomy specimen due to its unique biological behaviour as explained previously and a case is made for excising residual masses <1 cm.

Seminoma: in general, surgery is rarely indicated in metastatic seminoma post chemotherapy. An FDG-PET scan has a high negative predictive value in patients with residual masses. The possibility of necrosis in post-chemotherapy seminoma masses <3 cm in size are very high and surgery is not a standard of care in these patients. For masses >3 cm in size, an FDG-PET scan is advised at least 6 weeks after completion of chemotherapy. Progression or persistence of β-hCG is an indication for second-line chemotherapy. RPLND is reserved as a last resort after SMDT discussions and appraisal of options including radiotherapy. A case can be made for undertaking this surgery in very specialized and small number of centres due to intense fibrosis and severe induration that is invariably present in such patients.

Expert comment Surgical decision-making in the MDT 2

Timing

RPLND should be performed within 6–8 weeks of completion of chemotherapy. Delays in surgery lead to inferior survival and the possibility of needing reinduction chemotherapy.[12,13]

Patients can present with metastasis at various sites—particularly the retroperitoneum and lungs. The management is personalized to each patient and there is a variation in policy at different testis centres but, in general, the following factors need to be taken into account:

- There is a histopathological discordance:
  - Of 20% between lung metastasis in both lungs but this can be as low as 5% if necrosis is found at first lung resection and tumour markers normal[14,15]
  - Of approximately 10% between retroperitoneal and lung resection when necrosis only is present in the retroperitoneum.[16]
- If RPLND is performed first then the histology can be used to determine the need for thoracotomy. The reverse strategy is unlikely to be sufficiently predictive.

Expert comment Surgical decision-making in the MDT 3

Procedure

It is not justifiable to carry out a lumpectomy and a decision has to be made regarding performing a bilateral RPLND (the case presented here), right or left template RPLND, or a bilateral nerve-sparing RPLND. The type of dissection is determined at the SMDT and is based on the location and extent of the residual disease. Radical dissection must not be compromised but a nerve-sparing template dissection should be considered where appropriate to lessen risk of ejaculatory dysfunction.

Post-chemotherapy RPLND is usually challenging and the surgical approach to the residual masses depends on their location—in particular, the involvement of retrocrural area and presence of significant disease above the renal hilum. It is possible to determine the extent of resection in terms of the need for a nephrectomy or aortic/IVC excision and graft replacement or liver resection or psoas excision. The surgical team should be equipped and prepared to do this at specialized centres capable of multidisciplinary surgery.[17]

Preoperatively, the patient had lost 8 kg in weight with a body mass index of 17.2; he was seen by a dietician and commenced on total parenteral nutrition to try and prevent further weight loss and maintain his physical condition. He struggled with pain and had developed an opioid dependence, which was very challenging to manage on the ward. The pain team were involved early and his pain was managed with pregabalin and modified-release morphine.

Postoperatively, the patient was managed on the high dependency unit and then stepped down to ward level care on the 'young oncology unit'. There were significant challenges managing his postoperative pain and, despite involvement of the pain team, the patient remained on high-dose opioids for many months after discharge.

Expert comment Operative note: bilateral RPLND to achieve radical excision

Following an epidural, general anaesthetic, and insertion of central and arterial lines, the abdomen was opened with a midline incision. The colon was completely mobilized and dissection commenced with the coeliac axis and the superior mesenteric artery freed from the adjacent cystic structure. The third part of the duodenum was tethered to the mass and partially released. The splenic vein was then identified and the left renal vein carefully dissected along its length and a significant component of the mass separated from the left renal hilum. Painstaking mobilization was required to separate the superior aspect of the mass from the proximal aorta and left and right renal arteries. The aortal and IVC were completely dissected and encircled proximally so that they could be controlled. Similar dissection was carried out distally at the iliac vessels to allow control if needed.

The IVC was plastered onto the left side of the mass and careful dissection was undertaken with the right renal vein preserved. Meticulous ligation of multiple right- and left-sided lumbar veins was required to fully release the IVC.

The circumferential mass was gradually released from the aorta, with three sets of lumbar arteries ligated. Due to the sheer bulk of the mass, it could not be removed en bloc so was split in line with the inferior mesenteric artery. This allowed a more controlled separation of the right side of the mass from the aorta, spine, and psoas and the right side of the mass could be removed.

The lower third of the aorta was densely plastered to the mass and a plane had to be painstakingly developed. The inferior mesenteric artery was transfixed and divided at its origin to allow mobilization. The mass was densely adherent to the left and right iliac veins and compressing them. Lengthy dissection was undertaken to allow control of these vessels in case of bleeding. The masses were excised on both sides in this bilateral template.

The inter aortocaval aspect of the mass was mobilized and the right hilum preserved. Posterior mobilization of the left side mass could then be completed and it was excised with no further visible disease. Haemostasis was carefully checked and minor bleeding points managed with Prolene® sutures. Lymph fluid leakage was underrun with Monocryl®, the colon replaced, and posterior retroperitoneum reconstructed. A drain was inserted and the abdomen closed.

The final histology report described an extensive conglomerate of five masses in one resection specimen weighing > 10 kg (Figure 19.4). The microscopic appearances were consistent with teratoma containing mature elements in the form of cysts lined by glandular and/or squamous epithelium in addition to fibromuscular stroma but with no evidence of neoplasia. This finding is typical of the growing teratoma syndrome (GTS).

Clinical tip Involvement of young person's services

A diagnosis of cancer and the impact of subsequent treatments (especially major surgery that may impact sexual function and fertility) can be very challenging psychologically for a young person. Their lives, expectations, and understanding may be quite different to older people. Involvement of psychological services and expertise on a 'young oncology unit' aimed at young people is therefore essential to provide support that may be outside of the surgeon's remit to provide.

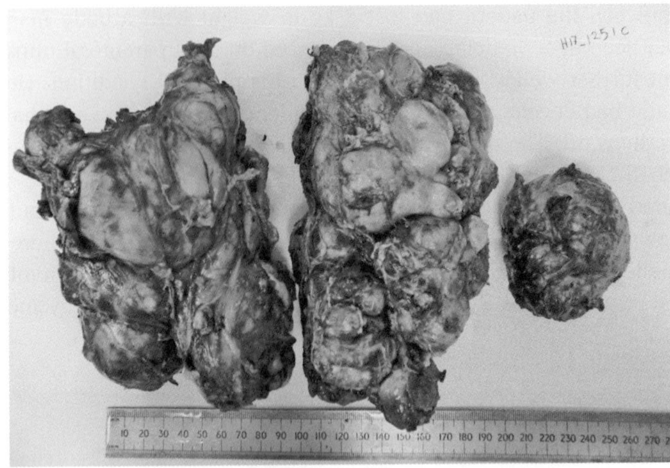

Figure 19.4 Resected retroperitoneal masses weighing >10 kg.

Expert comment Surgical planning of template dissections

Careful dissection, isolation, and protection of the structures forming the boundaries of the template resection (bifurcation of the aorta and dissection along common iliac vessel (right or left) inferiorly, ureter laterally, renal hilum superiorly, inferior mesenteric artery, and either the midpoint of the aorta or IVC for right and left template respectively) in every case is the safest approach. When these boundaries are defined and proximal and distal control of the IVC and aorta is established, then it is feasible to perform this operation with excellent outcomes. The fundamental surgical principles must not be compromised in those patients considered suitable for robot-assisted laparoscopic RPLND. A bilateral template includes both right- and left-sided templates and is more extensive.

Expert comment Holistic needs of testis cancer patients

All patients, of course, must be treated as individuals and patients with metastatic testis cancer require particularly careful management. They have typically built rapport with their specialist urologist, clinical oncologist, and specialist nurses throughout their journey. They are classically young, fit, and healthy individuals who have unexpectedly had their lives changed irrevocably. Having been through the trauma of diagnosis, potentially perceived emasculating orchidectomy, fertility concerns, and effects of chemotherapy, they are faced with the formidable prospect of RPLND. They require careful, considered, and individualized counselling with regard to their extent of surgery and associated risks. An MDT approach is essential and the role of additional services can be invaluable (see 'Clinical tip' box on young person's services).

Discussion

The GTS is a rare condition with a prevalence of only 2–8% in patients with metastatic NSGCT.[18] GTS is defined as an enlarging metastatic mass during or after completion of appropriate chemotherapy for NSGCT in the presence of reducing or normalized tumour markers.[19] It is most commonly found in the retroperitoneum but can also be observed in the mediastinum, lung, supraclavicular and inguinal lymph nodes, or a combination of these.[20] Radiological features on CT include evidence of enlarging masses with presence of calcification, fat, or cystic changes.[21] Histology of resected

GTS masses reveals benign mature teratoma with no residual viable malignant germ cell tumour.[22] GTS masses have the potential for rapid growth and high morbidity and mortality as they disrupt local anatomy or obstruct other organs and vessels.

Complete surgical resection is essential as the recurrence rates can be as high as 83% in patients with incomplete resection compared to 4% in patients with complete resection[18] and multiple surgeries maybe required to ensure complete resection.[23] Resection is also required to confirm the diagnosis and reduce the risk of malignant transformation. If the diagnosis of GTS is made during chemotherapy treatment, the proposed induction course should be completed as planned unless toxicity prevents this or if there is evolving emergency of a local effect of tumour growth (causing vessel or viscous compression).

Expert comment Role of FDG-PET/CT in post-chemotherapy residual retroperitoneal lymph node mass in NSGCT

The role of FDG-PET/CT in the evaluation of residual retroperitoneal lymph node mass after chemotherapy for metastatic seminoma has been well documented to diagnose residual viable tumour. In NSGCT, the role of FDG-PET/CT is less clear, with studies showing no significant improvement in accuracy of detecting viable tumour in residual masses over standard CT or serum tumour markers. Furthermore, it cannot clearly differentiate between teratoma, viable malignancy, or necrosis. In any case, significant residual or growing retroperitoneal masses should be resected completely and this further limits the role of FDG-PET/CT in these patients.

A final word from the expert

All patients diagnosed with testis cancer should go through a stepwise management process starting with mandatory preoperative estimation of tumour markers and discussions regarding fertility preservation, contralateral testis biopsy, and prosthesis insertion. A CT scan of the thorax, abdomen, and pelvis is important for staging the disease.

Following radical orchidectomy, it is important to assess the nadir values of serum AFP, β-hCG, and LDH to allocate an S category (S1, S2, or S3). Using the combined information from the site of the primary (testis or retroperitoneal primary or mediastinal), final histology (seminoma or non-seminomatous germ cell tumour), S category, and staging CT scan to determine extent/location of metastatic disease allows patients to be allocated to good, intermediate, or poor prognostic group as per the International Germ Cell Cancer Collaboration Group.[9] No seminoma patients are classified in the poor prognostic group.

Patients with residual masses after completion of chemotherapy should undergo RPLND at high-volume specialist surgical centres. Benefits of undertaking RPLND at designated specialized sites are significant and include lower morbidity and mortality, a higher chance of complete excision, and lower occurrence of infield recurrences. Adjunctive procedures such as nephrectomy, aortic/IVC excision and graft replacement, psoas excision, excision of retrocrural masses, bowel resection, and liver resections should be part of the armamentarium at these specialized sites.

The case presented here of a GTS exemplifies importance of the decision-making process at the testis SMDT meeting. The prognosis for GTS is excellent if diagnosed in a timely manner and treated with a radical surgical approach with complete resection of all residual disease. For complete resection, adjuvant procedures are necessary in 23–33% of cases including nephrectomy, bowel resection, and vascular procedures. This aspect has to be taken into consideration when planning surgical treatment of patients with GTS and patients should be treated in high-volume specialized centres.

Postpubertal type teratoma (not prepubertal) is derived from germ cell neoplasia and is a malignant tumour with a potential for significant metastasis. This is an interesting phenomenon as, in many other types of cancer, *in situ* neoplasia has low malignant/metastatic potential yet in germ cell neoplasia this is the reverse.

It must not be overlooked that GTS patients are usually young and otherwise fit and well. They have had extraordinary upheaval to their everyday working and personal lives, often with significant physical and psychological side effects from their previous surgery and systemic therapy. This necessitates a personalized approach to counselling about their often-formidable procedures and frequently requires significant support from all members of the MDT.

References

1. Laguna MP, Albers P, Algaba F, et al. EAU guidelines on testicular cancer. European Association of Urology. 2020. https://uroweb.org/wp-content/uploads/EAU-Guidelines-on-Testicular-Cancer-2020.pdf
2. Kliesch S, Behre HM, Jürgens H, Nieschlag E. Cryopreservation of semen from adolescent patients with malignancies. *Med Pediatr Oncol.* 1996;26(1):20–27.
3. Rives N, Perdrix A, Hennebicq S, et al. The semen quality of 1158 men with testicular cancer at the time of cryopreservation: results of the French National CECOS Network. *J Androl.* 2012;33(6):1394–1401.
4. Robinson R, Tait CD, Clarke NW, Ramani VA. Is it safe to insert a testicular prosthesis at the time of radical orchidectomy for testis cancer: an audit of 904 men undergoing radical orchidectomy. *BUJ Int.* 2016;117(2):249–252.
5. Dieckmann KP, Kulejewski M, Pichlmeier U, Loy V. Diagnosis of contralateral testicular intraepithelial neoplasia (TIN) in patients with testicular germ cell cancer: systematic two-site biopsies are more sensitive than a single random biopsy. *Eur Urol.* 2007;51(1):175–183.
6. Williamson SR, Delahunt B, Magi-Galluzzi C, et al. The World Health Organization 2016 classification of testicular germ cell tumours: a review and update from the International Society of Urological Pathology Testis Consultation Panel. *Histopathology.* 2017;70(3):335–346.
7. Moch H, Cubilla AL, Humphrey PA, Reuter VE, Ulbright TM. The 2016 WHO classification of tumours of the urinary system and male genital organs—part A: renal, penile, and testicular tumours. *Eur Urol.* 2016;70(1):93–105.
8. Zhang C, Berney DM, Hirsch MS, Cheng L, Ulbright TM. Evidence supporting the existence of benign teratomas of the postpubertal testis: a clinical, histopathologic and molecular genetic analysis of 25 cases. *Am J Surg Pathol.* 2013;37(6):827–835.
9. International Germ Cell Cancer Collaborative Group. International Germ Cell Consensus Classification: a prognostic factor-based staging system for metastatic germ cell cancers. *J Clin Oncol.* 1997;15(2):594–603.
10. De Wit R, Stoter G, Sleijfer DT, et al. Four cycles of BEP vs four cycles of VIP in patients with intermediate-prognosis metastatic testicular non-seminoma: a randomized study of the EORTC Genitourinary Tract Cancer Cooperative Group. European Organization for Research and Treatment of Cancer. *Br J Cancer.* 1998;78(6):828–832.
11. Honecker F, Aparicio J, Berney D, et al. ESMO Consensus Conference on testicular germ cell cancer: diagnosis, treatment and follow up. *Ann Oncol.* 2018;29(8):1658–1686.
12. Hendry WF, Norman AR, Dearnaley DP, et al. Metastatic nonseminomatous germ cell tumours of the testis: results of elective and salvage surgery for patients with residual retroperitoneal masses. *Cancer* 2002;94(6):1668–1676.
13. Sheinfeld J. The role of adjunctive postchemotherapy surgery for nonseminomatous germ-cell tumours: current concepts and controversies. *Semin Urol Oncol.* 2002;20(4):262–272.

14. Schirren J, Trainer S, Eberlein M, Lorch A, Beyer J, Bölükbas S. The role of residual tumor resection in the management of nonseminomatous germ cell cancer of testicular origin. *Thorac Cardiovasc Surg.* 2012;60(6):405–412.
15. Besse B, Grunenwald D, Fléchon A, et al. Nonseminomatous germ cell tumors: assessing the need for postchemotherapy contralateral pulmonary resection in patients with ipsilateral complete necrosis. *J Thorac Cardiovasc Surg.* 2009;137(2):448–452.
16. Steyerberg EW, Donohue JP, Gerl A, et al. Residual masses after chemotherapy for metastatic testicular cancer: the clinical implications of the association between retroperitoneal and pulmonary histology. Re-analysis of Histology in Testicular Cancer (ReHiT) Study Group. *J Urol.* 1997;158(2):474–478.
17. Wells H, Hayes MC, O'Brien T, Fowler S. Contemporary retroperitoneal lymph node dissection (RPLND) for testis cancer in the UK—a national study. *BJU Int.* 2017;119(1):91–99.
18. Spiess PE, Kassouf W, Brown GA, et al. Surgical management of growing teratoma syndrome: the M. D. Anderson cancer center experience. *J Urol.* 2007;177(4):1330–1334.
19. Logothetis CJ, Samuels ML, Trindade A, Johnson DE. The growing teratoma syndrome. *Cancer.* 1982;50(3):1629–1635.
20. Maroto P, Tabernero JM, Villavicencio H, et al. Growing teratoma syndrome: experience of a single institution. *Eur Urol.* 1997;32(3):305–309.
21. Panda A, Kandasamy D, Sh C, Jana M. Growing teratoma syndrome of ovary: avoiding a misdiagnosis of tumour recurrence. *J Clin Diagn Res.* 2014;8(1):197–198.
22. Gorbatiy V, Spiess PE, Pisters LL. The growing teratoma syndrome: current review of the literature. *Indian J Urol.* 2009;25(2):186–189.
23. Priod F, Lorge F, Di Gregorio M, et al. Recurrent masses after testicular cancer: growing teratoma syndrome. A case report and review of the literature. *Case Rep Oncol.* 2017;10(3):910–915.
24. British Association of Urological Surgeons. Retroperitoneal excision of abdominal lymph node (RPNLD). British Association of Urological Surgeons. July 2021. https://www.baus.org.uk/_userfiles/pages/files/Patients/Leaflets/RPLND.pdf
25. Hinton S, Catalano PJ, Einhorn LH, et al. Cisplatin, etoposide and either bleomycin or ifosfamide in the treatment of disseminated germ cell tumors: final analysis of an intergroup trial. *Cancer.* 2003;97(8):1869–1875.
26. Tran B, Ruiz-Morales JM, Gonzalez-Billalabeitia E, et al. Large retroperitoneal lymphadenopathy and increased risk of venous thromboembolism in patients receiving first-line chemotherapy for metastatic germ cell tumors: a study by the global germ cell cancer group (G3). *Cancer Med.* 2020;9(1):116–124.
27. Seidel C, Daugaard G, Tryakin A, et al. The prognostic impact of different tumor marker levels in nonseminomatous germ cell tumor patients with intermediate prognosis: a registry of the International Global Germ Cell Tumor Collaborative Group (G3). *Urol Oncol.* 2019;37(11):809.e19–809.e25.
28. Aide N, Comoz F, Sevin E. Enlarging residual mass after treatment of a nonseminomatous germ cell tumor: growing teratoma syndrome or cancer recurrence? *J Clin Oncol.* 2007;25(28):4494–4496.

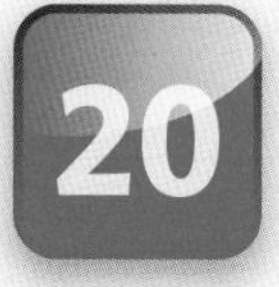

Metastatic testicular cancer: post-chemotherapy residual mass and cancer survivorship

Findlay MacAskill

Expert commentary Archie Fernando

Case history

A 34-year-old man was referred to the urology clinic via the '2-week wait' suspected cancer pathway for assessment of a scrotal lump. He had noticed the lump while in the shower about a month previously and was concerned that it might be increasing in size. There was no associated pain, history of trauma, or symptoms suggestive of infection. He was otherwise well. His past medical history included a previous appendicectomy aged 14 years and childhood asthma. There was no family history of testicular disease. On examination, a right testicular mass was easily palpable. There was no associated hydrocele and no lymphadenopathy. No abnormality was palpable in the left testis.

Ultrasound scanning confirmed a 5.2 × 3.4 × 2.7 cm heterogeneous right testicular mass with increased vascularity consistent with malignancy. The left testis was normal. Blood tests showed elevated tumour markers: alpha-fetoprotein (AFP) 101.6 ng/mL, beta human chorionic gonadotropin (β-hCG) 308 IU/mL, and lactate dehydrogenase (LDH) 275 U/L. Testosterone level was normal. A computed tomography (CT) scan of the thorax, abdomen, and pelvis showed a 7 cm retroperitoneal mass in the inter-aortocaval region likely to be metastatic testicular cancer (TC) (Figure 20.1). No other abnormality was detected.

Clinical tip Examination

Examination of the scrotum must always be carried out together with a general examination to find possible distant metastases, such as a supraclavicular node, a palpable abdominal mass, or gynaecomastia, which can be present in up to 10% of cases.[1]

(a)

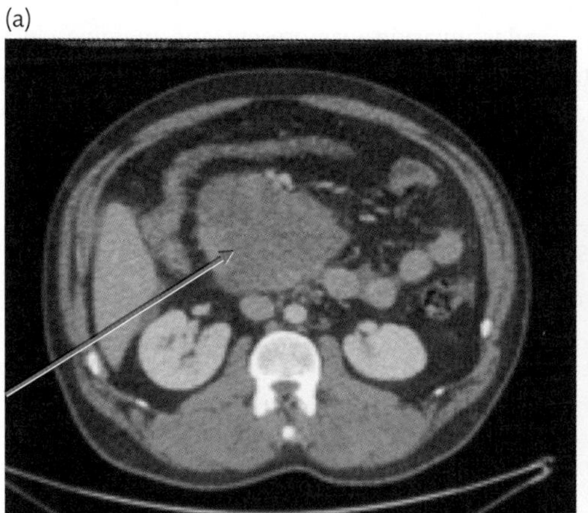

(b)

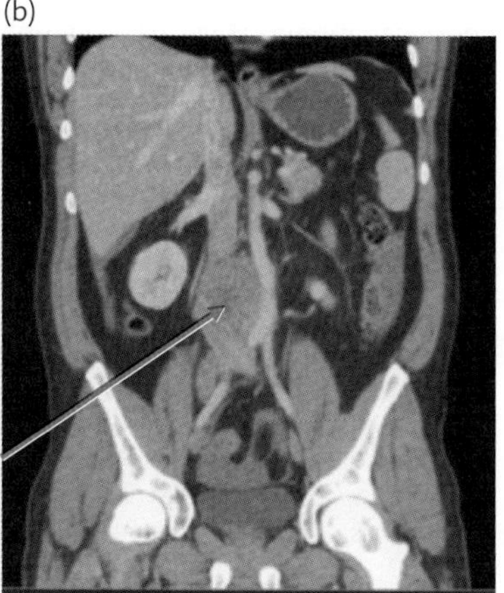

Figure 20.1 CT scan of the abdomen and pelvis shows a large inter-aortic mass in (a) axial and (b) coronal sections.

Learning point Tumour markers

Serum tumour markers help in the diagnosis and staging of testis cancer, and can also be used as prognostic factors both at the time of diagnosis and during treatment.[1]

Approximately 10% of TC is advanced (>stage III) at presentation and the majority of these have elevated tumour markers.[2] Increased AFP concentration suggests a diagnosis of non-seminomatous germ cell tumour (NSGCT) or mixed germ cell tumour (GCT).

Table 20.1 Adapted prognostic-based staging system for metastatic non-seminomatous germ cell cancer

Prognosis	Type	Criteria
Good	Non-seminoma (56%): 5-year PFS 89% 5-year survival 92%	All: 1. Testis/retroperitoneal primary 2. No non-pulmonary visceral metastases 3. AFP <1000 ng/mL 4. hCG <5000 IU/L 5. LDH <1.5 × ULN
Intermediate	Non-seminoma (28%): 5-year PFS 75% 5-year survival 80%	All: 1. Testis/retroperitoneal primary 2. No non-pulmonary visceral metastases 3. AFP 1000–10,000 ng/mL 4. hCG 5000–50,000 IU/L 5. LDH 1.5–10 × ULN
Bad	Non-seminoma (16%): 5-year PFS 41% 5-year survival 48%	All: 1. Testis/retroperitoneal primary 2. Non-pulmonary visceral metastases 3. AFP >10,000 ng/mL 4. hCG >50,000 IU/L 5. LDH >10 × ULN

PFS, progression-free survival; ULN, upper limit of normal.
International Germ Cell Collaborative Group (IGCCG).[4]

A multidisciplinary team decision was made to proceed to urgent right inguinal orchidectomy. Semen analysis was performed prior to orchidectomy showing mild oligospermia, with normal semen volume and pH, but sufficient quality sperm for banking. The patient was in a relationship and neither of them had any children. Following counselling of the patient and his girlfriend with regard to the likelihood of treatment impacting future fertility, they opted to cryopreserve semen prior to orchidectomy.

The patient underwent a right inguinal orchidectomy and prosthesis insertion without complication and made a swift recovery. Tumour markers 1 week following orchidectomy were AFP 54.2 ng/mL, β-hCG 1 IU/mL, LDH 217 U/L. Histological examination of the orchidectomy specimen revealed a NSGCT with 40% yolk sac, 40% embryonal, and 20% choriocarcinoma, stage pT2. Lymphovascular invasion was present and margins clear of tumour. Histological analysis and tumour markers placed him in the good prognosis group (Table 20.1). The multidisciplinary team decision was to proceed with three cycles of bleomycin, etoposide, and cisplatin (BEP) chemotherapy, once he had recovered fully.

Learning point Prompt orchidectomy

In cases of metastatic TC at presentation, proceed directly to orchidectomy unless unwell, multiple lung metastases, AFP >1000 ng/mL, hCG >5000 IU/mL, or renal obstruction.

Expert comment Semen analysis

Semen analysis should be included in initial diagnostics because up to 50% of men with TC have impaired spermatogenesis, 29% have oligospermia, and 11% azoospermia[3]; both cancer and its treatment can have an effect on spermatogenesis.

Onco-testicular sperm extraction (onco-TESE) can be offered to patients who are azoospermic at presentation.

Learning point Chemotherapy for NSGCT

Chemotherapy for NSGCT is based on prognostic category:

- Good prognosis: three cycles of BEP. A 5-day regimen is recommended as 3-day regimen was found to be associated with increased toxicity despite equal efficacy.[7]
- Intermediate prognosis: four cycles of BEP.
- Poor prognosis: four cycles of BEP with consideration of switching to a more dose-intensive regimen if there is poor marker decline after the first cycle.

A three-cycle BEP regimen should be administered at 21-day intervals with delay only in cases where patients develop fever with associated granulocytopenia (<1000/mm^3) or thrombocytopenia (<100,000/IU).

Two weeks after his right orchidectomy and prosthesis insertion, the patient commenced chemotherapy. The dosing regimen used was cisplatin 20 mg/m^2 days 1–5 with hydration; etoposide 100 mg/m^2 days 1–5; and bleomycin 30 mg days 1, 8, and 15; with a 21-day interval between the start of cycles. He tolerated chemotherapy relatively well with only mild side effects which included nausea, hair loss, and anaemia. His tumour markers were checked between cycles. Following the first cycle: AFP 30.6 ng/mL, β-hCG < 1 IU/mL, and LDH 228 U/L. Following the third cycle: AFP, β-hCG, and LDH all normalized.

Expert comment Serum tumour markers during chemotherapy

Serum tumour markers should decline during chemotherapy to indicate therapeutic effect. Persistence of tumour markers during chemotherapy has adverse prognostic value.[8,9] Switching to more dose-intensive regimens in poor-risk NSGCT patients with slow marker decline following the first cycle of BEP may reduce progression-free survival, although not overall survival.[10] Poor-risk patients should be treated within a clinical trial in a high-volume reference centre where possible.[11,12]

Current trials

- Phase III BEP (P3BEP): phase III trial of accelerated versus standard BEP for intermediate- or poor-risk patients.
- TIGER: phase III trial of salvage chemotherapy comparing conventional-dose chemotherapy using paclitaxel, ifosfamide, and cisplatin with high-dose chemotherapy using mobilizing paclitaxel plus ifosfamide followed by high-dose carboplatin and etoposide as first treatment in relapsed or refractory GCTs.

Six weeks post chemotherapy, a CT scan was carried out to assess treatment response (Figure 20.2). This showed a good response with the retroperitoneal mass reducing in size to 1.6 cm with no other areas of disease involvement.

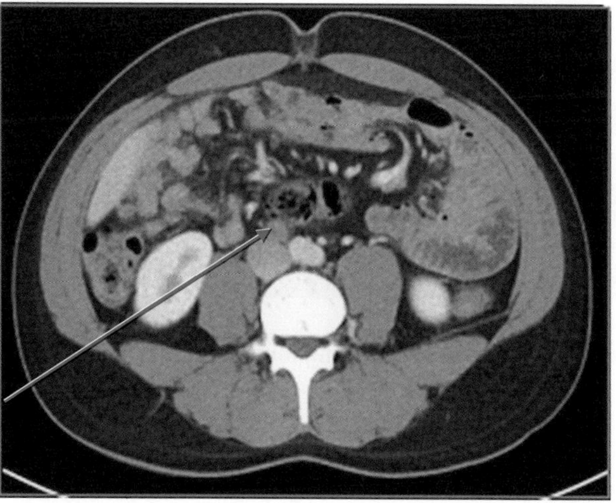

Figure 20.2 CT scan showing a persistent 1.6 cm inter-aortic mass.

Expert comment Uncertainty about metastatic disease

In cases where there is uncertainty about the presence of metastatic disease (e.g. lymph nodes <2 cm in size with normal tumour markers), reimaging after a 6–8-week period of surveillance or ultrasound- or CT-guided biopsy should be considered prior to treatment. There is insufficient evidence to support the use of positron emission tomography to clarify the situation in this setting.

Learning point First-line treatment of metastatic GCTs

The first-line treatment of metastatic GCTs depends on:

- The histology of the primary tumour
- Prognostic groups as defined by the International Germ Cell Cancer Collaborative Group based on 5202 non-seminoma and 660 seminoma cases (Table 20.1)[4]
- Marker decline during the first cycle of chemotherapy in 'poor prognosis' patients.

Clinical tip Contraindication to bleomycin

If bleomycin is contraindicated (interstitial pneumonitis, lung fibrosis; chronic lung disease; liver dysfunction; renal failure) then four cycles of etoposide and cisplatin should be used although there is some evidence that this regimen is inferior to BEP.[4–6]

The patient was extremely disappointed with the news that there was a residual mass present following chemotherapy. It was explained to him that the management of this residual mass presents a clinical dilemma as it is difficult to be certain whether the residual mass contains any viable tumour or is simply 'dead tissue' following successful treatment with chemotherapy. He became tearful during the consultation and wished to defer further discussion to later in the week. An interim appointment with the in-hospital counselling support service was arranged and a follow-up review in 3 days.

Learning point Residual masses post chemotherapy

Post chemotherapy mass in NSGCT is[13]:

- Fifty per cent fibrosis/necrosis
- Forty per cent teratoma: resistant to chemotherapy; can grow causing organ compression; 3–6% transformation to malignant neoplasms such as sarcoma, adenocarcinoma, or primitive neuroendocrine cancer
- Ten per cent residual GCT.

Future directions MicroRNA-371a-3p biomarker

In 2011, a novel serum microRNA biomarker was proposed. Micro-RNAs are small non-coding RNAs involved in gene expression. Serum levels of micro-RNA-371a-3p (M371 test) in patients with stage I, metastatic, and relapsed TC were compared to classical biomarkers and to male controls. It showed significantly higher sensitivity and specificity, 90.1% and 94% respectively, with a positive predictive value of 97.2%.[15] micro-RNA-371a-3p was also significantly associated with clinical stage, primary tumour size, and response to treatment. Furthermore, micro-RNA-371a-3p showed elevated levels in relapsed cases, which normalized following successful treatment. This novel biomarker could greatly improve diagnosis and surveillance in TC, and may help predict the presence of viable tumour in borderline cases of extra-testicular disease both at diagnosis and after chemotherapy.[15]

Expert comment Residual masses post chemotherapy

- Predicting histology of post-chemotherapy masses is challenging. While useful in seminomas >3 cm, positron emission tomography scanning in NSGCT is only 70% sensitive and 48% specific for GCT.[14]
- Even features such as absence of teratoma in orchidectomy specimen, marker normalization, and small size of mass (<5 mm) cannot reliably exclude viable tumour.[16]
- In cases where the residual NSGCT mass is >1 cm, surgical resection is recommended.[17] However, some lesions slightly >1 cm may continue to reduce further in size.
- In residual NSGCT masses <1 cm, recommendation is less clear. Although these may contain viable tumour, >70% contain fibronecrotic tissue only.[18]
- Surveillance is therefore an option in these cases especially with normal tumour markers. With observation in these cases there is a 9% life-long risk of recurrence with a 70% chance of subsequent cure.[19]

On his next visit 3 days later, following multidisciplinary team discussion, the patient was offered the options of surveillance with a 6-week interval scan versus surgical resection of the residual mass. The pros and cons of each option were discussed at length. The patient felt uncomfortable with surveillance but was also anxious about major surgery. After evaluation of all involved areas present on the initial and post-treatment CT scans he was deemed suitable for minimally invasive robotic-assisted retroperitoneal lymph node dissection (RPLND) involving a unilateral right-sided nerve-sparing template. Following discussion of what surgery involved and the associated risks, and a further day to confer with his family, he opted to have surgery.

Future directions RPLND

Post RPLND 'dry ejaculation' is due to the resection of sympathetic nerves entering the superior hypogastric plexus and lumbar splanchnic nerves during surgery. The original 'bilateral template RPLND' includes supra-hilar and infra-iliac dissection resulting in dry ejaculation in almost all patients (Figure 20.3a). Dry ejaculation rates reduced to approximately 75% with 'modified RPLND' sparing the contralateral iliac region below the iliac bifurcation (Figure 20.3b). 'Unilateral template RPLND' confined to the ipsilateral side of the aortic midline below the inferior mesenteric artery (Figure 20.3c, d) was then developed, preserving ejaculation in >80%.[20] Donohue et al. subsequently introduced 'nerve-sparing RPLND' where the sympathetic nerve fibres were carefully dissected out, identified, and preserved.[21] The 10-year recurrence-free and overall survival of unilateral and nerve-sparing RPLND in appropriately selected cases, even post chemotherapy, is the same as with bilateral RPLND with significantly higher rates of preserved ejaculation (>85% compared to <20%).[20–22] The first laparoscopic RPLND in 1992 marked an initiative to reduce surgical morbidity for TC patients. Following the first robotic-assisted laparoscopic RPLND (R-RPLND) in 2006, experienced high-volume centres have shown comparable oncological outcomes of R-RPLND with reduced peri- and postoperative morbidity in the primary setting.[23]

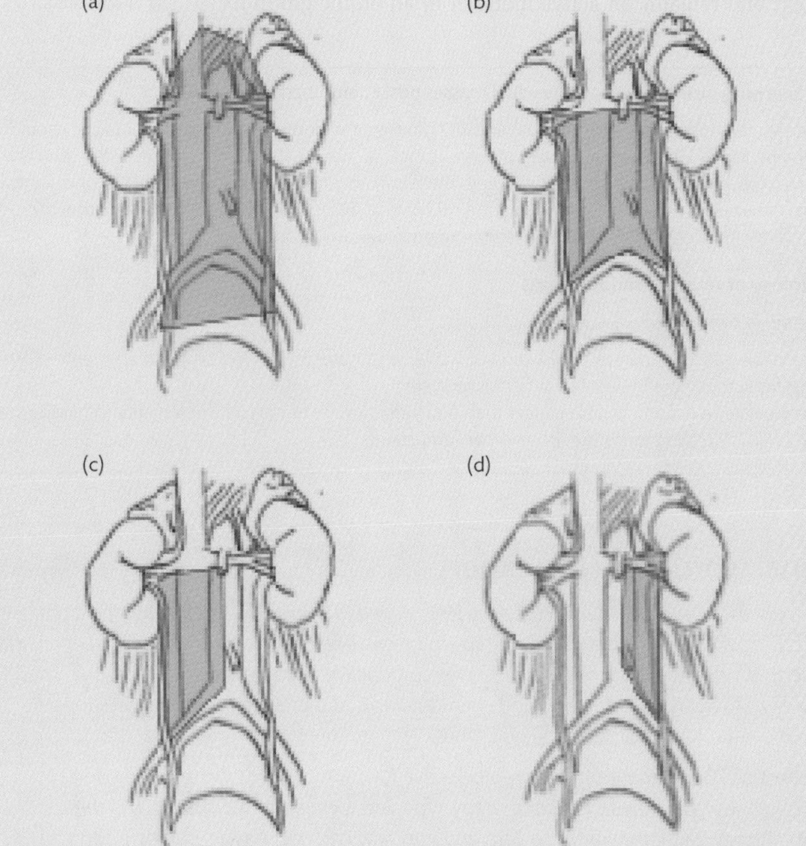

Figure 20.3 RPLND templates. (a) Standard bilateral; (b) modified bilateral; (c) unilateral modified, right; (d) unilateral modified, left.

Expert comment RPLND

RPLND in TC is challenging surgery with up to 30% of patients requiring additional procedures such as nephrectomy, muscle resection, and vascular reconstructive surgery. RPLND should therefore be performed in specialist centres. Centralization of surgery has reduced mortality from 6% to 0.8% and local recurrence from 16% to 3%.[25] Resection of residual masses of seminoma is rarely indicated, as surgery is extremely difficult due to intense fibrosis.

Furthermore, there is a small but steadily increasing body of evidence that post-chemotherapy R-RPLND in selected cases of small post-chemotherapy masses is safe both surgically and oncologically if performed in specialist high-volume centres.[24]

Surgery was performed using a robotic-assisted laparoscopic technique by a two-consultant surgical team. The residual mass was adherent to the inferior vena cava. Resection of the mass resulted in a small cavotomy which required repair. Lymphatics were cauterized or clipped throughout the RPLND to reduce risk of postoperative lymph leak. The operating time was 3 hours and blood loss 280 mL. The patient was quite uncomfortable on the night of surgery but felt well the next day. There was 120 mL of serous fluid in the abdominal drain so the drain was left for a further 24 hours to monitor for a lymphatic leak. He was very well on day 2 with only 10 mL in the drain so the drain was removed and he was discharged home.

Histology of the surgical specimen showed 14 nodes with some evidence of necrosis but no viable tumour seen. When the patient returned for his postoperative visit he was well and with minimal pain. His erections and ejaculation were normal. He was delighted with the pathological finding of no viable tumour. He therefore required no further treatment and was placed on surveillance. He continued with counselling support and remains an active member of an online group for TC survivors.

Learning point Surgery for residual masses post chemotherapy

When surgery is performed for residual masses following chemotherapy, 'lumpectomy' alone should not be performed. All areas of primary metastatic disease sites must be completely resected usually within 6 weeks of completing chemotherapy. There is increasing evidence supporting the oncological safety of template dissections rather than radical bilateral dissections which allow preservation of ejaculatory function[20-22] without compromising oncological outcomes.

Histology of resected residual mass

If histology of the resected residual mass shows:

- No viable cancer or complete resection of viable cancer present in <10% of the total volume of the specimen then no additional treatment is indicated
- Incomplete resection of viable cancer then two further cycles of cisplatin- based chemotherapy may be given in certain groups (e.g. poor-prognosis patients).[14]

A final word from the expert

TC is a disease of survivors. Given the excellent prognosis (survival rates >95%) of most patients with TC, focus on high-quality survivorship—future well-being—at each stage of TC management is crucial. Efforts should be made to preserve reproductive and hormonal function; minimize morbidity of surgery, radiotherapy, and chemotherapy; and provide psychological support, without compromising oncological outcomes.

The effect of TC treatment on male reproductive function depends on several factors, including age at the time of cancer therapy, type and location of the cancer, and the treatment(s) given. Both hypogonadism and infertility can occur as a result of TC and its treatments. Primary assessment should therefore include both semen analysis and serum hormone testing.[26,27]

Testis-sparing surgery may be suitable in cases of synchronous bilateral testicular tumours, metachronous contralateral tumours, or tumour in a solitary testis. Tumour volume should be <30% of overall testicular volume and oncological surgical rules respected. Onco-TESE (*ex vivo* testicular sperm extraction from the affected testicle at the time of orchidectomy) can be offered to patients who are azoospermic and have an abnormal or absent contralateral testis to preserve future fertility.[26]

Biochemical hypogonadism is prevalent in 5–13% of patients following orchidectomy and 11–27% following chemotherapy.[27] Hormone levels should be checked at diagnosis and after all treatments, and testosterone replacement offered. Patients should also be made aware of the symptoms of hypogonadism such as fatigue and low libido.

The peri- and postoperative morbidity of RPLND is considerable. Many patients develop retrograde ejaculation due to damaged superior hypogastric and lumbar splanchnic nerves resulting in loss of ejaculation and the ability to conceive naturally. The use of unilateral and nerve-sparing RPLND in appropriate cases, the utilization of minimally invasive techniques where appropriate, and the centralization of this complex operation to high-volume specialist centres has significantly reduced morbidity, mortality, and long-term sequelae.[14,21–25]

Long-term side effects of chemotherapy for TC can include hearing loss, gastric symptoms, lung damage, and peripheral neuropathy. Current chemotherapy regimens aim to minimize these; for example, administration of cisplatin over 5 days instead of 3 days reduces incidence of hearing impairment and tinnitus.[7] A large multinational prospective trial has shown that delivery of chemotherapy in high-volume centres is associated with better outcomes: higher cumulative doses, lower toxicity and treatment-related mortality, and more frequent use of post-chemotherapy resection of residual masses.[28]

Finally, although TC is highly 'curable', this does not lessen the emotional toll on patients, the effects of which should not be underestimated. The levels of psychological distress reported by TC survivors is between 9% and 27%.[29] Psychosocial morbidity includes uncertainty about the future, feelings of inadequacy, fear of stigmatization, anxiety, depression, and symptoms of post-traumatic stress disorder. Comprehensive TC services should offer easy access to counselling and actively encourage involvement in TC communities to ensure that TC survivors have a good quality of life after cure.

References

1. Kim W, Rosen MA, Langer JE, Banner MP, Siegelman ES, Ramchandani P. US MR imaging correlation in pathologic conditions of the scrotum. *Radiographics.* 2007;27(5):1239–1253.
2. Northern Ireland Cancer Registry, Queens University Belfast. *Incidence by stage 2010–2014.* Belfast: Northern Ireland Cancer Registry; 2016.
3. Howard GC, Nairn M; Guideline Development Group. Management of adult testicular germ cell tumours: summary of updated SIGN guideline. *BMJ.* 2011;342:d2005.
4. Baniel J, Roth BJ, Foster RS, Donohue JP. Cost- and risk-benefit considerations in the management of clinical stage I non-seminomatous testicular tumors. *Ann Surg Oncol.* 1996;3(1):86–93.
5. Giannatempo P, Greco T, Mariani L, et al. Radiotherapy or chemotherapy for clinical stage IIA and IIB seminoma: a systematic review and meta-analysis of patient outcomes. *Ann Oncol.* 2015;26(4):657–668.
6. Weissbach L, Bussar-Maatz R, Flechtner H, Pichlmeier U, Hartmann M, Keller L. RPLND or primary chemotherapy in clinical stage IIA/B non-seminomatous germ cell tumors: results of a prospective multicenter trial including quality of life assessment. *Eur Urol.* 2000;37(5):582–594.

7. Krege S, Boergermann C, Baschek R, et al. Single agent carboplatin for CS IIA/B testicular seminoma. A phase II study of the German Testicular Cancer Study Group (GTCSG). *Ann Oncol.* 2006;17(2):276–280.
8. Brierley JE, Gospodarowicz MK, Wittekind C, eds. *TNM Classification of Malignant Tumours*. 8th ed. Chichester: Wiley-Blackwell; 2017.
9. Peyret C. Tumeurs du testicule. Synthèse et recommandations en onco-urologie. [Testicular tumours. Summary of onco-urological recommendations.] *Prog Urol.* 1993;2:60–64.
10. Mead GM, Stenning SP. The International Germ Cell Consensus Classification: a new prognostic factor based staging classification for metastatic germ cell tumours. *Clin Oncol (R Coll Radiol).* 1997;9(4):207–209.
11. Zengerling F, Hartmann M, Heidenreich A, et al. German second-opinion network for testicular cancer: sealing the leaky pipe between evidence and clinical practice. *Oncol Rep.* 2014;31(6):2477–2481.
12. Chung PW, Gospodarowicz MK, Panzarella T, et al. Stage II testicular seminoma: patterns of recurrence and outcome of treatment. *Eur Urol.* 2004;45(6):754–759.
13. Gillessen S, Powles T, Lim L, Wilson P, Shamash J. Low-dose induction chemotherapy with Baby-BOP in patients with metastatic germ-cell tumours does not compromise outcome: a single-centre experience. *Ann Oncol.* 2010;21(8):1589–1593.
14. Laguna MP, Albers P, Algaba F, et al. EAU guidelines on testicular cancer. European Association of Urology. 2020. https://uroweb.org/wp-content/uploads/EAU-Guidelines-on-Testicular-Cancer-2020.pdf
15. Dieckmann KP, Radtke A, Geczi L, et al. Serum levels of microRNA-371a-3p (M371 test) as a new biomarker of testicular germ cell tumors: results of a prospective multi-centric study. *J Clin Oncol.* 2019;37(16):1412–1423.
16. Oldenburg J, Alfsen GC, Lien HH, Aass N, Waehre H, Fossa SD. Post-chemotherapy retroperitoneal surgery remains necessary in patients with non-seminomatous testicular cancer and minimal residual tumor masses. *J Clin Oncol.* 2003;21(17):3310–3317.
17. Hartmann JT, Candelaria M, Kuczyk MA, Schmoll HJ, Bokemeyer C. Comparison of histological results from the resection of residual masses at different sites after chemotherapy for metastatic non-seminomatous germ cell tumours. *Eur J Cancer.* 1997;33(6):843–847.
18. Carver BS, Shayegan B, Serio A, Motzer RJ, Bosl GJ, Sheinfeld J. Long-term clinical outcome after post-chemotherapy retroperitoneal lymph node dissection in men with residual teratoma. *J Clin Oncol.* 2007;25(9):1033–1037.
19. Ehrlich Y, Brames MJ, Beck SD, Foster RS, Einhorn LH. Long-term follow-up of cisplatin combination chemotherapy in patients with disseminated non-seminomatous germ cell tumors: is a post-chemotherapy retroperitoneal lymph node dissection needed after complete remission? *J Clin Oncol.* 2010;28(4):531–536.
20. Hiester A, Nini A, Fingerhut A, et al. Preservation of ejaculatory function after postchemotherapy retroperitoneal lymph node dissection (PC-RPLND) in patients with testicular cancer: template vs. bilateral resection. *Front Surg.* 2018;5:80.
21. Donohue JP, Foster RS. Retroperitoneal lymphadenectomy in staging and treatment. The development of nerve-sparing techniques. *Urol Clin North Am.* 1998;25(3):461–468.
22. Heidenreich A, Pfister D, Witthuhn R, Thüer D, Albers P. Post-chemotherapy retroperitoneal lymph node dissection in advanced testicular cancer: radical or modified template resection. *Eur Urol.* 2009;55(1):217–224.
23. Stepanian S, Patel M, Porter J. Robot-assisted laparoscopic lymph node dissection for testicular cancer: evolution of the technique. *Eur Urol.* 2016;70(4):661–667.
24. Schwen ZR, Gupta M, Pierorazio PM. A review of the outcomes and technique for robotic-assisted laparoscopic retroperitoneal lymph node dissection for testicular cancer. *Adv Urol.* 2018;3:140–145.
25. Flechon A, Tavernier E, Boyle H, Meeus P, Rivoire M, Droz JP. Long term oncological outcome after post-chemotherapy retroperitoneal lymph node dissection in men with metastatic non-seminomatous germ cell tumour. *BJU Int.* 2010;106(6):779–785.

26. Moody JA, Ahmed K, Yap T, Minhas S, Shabbir M. Fertility management in testicular cancer: the need to establish a standardised and evidence-based patient-centric pathway. *BJU Int.* 2019;123(1):160–172.
27. Oldenburg J. Hypogonadism and fertility issues following primary treatment for testicular cancer. *Urol Oncol.* 2015;33(9):407–412.
28. Feuer EJ, Sheinfeld J, Bosl GJ. Association between number of patients treated and patient outcome in metastatic testicular cancer. *J Nat Cancer Inst.* 1999;91(10):816–818.
29. Fleer J, Hoekstra HJ, Sleijfer DT, Hoekstra-Weebers JE. Quality of life of survivors of testicular germ cell cancer: a review of the literature. *Support Care Cancer.* 2004;12(7):476–478.

SECTION 9

Functional, female, and neurourology

CASE

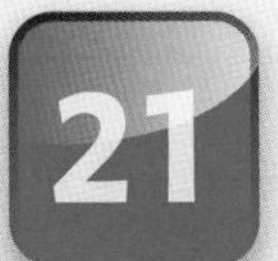

Benign prostatic enlargement and acute urinary retention

Emma Papworth, Joseph Jelski, and Hashim Hashim

Expert commentary Hashim Hashim

Case history

A 60-year-old man presents to the urology outpatient department complaining of lower urinary tract symptoms (LUTS). On questioning, he describes mixed storage and voiding symptoms, including urinary frequency, urgency, nocturia, and reduced flow. He denies any episodes of urinary incontinence. He completes an International Prostate Symptom Score (IPSS) questionnaire with a score of 19 demonstrating moderate symptom severity. His bother score is 6.

Breakdown of his IPSS score:

- Incomplete emptying 3; frequency 3; intermittency 2; urgency 3; weak stream 3; straining 2; nocturia 3.
- Voiding/storage ratio >1, indicating a slight predominance of voiding symptoms.[1]

Clinical tip Assessment of male LUTS

There are a number of validated tools for the assessment of male LUTS including the IPSS and the International Consultation on Incontinence Modular Questionnaire for Male Lower Urinary Tract Symptoms (ICIQ-MLUTS). The most commonly used is the IPSS, which has been shown to be reliable and reproducible.

IPSS:

- Seven questions on symptoms and one question on quality of life.
- Max score: 35.
- Mild: 0–7; moderate: 8–19; severe: 20–35.

ICIQ-MLUTS:

- Twenty-four questions, individual bother score for each symptom.

When using the IPSS, missing the symptoms of hesitancy and urgency urinary incontinence (UUI) may significantly affect the management, and hence affect the clinical outcome. These symptoms are better detected by the ICIQ-MLUTS questionnaire. The ability to assess bother associated with individual symptoms using the ICIQ-MLUTS enables treatment to be individualized and enables a more patient-centred approach to the assessment of male LUTS.

A frequency/volume chart confirms consumption of between four and five cups of coffee each day with frequent small-volume voids and no evidence of leaking or

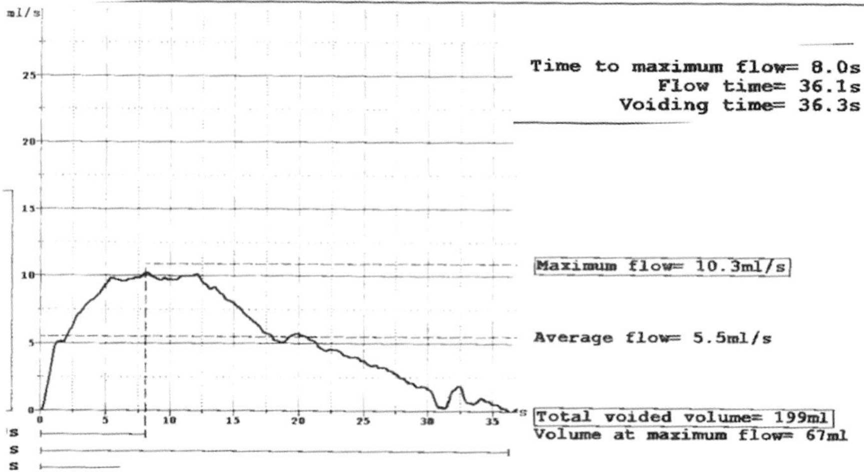

Figure 21.1 Uroflowmetry.

nocturnal polyuria. A flow test performed in clinic reveals a reduced maximum flow rate (Qmax) of 10 mL/s with a voided volume of 199 mL and a post-void residual of 80 mL (Figure 21.1). Digital rectal examination reveals a mildly enlarged, benign-feeling prostate with a prostate-specific antigen level of 2.8 ng/mL.

Clinical tip Uroflowmetry

To prepare for a flow test, a patient will need to have a comfortably full bladder, usually needing to consume between 500 and 1000 mL of fluid prior to attending. The test can take up to 2–3 hours. Flows are only useful if a there is at least 150 mL in the bladder. Some patients are unable to fill to significant volumes and this is important to know prior to starting the test and will be evident on the bladder diary. The International Continence Society 'Good Urodynamics Practice' guidelines[2] recommend one representative flow. In practice, patients are usually asked to do two flows to ensure that an adequate and representative flow is obtained. Patients should be asked if the flow was illustrative of their day-to-day flow, if not then it should be repeated.

The patient should be told to avoid compressing/squeezing the urethra during voiding in order to limit the 'squeeze artefact', and should not allow 'wandering/cruising' around the funnel, which may lead to an inaccurate result.

A flow test should be visually reviewed to ensure that any spurious results are identified (do not rely on the electronic printed report only). If there is considerable doubt as to the veracity of the test, pressure–flow studies are indicated after failure of medical and conservative therapy.

Learning point Flow rates

Of men with a Qmax <10 mL/s, about 90% will be obstructed on pressure–flow urodynamic criteria. The remaining proportion of patients will have a low-pressure, low-flow situation with reduced contractility—detrusor underactivity.[3]

Of men with a flow rate of >15 mL/s, 75% will not have bladder outlet obstruction (BOO).[3] The remainder with good flow may have a high-pressure high flow situation where increased detrusor work compensates for a degree of obstruction. A reduced flow rate is a risk factor for symptomatic progression to urinary retention (UR).

The patient's general practitioner had tried an alpha-1 antagonist (tamsulosin 400 mcg once a day); however, the patient had stopped taking this due to retrograde ejaculation.

Evidence base Medical therapy for LUTS

Monotherapy with alpha antagonists/blockers is recommended for all men with uncomplicated LUTS. Meta-analysis of alpha-blocker trials has demonstrated a reduction in symptoms of 30–40% and a durable improvement in flow rates of 16–25%.[4]

Finasteride (5-alpha reductase inhibitor) does not appear to be as effective as a single agent; however, data have shown the importance of this drug in reducing disease progression. The PLESS study shows a reduction in UR (57%) and the need for a transurethral resection of the prostate (TURP; 55%) over 4 years.[5]

Results from the MTOPS[6] and CombAT[7] studies have demonstrated significant benefit from combination therapy with an alpha antagonist and 5-alpha reductase inhibitor.

BAUS guidelines[8] recommend the use of combination treatment for those with bothersome LUTS, prostatic obstruction, and risk factors for progression.

Following initial consultation, management of the patient's storage symptoms are prioritized as these were reported to be the most bothersome to his quality of life. To manage his overactive bladder (OAB) symptoms, the patient is advised to reduce consumption of bladder irritants including caffeinated drinks, bearing in mind the small proportion of caffeine in decaffeinated preparations. The patient is also given bladder re-training advice to include prolongation of time between voids and the technique of double voiding to aid bladder emptying. Fluid manipulation and reduction of fluid by 25% is advised as long as the patient drinks >1 L a day.[9] If conservative measures fail, use of an anticholinergic/antimuscarinic or beta-3 agonist medications is recommended. Various antimuscarinic preparations are available which can be trialled according to efficacy and degree to which the patient experiences side effects.

Unfortunately, the patient goes on to develop a urinary tract infection and presents in UR. He is catheterized, restarted on tamsulosin, and goes on to successfully void following a trial without catheter one week later.

Learning point OAB

- OAB occurs in both men and women. It is a symptom complex expressed by the patient and should not be confused with detrusor overactivity, which is a urodynamic diagnosis.
- About 80% of men who have OAB will have detrusor overactivity and about 55% of women.[10]
- OAB can coexist with other common conditions such as benign prostatic obstruction (BPO), stress incontinence, and nocturnal polyuria.

Learning point Risk factor for acute urinary retention

A number of risk factors for acute urinary retention (AUR) have been identified as shown in Table 21.1.[11]

Table 21.1 Risk factors for acute urinary retention

Risk factor	AUR relative risk
PSA >1.4 ng/mL	2.0
Prostate volume >30 mL	3.0
IPSS >7	3.2
Qmax <12 mL/s	3.9
Age >70 vs 40–49 years	10–11

In view of this episode of UR and ambiguity as to the causality of symptoms, urodynamics were requested at this stage (Figure 21.2).

Evidence base UPSTREAM study

Symptom outcomes are non-inferior when invasive urodynamics is included in the assessment of male LUTS but further analysis is needed to determine the group of patients for whom urodynamics is useful. The UPSTREAM study did, however, show that patients reported satisfaction with understanding their underlying condition if urodynamics were performed prior to surgery.[12]

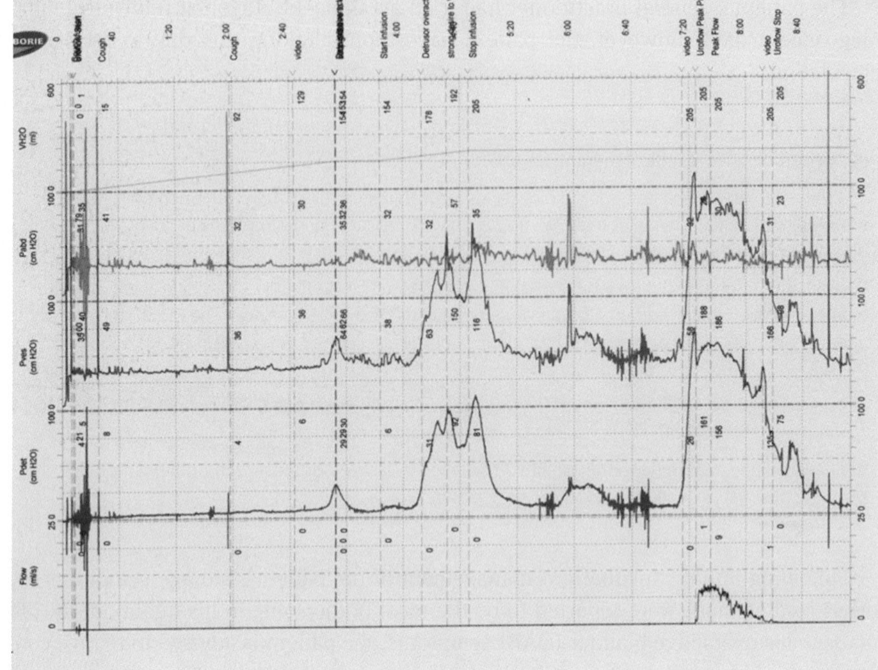

Figure 21.2 The UDS reveals a mixed picture with proven detrusor overactivity but also evidence of bladder outlet obstruction.

Learning point Urodynamics

BOO is a urodynamic diagnosis, which can only be measured through the concomitant measurement of urinary flow and detrusor pressure. It represents a high-pressure, low-flow situation.

The International Continence Society nomogram categorizes patients as obstructed, unobstructed, or equivocal (Figure 21.3).

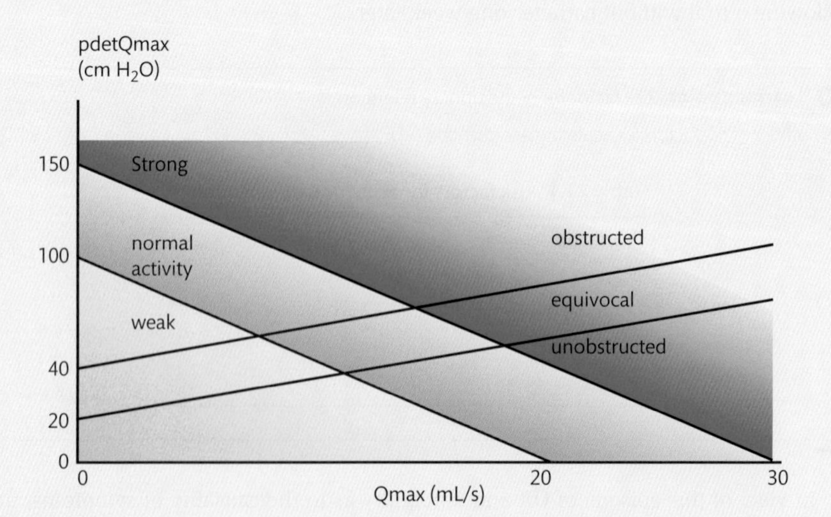

Figure 21.3 Composite obstruction (BOOI) and contractility (BCI) nomogram. Pdet, detrusor pressure; PdetQmax, detrusor pressure at maximum flow rate; Qmax, maximum flow rate.

The Bladder Outflow Obstruction Index (BOOI) gives a single numeric value through the equation:

$$PdetQmax - (2 \times Qmax) = BOOI$$

where:

- >40 = obstructed
- 20–40 = equivocal
- <20 = unobstructed.

The Bladder Contractility Index (BCI) can be calculated through the following equation:

$$BCI = PdetQmax + (5 \times Qmax)$$

where:

- <100 = detrusor underactivity
- >100 = normal
- >150 = strong.

In view of the confirmed evidence of BOO, recent UR, and urinary tract infection, the patient was offered a TURP. Following a detailed consent process including the risk of 20–25% of urgency incontinence, the patient was listed for surgery. At TURP a high bladder neck and middle lobe were noted. Postoperatively, the patient successfully passed a trial without catheter.

Three months later, the patient is reviewed in clinic. Flow tests showed an improved flow rate of 25 mL/s and minimal post-void residual. Unfortunately, however, the patient continues to suffer with bothersome urgency and frequency with occasional episodes of urgency incontinence.

He is commenced on a second-line anticholinergic, with advice to trial mirabegron (beta-3 agonist) if there was no significant improvement in symptoms over a 4-week period. Subsequent review 6 months postoperatively confirms satisfactory improvement in symptoms following the initiation of mirabegron.

Expert comment OAB symptoms post TURP

Previous research has shown that OAB occurs in 50–75% of men with BPO. After prostatectomy, evidence shows that 62% of patients with OAB preoperatively will have a normal cystometry postoperatively. However, 19% continue to experience storage symptoms post prostatectomy, and the more elderly the patient, the less likely these symptoms are to resolve. It is therefore important to counsel patients appropriately preoperatively regarding the possibility of persistent OAB symptoms requiring treatment following TURP. OAB symptoms resolve in 70% of men with BOO post TURP.[13] Persistent storage symptoms appear to be more marked in men aged >80 years.

Learning point International Continence Society definitions

- **Urgency**: complaint of sudden, compelling desire to pass urine, which is difficult to defer.
- **OAB**: urinary urgency, usually with increased daytime frequency and nocturia, with or without urgency urinary incontinence, in the absence of any other pathology.
- **BPH**: benign prostatic hypertrophy/hyperplasia—enlargement of the prostate caused by prostatic cell hyperplasia/ hypertrophy (a histological diagnosis).
- **BPE**: benign prostatic enlargement—enlargement of the prostate discovered on rectal examination.
- **BOO**: bladder outflow obstruction. A diagnosis based on urodynamic investigations (pressure-flow studies ± imaging ± electromyography), generally (but not always) with relevant symptoms and signs, manifest by an abnormally slow urine flow rate, with evidence of abnormally high detrusor voiding pressures and abnormally slow urine flow during pressure-flow studies, with or without

a high post-void residual. BOO can be functional (bladder neck obstruction, detrusor sphincter dysfunctions, or pelvic floor overactivity) or mechanical (prostatic enlargement, sphincter sclerosis, urethral stricture, meatal stenosis).

- **BPO**: benign prostatic obstruction.
- **DO**: detrusor overactivity. Urodynamic observation characterized by involuntary detrusor contractions during the filling phase that may be spontaneous or provoked.
- **DUA**: detrusor underactivity. A diagnosis based on urodynamic investigations, generally (but not always) with relevant symptoms and signs, manifest by low detrusor pressure or short detrusor contraction in combination with a low urine flow rate resulting in prolonged bladder emptying and/or a failure to achieve complete bladder emptying within a normal time span (a high post-void residual may be present).

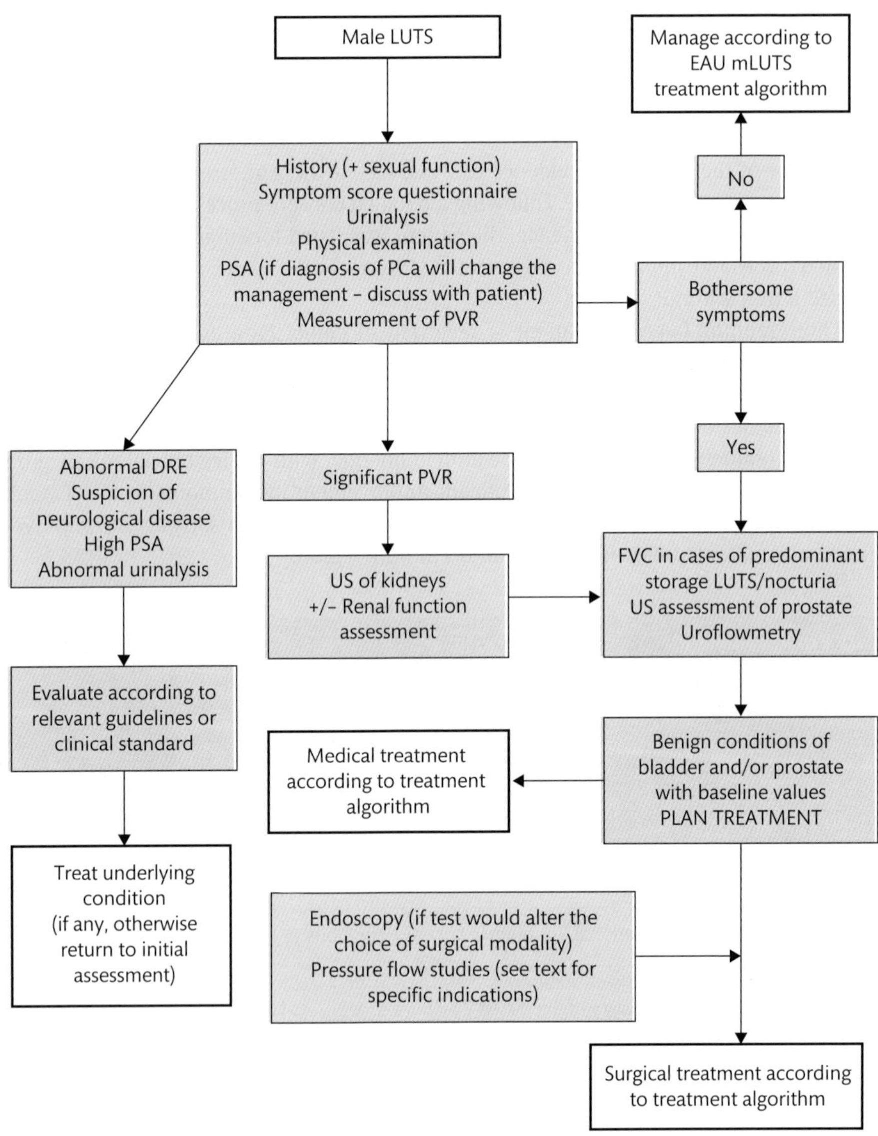

Figure 21.4 Assessment algorithm of LUTS in men aged 40 years or older. DRE, digital rectal examination; FVC, frequency voiding chart; LUTS, lower urinary tract symptoms; PCa, prostate cancer; PSA, prostate specific antigen; PVR, post-void residual; US, ultrasound.

Adapted from EAU Guidelines on Management of Non-Neurogenic Male Lower Urinary Tract Symptoms (LUTS), incl. Benign Prostatic Obstruction (BPO) 2020.

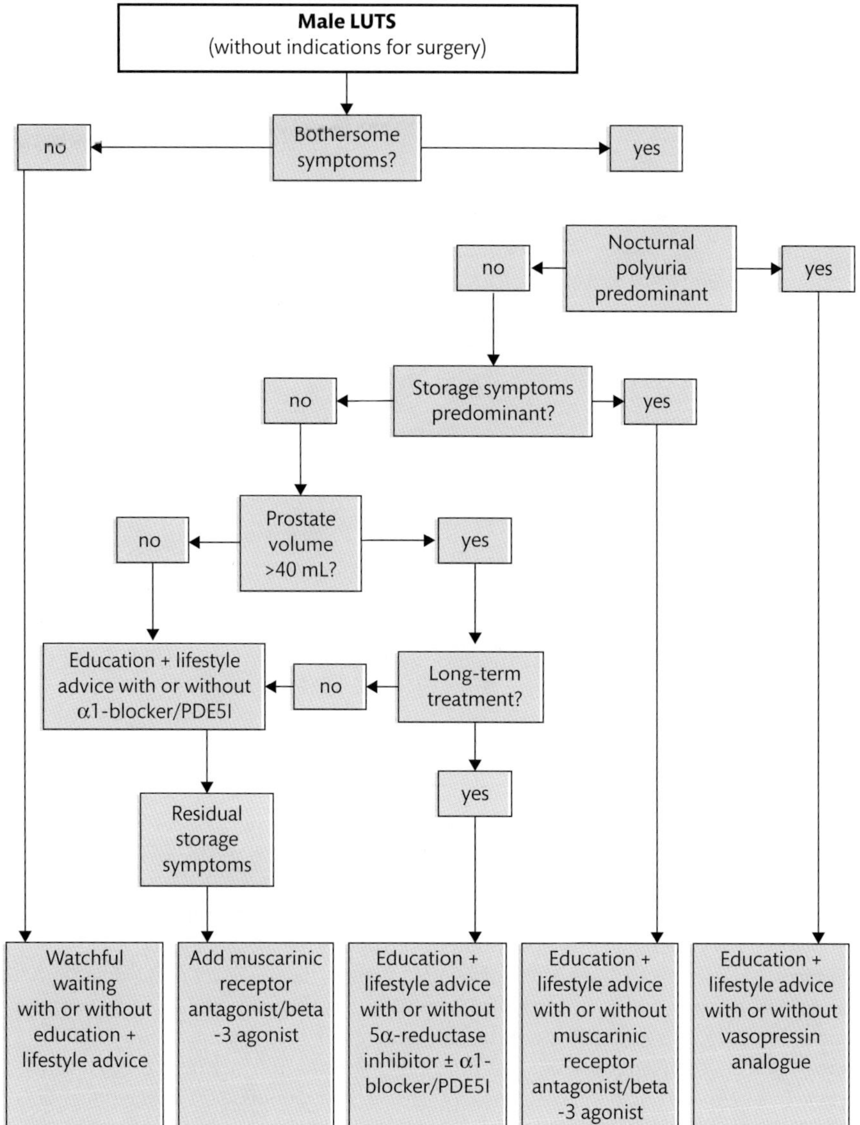

Figure 21.5 Treatment algorithm of male LUTS using medical and/or conservative treatment options. Treatment decisions depend on results assessed during initial evaluation. Note that patients' preferences may result in different treatment decisions. PDE5i, phosphodiesterase 5 inhibitor.

Adapted from EAU Guidelines on Management of Non-Neurogenic Male Lower Urinary Tract Symptoms (LUTS), incl. Benign Prostatic Obstruction (BPO) 2020.

Expert comment Surgical options for male LUTS

Although LUTS medical management has improved the number of patients requiring surgical management, many of these medications have significant side effects.

Surgical management is now evolving at a pace with multiple new therapies being approved by the National Institute for Health and Care Excellence (NICE); these should be seen as possible interim treatments that may delay or prevent the need for a TURP or holmium laser enucleation of the prostate (HoLEP) procedure.

One such treatment is UroLift which, following results from the BPH-6 study,[14] has been approved by NICE for clinical use. The study confirmed improved preservation of ejaculatory function in comparison to TURP in addition to improved quality of recovery with acceptable improvement in symptoms but objective flow measurements which are less than TURP. Limitations, however, included small sample size and relatively stringent inclusion criteria, for example, prostate size <60 mL and no evidence of a median lobe. Revision rate is about 13% at 5 years.[15]

Prostatic artery embolization is another technique increasing in popularity for the treatment of BPO. This interventional radiological technique involves direct injection of particles into prostatic arteries leading to devascularization of prostatic nodules. This is a technically challenging procedure shown to have good outcomes in the UK-ROPE study.[16] The complication rate was low, and the procedure appeared clinically effective, producing a median 15-point IPSS score improvement 12 months post procedure. The procedure takes about 2–3 hours under local anaesthesia. A preoperative CT arteriogram is usually required.

The Rezum system has also shown promise in relieving LUTS with preservation of ejaculatory function. The system employs thermal energy in the form of water vapour delivered to the prostate tissue via the transurethral route. Initial studies have shown acceptable improvement in IPSS scores with a recurrent treatment rate of 4.4% at 4 years. Again, this is limited to smaller prostate <80 mL in size.

A trial in the UK will hopefully be conducted comparing these minimally invasive therapies funded by the National Institute for Health Research.[17]

The use of laser techniques in the management of BPO is increasing in prevalence with HoLEP being recommended by NICE guidelines in 2010.[18] Greenlight laser has also been approved.[19] An important trial in the consideration of laser prostatectomy is the UNBLOCS trial, a level 1 evidence randomized controlled trial inclusive of 410 men. The trial compared thulium laser vaporesection of the prostate (ThuVARP) to TURP, and confirmed similar outcomes in terms of IPSS but with TURP being superior in terms of improving Qmax. ThuVARP had a short learning curve, potentially increasing the appeal and reproducibility of this laser technique compared to others.

A final word from the expert

Male LUTS can be divided into storage, voiding, and post-micturition symptoms. These symptoms usually coexist and storage symptoms are usually the most bothersome and prevalent. It is important to assess these patients accurately, starting with a detailed history and focused clinical examination. Asking the question 'Which is your most bothersome symptom?' is often very helpful as treatment is directed at that symptom first. Once the history and examination are completed, baseline assessment is performed. This includes a 3-day bladder diary, a quality-of-life questionnaire, urine dipstick, free flow rate, and post-void residual. Other investigations such as cystoscopy, blood tests, and renal tract ultrasound scan are indicated if there are 'red flag' signs such as haematuria, increased residuals, abnormal rectal examination, and so on.

Conservative treatment is initially initiated in the form of bladder training, pelvic floor exercises, and fluid manipulation in the case of OAB; leg elevation, compression stockings, and exercise if there is nocturia with peripheral oedema; and double voiding if residual is slightly elevated.

After 6 weeks to 3 months, if these don't help symptoms then medication is initiated. If there are OAB symptoms which are most bothersome then antimuscarinics can be tried. Usually, two different types are tried at maximum dose for a minimum of 4 weeks each. If these fail, then mirabegron is tried for a minimum of 6 weeks. Patients need to be warned about the risks of all these medications including cognitive impairment, dry mouth, blurred vision, and constipation with antimuscarinics and headaches and palpitations with mirabegron due to hypertension. If the voiding symptoms are bothersome then men can be tried on an alpha blocker with or without a 5-alpha reductase inhibitor, remembering that the latter can take 3–6 months to give maximum benefit. These can be given at the same time as antimuscarinics depending on symptom bother. Antimuscarinics are contraindicated in patients with a post void residual of 150 mL due to the risk of causing retention.

If medical therapy fails, then urodynamics is indicated if it is going to change management and help in counselling the patient about potential options, thus giving the patient a more informed choice about their treatment.

Refractory OAB can be treated by onabotulinum toxin A into the bladder or sacral neuromodulation. Rarely, augmentation cystoplasty is performed. For the BOO due to prostatic enlargement, treatment can either be using minimally invasive techniques (Urolift, Rezum, prostatic artery embolization) or transurethral prostatectomy (monopolar TURP, bipolar TURP, HoLEP, Green light, ThuVARP). All options essentially have to be offered to patients and ultimately it is their choice to choose, with patients being referred to other centres if the operation they wish to have is not available locally. It has to be remembered, though, that the majority of these new treatments have no long-term data compared to TURP, which has been around for at least 30 years and has withstood the test of time!

References

1. Liao CH, Chung SD, Kuo HC. Diagnostic value of International Prostate Symptom Score voiding-to-storage subscore ratio in male lower urinary tract symptoms. *Int J Clin Prac.t* 2011;65(5):552–558.
2. Rosier P, Schaefer W, Lose G, et al. International Continence Society good urodynamic practices and terms 2016: urodynamics, uroflowmetry, cystometry, and pressure-flow study. *Neurourol Urodyn.* 2017;36(5):1243–1260.
3. Abrams P, Bruskewitz R, De La Rosette J, et al. The diagnosis of bladder outlet obstruction: urodynamics. In: Cockett ATK, Khoury S, Aso Y, et al., editors. Proceedings, the 3rd International Consultation on BPH. *World Health Organization* 1995;299–367.
4. Chapple CR, Wyndaele JJ, Nordling J, et al. Tamsulosin, the first prostate-selective alpha 1A-adrenoceptorantagonist: a meta-analysis of two randomized, placebo-controlled, multicentre studies in patients with benign prostatic obstruction (symptomatic BPH). *Eur Urol.* 1996;29(2):155–167.
5. Roehrborn CG, McConnell JD, Lieber M, et al. Serum prostate-specific antigen concentration is a powerful predictor of acute urinary retention and need for surgery in men with clinical benign prostatic hyperplasia. PLESS Study Group. *Urology.* 1999;53(3):473–480.
6. McConnell JD, et al. The long-term effect of doxazosin, finasteride, and combination therapy on the clinical progression of benign prostatic hyperplasia. *N Engl J Med.* 2003;349(25):2387–2398.
7. Roehrborn CG, Siami P, Barkin J, et al. The effects of dutasteride, tamsulosin and combination therapy on lower urinary tract symptoms in men with benign prostatic hyperplasia and prostatic enlargement: 2-year results from the CombAT study. *J Urol* 2008;179(2):616–621.
8. Speakman MJ, Kirby RS, Joyce A, Abrams P, Pocock R; British Association of Urological Surgeons. Guideline for the primary care management of male lower urinary tract symptoms. *BJU Int* 2004;93(7):985–990.
9. Hashim H, Abrams P. How should patients with an overactive bladder manipulate their fluid intake? *BJU Int.* 2008;102(1):62–66.
10. Hashim H, Abrams P. Is the bladder a reliable witness for predicting detrusor overactivity? *J Urol.* 2006;175(1):191–194.
11. Roehrborn CG. Definition of at-risk patients: baseline variables. *BJU Int.* 2006;97(Suppl 2):7–11.

12. Lewis AL, Young GJ, Selman LE, et al. Urodynamics tests for the diagnosis and management of bladder outlet obstruction in men: the UPSTREAM non-inferiority RCT. *Health Technol Assess.* 2020;24(42):1–122.
13. Gormley EA, Griffiths DJ, McCracken PN, Harrison GM, McPhee MS. Effect of transurethral resection of the prostate on detrusor instability and urge incontinence in elderly males. *Neurourol Urodyn.* 1993;12(5):445–453.
14. Sønksen J, Barber NJ, Speakman MJ, et al. Prospective, randomized, multinational study of prostatic urethral lift versus transurethral resection of the prostate: 12-month results from the BPH6 study. *Eur Urol.* 2015;68(4):643–652.
15. Roehrborn CG, Barkin J, Gange SN, et al. Five year results of the prospective randomized controlled prostatic urethral L.I.F.T. study. *Can J Urol.* 2017;24(3):8802–8813.
16. Ray AF, Powell J, Speakman MJ, et al. Efficacy and safety of prostate artery embolization for benign prostatic hyperplasia: an observational study and propensity-matched comparison with transurethral resection of the prostate (the UK-ROPE study). *BJU Int.* 2018;122(2):270–282.
17. HTA 19/39 Commissioning Brief—Minimally invasive operative interventions for bladder outlet obstruction due to benign prostatic hyperplasia. May 2019.
18. National Institute for Health and Care Excellence. Lower urinary tract symptoms in men: management. Clinical guideline [CG97]. May 2010, updated June 2015. National Institute for Health and Care Excellence. https://www.nice.org.uk/guidance/cg97
19. National Institute for Health and Care Excellence. GreenLight XPS for treating benign prostatic hyperplasia. Medical technologies guidance (MTG29). June 2016. National Institute for Health and Care Excellence. https://www.nice.org.uk/guidance/mtg29

CASE

22 Chronic retention, renal failure, and diuresis

Cherrie Ho and James Jenkins

Expert commentary Marcus Drake

Case history

A 74-year-old gentleman was referred to the urology department by his general practitioner with impaired renal function, discovered as part of an annual check-up. At the point of referral, an abdominal ultrasound had been arranged which demonstrated bilateral hydroureter, moderate to gross hydronephrosis (Figure 22.1), and a post-micturition volume of 2640 mL.

Learning point Definitions of urinary retention

Definitions of retention have been set out by the International Continence Society in the recent standardization for male lower urinary tract symptoms (LUTS).[1] This states that urinary retention is the complaint of the inability to empty the bladder completely. The two main types of retention are as follows:

- **Acute urinary retention** (AUR) is the complaint of a rapid onset, usually painful suprapubic sensation (from a full bladder) due to inability to void (non-episodic), despite persistent intensive effort.
- **Chronic urinary retention** (CUR) is the chronic or repeated inability to empty the bladder, despite the ability to pass some urine. This may result in the frequent passage of small amounts of urine or urinary incontinence and a distended bladder.

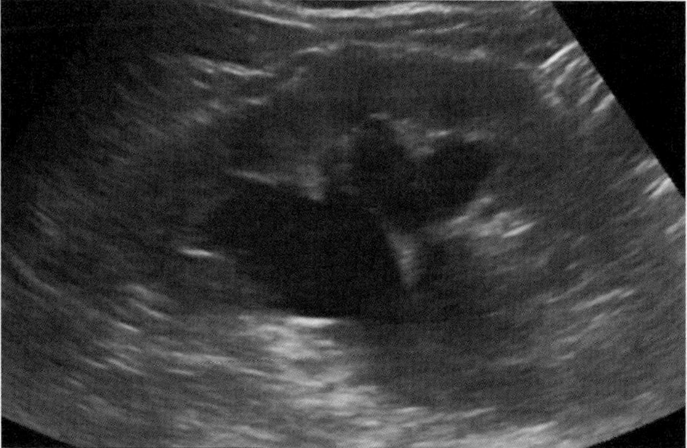

Figure 22.1 Ultrasound scan illustrating hydronephrotic kidney, with slight loss of parenchyma.

Expert comment Post-void residual and hydronephrosis

There is no consensus as to a volume threshold to define urinary retention,[2] but a post-void residual (PVR) of >300 mL is often used as evidence of CUR.[3] This may be an innocuous incidental observation for some people. However, if it is associated with hydronephrosis, the implications for renal function are concerning. Accordingly, CUR can be subdivided into high-pressure chronic retention (HPCR) or low-pressure chronic retention (LPCR), referring to the detrusor pressure at the end of voiding,[4,5] that is, the lowest pressure in the bladder at any time in the micturition cycle. Patients with LPCR have a poorly contractile bladder and do not typically develop hydronephrosis. HPCR usually occurs in association with bladder outlet obstruction (BOO), so it is associated with poor urinary flow rates despite the high pressure. The constantly raised bladder pressure impairs ureteric emptying, with consequent bilateral hydronephrosis, and potential for renal impairment. Formally these definitions are based on urodynamic findings; however, new-onset enuresis (bed-wetting), a palpable bladder, and radiologically demonstrated dilatation of the upper tract strongly indicates HPCR.

On questioning, the patient described a sense of incomplete bladder emptying for several years and occasional nocturnal enuresis, but reported a reasonable urinary flow rate. His medical history was that of hypertension and a previous left hip replacement only, and he was otherwise fit and active. His medications were mirabegron, sildenafil, atorvastatin, and amlodipine. He was a retired truck driver and an ex-smoker.

Expert comment Overactive bladder drugs and urinary retention

Antimuscarinics are the first-line drug treatment for symptoms of overactive bladder syndrome (OAB). They inhibit muscarinic receptors, and work by blocking the effect of the low-level acetylcholine release during the storage phase of the micturition cycle. In theory, they can block neuromuscular transmission in many autonomic organs. In the bladder, this could mean inhibiting the nerve signals driving the bladder contraction for voiding. However, at the very low doses used clinically in OAB they have minimal effect on voiding for normal people. In people with a high PVR, they may be best avoided in case of unwanted additional suppression of detrusor muscle voiding function, and hence further impaired bladder emptying. The European Association of Urologists recommends avoiding the use of antimuscarinics in men with PVR >150 mL. Abrams and colleagues demonstrated a modest increase in PVR, but no effect on AUR in men with mild to moderate BOO treated with an antimuscarinic.[6] Similarly, the NEPTUNE study demonstrated low rates of AUR when combining antimuscarinics with alpha-1 adrenergic blockers (tamsulosin) in men with mixed storage and voiding symptoms.[7] Beta-3 agonists (such as mirabegron) are another medication used in OAB. The mechanism is different from antimuscarinics, as they work by eliciting detrusor muscle relaxation directly. In theory, they may introduce the same risk of increasing PVR in men with already impaired voiding. However, they apparently have limited impact on PVR in observational evaluation.[8] In the current case, there is a reasonable chance that mirabegron had originally been started due to increased urinary frequency on the assumption that OAB was the cause, whereas the reality may have been that CUR was already present and causing frequent small voids. Accordingly, mirabegron was discontinued.

Clinical tip Initial investigations for urinary retention

- **Routine urinalysis**: to exclude urinary tract infection.
- **Routine blood tests**: to establish baseline and risk factors, notably renal function and full blood count.
- **Renal ultrasound**: indicated in patients with abnormal renal function and those with high-volume retention.
- **Abdominal imaging**: if diagnosis is uncertain. Intra-abdominal pathology (e.g. perforated bowel, abdominal aortic aneurysm) and ascites can mistakenly be referred into hospital as urinary

retention. Patients should be re-examined soon after catheterization to confirm resolution of symptoms and to exclude any serious underlying causes.
- **Prostate-specific antigen**: not routinely recommended during the acute episode, due to difficulty interpreting an elevated value.

Clinical examination revealed a distended bladder, which was palpable to the level of the umbilicus. Digital rectal examination revealed normal anal tone and an enlarged but benign-feeling prostate.

The patient was admitted to the urology ward following insertion of a Ch14 Foley urethral catheter in the emergency urology clinic. An initial 3500 mL of straw-coloured urine was drained in the first 2 hours. Hourly urine output monitoring was undertaken, showing a diuresis with an average urine output of 500 mL per hour and he required supplementary intravenous fluids. He received 3 L of Hartmann's solution over 15 hours with careful fluid input and output monitoring.

Expert comment Potential neurological factors

A rare potential cause of CUR is neurological lower urinary tract dysfunction. In an emergency setting, spinal cord compression can present with non-painful urinary retention, due to impaired motor and sensory function. Two crucial potential causes are central prolapsed intervertebral disc and bony metastases (of which advanced prostate cancer is a notable cause[9]). A history of back pain, and physical examination identifying saddle anaesthesia (reduced perianal, perineal, and genital skin sensation) and decreased anal sphincter tone on digital rectal examination are crucial. If spinal cord or cauda equina compression is suspected, immediate magnetic resonance imaging must be undertaken for further assessment in the emergency context. This is to identify if cord compression is present, and identify the cause. If identified, same-day treatment (disc prolapse surgery or radiotherapy to a metastasis) is needed in order to minimize progression of the neurological problem, including the potential development of paraplegia.

Clinical tip Initial treatment of urinary retention

- **AUR**: urgent catheterization of the bladder should be carried out by a competent clinical practitioner. Urine volume drained in the first 15 minutes must be accurately recorded to enable distinction between acute and acute-on-chronic retention (i.e. a person with preceding CUR who becomes unable to void at all, leading to emergency presentation).
- **CUR**: early catheterization is indicated principally if there is renal dysfunction and/or hydronephrosis. If there is no renal dysfunction, catheterization can be avoided, but early listing for definitive treatment should be planned.

Expert comment Haematuria after catheterization

Haematuria is a well-recognized complication following catheterization for CUR. This is caused by the decompression of a urinary tract that has undergone structural changes including bladder hypertrophy leading to weakening of surface capillaries. Decompression haematuria usually settles within 48–72 hours, but it can be severe, sometimes requiring bladder washouts via the catheter. Historically, gradual decompression (or intermittent clamping of the catheter) had been the practice in many urological units in attempt to reduce the incidence of bleeding. In fact, it has since been demonstrated that attempts to reduce the speed of bladder decompression make minimal difference to the chance of bleeding. In one randomized trial, haematuria occurred in 11% of people undergoing gradual decompression and the same with rapid decompression; six patients in the former group and four in the latter required further treatment.[10] Accordingly, the policy currently is to catheterize on unimpeded free drainage, but maintain observation to identify any problems arising early.

Learning point Post-obstructive diuresis

Post-obstructive diuresis (POD) can be defined as the production of >200 mL/hour of urine for two consecutive hours, or >3000 mL over 24 hours. While it should be anticipated in all those newly catheterized for HPCR, Hamdi and colleagues noted it is increasingly likely in those with raised serum creatinine or bicarbonate levels, or bladder residuals in excess of 1500 mL at presentation.[11] POD in the initial setting may be considered a physiological process allowing the offloading of excess water, electrolytes, and toxins. This is driven by an osmotic diuresis related to the accumulation of salts and metabolites, such as urea, though persistent renal failure. In isolation, it is a self-limiting process. However, because the diuresis is driven by the elimination of excess solutes, rather than being a homeostatic control of water levels, excessive water loss can result. A pathologically intractable POD with excessive fluid loss and salt wasting continuing beyond homeostasis may be observed in some patients, and they may struggle to maintain adequate intravascular volume. Furthermore, once obstruction is relieved, the ability to eliminate the accumulated toxins may give rise to osmotic diuresis. In these patients, excessive fluid replacement may delay renal recovery, and close monitoring for volume depletion, hypokalaemia, hypo/hypernatraemia, and hypomagnesaemia must be observed.

The patient's initial blood test on admission showed that his sodium level was 143 mmol/L, potassium 4.4 mmol/L, urea 5.3 mmol/L, creatinine 169 μmol/L, and estimated glomerular filtration rate (eGFR) 34 mL/min/1.73 m^2 (Table 22.1). Liver function tests and full blood count were normal.

The patient's renal function stabilized over the course of 24 hours and he was discharged following the resolution of his diuresis.

Learning point Renal failure

The high renal pelvis pressures found in HPCR result in protracted partial obstruction of the kidneys. The pathophysiology of obstructive nephropathy relates to both reduction in renal blood flow and progressive histopathological changes. Pathophysiological processes result in tubular dysfunction, particularly loss of the medullary concentration gradient, with downregulation of sodium transporters in the thick ascending loop of Henle. Consequently, there may be inability to concentrate urine, decreased sodium reabsorption due to abnormal renal tubule sodium transporter expression, and insensitivity to antidiuretic hormone. The extent and nature of these changes relate to the timespan of renal obstruction and severity of resulting pressure rises. While changes to renal blood flow may resolve promptly, renal scaring can lead to thinning of the renal cortex and medulla, which may never resolve entirely to baseline function.

Table 22.1 Trend of creatinine, urea, and eGFR

Date	Creatinine	Urea	eGFR
18/01/2016	98	2.6	66
27/02/2017	111	3.5	57
16/04/2018	114	4.5	55
27/08/2019	149	5.8	43
03/09/2019	154	4.9	38
10/10/2019 (catheter insertion)	169	5.3	34
11/10/2019	145	5.2	41
18/10/2019	132	4.6	45
30/10/2019	125	4.8	49

Learning point Fluid replacement

Strict monitoring of fluid balance (recording hourly fluid intake and urine output), lying and standing blood pressure (to detect postural hypotension), and daily weight are crucial in the management of POD. The treatment of POD should be directed at replacing electrolytes and correction of intravascular volume. In addition, daily measurements of urea, creatinine, and electrolytes help ascertain resolution of any acute kidney injury and monitor restoration of safe levels of salts. Many people will cope simply with oral fluid intake. Intravenous fluids (normal saline) are needed for patients with postural drop in blood pressure, haemodynamic instability, or electrolyte disturbances, or those who are unable to maintain required fluid intake orally.[12] In about 10% of cases, careful fluid replacement is required due to excess diuresis.[13] Intravenous fluid support should be normal saline and limited to no more than 75% of the prior 1–2-hour urine production,[14] to avoid perpetuating diuresis.[15] A urine specific gravity of 1.020 or more indicates that the kidneys are concentrating the urine, implying a return of function which anticipates resolution of the period of diuresis. If the specific gravity is <1.010, the kidneys are not concentrating the urine. These people may need ongoing fluid replacement, since they may lose disproportionately large fluid and salt, and hence be at risk of volume depletion.

Expert comment Therapy considerations

The management of patients with CUR should be directed at dealing with reversible causes of voiding dysfunction. In patients presenting with CUR but with normal renal function, it is best to avoid catheterization where possible, given the potential for associated complications (e.g. catheter-associated infection, trauma, bladder stone formation, and retained foreign bodies). Instead, intervention to relieve BOO should be considered as a priority. Urodynamics (in men who can void) can identify the chance of benefit from transurethral resection of prostate (TURP). Detrusor pressure at maximum cystometric capacity is indicative,[5] and 25 cmH_2O is a threshold to distinguish low-pressure CUR from high-pressure CUR. High-pressure CUR is an indication for TURP, with priority scheduling to avoid ongoing renal dysfunction risk. In patients with low pressure retention, an underactive detrusor is often found, and neither LUTS nor flow rate are likely to improve after TURP in this subset of patients.[16] Hence, urodynamic workup helps to determine who stands to benefit from surgical treatment. If a man has an indwelling catheter (having failed trial without catheter and ISC training), urodynamics is unreliable. In this situation, he should be considered for TURP once his general health allows surgical intervention; to ensure informed consent, counselling must discuss the risks of surgery, and it should be made clear that it is not certain that voiding will be restored. Potentially this could represent consequences of accumulating detrusor deterioration over time.[17] Patients with LPCR in particular frequently fail to void completely after BOO surgery, and for catheterized patients it is impractical to undertake urodynamics in order to identify whether LPCR applies.

The patient returned for a bipolar TURP under general anaesthetic 8 weeks following his initial presentation and was found to have a moderately enlarged prostate with a heavily trabeculated bladder during the procedure. Total resection time was < 60 minutes and tissue fragments together weighed a total of 50 g. Histopathology of the resected prostatic chips showed benign hyperplasia only. He was discharged the same day and was scheduled to return for a trial without catheter 1 week later.

During his trial without catheter appointment, he only managed to void very small volumes with a large PVR of 900 mL. He was taught to perform intermittent self-catheterization (ISC).

At a telephone consultation 4 months following his TURP and unsuccessful trial without catheter, the patient reported that he was well established on ISC. His PVR had reduced down to 600 mL and he managed to pass urine throughout the day. He was advised to continue with twice-daily ISC and he was discharged back to his general practitioner's care.

Expert comment Unsuccessful surgery

Urinary retention post TURP could be secondary to inadequate resection, poor bladder contractility, and/or presence of a large bladder diverticulum. Failure to void following prostatectomy is reported to occur in 0.5–11% of cases.[18] The diagnosis of poor bladder contractility/detrusor underactivity may not be apparent prior to BOO surgery. Urodynamic studies and cystoscopy may be considered postoperatively if the cause of persisting urinary retention is not clear. If detrusor underactivity is the cause, clean intermittent self-catheterization (CISC) should be considered as the long-term management. Once detrusor underactivity has been excluded, inadequate resection can be redressed by repeat resection of prostatic tissue typically at or just proximal to the verumontanum. Careful resection should be carried out when removing these tissues to avoid the adjacent external sphincter, which is crucial to avoid stress urinary incontinence.

Evidence base Role of intermittent self-catheterization

A chronic PVR may perpetuate voiding dysfunction by placing the detrusor into an overstretched configuration, and escalating PVR conceivably can progressively reduce contractility. To determine whether a preliminary period of CISC improves bladder contractility and surgical outcome in men with CUR, a two-centre randomized trial evaluated the role of CISC.[3] Forty-one men scheduled for TURP with LUTS, an International Prostate Symptom Score of >7, benign prostatic enlargement, and a persistent PVR of >300 mL were evaluated. Seventeen were randomized to immediate TURP and 24 to CISC. There was a significant improvement in International Prostate Symptom Score and quality of life at 6 months in both groups. In the CISC group, there was a significant improvement in voiding and end-filling pressures, suggesting some improvement of bladder function. Both CISC and immediate TURP were reported to improve LUTS and quality of life. A preliminary period of CISC before TURP for men with CUR and low voiding pressure may be valuable. This would particularly apply in men who need workup to improve fitness for surgery, or who face protracted recovery from severe renal dysfunction. No one CISC catheter type appears to bring a clinical advantage, so choice depends on patient preference and cost.[19]

Evidence base Definitive management

Most investigators suggest surgical treatment to avoid permanent indwelling or intermittent catheterization. Most studies suggest a patient with CUR benefits from BOO surgery, and many authors suggested surgery may be more effective in HPCR patients than those with LPCR.[20] The authors of a retrospective series reported disappointing long-term symptomatic or urodynamic outcomes from TURP in men shown to have detrusor underactivity prior to surgery.[16] In a randomized trial, Ghalayini and colleagues found a significant improvement in symptoms and quality of life at 6 months for both immediate TURP and CISC ($p < 0.001$).[3] The authors concluded CISC is useful in ensuring bladder function recovery in men with CUR, and both CISC and immediate TURP are effective for relieving LUTS with better quality of life. The CLasP study showed lower-power laser coagulation and TURP were both effective for relieving LUTS, improving health-related quality of life, and decreasing PVR.[21] For photoselective vaporization prostatectomy, Monoski and colleagues found that patients without detrusor overactivity (DO) or detrusor underactivity preoperatively improved most, with significantly lower symptoms.[22]

A final word from the expert

CUR clearly reflects a protracted process in which a very slow clinical progression means that an affected individual does not seek medical attention. This results in a cumulative effect on the physiology of the whole urinary tract that ultimately can result in considerable dysfunction, both in the kidneys and the bladder. Fortunately, for the case described, renal function was not profoundly affected, so that renal impairment was mild and the clinical pathway was comparatively smooth. Severe cases are unusual in modern practice, but an extreme case can have such bad renal dysfunction and toxin/salt accumulation that they may even diurese at a rate of 20 L per 24 hours. This may only begin 48 hours after catheterization, so early discharge from hospital of someone with badly deranged renal function may be dangerous, as they may rapidly become dehydrated once the full diuresis becomes established. These patients may have to stay in hospital for a few days until the diuresis rate drops to a level they can conceivably match with ordinary fluid consumption. This sort of patient probably has not looked after himself in a healthy way for a long time, so discharge can be difficult, as their home circumstances may have been somewhat neglected. Once renal function has stabilized, there will generally considerable recovery compared with admission values, but usually not to baseline function. More severe and protracted renal dysfunction obviously leads to less noteworthy recovery after catheterization.

Once identified, a patient with CUR needs to get timely definitive management:

- For someone with CUR and normal renal function, no catheter is needed, and a pathway of early urodynamics and thence interventional treatment (for HPCR) is appropriate. Where LPCR is identified, ISC may be considered in the hope of improving residual voiding function.
- For someone with CUR presenting with abnormal renal function, a catheter is needed only as long as it takes to bring renal function to its best level. Many of these men can then be switched to ISC, enabling urodynamics and interventional treatment (for HPCR) if appropriate.
- Where LPCR is identified, ISC may be considered in the hope of improving residual voiding function. This may also have to be the care for someone with HPCR who is not fit for interventional treatment, or is unwilling to accept it.

In each case, follow-up is needed, regardless of treatment modality. This can be in the urology clinic, but regular renal function assessment can safely be established in primary care, provided clear indicators for ultrasound assessment and re-referral are communicated.

These are rather complex patients, since they reflect a severe form of lower urinary tract dysfunction which affects overall health and fitness. Nonetheless, basic principles can be applied to give a reasonable chance of restoring adequate voiding for most men affected.

References

1. D'Ancona C, Haylen B, Oelke M, et al. The International Continence Society (ICS) report on the terminology for adult male lower urinary tract and pelvic floor symptoms and dysfunction. *Neurourol Urodyn*. 2019;38(2):433–477.
2. Kaplan SA, Wein AJ, Staskin DR, Roehrborn CG, Steers WD. Urinary retention and post-void residual urine in men: separating truth from tradition. *J Urol*. 2008;180(1):47–54.
3. Ghalayini IF, Al-Ghazo MA, Pickard RS. A prospective randomized trial comparing transurethral prostatic resection and clean intermittent self-catheterization in men with chronic urinary retention. *BJU Int*. 2005;96(1):93–97.
4. George NJ, O'Reilly PH, Barnard RJ, Blacklock NJ. High pressure chronic retention. *Br Med J (Clin Res Ed)*. 1983;286(6380):1780–1783.
5. Abrams PH, Dunn M, George N. Urodynamic findings in chronic retention of urine and their relevance to results of surgery. *Br Med J*. 1978;2(6147):1258–1260.
6. Abrams P, Kaplan S, De Koning Gans HJ, Millard R. Safety and tolerability of tolterodine for the treatment of overactive bladder in men with bladder outlet obstruction. *J Urol*. 2006;175(3 Pt 1):999–1004.
7. Drake MJ, Oelke M, Snijder R, et al. Incidence of urinary retention during treatment with single tablet combinations of solifenacin + tamsulosin OCAS for up to 1 year in adult men with both storage and voiding LUTS: a subanalysis of the NEPTUNE/NEPTUNE II randomized controlled studies. *PLoS One*. 2017;12(2):e0170726.

8. Nitti VW, Rosenberg S, Mitcheson DH, He W, Fakhoury A, Martin NE. Urodynamics and safety of the beta(3)-adrenoceptor agonist mirabegron in males with lower urinary tract symptoms and bladder outlet obstruction. *J Urol.* 2013;190(4):1320–1327.
9. Ziu E, Viswanathan VK, Mesfin FB. *Cancer, Spinal Metastasis*. Treasure Island, FL: StatPearls; 2020.
10. Boettcher S, Brandt AS, Roth S, Mathers MJ, Lazica DA. Urinary retention: benefit of gradual bladder decompression—myth or truth? A randomized controlled trial. *Urol Int.* 2013;91(2):140–144.
11. Hamdi A, Hajage D, Van Glabeke E, et al. Severe post-renal acute kidney injury, post-obstructive diuresis and renal recovery. *BJU Int.* 2012;110(11 Pt C):E1027–E1034.
12. Shah A, Ellis G, Kucheria R. A guide for the assessment and management of post-obstructive diuresis. *Urol News.* 2015;19:3.
13. Kalejaiye O, Speakman M. Management of acute and chronic retention in men. *Eur Urol Suppl.* 2009;8:523–529.
14. Leslie SW, Sajjad H, Sharma S. *Postobstructive Diuresis*. Treasure Island, FL: StatPearls; 2020.
15. Baum N, Anhalt M, Carlton CE Jr, Scott R Jr. Post-obstructive diuresis. *J Urol.* 1975;114(1):53–56.
16. Thomas AW, Cannon A, Bartlett E, Ellis-Jones J, Abrams P. The natural history of lower urinary tract dysfunction in men: minimum 10-year urodynamic followup of transurethral resection of prostate for bladder outlet obstruction. *J Urol.* 2005;174(5):1887–1891.
17. Cathcart P, van der Meulen J, Armitage J, Emberton M. Incidence of primary and recurrent acute urinary retention between 1998 and 2003 in England. *J Urol.* 2006;176(1):200–204.
18. Reynard JM, Shearer RJ. Failure to void after transurethral resection of the prostate and mode of presentation. *Urology.* 1999;53(2):336–339.
19. Health Quality Ontario. Intermittent catheters for chronic urinary retention: a health technology assessment. *Ont Health Technol Assess Ser.* 2019;19(1):1–153.
20. Negro CL, Muir GH. Chronic urinary retention in men: how we define it, and how does it affect treatment outcome. *BJU Int.* 2012;110(11):1590–1594.
21. Gujral S, Abrams P, Donovan JL, et al. A prospective randomized trial comparing transurethral resection of the prostate and laser therapy in men with chronic urinary retention: the CLasP study. *J Urol.* 2000;164(1):59–64.
22. Monoski MA, Gonzalez RR, Sandhu JS, Reddy B, Te AE. Urodynamic predictors of outcomes with photoselective laser vaporization prostatectomy in patients with benign prostatic hyperplasia and preoperative retention. *Urology.* 2006;68(2):312–317.

CASE

23 Urge urinary incontinence

Pravisha Ravindra

Expert commentary Richard Parkinson

Case history

A 48-year-old woman was referred to the specialist continence nurse clinic by her general practitioner with 'urinary incontinence'. A careful history was taken, which established that her incontinence was usually preceded by an urgent desire to pass urine. She also occasionally leaked when she went to the gym, particularly doing high-intensity exercise. The patient complained of having to pass urine frequently (both during the day and overnight) and having to rush to the toilet. She reported occasions where she had leaked when she had not managed to find a toilet in time. The nurse made a diagnosis of urge-predominant mixed urinary incontinence (UI) and determined that the stress urinary incontinence (SUI) was not a bothersome problem.

Learning point Definition of urinary symptoms

The International Continence Society defines the following symptoms as:

- **Urgency**: the complaint of a sudden, compelling desire to pass urine which is difficult to defer.
- **Daytime frequency**: number of micturitions during daytime (awake hours, including first void after waking up from sleep and last void before sleep). Up to eight can be considered normal.
- **Nocturia**: the number of times urine is passed during the main sleep period. Once is normal.
- **Urge urinary incontinence (UUI)**: complaint of involuntary loss of urine associated with urgency.[1]

The patient had taken to wearing pads, getting through three or four pads in a 24-hour period. In the preceding 12 months, she had experienced symptoms of a urinary tract infection (UTI) twice. During one of these episodes, she had noticed some pink urine that resolved as the dysuria resolved. Her fluid intake consisted of four cups of tea, two cups of coffee, and two glasses of water a day. She denied any voiding dysfunction.

Her past medical history included a laparoscopic sterilization. Her body mass index was 31 kg/m^2. Obstetric history included two normal vaginal deliveries. She was sexually active and had noticed some mild dyspareunia in recent months. She had no drug history and was otherwise fit and well. She was an ex-smoker and had no significant family history.

On examination, her abdomen was soft and non-tender. There was no palpable bladder. Examination of the external genitalia showed vaginal atrophy, no evidence of pelvic organ prolapse, with a small urine leak on coughing. Urine dip revealed microscopic haematuria and no evidence of a UTI. A post-void residual bladder scan was minimal.

Clinical tip History taking

A careful history taking will often indicate the diagnosis. Key features that should be specifically questioned for include:

- Storage symptoms:
  - Frequency
  - Urgency
  - UUI—volume, frequency
  - SUI—volume, frequency
- Voiding dysfunction
- Pad usage—quantified
- Fluid intake—what type, how much
- Red flags—see 'Expert comment' box on red flags
- Obstetric history
- Sexual function/dysfunction
- Quality of life
- Patient expectations.

In the first instance, due to the presence of microscopic haematuria, the patient was referred to the haematuria clinic. A flexible cystoscopy and a renal tract ultrasound scan were performed, which were unremarkable.

The patient was asked to complete a 3-day bladder diary and symptom and quality-of-life questionnaires. The patient's bladder diary revealed a daytime frequency of eight, nocturia three, and two or three incontinence episodes per day. Her scores on the International Consultation on Incontinence Questionnaire (ICIQ) modules on overactive bladder (OAB) and UI were 14 and 18, respectively. The specialist continence nurse diagnosed the patient with OAB syndrome.

Expert comment Red flags

Certain features should trigger early referral and/or further investigation by a urologist. These include:

- Haematuria or sterile pyuria
- Bladder pain
- Incomplete bladder emptying, voiding dysfunction
- Neurological symptoms such as perineal numbness or leg weakness
- Persistent UTIs.

Clinical tip Symptom and quality-of-life questionnaires

It is important to quantify a patient's symptoms and establish the impact that the symptoms have on their quality of life using a validated questionnaire. This enables accurate assessment and objective comparison following treatment. The ICIQ modules on OAB and UI have both been awarded 'Grade A' for their validity, reliability, and responsiveness. The ICIQ-OAB consists of four questions on frequency, nocturia, urgency, and UUI, being scored overall from 0 to 16 (greater values indicating greater severity). The ICIQ-UI also consists of four items on frequency or UI, amount of leakage, overall impact of UI, and a self-diagnostic item. This is scored from 0 to 21.[2]

Learning point OAB syndrome

The International Continence Society defines OAB syndrome as urinary urgency, usually accompanied by increased daytime frequency and/or nocturia, with UI (OAB-wet) or without (OAB-dry), in the absence of a UTI or other detectable disease.[1] It is a very common condition, and the prevalence of bothersome symptoms has been reported in 10–14% of men and 22–33% of women. The incidence has been shown to increase with age.[3] Other risk factors for UI in general include obesity, parity, mode of delivery, family history, ethnicity, and smoking. The condition has both physical and mental health implications as a consequence of sleep deprivation, falls, skin breakdown due to incontinence, and overall lower quality of life. Patients have also reported limiting social activities and detrimental job performance as a result.[4]

Advice was given on fluid management, including cutting out caffeinated drinks and avoiding drinks after 8 pm, although the evidence for this is equivocal.[5] Performance of pelvic floor exercises was supervised and advised three times a day along with bladder retraining. Weight loss was encouraged. In view of the vaginal atrophy, a topical oestrogen cream was prescribed.

Evidence base Topical oestrogen therapy

A 2012 Cochrane review looked at 34 trials with over 19,000 women with stress, mixed, or urge incontinence[6]; 9599 women received oestrogen therapy, of whom 1464 received local vaginal oestrogen administration. The latter showed improvement of UI, and fewer voids with less frequency and urgency. There were no serious adverse events reported although some patients reported vaginal spotting, breast tenderness, or nausea. The review was unable to reach conclusions on the period after oestrogen therapy ceased. The majority of guidelines now recommend a trial of vaginal oestrogen therapy for post- or perimenopausal women with UI.

A urologist review was arranged for 3 months' time. The patient was pleased because her mild SUI had significantly improved, as had some of her daytime frequency.

She still experienced urgency and had episodes of UUI. She had cut out caffeinated and evening drinks. At this point, the urologist suggested a trial of pharmacotherapy. In the first instance, as per the National Institute for Health and Care Excellence guidelines, he suggested an anticholinergic with the lowest acquisition cost for 6 weeks. If this was ineffective, an alternative anticholinergic could be trialled. She was counselled on the possible risks of dry mouth, blurred vision, and constipation. Her general practitioner was advised to add in a beta-3 agonist such as mirabegron if the patient felt that her symptoms had not improved fully. A follow-up appointment was suggested for 4–6 weeks after initiating therapy.

Evidence base Discontinuation of anticholinergics

A systematic review has demonstrated that oxybutynin had the highest rate of treatment discontinuation due to side effects.[7] Retrospective data have suggested that the median time to discontinuation of antimuscarinic medication was 30–78 days (compared to 169 days for mirabegron).[8]

Evidence base Mirabegron as combination therapy

There have been a number of trials looking at the use of mirabegron in combination therapy for overactive bladder. The Symphony trial (A Study to Evaluate the Efficacy, Safety and Tolerability of Mirabegron and Solifenacin Alone and in Combination for the Treatment of Overactive Bladder) was a multinational, multi-arm, phase II, double-blind randomized controlled trial with OAB patients using solifenacin and mirabegron in different dose combinations, as monotherapy or placebo. Combination therapy (in any dose combination) was found to be significantly more effective than solifenacin 5 mg monotherapy. The SYNERGY (Efficacy and Safety of Combinations of Mirabegron and Solifenacin Compared with Monotherapy and Placebo in Patients with Overactive Bladder) study was a phase III trial, with more patients, with similar arms. This confirmed the superiority of combination therapy (mirabegron 50 mg/solifenacin 5 mg) and mirabegron 50 mg monotherapy when compared to solifenacin 5 mg. The BESIDE study (Efficacy and Safety of Mirabegron Add-On Therapy to Solifenacin in Incontinent Overactive Bladder Patients with an Inadequate Response to Initial 4-week Solifenacin Monotherapy: A Randomized Double-Blinded Multicentre Phase 3B Study) looked at patients who had failed solifenacin 5 mg monotherapy; it demonstrated that combination therapy was non-inferior to solifenacin 10 mg, but the former resulted in fewer side effects.[9] It is important to note that the manufacturers of mirabegron funded all three trials.

Expert comment Contraindications to medical treatment

- Caution should be exercised when using vaginal oestrogen therapy in those with a previous history of breast cancer.
- Contraindications to anticholinergic use include myasthenia gravis, bladder outflow obstruction or urinary retention, severe ulcerative colitis, or gastrointestinal obstruction. Untreated narrow-angle glaucoma is also a contraindication, but this is rare (the more common open-angle glaucoma is not an issue).
- Contraindications to beta-3 agonist use include severe renal or hepatic disease as well as uncontrolled hypertension.

The patient voiced concerns about the link between anticholinergics and dementia but was reassured by a discussion about the evidence.

Evidence base Anticholinergic burden and dementia

There has been controversy about the link between anticholinergic medication and dementia risk. The evidence thus far has demonstrated an associative (not causative) link between anticholinergic use and an increased risk of dementia. This link was found to be cumulative both in association with other medication (as part of the anticholinergic burden, e.g. warfarin, furosemide) as well as length of exposure.[10] This is a distinct phenomenon to the well-established link between anticholinergics and acute-onset cognitive impairment in at-risk patients (the European Association of Urology guidelines recommend caution with long-term antimuscarinic treatment in elderly patients who have, or are at risk of cognitive impairment[11]).

Unfortunately, the patient did not have a significant improvement with medical therapy and so was referred back to the outpatient clinic. Due to her initial presentation of mixed urinary incontinence, formal urodynamic studies (UDS) were organized. This demonstrated a good bladder capacity of 600 mL, detrusor overactivity associated with urgency, and UUI and a good flow with no evidence of outlet obstruction (Figure 23.1). There was no demonstrable SUI despite provocation measures. The patient agreed that her symptoms had been successfully reproduced.

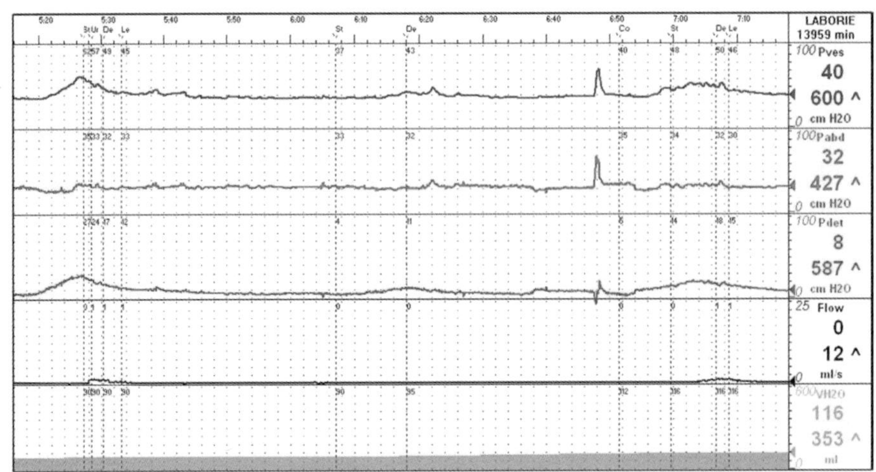

Figure 23.1 Urodynamic trace showing detrusor overactivity and associated urine leak.
Adapted from Ahmed M. Shaban, Marcus J. Drake, Hashim Hashim. The medical management of urinary incontinence. *Autonomic Neuroscience* Vol 152 Issue 1–2, pg4–10.

Expert comment The role of urodynamic studies

Most studies show that UDS do not reliably predict patient response to treatment; this is the case for pharmacotherapy,[12] sacral neuromodulation (SNM),[13] and intravesical botulinum toxin (BTX).[14] In diagnosing OAB syndrome, UDS have been shown to have a sensitivity of 75% and a specificity of 55%.[15] UDS have a role in helping to define bladder function, and any disparity between clinical symptoms and study results should prompt a review of the patient's symptoms. However, treatment should not be directed by the study results alone.

At this point, the patient was counselled about further management options—this included intravesical BTX, percutaneous tibial nerve stimulation (PTNS), SNM, or augmentation cystoplasty.

Expert comment Treatment options counselling

When counselling patients about treatment options, it is essential to discuss all the treatment options suitable for that patient in order for them to make an informed decision and to provide informed consent for treatment. It is also necessary to remind the patient that there is an option of no treatment. Failure to document a discussion of treatment options is a common reason for successful litigation.

Learning point Intravesical BTX

Botulinum toxin serotype A is used in the bladder in the form of onabotulinum toxin (Botox®, Allergan) or abobotulinum toxin (Dysport®, Ipsen). The toxin functions by inhibiting the release of acetylcholine vesicles at the presynaptic junction in peripheral nerve endings. This results in muscle paralysis, with clinical effects lasting 6–12 months when injected into the bladder. The original randomized, double-blind, placebo-controlled trial demonstrated significant reduction in all OAB parameters and a significant improvement in patient quality of life. There is strong evidence supporting its use in patients with idiopathic overactive bladder as well as neurogenic detrusor overactivity.[16,17] Recognized risks include bleeding, infection and need for intermittent self-catheterization (ISC).[18] Caution should be exercised in individuals with peripheral motor neuropathic diseases, amyotrophic lateral sclerosis, or neuromuscular junction disorders (such as myasthenia gravis or Eaton–Lambert syndrome) due to the increased risk of generalized muscle weakness, dysphagia, and respiratory compromise.

The patient was warned of a 5–10% risk of ISC with intravesical BTX injections. She did not feel that she would manage with ISC and therefore decided against this treatment. For this reason, she also ruled out augmentation cystoplasty, for which the risk of ISC is >50%. Unfortunately, PTNS was not offered in her local area and she was not willing to travel to have the procedure regularly. As such, she opted to have a trial of SNM.

Clinical tip Administration of intravesical BTX

BTX is normally supplied in powder form in a glass vial. Administration can be performed under local anaesthetic using a flexible cystoscope or a general/regional anaesthetic using a rigid cystoscope. The BTX is reconstituted using saline (usually 10–20 mL) injected into the vial and slow mixing to allow the powder to dissolve. Ten to twenty equally spaced injections are given into the detrusor muscle. There is no evidence that trigone sparing is necessary.

Learning point PTNS

An acupuncture needle is placed above the medial malleolus of the ankle with electrical stimulation applied for 30 minutes. This results in stimulation of the sacral micturition centre via S2–S4. These are normally done as weekly sessions for 12 weeks followed by monthly maintenance therapy. Efficacy has been estimated at around 60% (similar to tolterodine) although the majority of studies are small and follow-up is short (longest 3 years). There are no demonstrable adverse effects and no evidence to suggest that PTNS cures urge incontinence.[19]

Learning point Augmentation cystoplasty

A detubularized segment of bowel (traditionally ileum) is mobilized on its mesentery and attached to the bivalved bladder. The aim of this is to disrupt waves of detrusor overactivity spreading through the bladder, thereby reducing the symptoms of an overactive bladder. This procedure can also be used to treat small capacity bladder and neurogenic detrusor overactivity. In a case series of 51 patients undergoing augmentation cystoplasty for non-neurogenic urge incontinence, 53% were completely continent at 75.4 months.[20] Possible risks and complications include recurrent UTIs, stone formation, need for ISC, long-term renal impairment, and metabolic disturbance.

Learning point SNM

SNM is a two-stage procedure indicated for patients with refractory overactive bladder. The first stage involves a peripheral nerve evaluation or insertion of a permanent tined lead for a longer test phase. It is performed under fluoroscopic control with the electrode being placed in the S3 foramen. Patients then closely monitor and record their symptoms, while trying different intensities. In those who demonstrate a 50% or more improvement in their OAB symptoms, a permanent device is fitted. The device is MRI-compatible and depending on whether the patient opts for a recharge-free or rechargeable device, the battery can last between 5-15 years before a replacement is required. Studies have shown that 50% of patients demonstrated >90% improvement in urinary incontinence, 25% demonstrating a 50–90% improvement, and a further 25% demonstrating <50% improvement. Cure rates have been cited at 15%. This appears to be sustained at 4 years. Adverse events have been described in 50% of cases with revision rates of 33–41% cited.[21] An randomized controlled trial (ROSETTA trial: Refractory Overactive Bladder: Sacral Neuromodulation vs. Botulinum Toxin Assessment) comparing repeat BTX injections versus SNM suggested greater effectiveness of BTX; patient counselling is therefore key.[22]

The procedure was performed as a day case. A 2-week trial revealed >50% improvement in the patient's symptoms and she therefore opted to have a permanent device fitted. At her 3-month follow-up, the wound had healed well and the patient was happy with the result. She remained in close contact with the specialist nurse as a first point of contact if ever her symptoms changed in the future.

A final word from the expert

Urinary urgency has been demonstrated to be the most common bothersome lower urinary tract symptom in a large-scale population study. The same study also demonstrated that for individuals, UUI was the most bothersome symptom.[23] It is important to accurately characterize a patient's presenting complaint. The priority of the urologist is to determine whether the patient's symptoms point towards idiopathic OAB syndrome or another condition which could cause similar symptoms such as recurrent UTIs, bladder pain syndrome, bladder cancer, bladder stones, pelvic malignancy, sexually transmitted diseases, or previous pelvic radiotherapy.

Initial investigations should include a 3-day bladder diary, post-void bladder scan, and urine dipstick. Conservative management strategies can often reduce the bother patients experience from their symptoms—these include weight loss, fluid management (including cutting out caffeine), and pelvic floor exercises. Medical therapy such as topical vaginal oestrogen therapy, anticholinergics, and beta-3 agonists have reasonable efficacy although compliance is an issue. The role of UDS is controversial; it is usually only indicated if symptoms are refractory to medical treatment and there is no compelling evidence that it helps to select a treatment modality or predict response. It is generally helpful if a patient presents with mixed symptoms, there is an unclear diagnosis, poor history, associated voiding symptoms, or a background neurological condition.

Intravesical BTX is a very effective treatment although patients will need repeated treatments. PTNS offers similar efficacy to pharmacotherapy but requires a regular time commitment from the patient at the start as well as for maintenance sessions. It is not widely offered. SNS is a reasonably safe and minimally invasive treatment option but does require intensive commitment on behalf of the patient. Revision rates can be high. Augmentation cystoplasty should be reserved for the most refractory cases and in patients who are fit to undergo major surgery. They should be appropriately counselled about the high risk of ISC and other associated risks and complications. Invasive treatment modalities should be discussed within a multidisciplinary setting and all treatment options explored with the patient.

References

1. Bo K, Frawley HC, Haylen BT, et al. An International Urogynecological Association (IUGA)/International Continence Society (ICS) joint report on the terminology for the conservative and nonpharmacological management of female pelvic floor dysfunction. *Neurourol Urodyn.* 2017;36(2):221–244.
2. Avery K, Donovan J, Peters TJ, Shaw C, Gotoh M, Abrams P. ICIQ: a brief and robust measure for evaluating the symptoms and impact of urinary incontinence. *Neurourol Urodyn.* 2004;23(4):322–330.
3. Coyne KS, Sexton CC, Kopp ZS, Ebel-Bitoun C, Milsom I, Chapple C. The impact of overactive bladder on mental health, work productivity and health-related quality of life in the UK and Sweden: results from EpiLUTS. *BJU Int.* 2011;108(9):1459–1471.
4. Willis-Gray MG, Dieter AA, Geller EJ. Evaluation and management of overactive bladder: strategies for optimizing care. *Res Rep Urol.* 2016;8:113–122.
5. Robinson D, Hanna-Mitchell A, Rantell A, Thiagamoorthy G, Cardozo L. Are we justified in suggesting change to caffeine, alcohol, and carbonated drink intake in lower urinary tract disease? Report from the ICI-RS 2015. *Neurourol Urodyn.* 2017;36(4):876–881.
6. Cody JD, Jacobs ML, Richardson K, Moehrer B, Hextall A. Oestrogen therapy for urinary incontinence in post-menopausal women. *Cochrane Database Syst Rev.* 2012;10:CD001405.
7. Shamliyan T, Wyman JF, Ramakrishnan R, Sainfort F, Kane RL. Benefits and harms of pharmacologic treatment for urinary incontinence in women: a systematic review. *Ann Intern Med.* 2012;156(12):861–874.
8. Chapple CR, Nazir J, Hakimi Z, et al. Persistence and adherence with mirabegron versus antimuscarinic agents in patients with overactive bladder: a retrospective observational study in UK clinical practice. *Eur Urol.* 2017;72(3):389–399.
9. Allison SJ, Gibson W. Mirabegron, alone and in combination, in the treatment of overactive bladder: real-world evidence and experience. *Ther Adv Urol.* 2018;10(12):411–419.

10. Gray SL, Anderson ML, Dublin S, et al. Cumulative use of strong anticholinergics and incident dementia: a prospective cohort study. *JAMA Intern Med.* 2015;175(3):401–407.
11. Nambiar AK, Bosch R, Cruz F, et al. EAU guidelines on assessment and nonsurgical management of urinary incontinence. *Eur Urol.* 2018;73(4):596–609.
12. Malone-Lee JG, Al-Buheissi S. Does urodynamic verification of overactive bladder determine treatment success? Results from a randomized placebo-controlled study. *BJU Int.* 2009;103(7):931–937.
13. Brazzelli M, Murray A, Fraser C. Efficacy and safety of sacral nerve stimulation for urinary urge incontinence: a systematic review. *J Urol.* 2006;175(3):835–841.
14. Jackson BL, Burge F, Bronjewski E, Parkinson RJ. Intravesical botulinum toxin for overactive bladder syndrome without detrusor overactivity. *Br J Med Surg Urol.* 2012;5(4):169–173.
15. Colli E, Artibani W, Goka J, Parazzini F, Wein AJ. Are urodynamic tests useful tools for the initial conservative management of non-neurogenic urinary incontinence? A review of the literature. *Eur Urol.* 2003;43(1):63–69.
16. Rovner E, Kennelly M, Schulte-Baukloh H, Zhou J, Haag-Molkenteller C, Dasgupta P. Urodynamic results and clinical outcomes with intradetrusor injections of onabotulinumtoxinA in a randomized, placebo-controlled dose-finding study in idiopathic overactive bladder. *Neurourol Urodyn.* 2011;30(4):556–562.
17. Schurch B, de Seze M, Denys P, et al. Botulinum toxin type a is a safe and effective treatment for neurogenic urinary incontinence: results of a single treatment, randomized, placebo controlled 6-month study. *J Urol.* 2005;174(1):196–200.
18. Chapple C, Sievert KD, MacDiarmid S, et al. OnabotulinumtoxinA 100 U significantly improves all idiopathic overactive bladder symptoms and quality of life in patients with overactive bladder and urinary incontinence: a randomised, double-blind, placebo-controlled trial. *Eur Urol.* 2013;64(2):249–256.
19. Peters KM, Carrico DJ, Wooldridge LS, Miller CJ, MacDiarmid SA. Percutaneous tibial nerve stimulation for the long-term treatment of overactive bladder: 3-year results of the STEP study. *J Urol.* 2013;189(6):2194–2201.
20. Awad SA, Al-Zahrani HM, Gajewski JB, Bourque-Kehoe AA. Long-term results and complications of augmentation ileocystoplasty for idiopathic urge incontinence in women. *Br J Urol.* 1998;81(4):569–573.
21. van Kerrebroeck PE, van Voskuilen AC, Heesakkers JP, et al. Results of sacral neuromodulation therapy for urinary voiding dysfunction: outcomes of a prospective, worldwide clinical study. *J Urol.* 2007;178(5):2029–2034.
22. Amundsen CL, Richter HE, Menefee SA, et al. OnabotulinumtoxinA vs sacral neuromodulation on refractory urgency urinary incontinence in women: a randomized clinical Trial. *JAMA.* 2016;316(13):1366–1374.
23. Agarwal A, Eryuzlu LN, Cartwright R, et al. What is the most bothersome lower urinary tract symptom? Individual- and population-level perspectives for both men and women. *Eur Urol.* 2014;65(6):1211–1217.

24 Stress urinary incontinence

Rachel Barratt

Expert commentary Suzanne Biers

Case history

A 52-year-old woman presented with long-standing urinary incontinence (UI), progressively worsening over the last 18 months. Urinary leak while running had meant she had stopped exercising and had put on weight as a result, with a raised body mass index (BMI) of 34 kg/m^2. She also leaked on coughing, laughing, and occasionally without any obvious cause, and required three large pads per day which were often saturated. She denied associated lower urinary tract symptoms (LUTS). She had two children by normal vaginal delivery, and was now perimenopausal. Urinalysis was negative, post-void residual (PVR) was negligible, and 24-hour pad weight was significant at 70 g. Examination revealed mild vaginal atrophy, a demonstrable stress leak on cough, but no pelvic organ prolapse (POP), and pelvic floor power was 3 out of 5 (Table 24.1).

Expert comment Assessment of UI

Be vigilant and seek out 'red flag' symptoms when assessing patients with UI. These include haematuria, pain, recurrent urinary tract infections (UTIs), previous pelvic radiotherapy or surgery, and symptomatic POP. There is a small subset of women with 'complete' UI, with new or worsening incontinence who are 'never dry'. Maintain a high level of suspicion for vesicovaginal fistula in these cases. Congenital causes of persistent lifelong UI include duplex kidney with an ectopic ureter inserting into the distal urethra or vagina.

Pad weight tests are not routinely recommended, but 24-hour pad weights can be helpful in quantifying the severity of SUI[1]; >4.0 g is considered significant.[2] The International Consultation on Continence Questionnaire for Urinary Incontinence (ICIQ-UI) short form is a useful, validated, succinct questionnaire assessing frequency, volume, and bother from and triggers for UI, and is helpful in objectively recording symptoms at baseline and after intervention.[3]

Table 24.1 The Medical Research Council grading and Laycock's Modified Oxford Scale (adapted) are examples of systems utilized by pelvic floor physiotherapists to manually assess muscle strength, and both are graded on a scale from 0 to 5

MRC grading of muscle strength	Oxford grading system	Score
No contraction	No contraction	0
Flicker of movement	Flicker	1
Active movement with gravity eliminated	Weak	2
Active movement against gravity	Moderate	3
Active movement against gravity and resistance	Good (with lift)	4
Active movement against strong resistance	Strong	5

Adapted and used with the permission of the Medical Research Council (MRC), https://mrc.ukri.org/research/facilities-and-resources-for-researchers/mrc-scales/mrc-muscle-scale/; Laycock J. Incontinence. Pelvic floor re-education. *Nursing (Lond).* 1991 Jul 25–Aug 21;4(39):15–7. PMID: 1881640.

Learning point Conservative options for SUI

The starting point for any patient with SUI is a trial of conservative measures.

Weight loss

For patients with a BMI >30 kg/m^2, weight loss programmes achieving a loss of 5–10% body weight in overweight individuals result in symptom improvement in 47–65%.[4]

Oestrogen therapy

- Treatment with topical oestrogen therapy has been shown to be of use in postmenopausal patients.[5]
- Conversely, systemic oestrogen therapy (with conjugate equine oestrogens) can worsen pre-existing SUI or cause new SUI.[6]

Duloxetine medication

- Inhibits presynaptic reuptake of serotonin and norepinephrine in the sacral spinal cord, increasing the availability of these neurotransmitters to the postsynaptic pudendal motor neurons, and thus increasing the resting tone of the urethral striated sphincter.
- Systematic review has shown it is efficacious when compared to placebo, but has a high rate of gastrointestinal and nervous system side effects resulting in a high discontinuation rate.[7]
- Both National Institute of Health and Care Excellence (NICE) and European Association of Urology (EAU) guidelines do not recommend the use of duloxetine as a primary treatment, but it can be used in those who do not wish to embark on surgical therapy.[8,9]

Pelvic floor muscle training

Supervised pelvic floor muscle training (PFMT) has been shown to improve SUI by 20–87%, but there is a lack of evidence for sustained long-term benefit.[10] PFMT consists of supervision from a trained pelvic floor healthcare professional in identifying pelvic floor contraction and then performing eight to ten fast-twitch fibre exercises (quick hold and release) and eight to ten slow-twitch fibre recruiting exercises (hold for 10 seconds and release) performed three times per day.

Expert comment Topical oestrogen

Topical oestrogen therapies are available in pessary tablet, cream, and oestradiol-releasing vaginal ring pessary (Estring®) forms. Pelvic floor, urethral, and bladder tissues are sensitive to the effects of local oestrogen, and oestrogen receptors enhance the support mechanism of the pelvis through effects on synthesis and breakdown of collagen. Although topical oestrogens have minimal systemic absorption, advice should be taken from haematology and oncology experts if its use is considered in patients with prothrombotic conditions or a history of breast or endometrial cancer.

Evidence base Cochrane systematic review comparing the outcomes of PFMT versus no treatment on UI

A Cochrane review included 31 randomized or quasi-randomized trials, and involved 1817 women from 14 countries[11]:

- Symptomatic 'cure' of SUI was eight times more likely for patients receiving PFMT compared to no treatment (56% vs 6%).
- Symptomatic 'cure or improvement' of SUI was six times more likely for patients receiving PFMT compared to no treatment (74% vs 11%).
- PFMT were associated with significant improvement in both UI symptoms, quality of life scores and satisfaction, and reduced UI episodes by one per day.

Unfortunately, after 6 months of supervised PFMT and a slight reduction in BMI (now 32 kg/m^2) alongside a trial of topical oestrogen therapy, the patient's symptoms failed to improve. As the patient reported primary pure SUI, the decision was taken to not proceed with twin-channel urodynamic studies (UDS). She wished to pursue active treatment and was counselled on all (surgical) options, and provided with a patient decision aid and patient information leaflets.

Evidence base The role of urodynamics in uncomplicated primary SUI

Both NICE and EAU guidelines[8,9] do not recommend UDS for the patient with primary 'pure' SUI. Of note, this represents a very small number of patients (5.2%).[12] If there is any doubt in the diagnosis, voiding dysfunction, POP, urge-predominant mixed UI, or recurrent SUI, UDS should be offered.

Two randomized controlled trials have looked at the use of UDS for predominant SUI symptoms and the resulting surgical outcomes:

The Value of Urodynamic Evaluation (VALUE) study

This evaluated differences in treatment outcomes at 12 months in 630 women between standard 'office' evaluation and twin-channel UDS assessment[13]:

- Treatment success was 76.9% in the UDS group and 77.2% in the office evaluation group (non-inferior outcomes).
- Ninety-seven per cent with a clinical diagnosis of SUI had confirmed UDS SUI. UDS identified voiding dysfunction which had not been detected clinically in 10%, and excluded detrusor overactivity when it had been reported clinically in around 10–20% of patients.

The Value of Urodynamics Prior to Stress Incontinence Surgery 2 (VUSIS 2) study

This evaluated the strategy of immediate surgery for SUI versus tailoring therapy according to UDS findings in 578 women, and found no difference at 12 months follow-up.[14]

Clinical tip Options for primary SUI

For patients who wish to undergo surgery for primary SUI, all options can be offered after discussion in a specialist local pelvic floor multidisciplinary team (MDT) meeting. Alongside efficacy, the most important factor when counselling patients is the side effect profile of each procedure. Please note, mid-urethral synthetic tapes have not been in UK use since 2018.

Urethral bulking agents (i.e. Bulkamid®, Macroplastique®, Coaptite™)

- Success rates up to 50% cure (dry) and 70–80% improvement in SUI at 12 months.[15]
- Repeat treatment is required in 30–60% of patients.
- Risks include infection (UTI), bleeding, retention of urine <2%, urethral pain, *de novo* overactive bladder symptoms <1%.
- Benefits are that it is a 'minimally invasive' day-case procedure that can be performed under local anaesthetic.

Mid-urethral (synthetic) tapes

- Subjective success rates are 62–98% within 12 months, with no differences in success rates between retropubic and transobturator tapes[16]; longer-term success rates are 43–92%.
- Side effect profile, however, does differ:
  - Retropubic mid-urethral tape (MUT) is associated with a higher rate of bladder perforation (<5%), voiding dysfunction, and suprapubic pain (2%).
  - Transobturator MUT is associated with higher rates of groin pain (6%) but has a decreased risk of voiding dysfunction and visceral or vascular injury (<1%).
  - General risks include infection; bleeding; pain (suprapubic, pelvic, vaginal, thigh or groin pain, which can be chronic); injury to or extrusion of mesh into the bladder, urethra, or vagina; voiding dysfunction; and *de novo* overactive bladder symptoms. Vaginal mesh extrusion is <3% for both.

Autologous fascial sling

- Success rates for autologous fascial sling (AFS) are around 82%.[17]

- Specific risks include urinary retention and voiding dysfunction—this is more common as compared to MUT and colposuspension.

Colposuspension

- Aims to reposition the urethra and bladder neck in a normal anatomical position, and is helpful for type 2 (hypermobility) SUI.
- Subjective success rates at <12 months are 85–90%, deteriorating slightly to 79% after 5-year follow-up.[18]
- Specific risks include middle and posterior compartment POP in around 15%.

Evidence base Review of the comparative data on colposuspension, pubovaginal slings, and MUTs in the surgical treatment of female SUI

This systematic review and meta-analysis reports the findings of all comparative trials involving MUT for the surgical management of primary female SUI up until 2016, and includes 28 randomized controlled trials.[19]

Colposuspension versus MUT

- MUT had significantly higher cure rates compared to colposuspension (when laparoscopic colposuspension was included).
- Subjective success rates were 82% versus 74% for MUT and colposuspension respectively, and objective success rates 79.7% versus 67.8%.

MUT versus AFS

- Both techniques had similar efficacy and prevalence of complications.
- There was a trend towards a higher risk of bladder perforation with MUT and a higher incidence of reoperation with AFS.
- Patients treated with MUT had a statistically significant lower incidence of storage LUTs.

Retropubic versus transobturator MUT

- Retropubic MUT had statistically significant higher objective and subjective success rates compared to transobturator MUT (86% vs 84% and 78% vs 74%, respectively), although when any definition of cure was used, overall continence rates were not significantly different.
- Retropubic MUT had higher rates of bladder and vaginal perforation (4.8% vs 1.6%), UTI (10% vs 7.9%), and voiding symptoms (9.2% vs 5.6%).
- Vaginal erosion rates were reported to be higher in transobturator MUT (2.8% vs 1.8%).
- Other complications including storage symptoms, reoperation rates, and requirement for clean intermittent self-catheterization were found to be equivalent.

The case was discussed at the local hospital MDT meeting, and the patient elected to proceed with a retropubic MUT (tension-free vaginal tape). Postoperative recovery was uneventful, but she failed to attend follow-up, and was re-referred by her general practitioner 18 months later for persisting UI. The patient reported occasional urgency, but symptoms were still predominantly SUI. Her BMI had risen to 37 kg/m^2. She reported improvement from her retropubic MUT, but still required two pads per day and wanted to be dry. She had not experienced UTI, pelvic pain, or dyspareunia, and had no evidence of POP or mesh erosion on vaginal examination in clinic.

Clinical tip Surgery for primary SUI in women

NICE clinical guidelines on female UI management (NG123)[9] advise that women with primary SUI should be discussed at the local MDT meeting prior to offering surgery, and should be counselled on all options with the assistance of a patient decision aid. First-line surgical options include colposuspension, AFS, and MUT (retropubic route, bottom-to-top). For all indwelling synthetic products, a comprehensive database should be kept (on a national registry) including information on date and detail of the procedure, mesh, bulking agent or suture material used, manufacturer, product unique identification code, date, and detail of complications, and women should be given a copy of their data. Mesh complications should be reported to the Medicines and Healthcare products Regulatory Agency (MHRA). For women considering repeat continence surgery, their case should be discussed at a regional MDT meeting with specialists who deal with complex pelvic floor dysfunction (and mesh-related problems).

Expert comment Vaginal mesh surgery

This case predates the 'pause' on vaginal mesh surgery which was introduced in the UK in July 2018, and extended in March 2019, following the NHS England Independent Medicines and Medical Devices Safety Review. Recommendations that should be established for practice to resume include:

- Only undertake operations if appropriately trained and operating regularly
- Report every procedure to a national database
- Register of operations maintained
- Report complications via the MHRA
- Accreditation of specialist centres for SUI mesh procedures
- NICE guidelines on the use of mesh for SUI (published 2 April 2019).[9]

Clinical tip Key points in the clinical history for recurrent UI after surgery

For patients with recurrent UI following previous surgery for SUI, the following additional pertinent symptom information should be gathered:

- Urgency: approximately 10–15% of women will develop *de novo* detrusor overactivity, with or without incontinence.
- Incomplete bladder emptying and poor flow is suggestive of voiding dysfunction.
- Recurrent UTIs may be indicative of voiding dysfunction, retention of urine, or can be a feature of mesh or suture exposure in the urinary tract.
- Vaginal pain and dyspareunia may be early signs of mesh extrusion into the vagina.

Expert comment Investigation of recurrent UI

Investigation of recurrent UI should include urinalysis, PVR, a 3-day bladder diary, and UDS.[8,9] This helps to rule out associated voiding dysfunction or detrusor overactivity, and allows accurate determination of the type of SUI, whether this is predominantly intrinsic sphincter deficiency or urethral hypermobility in nature. Video UDS can be used to classify SUI (Table 24.2). An abdominal (Valsalva) leak point pressure <60 cmH_2O on UDS and a mean urethral closure pressure <30 cmH_2O on urethral pressure profile testing, both suggest intrinsic sphincter deficiency.

Table 24.2 Blaivas classification of SUI from video urodynamic studies

Type	Description
Type 0	Clinical report of SUI, but without clinical signs
Type I	Leakage that occurs during stress with <2 cm descent of the bladder base below the inferior margin of the symphysis pubis
Type 2	Leakage on stress accompanied by marked bladder base descent (>2 cm) that occurs only during stress (II_a) or is permanently present (II_b)
Type 3	Bladder neck and proximal urethra are already open at rest (with or without descent), also known as intrinsic sphincter deficiency

Evidence base Surgical options for recurrent SUI

Approximately 8–17% of women will require further surgery after primary SUI treatment.[20]

A systematic review and meta-analysis of randomized controlled trials for recurrent SUI by Agur et al. failed to show any difference in outcomes or complications for MUT (either retropubic or transobturator), AFS, or colposuspension.[21] Another systematic review by Nikilopoulous et al. looked at all studies on recurrent SUI, and reported pooled success rates of 68% for MUT (this decreased to 62% if the primary procedure had also been MUT), 76% for colposuspension, and 79% for AFS.[22] In comparison, urethral bulking agents had pooled success rates of 38%, and adjustable slings and other continence devices pooled success rates of 53%.[22] Bladder neck artificial urinary sphincters (AUS) can also be used in recurrent SUI setting, with success rates of 42–86%.[23]

Video UDS demonstrated SUI with a stable bladder and normal voiding (Figure 24.1). After case discussion at a specialist (regional) MDT meeting, and after counselling, the patient opted for an AFS, which she underwent along with removal of the vaginal component of her tape concurrently. At the 4-week postoperative review, she reported problems with one UTI and sensation of incomplete bladder emptying despite initially passing her trial without catheter as an inpatient. In clinic, uroflowmetry showed a Qmax of 11 mL/s for a voided volume of 180 mL, with a PVR of 250 mL. The patient was happy with her continence and agreed to manage the elevated residuals with clean intermittent self-catheterization twice daily, and subsequently UTIs resolved. She remained continent and happy with her result.

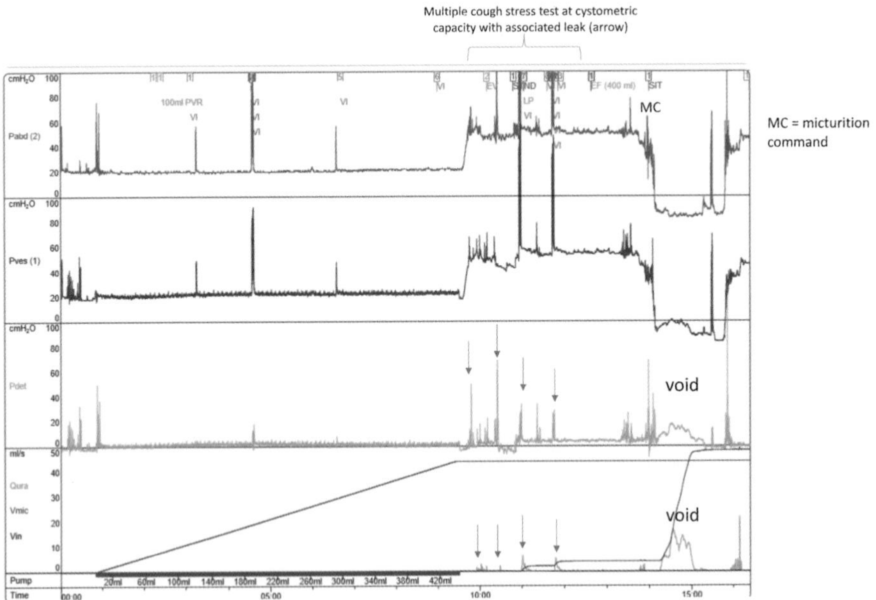

Figure 24.1 Twin-channel urodynamic trace demonstrating a stable detrusor during bladder filling, but SUI leaking on provocation with cough at bladder capacity. MC, micturition command.

Learning point Options for complex SUI cases

Options for complex SUI cases, when primary or secondary surgical procedures have failed, include bladder neck AUS insertion. The AMS 800™ is the only US Food and Drug Administration-approved AUS, although newer devices are available. The AUS can be inserted via an open abdominal or vaginal approach, laparoscopically or robotically, and has three components consisting of an inflatable cuff, a pump placed in the labia majora, and a pressure-regulating balloon placed in the extravesical space. Continence rates are 80% (ranging from 61% to 100%), but there is a recognized long-term deterioration in this with subsequent failure over time.

Complications

These include[24]:

- Infection of the device requiring explantation (up to 45%)
- Bleeding—requiring transfusion, embolization, or return to theatre in <2%
- Injury to bladder neck (44%) and vagina (25%)
- Erosion of device into urethra or vagina requiring explantation (up to 22%)
- Urethral atrophy resulting in recurrent incontinence
- Device failure requiring revision or replacement (up to 44%)
- Limited life expectancy of device—no long-term evidence in non-neuropathic women but estimated at 8–10 years in men.

'Last resort' surgical alternatives include urinary diversion with an ileal conduit formation or continent urinary diversion—either bladder neck closure or heterotopic neobladder formation combined with a continent catheterizable channel (Mitrofanoff or Monti).

A final word from the expert

Public concern regarding synthetic MUT

Following prominent patient group campaigns and Food and Drug Administration investigations from 2008 onwards, concerns have been raised over the complications and safety of synthetic MUT. Although current evidence suggests that synthetic MUTs are efficacious, when complications occur, they can significantly impair quality of life for patients. During a review into adverse events for primary SUI treated with synthetic MUT, the rate of complications in 92,000 patients was 9.8%, which is higher than previously recorded.[25] Currently, mesh procedures are not being offered in the UK, and specialist mesh centres are being commissioned, which as part of their role will offer specialist management of mesh complications.

Minimally invasive procedures

Advances in laparoscopic and robotic technology have led to the development of minimally invasive access for colposuspension as well as AUS insertion. Minimally invasive access has been shown to reduce intraoperative blood loss and decrease length of stay, but may also improve complication rates in other domains as experience in this area increases. Routine use of these techniques (in particular robotics) is hampered by the high cost of hardware and consumables required, and often render them economically unjustifiable.

Tissue engineering

Given the recent concerns regarding synthetic MUT and the inherent increased risk of harvesting autologous fascia, research is ongoing into producing biological materials to make slings. Research into electrospun poly-L-lactic acid and porcine small intestine submucosa shows they may be suitable scaffold materials for stem cells to 'seed' on, with proposed cells used in trials so far mainly consisting of adipose-derived stem cells. However, much more research is required before we will see biological derived slings entering clinical testing.[26]

References

1. Karantanis E, Allen W, Stevermuer TL, et al. The repeatability of the 24-hour pad test. *Int Urogynecol J Pelvic Floor Dysfunct.* 2005;16(1):63–68.
2. Painter V, Karantanis E, Moore KH. Does patient activity level affect 24-hr pad test results in stress-incontinent women? *Neurourol Urodyn.* 2012;31(1):143–147.
3. Avery K, Donovan J, Peters TJ, et al. ICIQ: a brief and robust measure for evaluating the symptoms and impact of urinary incontinence. *Neurourol Urodyn.* 2004;23(4):322–330.
4. Vissers D, Neels H, Vermandel A, et al. The effect of non-surgical weight loss interventions on urinary incontinence in overweight women: a systematic review and meta-analysis. *Obes Rev.* 2014;15(7):610–617.
5. Cody JD, Jacobs ML, Richardson K, et al. Oestrogen therapy for urinary incontinence in post-menopausal women. *Cochrane Database Syst Rev.* 2012;10:CD001405.
6. Steinauer JE, Waetjen LE, Vittinghoff E, et al. Postmenopausal hormone therapy: does it cause incontinence? *Obstet Gynecol.* 2005;106(5 Pt 1):940–945.
7. Li J, Yang L, Pu C, et al. The role of duloxetine in stress urinary incontinence: a systematic review and meta-analysis. *Int Urol Nephrol.* 2013;45(3):679–686.
8. Burkhard F, Bosch J, Cruz F, et al. Urinary incontinence. European Association of Urology. 2019. https://uroweb.org/guideline/urinary-incontinence/
9. National Institute for Health and Care Excellence. Urinary incontinence and pelvic organ prolapse in women: management. NICE guideline [NG123]. April 2019. National Institute for Health and Care Excellence. https://www.nice.org.uk/guidance/NG123
10. Bo K, Kvarstein B, Nygaard I. Lower urinary tract symptoms and pelvic floor muscle exercise adherence after 15 years. *Obstet Gynecol.* 2005;105(5 Pt 1):999–1005.
11. Dumoulin C, Hay-Smith EJC, Mac Habee-Seguin G. Pelvic floor muscle training versus no treatment, or inactive control treatments, for urinary incontinence in women. *Cochrane Database Syst Rev.* 2014;5:CD005654.
12. Agur W, Housami F, Drake M, et al. Could the National Institute for Health and Clinical Excellence guidelines on urodynamics in urinary incontinence put some women at risk of a bad outcome from stress incontinence surgery? *BJU Int.* 2009;103(5):635–639.
13. Nager CW, Brubaker L, Litman HJ, et al. A randomized trial of urodynamic testing before stress-incontinence surgery. *N Engl J Med.* 2012;366(21):1987–1997.
14. van Leijsen SAL, Kluivers KB, Mol BWJ, et al. Value of urodynamics before stress urinary incontinence surgery: a randomized controlled trial. *Obstet Gynecol.* 2013;121(5):999–1008.
15. Sokol ER, Karram MM, Dmochowski R. Efficacy and safety of polyacrylamide hydrogel for the treatment of female stress incontinence: a randomized, prospective, multicenter North American study. *J Urol.* 2014;192(3):843–849.
16. Ford AA, Rogerson L, Cody JD, et al. Mid-urethral sling operations for stress urinary incontinence in women. *Cochrane Database Syst Rev.* 2017;7:CD006375.
17. Blaivas JG, Purohit RS, Benedon MS, et al. Safety considerations for synthetic sling surgery. *Nat Rev Urol.* 2015;12(9):481–509.
18. Albo ME, Richter HE, Brubaker L, et al. Burch colposuspension versus fascial sling to reduce urinary stress incontinence. *N Engl J Med.* 2007;356(21):2143–2155.
19. Fusco F, Abdel-Fattah M, Chapple CR, et al. Updated systematic review and meta-analysis of the comparative data on colposuspensions, pubovaginal slings, and midurethral tapes in the surgical treatment of female stress urinary incontinence. *Eur Urol* 2017;72(4):567–591.

20. Albo ME, Litman HJ, Richter HE, et al. Treatment success of retropubic and transobturator mid urethral slings at 24 months. *J Urol.* 2012;188(6):2281–2287.
21. Agur W, Riad M, Secco S, et al. Surgical treatment of recurrent stress urinary incontinence in women: a systematic review and meta-analysis of randomised controlled trials. *Eur Urol.* 2013;64(2):323–336.
22. Nikolopoulos KI, Betschart C, Doumouchtsis SK. The surgical management of recurrent stress urinary incontinence: a systematic review. *Acta Obstet Gynecol Scand.* 2015;94(6):568–576.
23. Resus CR, Phe V, Dechartres A, et al. Performance and safety of the artificial urinary sphincter (AMS800) for non-neurogenic women with urinary incontinence secondary to intrinsic sphincter deficiency: a systematic review. *Eur Urol Focus.* 2020;6(2):327–338.
24. Peyronnet B, O'Connor E, Khavari R, et al. AMS-800 Artificial urinary sphincter in female patients with stress urinary incontinence: a systematic review. *Neurourol Urodyn.* 2018;38(Suppl 4):S28–S41.
25. Morling JR, McAllister DA, Agur W, et al. Adverse events after first, single, mesh and non-mesh surgical procedures for stress urinary incontinence and pelvic organ prolapse in Scotland, 1997-2016: a population-based cohort study. *Lancet* 2017;389(10069):629–640.
26. Chapple CR, Osman NI, Mangera A, et al. Application of tissue engineering to pelvic organ prolapse and stress urinary incontinence. *Low Urin Tract Symptoms.* 2015;7(2):63–70.

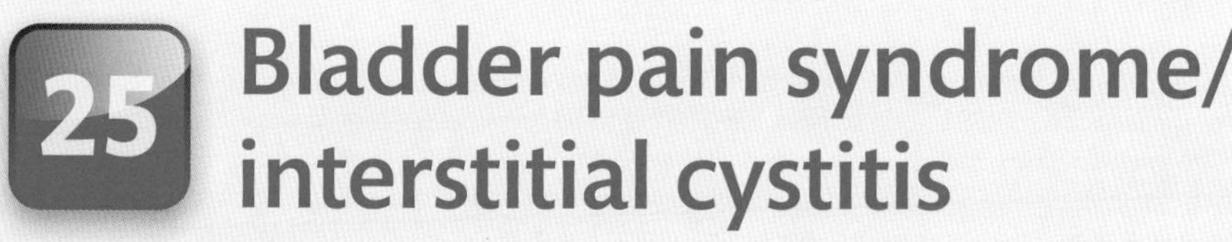

CASE 25

Bladder pain syndrome/ interstitial cystitis

Altaf Mangera

Expert commentary Altaf Mangera

Case history

A 49-year-old female describes a pain in her lower abdomen leading her to void every hour during the daytime and wake every 90 minutes at night to pass urine. She does not have any voiding symptoms such as reduced flow, straining, intermittency, and hesitancy. Her general practitioner referred her for assessment of her recurrent 'urinary tract infections' (rUTIs). She has had multiple urinary dipstick assessments by her general practitioner which sometimes show leucocytes and sometimes nitrites. Urine culture has been positive on two occasions in the last 18 months with *Escherichia coli* being grown by the laboratory. Other occasions mostly show no growth or mixed growth. When symptoms are 'bad', she has severe urgency and is incontinent in pads.

Clinical tip Differentiating between overactive bladder syndrome, rUTI, and bladder pain syndrome

The differential diagnoses for bladder pain syndrome (BPS)/interstitial cystitis (IC) are shown in Box 25.1. From a patient history, it can be difficult to differentiate between overactive bladder syndrome (OAB), rUTI, or BPS/IC. Urgency, the hallmark symptom of OAB, is described by the International Continence Society as 'a sudden compelling desire to void which is difficult to defer'. However, patients with BPS and rUTI will also exhibit this symptom. The excluding factor for OAB is the presence of pain which also accompanies BPS and rUTI. Typically, the pain in BPS was thought to occur with bladder filling and relief with voiding and in rUTI the pain is with voiding also known as dysuria. Infective symptoms such as a temperature, malaise, and offensive urine may point to rUTI but a good differentiating question would be 'Do antibiotics completely rid you of your symptoms?' Having symptom-free periods when antibiotics have taken effect and the presence of bacteria in the urine are strongly indicative of rUTI. BPS has a more chronic course with intermittent 'flare-ups', although there are no strict criteria on how long the symptoms need to go on for.

Box 25.1 Differential diagnoses for BPS/IC

- Overactive bladder.
- Urinary tract infection.
- Drug induced cystitis (i.e. ketamine).
- Tuberculous cystitis.
- Radiation cystitis.
- Bladder or ureteric calculi.
- Bladder cancer.
- Vulvodynia.
- Prostatitis.
- Endometriosis.
- Bowel disorders.
- Genital herpes.

The US National Institute of Diabetes and Digestive and Kidney Diseases (NIDDK) defines criteria for the research of BPS but these have been found to be too strict for everyday use. Therefore, different guideline panels have provided different definitions of BPS which typically rely on history, examination, cystoscopic findings, and exclusion of other conditions with overlapping symptoms. All guidelines agree that a pressure, pain, or discomfort needs to be felt in the pelvis with at least one other urinary symptom and other possible causes need to be excluded through thorough evaluation.[1] Cystoscopic examination either with or without hydrodistension should be considered either to exclude a competing pathology or to help subtyping of patients. Bladder capacity under anaesthetic is an independent predictor of severity and bladder treatment success along with the presence of Hunner's lesions (cracks in the lining of the bladder) which are thought to represent a separate subclassification.[2]

Expert comment Combination of diagnoses

Despite the individualized definitions of OAB, BPS, and rUTI, it can be difficult to tell them apart and some patients may present with a combination of problems. There is no reason why a patient with BPS may not have a UTI periodically and one would even argue it occurs more frequently than in those without BPS. An open mind is required when taking a history and the individual symptoms and their bother should be recorded. Other frequently encountered diagnoses in patients with BPS include inflammatory bowel disease, systemic lupus erythematosus, allergies to medications, irritable bowel syndrome, sensitive skin, and fibromyalgia.[3]

The patient is perimenopausal and does not have any bowel or gynaecological problems. She does suffer from anxiety and has also been told she has chronic fatigue syndrome which leads to a lot of tiredness.

Clinical tip Clinical assessment

Stress has been studied as a risk factor for BPS and flare-ups can occur during periods of heightened stress.[4] It is postulated that sympathetic dominance plays a role in inducing a hyperalgesic state.[5] Visceral hypersensitivity or more central hypersensitization are potential aetiological mechanisms and should be sought out in the history. Thus, careful assessment of the gynaecological, sexual, and bowel function needs to be undertaken. Exacerbating and relieving factors should be sought along with relationship to periods and food/drink. Pelvic floor muscle examination and trigger points need to be examined and, in men, prostate examination, paying particular attention to areas of tenderness, needs to be undertaken.

Learning point Investigations

As the urologist providing the specialist opinion, a urinary dipstick and midstream specimen of urine would be recommended to exclude a UTI and request a cystoscopy if red cells are present. Sterile pyuria may prompt the need to send samples to exclude tuberculosis and sexually transmitted infections.

A frequency volume chart is useful to show small functional bladder volumes and urinary frequency. The diagnosis of a specific bladder pain pathology is less likely if functional bladder volumes exceed 350 mL and with a frequency of fewer than eight/day. These were considered exclusions on the NIDDK criteria. A more objective measure of symptoms can be obtained with a visual analogue scale assessing pain severity or the use of a validated quality-of-life scoring tool such as the O'Leary–Sant Interstitial Cystitis Symptom Index (ICSI) and Problem index (ICPI).

The place of cystoscopy in the assessment of BPS is much debated. If there are any concerns picked up on the history or dipstick assessment then there should be no delay in obtaining the investigation which is generally done with a flexible cystoscope under local anaesthetic. On the other hand, a hydrodistension procedure with the opportunity to take a biopsy under a general anaesthetic would be more useful diagnostically and also has a potential therapeutic role. The timing of the hydrodistension procedure would follow after conservative measures have failed to improve the symptoms.

Clinical tip Performing a hydrodistension

It is important to standardize one's hydrodistension procedure. It is the author's practice to perform the procedure under general anaesthetic. The cystoscope should be inserted into the bladder and the water pressure set to 100 cm. A cystoscopy is undertaken looking for any urethral or bladder abnormalities including Hunner's lesions. The bladder is then filled until it reaches its capacity at 100 cmH_2O pressure. The cystoscopic inflow tap is left open so if any fluid leaks out around the cystoscope it can continue to fill. In women who have very weak sphincteric resistance, the urethra can be compressed against the cystoscope (if this is not done then the bladder may not fill as it all leaks around the cystoscope giving a false impression of a small-capacity bladder). The hydrodistension is held for 3 minutes. The anaesthetist is asked to report any changes in blood pressure or pulse which indicate a positive painful response under anaesthetic. After 3 minutes, the water inflow to the cystoscope is switched off and the bladder emptied into a measuring jug. The bladder capacity under anaesthetic with 100 cmH_2O pressure is recorded in the notes. The bladder is refilled and any glomerulations and their locations noted. Hunner's lesions may become more apparent after hydrodistension and are described as a circumscript, reddened mucosal area with small vessels radiating towards a central scar, with a fibrin deposit or coagulum attached to this area. This site ruptures with increasing bladder distension, with petechial oozing of blood from the lesion and the mucosal margins in a waterfall manner. A biopsy should only be taken after the hydrodistension and not before.

Learning point Intravesical instillations

Intravesical instillation of potassium chloride, as a diagnostic test for BPS, can be painful and has poor specificity for BPS and therefore is not widely performed.[6] It was postulated that an abnormal glycosaminoglycan layer allowed potassium ions to cross the epithelium leading to pain. However, this does not help in the diagnosis due to poor specificity and does not predict improvement with intravesical therapies designed to reline the glycosaminoglycan layer.[7] Similarly, the use of intravesical anaesthetic to localize the pain to the bladder and exclude an extravesical cause has been evaluated.[8] After instillation, if the pain improves or disappears then theoretically the bladder is implicated as the source of the pain. The test has not gained widespread acceptance due to the lack of robust data regarding its sensitivity and specificity.

Expert comment
Urodynamics

Urodynamics does not have a routine role in the assessment of BPS but may be utilized where there is ambiguity in the description of pain which may be described as a pressure to void by some patients. A detrusor overactive contraction may be responsible for such a sensation. Also, if voiding dysfunction is suspected, such as with a raised post-void residual, then urodynamics may be indicated.

Learning point Oral medications

The next line would be oral medications. Patients with central or organ-specific sensitization may benefit from amitriptyline or gabapentin. Pentosan polysulphate may be beneficial in some patients; however, a recent placebo-controlled randomized controlled trial (RCT) failed to show a significant difference to placebo.[9] Similarly, hydroxyzine has not shown significant benefit in a pilot RCT either.[10] Oral cyclosporine A was found to have a greater clinical response compared to pentosan polysulphate in one trial though with a higher side effect profile.[11] It requires close blood pressure and serum drug concentration monitoring, and has the potential for serious adverse events (e.g. nephrotoxicity and immunosuppression) and would thus not be used unless symptoms were severe.

Analgesic medication such as amitriptyline and gabapentin are also used by pain specialists in patients with a neuropathic-sounding pain possibly from a previous insult or surgical scarring. Amitriptyline has been found to be effective at reducing symptom scores in two RCTs when given at a dose >50 mg and is a recommended treatment for BPS/IC.[12,13] Gabapentin has not been studied in an RCT.

L-arginine when oxidized produces nitric oxide. A lack of nitric oxide has been proposed as a mechanism for BPS/IC. Two trials have not shown a clear benefit of L-arginine in improving

Expert comment
Patient education

Patient education is the most important aspect of BPS management. From the outset, patients should be told it is likely to be a chronic condition with flare-ups and -downs. Setting realistic expectations of improvements in quality of life are important. The optimal management should be multimodal and include behavioural, physical, and psychological techniques, and management should proceed in a step-wise manner, starting with the most conservative.

symptom and pain scores.[14,15] Sildenafil has been compared to placebo in a RCT of 48 women.[16] After 3 months it led to a >50% improvement in symptom scores and urodynamic parameters but not on the visual analogue scale scores.

Sequential antibiotic rotation has also been assessed in a small randomized study and only showed benefit in a small number of patients with many side effects.[17] There is also a risk of developing antibiotic resistance and so should not be utilized in patients.

Learning point Behavioural techniques

Behavioural techniques such as timed voiding, fluid modification, and bladder training are recommended as first line. Diet modification is recommended, that is, reducing acidic beverages, spicy foods, and alcohol which have been reported to exacerbate symptoms in up to 90% of patients with BPS. Physiotherapy is also recommended, especially for patients with pelvic floor dysfunction, and phenotype-directed multimodal management approaches (including stress management and psychotherapy) are suggested as first-line management options.

Learning point Intravesical therapies

Intravesical instillations of hyaluronic acid have shown efficacy in patients with BPS/IC.[18,19] In a study of 110 women, hyaluronic acid and chondroitin sulphate instillations were superior to DMSO in reducing pain intensity, and other endpoints such as quality-of-life scores were improved in both groups from baseline.[20] Pentosan polysulphate or lidocaine instillations have also been suggested to be useful in treating patients with BPS/IC in small studies.[21,22] Therefore, the European Association of Urology guidelines have recommended these intravesical therapies in patients with BPS/IC.

Learning point Other therapies

Botulinum toxin has shown mixed results in multiple RCTs and pooling of these data does suggest some overall benefit in improving symptoms cores, maximum cystometric capacity, and urinary frequency with an increase in post-void residue.[24] Similarly, sacral neuromodulation has shown benefit in patients with pelvic pain and in some with BPS/IC in improving pain and voiding symptoms.[25]

As with a lot of functional problems, radical surgery often forms a last resort and therefore the patients who go down this route tend to be the worst affected by their problems. A substitution cystoplasty either with a supratrigonal or subtrigonal cystoplasty is offered to those with exceptionally bad symptoms often demonstrated to have poor bladder capacity at hydrodistension under general anaesthetic. The alternative is a urinary diversion. In those undergoing a diversion without cystectomy, a cystectomy is required in 50% and therefore is recommended to be undertaken in the first instance. Patients must be warned that despite a total cystectomy, bladder pain may still persist. The literature contains mostly small series of patients having undergone surgery for BPS/IC with decent success rates reported.[26,27]

Learning point Acupuncture

Acupuncture is recommended by the East Asian, Royal College of Obstetricians and Gynaecologists, and Canadian Urological Association guidelines as a non-invasive option for motivated patients, and trigger-point injections with local anaesthetic are given a grade D recommendation by the Canadian Urological Association guideline panel as an option for patients with pelvic floor trigger-point pain.

Expert comment Bladder hydrodistension

Bladder hydrodistension and transurethral fulguration of Hunner's lesions are considered third-line options for the treatment of BPS after failure of the second-line therapies described above. Several case series have demonstrated long-term therapeutic benefit.[23]

Future directions Biomarkers

It is most likely that a number of different pathophysiological mechanisms and aetiological factors are responsible for BPS/IC and, as such, lumping together all patients with similar symptoms into one large category does not do the problem justice. Therefore, more work needs to be done in phenotyping and categorizing patients' symptoms, investigations, and test results. Further tests need to be developed to differentiate if the condition is inflammatory, diet related, related to loss of bladder lining, owing to neurosensitization (either central or peripheral), or as a result of other causes. With a better understanding of the underlying processes and biomarkers, better more targeted therapies can be developed.

A number of possible biomarkers have been studied to date including nerve growth factor which can induce bladder nociceptive responses, the proinflammatory cytokine tumour necrosis factor, and toll-like receptors, which play a role in the innate immune system. In addition, purinergic mechanisms may also contribute to the bladder dysfunction in BPS/IC as the P2X3 purinoceptor can drive sensitization of bladder afferents in response to ATP release from the urothelium. Thus, P2X3 antagonists have been proposed to reduce BPS/IC symptoms. These approaches are still in their infancy and with further research and development may be able to help patients with BPS/IC.

Expert comment Pathophysiology of bladder pain syndrome

The urothelial layer of the bladder was once thought of as being inert and impermeable. However, it is now recognized to receive, amplify, and transmit information about the extracellular environment either directly or through the lamina propria underneath (which contains interstitial cells) to the central nervous system.[28] Therefore, changes in the mucosal lining of the bladder may permit urine or toxic substances to pass to the deeper layers, irritating the underlying neurons leading to the symptoms commonly described.

In patients with pain symptoms of other organs, a central visceral hypersensitivity has been suggested which may involve dorsal horn neurons within the spinal cord leading to sensitization which may continue long after resolution of inflammation or pelvic insult. Alternatively, in those with widespread pain or associated fibromyalgia, functional magnetic resonance imaging shows functional connectivity involving sensorimotor and insular cortices, suggesting abnormal brain neuronal connectivity as a cause for the pain.[29]

A final word from the expert

It is important to place the patient at the centre of the consultation when assessing if they have BPS/IC. It is imperative to rule out other differential diagnoses. If other aetiologies are excluded and conservative measures fail to improve symptoms, then a cystodistension is useful both diagnostically and also may have therapeutic benefits. The bladder capacity is a good guide of the level of treatment indicated and a stepwise approach should be employed. It is important to educate your patient that most commonly this is a poorly understood life-long condition which needs managing and there is no quick-fix cure, although some patients do find long-term relief after certain interventions. Ultimately, we must try to do the best for each patient's quality of life and individualized management is necessary.

References

1. Malde S, Palmisani S, Al-Kaisy A, Sahai A. Guideline of guidelines: bladder pain syndrome. *BJU Int.* 2018;122(5):729–743.
2. Messing E, Pauk D, Schaeffer A, et al. Associations among cystoscopic findings and symptoms and physical examination findings in women enrolled in the Interstitial Cystitis Data Base (ICDB) Study. *Urology.* 1997;49(5A Suppl):81–85.
3. Alagiri M, Chottiner S, Ratner V, Slade D, Hanno PM. Interstitial cystitis: unexplained associations with other chronic disease and pain syndromes. *Urology.* 1997;49(5A Suppl):52–57.
4. Pierce AN, Christianson JA. Stress and chronic pelvic pain. *Prog Mol Biol Transl Sci.* 2015;131:509–535.
5. Williams DP, Chelimsky G, McCabe NP, et al. Effects of chronic pelvic pain on heart rate variability in women. *J Urol.* 2015;194(5):1289–1294.
6. Hanno P. Is the potassium sensitivity test a valid and useful test for the diagnosis of interstitial cystitis? Against. *Int Urogynecol J Pelvic Floor Dysfunct.* 2005;16(6):428–429.
7. Sairanen J, Tammela TL, Leppilahti M, Onali M, Forsell T, Ruutu M. Potassium sensitivity test (PST) as a measurement of treatment efficacy of painful bladder syndrome/interstitial cystitis: a prospective study with cyclosporine A and pentosan polysulfate sodium. *Neurourol Urodyn.* 2007;26(2):267–270.
8. Taneja R. Intravesical lignocaine in the diagnosis of bladder pain syndrome. *Int Urogynecol J.* 2010;21(3):321–324.
9. Nickel JC, Herschorn S, Whitmore KE, et al. Pentosan polysulfate sodium for treatment of interstitial cystitis/bladder pain syndrome: insights from a randomized, double-blind, placebo controlled study. *J Urol.* 2015;193(3):857–862.

10. Sant GR, Propert KJ, Hanno PM, et al. A pilot clinical trial of oral pentosan polysulfate and oral hydroxyzine in patients with interstitial cystitis. *J Urol.* 2003;170(3):810–815.
11. Sairanen J, Tammela TL, Leppilahti M, et al. Cyclosporine A and pentosan polysulfate sodium for the treatment of interstitial cystitis: a randomized comparative study. *J Urol.* 2005;174(6):2235–2238.
12. Foster HE Jr, Hanno PM, Nickel JC, et al. Effect of amitriptyline on symptoms in treatment naive patients with interstitial cystitis/painful bladder syndrome. *J Urol.* 2010;183(5):1853–1858.
13. van Ophoven A, Pokupic S, Heinecke A, Hertle L. A prospective, randomized, placebo controlled, double-blind study of amitriptyline for the treatment of interstitial cystitis. *J Urol.* 2004;172(2):533–536.
14. Cartledge JJ, Davies AM, Eardley I. A randomized double-blind placebo-controlled crossover trial of the efficacy of L-arginine in the treatment of interstitial cystitis. *BJU Int.* 2000;85(4):421–426.
15. Korting GE, Smith SD, Wheeler MA, Weiss RM, Foster HE Jr. A randomized double-blind trial of oral L-arginine for treatment of interstitial cystitis. *J Urol.* 1999;161(2):558–565.
16. Chen H, Wang F, Chen W, et al. Efficacy of daily low-dose sildenafil for treating interstitial cystitis: results of a randomized, double-blind, placebo-controlled trial—treatment of interstitial cystitis/painful bladder syndrome with low-dose sildenafil. *Urology.* 2014;84(1):51–56.
17. Warren JW, Horne LM, Hebel JR, Marvel RP, Keay SK, Chai TC. Pilot study of sequential oral antibiotics for the treatment of interstitial cystitis. *J Urol.* 2000;163(6):1685–1688.
18. Kallestrup EB, Jorgensen SS, Nordling J, Hald T. Treatment of interstitial cystitis with Cystistat: a hyaluronic acid product. *Scand J Urol Nephrol.* 2005;39(2):143–147.
19. Nordling J, Jorgensen S, Kallestrup E. Cystistat for the treatment of interstitial cystitis: a 3-year follow-up study. *Urology.* 2001;57(6 Suppl 1):123.
20. Cervigni M, Sommariva M, Tenaglia R, et al. A randomized, open-label, multicenter study of the efficacy and safety of intravesical hyaluronic acid and chondroitin sulfate versus dimethyl sulfoxide in women with bladder pain syndrome/interstitial cystitis. *Neurourol Urodyn.* 2017;36(4):1178–1186.
21. Daha LK, Lazar D, Simak R, Pfluger H. The effects of intravesical pentosanpolysulfate treatment on the symptoms of patients with bladder pain syndrome/interstitial cystitis: preliminary results. *Int Urogynecol J Pelvic Floor Dysfunct.* 2008;19(7):987–990.
22. Henry RA, Morales A, Cahill CM. Beyond a simple anesthetic effect: lidocaine in the diagnosis and treatment of interstitial cystitis/bladder pain syndrome. *Urology.* 2015;85(5):1025–1033.
23. Niimi A, Nomiya A, Yamada Y, et al. Hydrodistension with or without fulguration of hunner lesions for interstitial cystitis: long-term outcomes and prognostic predictors. *Neurourol Urodyn.* 2016;35(8):965–969.
24. Wang J, Wang Q, Wu Q, Chen Y, Wu P. Intravesical botulinum toxin A injections for bladder pain syndrome/interstitial cystitis: a systematic review and meta-analysis of controlled studies. *Med Sci Monit.* 2016;22:3257–3267.
25. Mahran A, Baaklini G, Hassani D, et al. Sacral neuromodulation treating chronic pelvic pain: a meta-analysis and systematic review of the literature. *Int Urogynecol J.* 2019;30(7):1023–1035.
26. Mateu AL, Gutierrez RC, Mayordomo FO, Martinez B, V, Palou RJ, Errando SC. Long-term follow-up after cystectomy for bladder pain syndrome: pain status, sexual function and quality of life. *World J Urol.* 2019;37(8):1597–1603.
27. Kim HJ, Lee JS, Cho WJ, et al. Efficacy and safety of augmentation ileocystoplasty combined with supratrigonal cystectomy for the treatment of refractory bladder pain syndrome/interstitial cystitis with Hunner's lesion. *Int J Urol.* 2014;21(Suppl 1):69–73.
28. Birder L, Andersson KE. Urothelial signaling. *Physiol Rev.* 2013;93(2):653–680.
29. Kutch JJ, Ichesco E, Hampson JP, et al. Brain signature and functional impact of centralized pain: a multidisciplinary approach to the study of chronic pelvic pain (MAPP) network study. *Pain.* 2017;158(10):1979–1991.

CASE

26 Female urinary retention

Pravisha Ravindra

Expert commentary Nikesh Thiruchelvam

Case history

A 23-year-old woman presented to the emergency department with lower abdominal discomfort and inability to pass urine for the preceding 24 hours. She has no associated bowel symptoms or symptoms to suggest a urinary tract infection. She had a past medical history of anxiety and polycystic ovary syndrome. Past surgical history included a diagnostic laparoscopy for pelvic pain 18 months previously. Drug history consisted of sertraline 10 mg once daily and the combined oral contraceptive pill. Observations on arrival into the department were unremarkable apart from a mild tachycardia of 105 beats per minute. Routine bloods were sent; white cell count was marginally raised at 11.5×10^9/L but all others were normal. Bladder scan was performed and showed > 999 mL in the bladder. As such, a urethral catheter was inserted and a residual volume of 1.2 L was drained. The patient was then discharged and a trial without catheter was arranged in the community.

Learning point Definition and epidemiology

Urinary retention (UR) is defined by the International Continence Society as the complaint of the inability to pass urine despite persistent effort.[1] There are many causes of UR in a woman, although the condition itself is relatively uncommon when compared to men.

One Danish study cited an incidence of acute urinary retention (AUR) in women as 7 per 100,000 population.[2] The prevalence of the chronic condition is difficult to quantify as it generally requires a bladder scan to confirm the diagnosis. In a group of female patients presenting with lower urinary tract symptoms, 5% were found to have a post-void residual of >150 mL.[3] There is no consensus on the post-void residual threshold that defines UR with the American Urological Association guidelines specifying 300 mL.[4]

Learning point Voiding reflex

For normal voiding to take place, the voiding reflex is initiated in the pontine micturition centre. The hypogastric nerve relaxes the external urethral sphincter and the pudendal nerve relaxes the pelvic floor. Voiding then results when the detrusor muscle contracts under parasympathetic control. Disruption at any point along this pathway can result in incomplete emptying.

Learning point Causes of UR

The aetiology is diverse and its presentation can be classified into acute (transient) or chronic (recurrent). Commonly, the key differentiating factor between the two types is the presence of pain. Pain is commonly associated with AUR; however, there are special occasions in which AUR can be painless such as spinal cord compression or post anaesthetic (Table 26.1). The pathophysiology of the condition is twofold, consisting of reduced or absent bladder contractility or bladder outlet obstruction (or a combination of the two).

Table 26.1 Causes of female urinary retention

	Acute/transient	Chronic/recurrent
Bladder outlet obstruction	Pelvic organ prolapse Urethral diverticulum Urethral stenosis SUI surgery Urethral injury	Any of the acute causes if not rectified
Neurological	Spinal cord injury CES Nerve injury	Spinal cord injury CES Nerve injury
Abnormal bladder function	Bladder injury Overdistension Pelvic mass Constipation Post-partum Drugs, e.g. anticholinergics, anaesthetic agents	Overdistension Diabetes mellitus Age Multiple sclerosis
Functional		Dysfunctional voiding Detrusor sphincter dyssynergia Fowler's syndrome Hinman's syndrome

Learning point UR: anatomical distortion

In the case of distortion, extrinsic or intrinsic compression such as pelvic organ prolapse, urethral diverticulum, or pelvic mass (including constipation), UR may resolve once this has been rectified. There may not be complete bladder recovery, depending on the chronicity of the condition and some patients may always be reliant on some degree of catheterization. Obstruction may also occur as a consequence of surgery for stress urinary incontinence (SUI); the need for and timing of any division of tape or sling is controversial.[5] The incidence of urethral stenosis has been quantified at 4–13%.[6] Risk factors include prolonged catheterization, pelvic irradiation, childbirth, pelvic fracture, and surgery for urethral diverticulum or SUI. If stenosis is recurrent despite urethral dilatation, there are encouraging results with female substitution urethroplasty.[7]

Learning point UR: drug induced

Most commonly this can be because of anticholinergic use. If a specific culprit is identified, often stopping the drug improves bladder function.[8] This is similar if thought to be anaesthetic-induced postoperatively or postpartum. It is important this is diagnosed early in order to avoid overdistension injuries that may render the retention a chronic problem. Use of epidural anaesthesia has been linked to a greater risk of UR as has greater opioid use in orthopaedic surgery.[9,10]

Learning point UR: nerve injury

This could occur anywhere along the neural pathway from higher-level disorders (such as stroke), lower-level disorders such as traumatic nerve injury or cauda equina syndrome (CES), or a global neurological disorder such as ageing, diabetes mellitus, or multiple sclerosis. The prevalence of common conditions such as diabetes is on the increase and there is evidence to show that this can be a contributing factor to detrusor underactivity, as can age.[11,12] Detrusor sphincter dyssynergia can be a consequence of new or long-standing spinal cord injury or multiple sclerosis and has a characteristic pattern on urodynamic studies. Nerve injury could occur as a result of trauma or intraoperatively. Most commonly, this can be as a result of colorectal, obstetric, or gynaecological surgery.

Learning point Detrusor sphincter dyssynergia

In detrusor sphincter dyssynergia, detrusor contraction occurs simultaneously with urethral striated muscle contraction, preventing voiding.

Expert comment Management of female AUR

Initial management of these patients consists of bladder drainage, correction of any underlying cause if possible, and then, if still unresolved, a long-term bladder drainage strategy. To complicate matters further, the condition can be multifactorial. It is important to undertake a flexible cystoscopy to exclude anatomical causes, as outlined in Table 26.1. Every effort should be made to identify if there is a transient cause at play and attempt to resolve this. AUR is more likely to be reversible when compared with chronic UR as there is a greater chance that normal bladder function can be preserved, particularly if the condition presents early and is managed appropriately. A careful history should be taken; in most cases, the cause may be very apparent from this (e.g. postoperative AUR). Thorough abdominal, pelvic, gynaecological, and neurological examinations are mandated. If there is a clear transient cause identified, no further investigations may be required.

Two weeks later, the same patient presented again to the emergency department. Her successful trial without catheter was performed 3 days after her emergency department attendance but her symptoms had recurred. Bladder scan again revealed >999 mL in the bladder and a urethral catheter was inserted. This time, the residual volume was 1.4 L. On this occasion, she was referred to and admitted under the urology team. During her admission, she had an hourly input/output chart and daily weights. A full neurological and gynaecological examination was carried out with consent and no abnormalities were found. There was no evidence of diuresis. An inpatient ultrasound scan of the abdomen and pelvis did not reveal any pelvic masses or hydronephrosis. A urine sample from the catheter was sent for microscopy but there was no growth.

Clinical tip Assessment of female UR

A thorough neurological examination should be documented including negative findings. Back pain in spinal cord compression can be insidious; other associated symptoms include sciatica, saddle anaesthesia, lower limb weakness, and faecal incontinence. Although CES is a rare condition, it has a significant medicolegal profile; 50–70% of patients with CES have UR on presentation. In a case series of 33 patients, the mean duration of bladder symptoms was 3.6 days and 79% of patients had full bladder function recovery with prompt diagnosis.[15]

The patient underwent a successful trial without catheter the following day and prior to discharge was taught clean intermittent self-catheterization (CISC). The patient found the process very uncomfortable but was able to perform it. Outpatient investigations and follow-up were organized.

Clinical tip Bladder drainage

Initial bladder drainage of patients in UR could be performed with a urethral catheter (indwelling or intermittent) or an indwelling suprapubic catheter (SPC). The benefit of intermittent catheterization or suprapubic catheterization is the ease with which a return to normal voiding can be assessed.[16] It is possible to encourage normal filling and emptying while ensuring the upper tracts are protected. Indwelling catheters are comparatively associated with a higher morbidity.[17] Patient factors such as manual dexterity and patient preference should also be considered.

Expert comment Recurrent or unresolving UR

If the UR is recurrent or unresolving despite correction of a suspected transient cause, further investigations may be required. Although the cause may be apparent from the history, video urodynamic studies (VUDS) are often indicated to exclude any other features or signs that may impact future management such as detrusor overactivity or SUI. A flexible cystoscopy, while not mandated, could exclude any intrinsic cause in the bladder (which is rare but not impossible in a young patient) as well as assess the calibre of the urethra.

The patient attended for flexible cystoscopy 2 weeks later. She admitted to having two further episodes of difficulty passing urine that she managed to resolve using

Learning point UR: infection

Urinary tract infections are very common, affecting >75% of women at some point in their lives. Uncommonly, this can affect the bladder to the degree that UR occurs. In these cases, decompression of the bladder for a period of time while treatment of the urinary tract infection is completed is sufficient for normal bladder function to resume.[13]

Learning point UR: dysfunctional voiding

This term refers to a spectrum of disorders involving an intermittent and/or fluctuating flow rate owing to involuntary intermittent contractions of the periurethral striated muscle during voiding in neurologically normal individuals.[1] Patients with Fowler's syndrome are a particular subset. Another example is Hinman's syndrome (non-neurogenic neurogenic bladder) that comprises a vicious cycle of voiding dysfunction, urinary tract infection, and urinary incontinence associated with psychosocial problems.[14]

Expert comment Suspicion of CES

If there is any suspicion of CES, a neurosurgical opinion should be sought and magnetic resonance imaging organized. CES is a neurosurgical emergency and so the magnetic resonance imaging should be undertaken and acted upon on the same day.

CISC. She consented to the procedure but found insertion of the cystoscope very uncomfortable and the urologist performing the procedure commented on how tightly the urethra gripped the scope. No abnormalities were seen in the bladder. Unfortunately, following the procedure, the patient went into UR and on this occasion was unable to self-catheterize, as it was too painful. She also would not allow an indwelling urethral catheter to be inserted. Because of the fact that she had > 999 mL on bladder scan, a SPC was inserted under ultrasound guidance.

The patient attended for VUDS 3 weeks later. The SPC was clamped but the patient was unable to void and perform a free flow study. The bladder was filled at a standard rate to 800 mL, with no filling sensation or urge to void felt by the patient until the bladder came close to capacity. There was no evidence of detrusor overactivity or stress incontinence. The patient was then unable to void with no rise in detrusor pressure seen. The urologist then went on to perform urethral pressure profilometry using the standard Brown–Wickham method. This demonstrated a mean maximum urethral closure pressure of 102 cmH_2O.

Clinical tip Fowler's syndrome

A patient with Fowler's syndrome may complain of pain on insertion of a catheter or flexible cystoscope. Classically, operators comment on how the urethra grips the scope or catheter on withdrawal.

Learning point Urethral pressure profilometry

Brown and Wickham described their method for measuring urethral pressure profiles using a water-perfusion catheter system in 1969. The most commonly used technique today involves withdrawing an 8-French urethral catheter at 2 mm/s while infusing saline at 2 mL/min.[18] The expected mean maximum urethral closure pressure is calculated using the formula of 92 minus age (in years), based on work by Edwards and Malvern.[19] Further analysis in this area has demonstrated variation based on clinical diagnosis, age, and sex[20–22] (Table 26.2).

Table 26.2 Expected maximum urethral closure pressure based on sex and diagnosis

Diagnosis	Expected maximum urethral closure pressure in cmH_2O
Normal (healthy individuals)	Premenopausal women: 60 Postmenopausal women: 43.5 (Variation of ± 10–25 cmH_2O has been noted)
Hypotonic, consider intrinsic sphincter deficiency	<20
Hypertonic, consider obstruction	>75 in women >90 in men

At this point, the diagnosis of Fowler's syndrome was considered likely. The patient was seen back in the urology clinic by a consultant urologist with an interest in functional urology. The patient did not like the idea of carrying on long term with a SPC and wanted to know what options were available to try and void 'normally' again. The options presented to her included long-term CISC, a trial of sacral nerve stimulation (SNS), or the creation of a catheterizable continent channel such as a Mitrofanoff channel.

Learning point Fowler's syndrome

Classically, a patient with Fowler's syndrome is a young woman presenting with UR of >1 L with no obvious urological, gynaecological, or neurological cause found. There is a recognized association with polycystic ovarian syndrome in 40% of patients. VUDS show no rise in detrusor pressure on attempt to void. Further investigations include ultrasound estimation of sphincter volume (>1.8 mL) and sphincter electromyography (which shows repetitive complex discharges). The mean maximum urethral closure pressure in a patient with Fowler's syndrome is commonly >100 cmH_2O.[23]

Expert comment Fowler's syndrome

In Fowler's syndrome, an overactive sphincter may enlarge owing to continuous 'muscle activity', as measured by ultrasound sphincter volume. The aetiology of Fowler's syndrome is unclear but it is hypothesized to be a result of a hormonally sensitive channelopathy which produces a sustained striated urethral sphincter involuntary contraction.

Learning point Mitrofanoff procedure

Professor Paul Mitrofanoff described a continent supravesical antireflux appendicovesicostomy in 1980.[24] The appendix is harvested on its vascular pedicle and refashioned into a catheterizable continent channel which then passes into the bladder (or neo/augmented bladder) with antireflux properties (Figure 26.1). In patients with no appendix, a Yang–Monti procedure can be performed

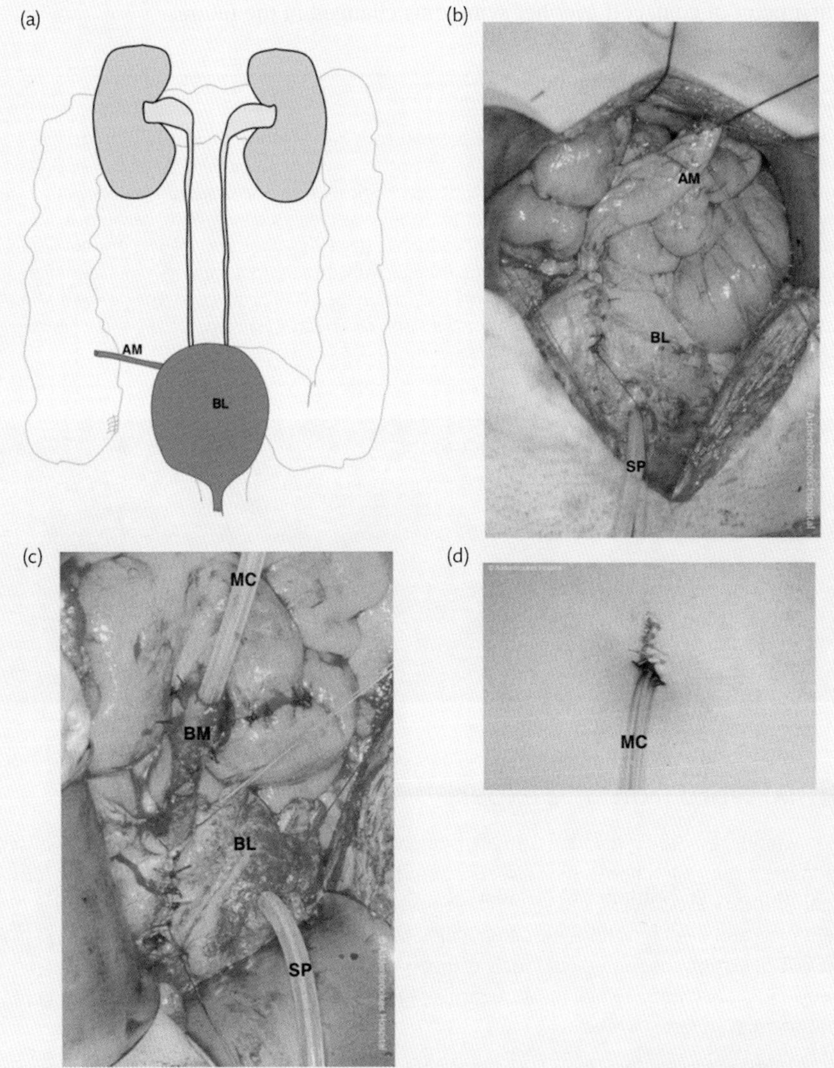

Figure 26.1 Mitrofanoff formation. (a) Diagrammatic representation of a Mitrofanoff catheterizable conduit. (b) Photograph taken during creation of a Mitrofanoff catheterizable conduit created using an appendix. (c) Photograph taken during creation of a Mitrofanoff catheterizable conduit created using small bowel. (d) Mitrofanoff stoma. AM, appendix Mitrofanoff; BL, bladder; BM, Monti small bowel Mitrofanoff; MC, Mitrofanoff catheter; SP, suprapubic catheter.

using small bowel as the channel.[25] Studies have reported continence rates ranging from 88% to 98% with medium-long-term follow-up.[26] The risk of complications is high, particularly with stomal stenosis which may require recurrent dilatation.[27]

The patient opted for a trial of SNS that was carried out as a day-case procedure. Supported by the clinical nurse specialists, the patient worked through different programmes to assess the effect on her voiding, finally settling on one that was successful. As a result, a permanent device was inserted. At her 3-month follow-up, the wound had healed well and the patient felt that her voiding was back to normal and was happy with the result. She remained in close contact with the specialist nurse as a first point of contact if ever her symptoms changed in the future.

Evidence base SNS success rates

The introduction of SNS in the treatment of patients with Fowler's syndrome was a game changer, avoiding the need for major surgery. Studies have found an overall success rate around 70%; however, the revision rate can be high (>40%).[28,29] Success rates are lower in non-Fowler's syndrome patients and the role of SNS in neuropathic patients is unclear.

Learning point Sacral neuromodulation

Sacral neuromodulation or SNS involves the percutaneous insertion of a stimulating lead into the S3 foramen. Indications for use include overactive bladder that is resistant to medication, faecal incontinence, and UR with no clear structural or neurological cause. The procedure is done with the patient prone under a general anaesthetic (or local anaesthetic/sedation) and often in two stages: stage 1 involves the insertion of a test lead, while stage 2 involves a permanent implant if stage 1 successfully resolves the patient's symptoms. Patients work through 'programmes' that have different strengths and patterns of electrical stimulation to optimize their voiding function. The device is MRI compatible and depending on whether the patient opts for a rechargeable or recharge-free device, the battery can last approximately 5-15 years.

Expert comment Mechanism of SNS

It is unclear how SNS works to allow voiding in patients with voiding dysfunction. It may work at a local spinal level via a gating mechanism to restore coordination of sphincter relaxation or a central level through restoration of activity associated with brainstem autoregulation and attenuation of cingulate activity.

Expert comment Long-term management

Longer-term management strategies such as SNS or a continent catheterizable channel will have to carefully take into account the patient's ideas, concerns, and expectations. Some patients may prefer an indwelling urethral catheter or SPC, while these options may not be acceptable to other patients. Some patients may lack the manual dexterity to perform CISC, may not wish to, or find the procedure too uncomfortable. There are many ways of optimizing patient adherence to CISC and continence nurse input is key.[30] A multidisciplinary approach involving specialist continence nurses, urologists, urogynaecologists, pelvic floor physiotherapists, and even a psychologist (in the case of any psychosocial issues) is recommended prior to embarking on any major invasive surgery.

A final word from the expert

UR in women, especially in young women, is uncommon. These patients, especially the Fowler's syndrome group, often have a high level of comorbidity with patients often having some form of pain, functional disorders, and/or psychological symptoms. Assessment should include anatomical and functional tests, including magnetic resonance imaging, pelvic ultrasound and VUDS. Further specialized tests such as urethral sphincter ultrasound, urethral sphincter electromyography, and urethral pressure profiles rarely alter management and should be kept for academic interest.

The ideal management for female UR is intermittent self-catheterization. If the patient is not able to tolerate this, then options include SNS if suitable, long-term suprapubic catheterization, and Mitrofanoff cutaneous catheterizable continent conduit. These latter three options are very useful when they work well but this not often the case. SNS devices can stop working, can cause pain, and patients need regular review and reprogramming. The device is expensive for the National Health Service and there is a high rate of revision. Mitrofanoff channels also have a high surgical revision rate, up to 50%, because of difficulty catheterizing at the skin level, along the channel, or as the catheter enters the bladder or because of leakage. SPCs can cause pain, bypassing, urinary tract infections, and need regular changing. They are also unpopular because of cosmetic reasons. A final option includes urinary diversion into an ileal conduit with lifelong use of a stoma bag to collect the urine (an incontinent diversion).

It is also important to consider female bladder outlet obstruction in women with UR. A helpful diagnostic tool is calculating the bladder outlet obstruction index based on urodynamic study parameters.[31] Urethral stenosis is an uncommon cause that can be successfully treated by a female urethroplasty in some women.

Pharmacotherapy has been tried to promote bladder emptying either by promoting bladder contraction as muscarinic agonists (such as bethanechol and carbachol) or by drugs that prevent the breakdown of the neurotransmitter acetylcholine (and so potentiate muscle contraction) using cholinesterase inhibitors such as distigmine, pyridostigmine, and neostigmine. Unfortunately, these drugs have been shown to have little clinical efficacy in treating UR and, due to their non-specific actions, have caused marked side effects, such as nausea, vomiting, diarrhoea, visual impairment, headaches, bronchospasms, and cardiovascular events.

Due to poor-quality evidence (largely retrospective data and poor sample sizes in heterogeneous populations), there are no guidelines on assessing and treating this difficult group of patients. As such, it is important these patients are managed in a tertiary urological environment utilizing a multidisciplinary team approach.

References

1. Bo K, Frawley HC, Haylen BT, et al. An International Urogynecological Association (IUGA)/International Continence Society (ICS) joint report on the terminology for the conservative and nonpharmacological management of female pelvic floor dysfunction. *Neurourol Urodyn.* 2017;36(2):221–244.
2. Klarskov P, Andersen JT, Asmussen CF, et al. Acute urinary retention in women: a prospective study of 18 consecutive cases. *Scand J Urol Nephrol.* 1987;21(1):29–31.
3. Groutz A, Gordon D, Lessing JB, Wolman I, Jaffa A, David MP. Prevalence and characteristics of voiding difficulties in women: are subjective symptoms substantiated by objective urodynamic data? *Urology.* 1999;54(2):268–272.
4. Stoffel JT, Peterson AC, Sandhu JS, Suskind AM, Wei JT, Lightner DJ. AUA white paper on nonneurogenic chronic urinary retention: consensus definition, treatment algorithm, and outcome end points. *J Urol.* 2017;198(1):153–160.
5. Mevcha A, Drake MJ. Etiology and management of urinary retention in women. *Indian J Urol.* 2010;26(2):230–235.
6. Nitti VW, Tu LM, Gitlin J. Diagnosing bladder outlet obstruction in women. *J Urol.* 1999;161(5):1535–1540.
7. West C, Lawrence A. Female urethroplasty: contemporary thinking. *World J Urol.* 2019;37(4):619–629.
8. Verhamme KM, Sturkenboom MC, Stricker BH, Bosch R. Drug-induced urinary retention: incidence, management and prevention. *Drug Saf.* 2008;31(5):373–388.
9. Olofsson CI, Ekblom AO, Ekman-Ordeberg GE, Irestedt LE. Post-partum urinary retention: a comparison between two methods of epidural analgesia. *Eur J Obstet Gynecol Reprod Biol.* 1997;71(1):31–34.
10. Gallo S, DuRand J, Pshon N. A study of naloxone effect on urinary retention in the patient receiving morphine patient-controlled analgesia. *Orthop Nurs.* 2008;27(2):111–115.

11. Pfisterer MH, Griffiths DJ, Schaefer W, Resnick NM. The effect of age on lower urinary tract function: a study in women. *J Am Geriatr Soc.* 2006;54(3):405–412.
12. Kaplan SA, Te AE, Blaivas JG. Urodynamic findings in patients with diabetic cystopathy. *J Urol.* 1995;153(2):342–344.
13. Selius BA, Subedi R. Urinary retention in adults: diagnosis and initial management. *Am Fam Physician.* 2008;77(5):643–650.
14. Hinman F Jr. Nonneurogenic neurogenic bladder (the Hinman syndrome)—15 years later. *J Urol.* 1986;136(4):769–777.
15. Gleave JR, MacFarlane R. Prognosis for recovery of bladder function following lumbar central disc prolapse. *Br J Neurosurg.* 1990;4(3):205–209.
16. Hakvoort RA, Thijs SD, Bouwmeester FW, et al. Comparing clean intermittent catheterisation and transurethral indwelling catheterisation for incomplete voiding after vaginal prolapse surgery: a multicentre randomised trial. *BJOG.* 2011;118(9):1055–1060.
17. Welford K. Comparing indwelling and intermittent catheterisation. *Nurs Times.* 2010;106(40):Suppl 6–7.
18. Brown M, Wickham JE. The urethral pressure profile. *Br J Urol.* 1969;41(2):211–217.
19. Edwards L, Malvern J. The urethral pressure profile: theoretical considerations and clinical application. *Br J Urol.* 1974;46(3):325–335.
20. Corcos J, Schick E. *The Urinary Sphincter.* New York: Marcel Dekker; 2001.
21. Sorensen S, Waechter PB, Constantinou CE, Kirkeby HJ, Jonler M, Djurhuus JC. Urethral pressure and pressure variations in healthy fertile and postmenopausal women with reference to the female sex hormones. *J Urol.* 1991;146(5):1434–1440.
22. Mahfouz W, Al Afraa T, Campeau L, Corcos J. Normal urodynamic parameters in women: part II—invasive urodynamics. *Int Urogynecol J.* 2012;23(3):269–277.
23. Swinn MJ, Fowler CJ. Isolated urinary retention in young women, or Fowler's syndrome. *Clin Auton Res.* 2001;11(5):309–311.
24. Mitrofanoff P. [Trans-appendicular continent cystostomy in the management of the neurogenic bladder.] *Chir Pediatr.* 1980;21(4):297–305.
25. Monti PR, Lara RC, Dutra MA, de Carvalho JR. New techniques for construction of efferent conduits based on the Mitrofanoff principle. *Urology.* 1997;49(1):112–115.
26. Harris CF, Cooper CS, Hutcheson JC, Snyder HM, 3rd. Appendicovesicostomy: the Mitrofanoff procedure-a 15-year perspective. *J Urol.* 2000;163(6):1922–1926.
27. Thomas JC, Dietrich MS, Trusler L, et al. Continent catheterizable channels and the timing of their complications. *J Urol.* 2006;176(4 Pt 2):1816–1820.
28. Swinn MJ, Kitchen ND, Goodwin RJ, Fowler CJ. Sacral neuromodulation for women with Fowler's syndrome. *Eur Urol.* 2000;38(4):439–443.
29. De Ridder D, Ost D, Bruyninckx F. The presence of Fowler's syndrome predicts successful long-term outcome of sacral nerve stimulation in women with urinary retention. *Eur Urol.* 2007;51(1):229–233.
30. Seth JH, Haslam C, Panicker JN. Ensuring patient adherence to clean intermittent self-catheterization. *Patient Prefer Adherence.* 2014;8:191–198.
31. Solomon E, Yasmin H, Duffy M, Rashid T, Akinluyi E, Greenwell TJ. Developing and validating a new nomogram for diagnosing bladder outlet obstruction in women. *Neurourol Urodyn.* 2018;37(1):368–378.

CASE

27 Neurogenic bladder

Hazel Ecclestone and Rizwan Hamid

Expert commentary Julian Shah

Case history

A 49-year-old man with spinal dysraphism presented to outpatients in a spinal injury centre, after being referred from his local hospital. His presenting complaint was recurrent urinary tract infections (UTIs) and epididymo-orchitis; however, his follow-up at his local hospital had been somewhat erratic. He had been doing clean intermittent self-catheterization (CISC) since childhood, up to five times a day; he stated, however, that of late he had been somewhat non-compliant with this regimen. He reported primarily voiding off urgency and by straining, but suffered with considerable urinary incontinence, necessitating the wearing of pads. He had no formal bowel regimen and complained of significant constipation. His serum creatinine level was significantly raised on referral to our institution at 250 mmol/L. We were unable to establish the chronicity of this due to the patient's non-attendance previously.

Evaluation

He underwent baseline investigations including ultrasound of the renal tract, video urodynamics (video cystometrography (VCMG)), and a mercaptoacetyltriglycine (MAG3) renogram. The images from these are shown in Figure 27.1.

As the patient did not demonstrate reflux into the ureters on VCMG, this raised the possibility of obstruction at the vesicoureteric junction (VUJ). The MAG3 renogram confirmed this was the case, as even with the bladder taken out of the equation (with an indwelling catheter), there was still a standing column down to the VUJ signifying high-grade obstruction.

Evidence base Safe bladder pressure on urodynamics

The cut off for 'safe bladder pressures' on urodynamics is reported as a detrusor leak point pressure (DLPP) of <40 cmH_2O. This number comes from the McGuire et al. study of 42 myelodysplastic children that found in those whose DLPP was <40 cmH_2O a 0% incidence of deterioration of the upper tract (reflux on video urodynamics), whereas 15% of those with DLPP >40 cmH_2O had radiographic evidence of reflux into the upper tracts.[1]

Learning point Grading system for vesicoureteral reflux on voiding cystourethrography, according to the International Reflux Study Committee

- **Grade I**: reflux does not reach the renal pelvis; varying degrees of ureteral dilatation.
- **Grade II**: reflux reaches the renal pelvis; no dilatation of the collecting system; normal fornices.
- **Grade III**: mild or moderate dilatation of the ureter, with or without kinking; moderate dilatation of the collecting system; normal or minimally deformed fornices.
- **Grade IV**: moderate dilatation of the ureter with or without kinking; moderate dilatation of the collecting system; blunt fornices, but impressions of the papillae still visible.
- **Grade V**: gross dilatation and kinking of the ureter, marked dilatation of the collecting system; papillary impressions no longer visible; intraparenchymal reflux.[2]

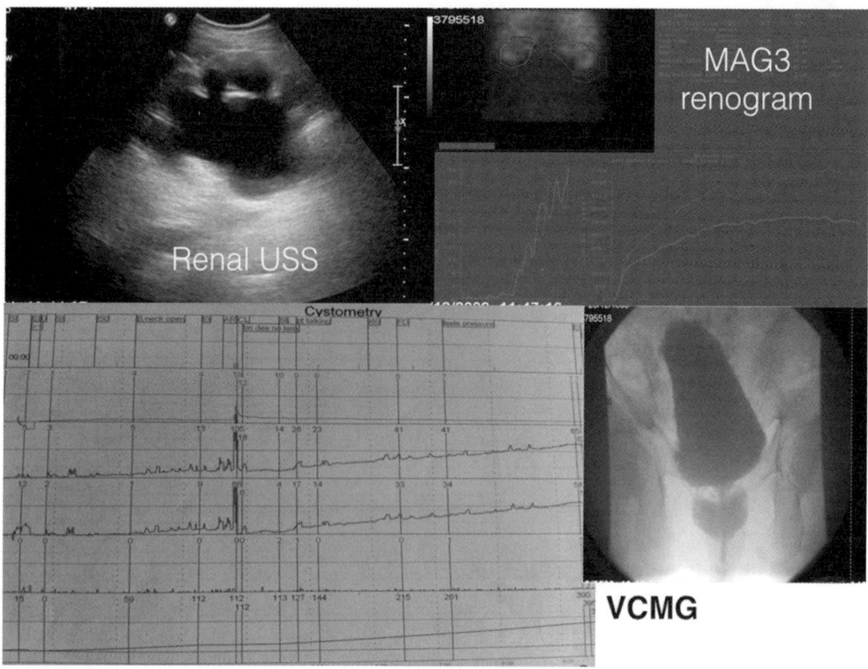

Figure 27.1 Baseline investigations including ultrasound scan (USS) of the renal tract, video urodynamics (VCMG), and a MAG3 renogram. Investigations revealed severe bilateral hydroureteronephrosis down to the vesicoureteric junction (VUJ) on ultrasound. The MAG3 renogram showed bilateral ureteric obstruction down to the VUJ with an empty bladder (MAG3 performed with indwelling catheter *in situ*). Video urodynamics revealed a very poorly compliant bladder, with images confirming a dilated posterior urethra with evidence of prostatic reflux (likely contributing to his recurrent epididymo-orchitis). No reflux was observed into the upper tracts despite bladder pressures being >60 cmH_2O at end fill (detrusor leak point pressure >60 cmH_2O).

Expert comment Presentation and investigations

This case sets out a reflection of what is the neglect of the long-term management of a patient with a spina bifida. This condition can cause significant problems for the urinary tract. The neuropathic bladder if left without management will deteriorate to the point at which the kidneys can suffer from hydronephrosis and then lead to renal failure. The fact that the patient to some extent had not been compliant with treatment contributed to the endpoint but appropriate medical therapy and reiteration of the importance of follow-up is important for any patient, particularly as they age with this condition.

His presentation is typical with recurrent infection leading to epididymo-orchitis. His intermittent catheterization regimen had begun to become erratic rather than consistent and he was voiding by straining. This should not be the case when there is a significant bladder dysfunction unless urodynamic studies have confirmed that the patient has a 'safe' bladder. It would seem from the presentation that he had not had urodynamic studies for some considerable time.

The investigations that were undertaken were entirely along standard lines, that is, a scan of the urinary tract and a MAG3 renogram to look at renal function and drainage and then urodynamic studies to look at the pressures within the bladder with video imaging to assess the appearance of the bladder. It can be seen that his bladder is poorly compliant with high end filling pressure and the bladder has the classical fir tree shape with an undermined prostate due to high pressure because of external sphincter dyssynergia.

Management options

The primary aim of the urologist is to protect the upper tracts and prevent further renal deterioration following previously inadequate bladder management. The patient, however, had somewhat different aims, in that he wished to be infection free and 'dry' in addition to being as 'normal' as possible. This case of a poorly compliant high-pressure bladder is further complicated by the anatomical obstruction at the VUJ. The management options are discussed in detail in the following boxes.

Clinical tip European Association of Urology guidelines on the primary aims for treatment of neurourological symptoms, and their priorities

- Protection of the upper urinary tract.
- Achievement (or maintenance) of urinary continence.
- Restoration of lower urinary tract function.
- Improvement of the patient's quality of life.[3]

Learning point Conservative/medical techniques to reduce bladder pressure

- **Increase frequency of self-catheterization and add anticholinergics**. The main advantage being minimal side effects and may improve UTIs, but patient may still be incontinent. The main disadvantage is that it doesn't address the underlying cause of ureteric obstruction and will not significantly increase his reduced capacity bladder.
- **Indwelling catheter—urethral or suprapubic**. This would not reduce frequency of UTIs, would not deal with ureteric obstruction, but may be a reasonable option in older patients not fit for significant intervention or if the patient is refusing other forms of intervention.

Learning point Minimally invasive therapies to reduce bladder pressure

- **Intradetrusor onabotulinum toxin A**. This may temporize things, but the bladder capacity will remain small and the compliance may not improve. There will be an increased frequency of self-catheterization due to the reduced functional capacity. The patient will also still need further intervention for ureteric obstruction. Furthermore, repeat injections would be required and it would be difficult to time the duration of injections appropriately to ensure the bladder pressures remain safe for adequate kidney drainage. Additionally, lifelong repeated injections would be necessary.
- **External sphincterotomy**. This is irreversible destruction of the external urethral sphincter with the aim of ensuring permanent incontinence. This could make the bladder 'safe' but with the consequence of the patient requiring permanent sheath drainage. Additionally, this would again not deal with ureteric obstruction.

Learning point Major surgery to reduce bladder pressure

- **Augmentation cystoplasty** (increasing the bladder capacity with the addition of bowel). The advantage is this will almost certainly improve bladder compliance, reduce bladder pressure, increase bladder capacity, improve incontinence, and reduce frequency of CISC. The ureteric obstruction can also be dealt with at the same time with bilateral ureteric re-implantations. However, there are a number of short- and long-term complications associated with the addition of bowel mucosa into the urinary tract (listed in Table 27.1).[4–6]
- **Urinary diversion**. An ileal conduit would remove the 'dangerous bladder' from the equation with the added benefit of treating the ureteric obstruction; however, continence and 'normality' would be sacrificed.

Table 27.1 Complications of urinary tract reconstruction with bowel

Immediate	Early	Late
Death (0–3.2%) Bleeding requiring return to theatre (0–3%)	Bowel/urine leak (2–10%) Intestinal obstruction (3–5.7%) Ventriculoperitoneal shunt infection (0–20%)	Voiding dysfunction/need for CISC (60%) Mucus (10–90%) Mucus retention (15%) Deterioration in renal function (0–15%) Incontinence: day (10%) Incontinence: night (10–47%) Biochemical abnormality (metabolic hyperchloraemic acidosis): biochemical (100%), overt acidosis (0–19%) Malignancy (0.6%) Stones (10%) Impaired bowel function (15%) Rupture (1.9%)

Learning point Techniques to deal with ureteric obstruction

Minimally invasive

- **Ureteric stents**. This is unlikely to be successful in this 'unsafe' system without a significant increase in frequency of CISC as bladder pressures in 'dangerous' bladders range from <200 mL capacity. They would also require lifelong changes and increase the risk of UTI as there would be a foreign body in the urinary tract.
- **Percutaneous nephrostomies**. The advantage would be to overcome the ureteric obstruction, and take the unsafe bladder out of the equation, but they would require lifelong regular changes, and would have deleterious effects on the patient's quality of life.

Major surgery

- **Ureteric reimplantation**. This has the advantage that it bypasses the anatomical obstruction; however, it is imperative that the reservoir the ureters have been implanted into is a low-pressure system.

Expert comment Management options

In this case, the first treatment is to place a catheter to drain the bladder and then wait for a couple of weeks to see whether or not the hydronephrosis reverts. If the hydronephrosis improves, then we know that the problem lies at the external sphincter mechanism. If the hydronephrosis remains, it is almost certain that the patient has developed bladder wall thickness obstruction. The management of each of these aspects of his condition have been outlined previously in this case.

Definitive management performed

All the options were discussed with the patient with risks and benefits of each intervention.

The patient opted for the operative intervention and underwent bilateral ureteric re-implantation and double clam ileocystoplasty.

This was undertaken by open procedure. A laparotomy was performed. The bladder was bivalved sagittally and a 25 cm piece of terminal ileum 30 cm from the ileocaecal junction was isolated. This was detubularized and folded back on itself to make a cup and attached to the bladder as described in Figure 27.2.[7] In addition, bilateral ureteric

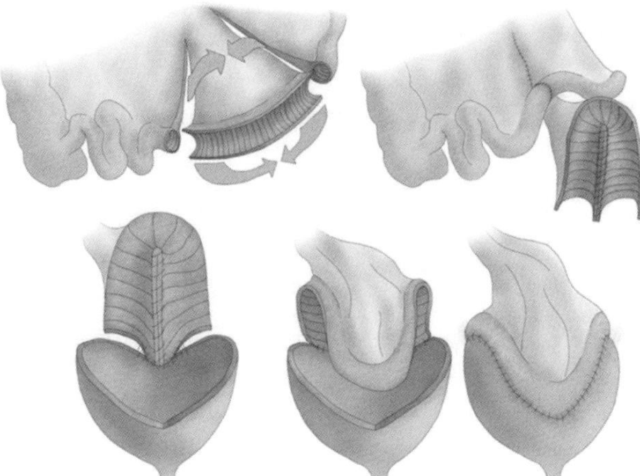

Figure 27.2 Clam ileocystoplasty—operative description. The bladder was bivalved sagittally and a piece of ileum was isolated, detubularized, and folded back on itself to make a cup and attached to the bladder.[7]

re-implantation was undertaken in the posterior bladder plate without the need for tapering the ureters in a non-refluxing manner.

He made an excellent postoperative recovery, his creatinine postoperatively improved to 220 mmol/L, and he was discharged home after about a week in the hospital. He had his JJ stents and suprapubic catheter removed at 6 weeks and restarted the CISC regimen.

Learning point Hydronephrosis and lower urinary tract dysfunction

- Hydronephrosis in patients with neuropathic bladders are usually due to abnormal lower urinary tract function.
- Neuropathic bladders may store urine at high pressure, causing secondary vesicoureteric reflux and subsequent deterioration in renal function.
- Long-standing neurourological lower urinary tract dysfunction can cause hypertrophy of the bladder wall/detrusor attempting to overcome increased outlet resistance; however, this hypertrophy can obstruct the ureters at the VUJ, and cause an anatomical obstruction with subsequent deterioration in renal function.
- If the cause of hydronephrosis and renal failure is purely due to reflux, reducing storage pressure often reverses or halts renal deterioration. However, it is important to identify VUJ obstruction as in this case reducing bladder pressure will not resolve the hydronephrosis in this situation.

Expert comment Management and follow-up

It is clear from the investigations and from the discussion that this gentleman had bilateral ureteric obstruction due to a thick bladder wall and that the only solution to his problem would be either a urinary diversion or a bladder reconstruction with ureteric reimplantation. As he wished to be 'bag free', the double-clam augmentation ileocystoplasty with bilateral ureteric reimplantation was entirely the appropriate approach to management.

The initial outcome from his surgery was that the bladder became 'normal' in terms of compliance. He was performing intermittent self-catheterization to drain his bladder.

It was more likely than not that his deterioration in renal function which remained was due to chronic renal disease caused by chronic (but relived) obstruction. The MAG3 renogram showed a rising curve in one kidney and a flat curve in the other, consistent with what could be obstruction but not confirmed by the nephrostogram. It was therefore appropriate for him to continue with the conservative management and to check his serum creatinine levels, which will be an indicator of any deterioration in renal function. Intervention was not necessary or appropriate.

His follow-up should now continue with measurement of his serum creatinine level every 3 months and careful supervised follow-up in a specialist centre with scans of the urinary tract every year with an annual video urodynamic study to ensure that his bladder pressures remain low. It is more likely than not that this will be the case.

Whether or not he will require renal replacement therapy very much depends upon any further deterioration in his renal function.

Follow-up

At the 3-month postoperative appointment, the patient was clinically much improved. He was dry with no reported urgency. He had no further UTIs. He was very satisfied with the outcome of his operation. However, his serum creatinine level remained at 228 mmol/L.

A VCMG (Figure 27.3a) revealed a good-capacity 'safe' bladder with normal compliance. The screening images (Figure 27.3b) show a much-improved capacity, storing urine at low pressure, without any prostatic reflux.

He had follow-up MAG3 renograms (Figure 27.4) which again showed poor drainage bilaterally, but without standing columns in the ureters. His creatinine level settled to a nadir of 223 mmol/L.

Unfortunately, 3 months later, he had a UTI and his creatinine concentration further increased to 305 mmol/L. The infection did settle with antibiotics but the serum creatinine only decreased to 280 mmol/L. After discussing his imaging and trend in serum creatinine, a decision was taken to insert bilateral nephrostomies and his creatinine concentration further reduced to 250 mmol/L. Subsequent nephrostograms, however, showed no evidence of definite obstruction or significant standing columns. The uroradiologists reported bilateral baggy systems probably secondary to chronic obstruction.

Since he had bilateral nephrostomies in place, it was decided to undertake a Whitaker test. This was performed and was reported as equivocal. The nephrostomies were clamped, and subsequently removed without further deterioration in renal function.

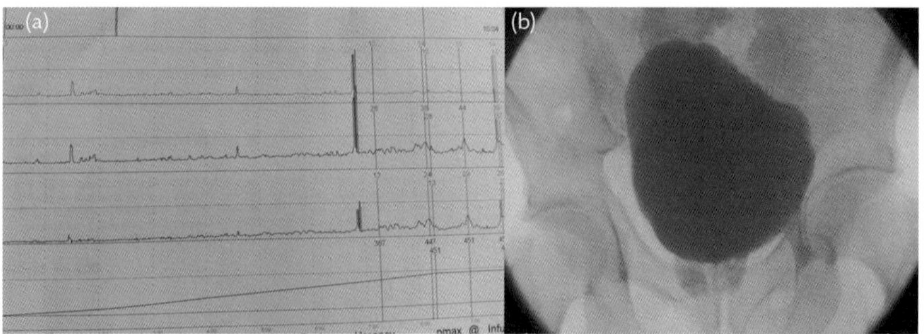

Figure 27.3 Video cystometrogram. There is a good capacity bladder with normal compliance without any reflux.

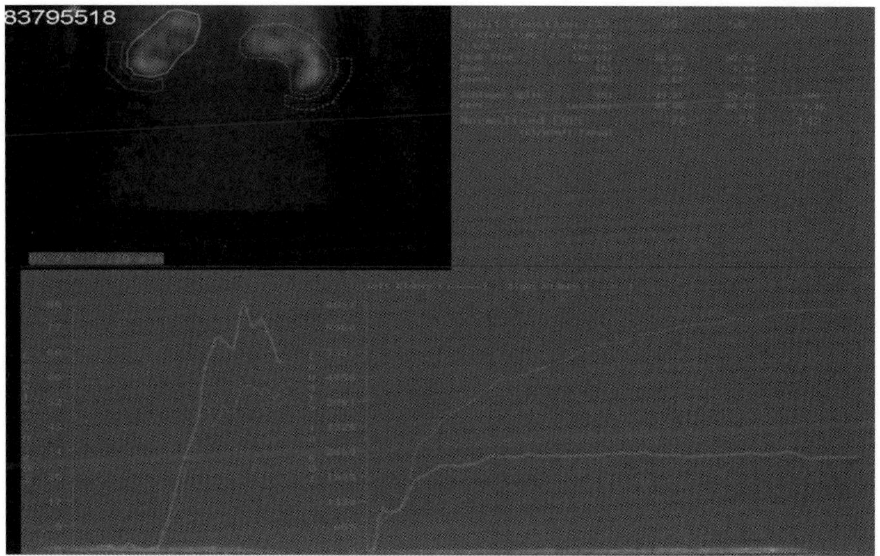

Figure 27.4 MAG3 renogram. There is poor drainage bilaterally, but without standing columns in the ureters.

He continues under follow-up with the nephrologists with a creatinine level that hovers between 230–270 mmol/L depending if he gets a UTI. He is extremely satisfied with the outcome, is continent, performing CSIC, and although he gets UTIs, they are quite infrequent.

His nephrologists were of the opinion that he has a degree of intrinsic renal disease and though at present there is no evidence of a significant obstruction, any insult to his renal tract including UTI could lead to a rise in his serum creatinine level. He has been informed that it is likely he would need renal replacement therapy in the future though the timings are difficult to quantify.

Learning point Whitaker test

A urethral pressure-sensing catheter is introduced, and infusion of saline into the renal pelvis is commenced at 10 mL/min. The pressure in the renal pelvis region is subtracted from the bladder pressure. The resultant pressure is then analysed according to the following values to determine if ureteric obstruction is present:

- <15 cm: unobstructed.
- 15–22 cm: equivocal.
- >22 cm: obstructed.

The Whitaker test[8] has an advantage over nuclear medicine scans in those with very large hydronephrosis and those with severe renal impairment as it does not rely on glomerular filtration for excretion.

Monitoring

The optimal follow-up for patients such as these has never been categorically defined. Certainly, patients with spinal cord lesions (such as myelodysplasia and spinal cord injury) are at higher risk of upper tract deterioration than other neurological conditions.

Table 27.2 Comparison of British versus European guidelines in neurourology follow-up

	Surveillance	
	NICE	EAU
High-risk patients	Lifelong follow-up [Clinical review interval not stated] US every 1–2 years UDS—consider surveillance regimen Do not rely on serum creatinine to monitor renal function	Lifelong follow-up Clinical review annually US at least once every 6 months UDS—mandatory baseline investigation and should be performed at regular intervals Perform regular urinalysis Annual blood chemistry
Lower-risk patients	Lifelong follow-up and ongoing risk stratification If a patient become high risk–for surveillance as above	Lifelong follow-up Follow-up at least every 2 years Regular urinalysis Significant clinical change should prompt urgent intervention

EAU, European Association of Urology: NICE, National Institute for Health and Care Excellence; UDS, urodynamic studies; US, ultrasound.

The follow-up should therefore be lifelong. There is a difference in opinion as to what investigations, and at what interval, are indicated in national and international guidelines. Table 27.2 summarizes the main similarities and differences in British and European guidelines.[9]

We adopted a follow-up protocol for this gentleman, with annual VCMG and ultrasound scans and MAG3 as indicated, or earlier if there is a clinical change. He remains well 5 years post cystoplasty with no further deterioration in his biochemical renal function.

A final word from the expert

Inappropriate bladder management in patients with neurological conditions can not only lead to a poor quality of life due to infections and incontinence, but can also lead to irreversible deterioration in kidney function leading to renal failure. As a consequence, the aims of the treatment are generally different from the physician's perspective when compared to the patient's perspective. The patient's priorities are often 'normality' and continence, with the physician's main concern being protection of the upper tracts and maintenance or improvement of renal function.

There are a number of management options in these complex cases. However, none of the treatments offer a 'perfect' solution. It is not unusual that the patient will trade one set of problems for another and hence very careful counselling needs to be undertaken to establish what the patient's wishes and desires are and these need to be married to the long-term optimization of the urinary tract. It is extremely important to tailor the definitive therapy according to the individual circumstances. It would not be unusual to have some 'compromises' in deciding the management options to achieve a practical solution.

All major surgical options, including cystoplasty, are major undertakings that require a motivated patient who is willing and able to comprehend the implications of this surgery not only on the urinary tract but also on bowel function, and understand the need to perform intermittent catheterization. Additionally, the patient needs to sign up to lifelong follow-up, understanding the significant morbidity of this surgery but expecting to have the potential benefits in the long term.[5]

References

1. McGuire EJ, Woodside JR, Borden TA, Weiss RM. Prognostic value of urodynamic testing in myelodysplastic patients. *J Urol.* 1981;126(2):205–209.
2. Lebowitz RL, Olbing H, Parkkulainen KV, Smellie JM, Tamminen-Möbius TE. International system of radiographic grading of vesicoureteric reflux. *Pediatr Radiol.* 1985;15(2):105–109.
3. Blok B, Castro-Diaz D, Del Popolo G, et al. Neuro-urology. European Association of Urology. 2019. https://uroweb.org/guideline/neuro-urology/
4. Biers SM, Venn SN, Greenwell TJ. The past, present and future of augmentation cystoplasty. *BJU Int.* 2012;109(9):1280–1293.
5. Hoen LT, Ecclestone H, Blok BF, et al. Long-term effectiveness and complication rates of bladder augmentation in patients with neurogenic bladder dysfunction: a systematic review. *Neurourol Urodyn.* 2017;36(7):1685–1702.
6. British Association of Urological Surgeons. Enlargement of the bladder with a piece of bowel. British Association of Urological Surgeons. 2019. https://www.baus.org.uk/_userfiles/pages/files/Patients/Leaflets/Enterocystoplasty.pdf
7. Greenwell TJ, Venn SN, Mundy AR. Augmentation cystoplasty. *BJU Int.* 2001;88(6):511–525.
8. Whitaker RH. Methods of assessing obstruction in dilated ureters. *Br J Urol.* 1973;45(1):15–22.
9. Ecclestone H, Hamid R. A comparison of UK versus European guidelines in neuro-urology. *J Clin Urol.* 2018;11(2):109–114.

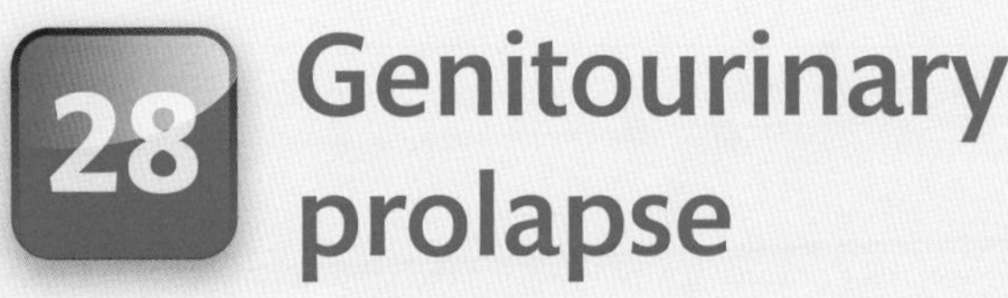

CASE 28 Genitourinary prolapse

Priyanka H. Krishnaswamy

Expert commentary Swati Jha

Case history

A 57-year-old lady was referred to the gynaecology clinic by her general practitioner as she could feel a reducible lump per vagina. She was medically fit and well, having had two normal vaginal deliveries in the past and no history of abdominal or pelvic surgeries. She was told by her general practitioner during a routine smear test 5 years ago that she may have a prolapse but did not want to be referred then as she had no symptoms. In the past 6 months she felt a lump vaginally when she walked and ran. In the recent 3 months, she became aware of this when she wiped herself in the toilet and felt that the lump got in the way during sex. She did not have any pain or abdominal, bowel, or bladder problems.

Learning point Definition of pelvic organ prolapse

Pelvic organ prolapse (POP; Latin: *prolapsus*, 'a slipping forth') is the downward displacement of pelvic organs into or beyond the vagina due to loss of the normal support mechanism[1] which is an increasingly common problem seen in the ageing population. Although as many as 50% of women older than age 50 have some degree of POP,[2] <20% seek treatment.[3] This may result from a number of causes, including a lack of symptoms, embarrassment, or misperceptions about available treatment options.

Types of uterovaginal prolapse are classified anatomically (Figure 28.1).[1]

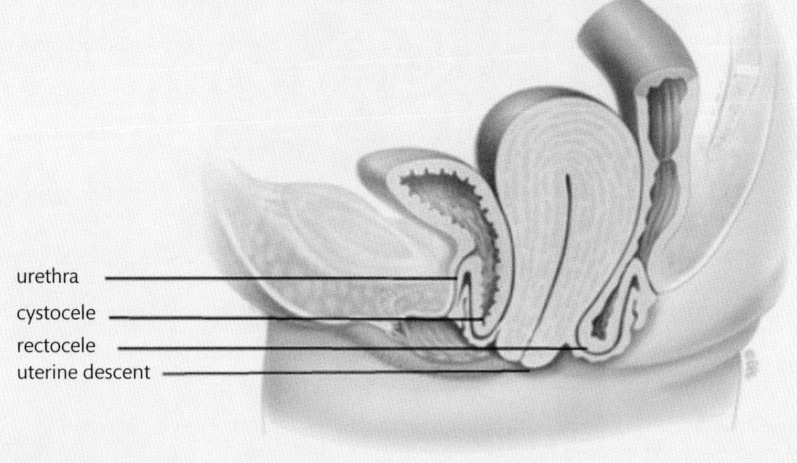

Figure 28.1 Uterovaginal prolapse.

Adapted with permission from Haylen BT, Maher CF, Barber MD, Camargo S, Dandolu V, Digesu A, et al. An International Urogynecological Association (IUGA)/International Continence Society (ICS) joint report on the terminology for female pelvic organ prolapse (POP). *International Urogynecology Journal* 2016;27:165–94.

Uterine/cervical prolapse is generally the result of poor apical support, which allows downward protrusion of the cervix and uterus towards the introitus.

Anterior vaginal wall prolapse:

- **Urethrocele** is prolapse of the lower anterior vaginal wall, involving the urethra only.
- **Cystocele** is prolapse of the upper anterior vaginal wall, involving the bladder.
- **Cystourethrocele** when there is prolapse of the urethra as well as the bladder.
- **Anterior enterocele** is a herniation of the peritoneum and abdominal contents through the anterior vaginal wall, most commonly after reconstructive surgery.

Posterior vaginal wall prolapse:

- **Rectocele** is prolapse of the lower posterior wall of the vagina involving the anterior wall of the rectum.
- **Enterocele** is prolapse of the upper posterior wall of the vagina involving loops of small bowel.

Vaginal vault prolapse involves a descent of the vaginal vault after a hysterectomy.

Learning point Anatomy of the pelvic organs

The normal position, support, and suspension of the pelvic organs rely on an interdependent system of bony, muscular, and connective tissue elements.

- **The lordosis of the lumbosacral region of the spine** places the posterior aspect of the pelvic inlet (sacral promontory) 60° above its anterior aspect (pubic symphysis). Posterior angulation of the vagina, which is enhanced by rises in abdominal pressure causing closure of the 'flap valve' as well, prevents downward prolapse of the uterus and vagina.
- **The muscles of the pelvic diaphragm** (Figure 28.2) form a basin or covering of the pelvic outlet and are often grouped together as the levator ani. The thickenings of the parietal fascia of the bellies of the iliococcygeus muscles are known as the arcus tendineus fascia pelvis (fascial arches)

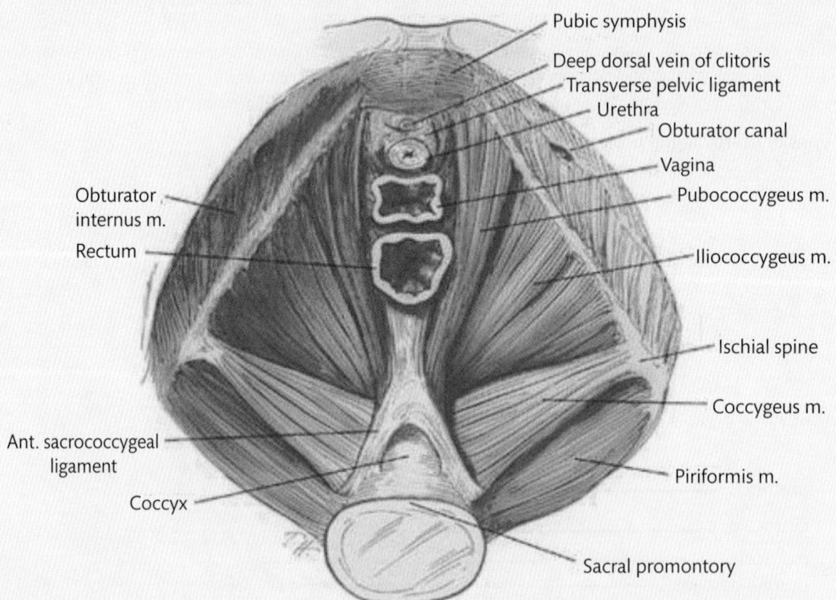

Figure 28.2 A view into the pelvic floor that illustrates the muscles of the pelvic diaphragm and their attachments to the bony pelvis.

Reproduced with permission from Berek J S. *Berek and Novak's Gynecology*. 15th ed. USA: Lippincott Williams and Wilkins; 2012.

or white lines. These lines are the lateral attachment points for the pubocervical septum and apical rectovaginal septum and serve the function of mid-vaginal lateral support.

- **The connective tissues of the pelvis** include the deep endopelvic connective tissue which consists of three pairs of ligaments: uterosacral ligaments, transverse cervical ligaments and pubocervical ligaments; two septae: pubocervical fascia and rectovaginal fascia; and one pericervical ring which connects all the above-mentioned tissues.

Expert comment Classification of POP

The Pelvic Organ Prolapse Quantification (POP-Q) method[5] is the internationally accepted standard and is the classification system of choice of the International Continence Society, the American Urogynecologic Society, and the Society of Gynecologic Surgeons. It has proven inter-observer and intra-observer reliability and is the most commonly cited system in the medical literature (Figure 28.3).

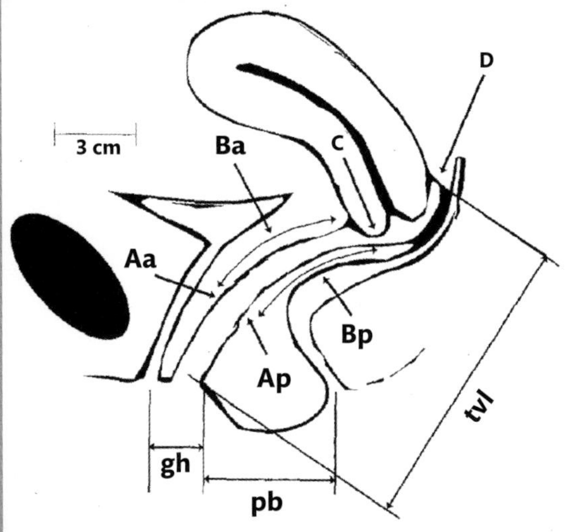

Figure 28.3 The nine specific sites of measurement used in the POP-Q system. Aa, point on the anterior vaginal wall that is 3 cm away from the external urethral meatus; Ap, point on the posterior vaginal wall that is 3 cm away from the hymen; Ba, most dependent/distal point on the anterior vaginal wall; Bp, most dependent/distal point on the posterior vaginal wall; C, distance of the cervix/vaginal cuff (after hysterectomy); D, distance of the posterior fornix (representing the Pouch of Douglas), absent after a hysterectomy; gh, length of the genital hiatus; pb, length of the perineal body; tvl, total vaginal length.

Reproduced with permission from Bump RC, Mattiasson A, Bø K, et al. The standardization of terminology of female pelvic organ prolapse and pelvic floor dysfunction. *Am J Obstet Gynecol* 1996;175:10.

Clinical tip Evaluation of POP

- **Comprehensive history**: including prolapse, urinary, bowel, and sexual history. Use of a standardized and validated quality-of-life assessment questionnaire which is a useful audit and research tool that helps with patient-centred assessment and goals.[6]
- **Examination**: palpation of the abdomen is done first to exclude an abdominal mass or ascites. A Sims speculum is used to systematically identify each component of the prolapse. The position of the cervix or the vault (after a hysterectomy), is also determined and a bimanual pelvic examination performed. A rectal examination may be required to differentiate between a rectocele and an enterocele.
- The mechanical strength of the pelvic diaphragm is directly correlated with the ability to voluntarily contract these muscles. Muscle activity is subjectively graded from 0 to 5 using the Modified Oxford score (0, no contraction; 1, flicker; 2, weak; 3, moderate; 4, good (with lift); 5, strong).[7] If no muscle activity is detected, a more formal neurological and medical workup should be considered.

Learning point DeLancey's supports

DeLancey helps explain the levels of normal uterovaginal support.[4]

- **Level 1:** the cervix and upper third of the vagina are supported by the transverse cervical and uterosacral ligaments.
- **Level 2:** the mid portion of the vagina is attached by the pubocervical and rectovaginal fascia (deep endopelvic connective tissue) to the arcus tendineus fascia pelvis.
- **Level 3:** the lower third of the vagina is supported by the pelvic diaphragm and the perineal body.

Learning point Aetiology of POP

Congenital

- Bladder exstrophy.
- Collagen defects (e.g. type IV Ehlers–Danlos syndrome, Marfan's syndrome).

Childbirth

- Trauma.
- Denervation.

Raised intra-abdominal pressure

- Chronic obstructive airway disease.
- Lifestyle: straining, constipation, heavy lifting, obesity, smoking.

Menopause

- Oestrogen deficiency.

Iatrogenic

- Pelvic surgery (i.e. hysterectomy).

Learning point Symptoms of POP

Non-specific

Bulge, pelvic pressure, lump protruding from the vagina, discomfort, dragging sensation in the vagina, laxity, dyspareunia, bleeding or infection, low back ache, rarely renal failure if with ureteric kinking in very large prolapse.

Specific

- Cystourethrocele: urinary frequency and urgency, incomplete bladder emptying leading to recurrent urinary tract infection, slow stream, stress urinary incontinence (SUI).
- Rectocele: incomplete bowel emptying, digitation, splinting, rectal urgency, passive anal incontinence.

Clinical tip Clinical examination

Perform examinations for investigation of a prolapse in the left lateral position using a Sims speculum and a sponge holder or tongue depressor.

Clinical tip Treatment options

Options for treatment for the various compartments of prolapse are discussed in detail in the 2019 National Institute for Health and Care Excellence (NICE) guidelines (NG 123).[8] Following diagnosis of the type of prolapse, patients should be given patient decision aids to allow them to decide which option they wish to pursue.[9]

Table 28.1 POP-Q score

+2	+2	+3
(Aa)	(Ba)	(C)
2	2	8
(gh)	(pb)	(tvl)
+1	0	−2
(Ap)	(Bp)	(D)

On examination with a Sims speculum, there was descent of the cervix up to 2 cm beyond the hymenal margin with a POP-Q score as demonstrated in Table 28.1 and with stage III POP.[5]

On discussion of options of management which included conservative management, use of vaginal pessary, or surgical management, this lady preferred to have surgery to correct the prolapse.

Learning point Options for management of prolapse

1. **Conservative management**: pelvic floor muscle training (PFMT) or pessary.
2. **Surgical management**.

Conservative management

PFMT

Generally, preventative measures should be the most widely applied techniques. Pelvic floor exercises, weight loss, treatment of chronic diseases including effective treatment of persistent cough, constipation, and cessation of smoking should be advised. Oestrogen therapy not only helps to prevent osteoporosis but also has positive effects on the various oestrogen-sensitive tissues of the pelvis.

Vaginal pessaries

Vaginal pessaries could be used, offering an excellent non-surgical option for women with prolapse with virtually no contraindications.

Learning point Vaginal pessaries

Pessaries are devices which are inserted into the vagina. They are offered to alleviate the symptoms of prolapse and delay or eliminate the need for surgery. Pessaries may help with bowel and bladder symptoms of prolapse. Kinking of the urethra due to the prolapse may cause voiding dysfunction leading to bladder neck obstruction. By correcting this, obstructive and urgency symptoms may be relieved. However, pessaries may also cause *de novo*/occult SUI due to the 'unkinking' of the urethro-vesical angle.

Two categories of pessaries, support and space filling, exist for prolapse. The ring and other support pessaries are typically recommended for stage I and II prolapse, whereas the space-filling pessaries are usually used for stage III and IV prolapse. After initial fitting, follow-up checks to look for vaginal excoriation and replacement of pessaries may be scheduled every 3–6 months. Minor, transient complications may be seen commonly including pessary expulsion, urinary incontinence, rectal pressure, vaginal discharge or bleeding, and mechanical pressure ulcers. Serious complications of pessary use can typically be avoided with regular follow-up examinations and are rare.

Learning point Surgical management of anterior compartment prolapse

Anterior colporrhaphy

The objective of this surgery is to plicate the layers of the pubocervical fascia in such a way as to reduce the central protrusion of the bladder and vagina.

Paravaginal defect/site-specific repair

Paravaginal defect is characterized by presence of rugae on the anterior vagina and absence of sulci on the lateral vagina due to the detachment of the endopelvic fascia from the lateral pelvic side wall. In these cases, repair is done by fixing (reattaching) the endopelvic fascia to the arcus tendineus fascia (white line) of the pelvis. This may be done laparoscopically, retropubically through the space of Retzius, or vaginally. Vaginal paravaginal repair did not appear to offer any advantage over midline colporrhaphy alone in terms of either maintenance of anatomical support or symptomatic improvement.[15]

Evidence base PFMT

A large multicentre randomized controlled trial (the Pelvic Organ Prolapse PhysiotherapY (POPPY) trial).[10] showed that one-to-one PFMT for prolapse is effective for the improvement of prolapse symptoms. Both the NICE and the American College of Obstetricians and Gynecologists list PFMT as a treatment option in women with all types of vaginal prolapse[11,12] and especially for POP-Q stage I–II vaginal prolapse.[13,14]

Learning point Surgical management of uterine prolapse

Historically, the treatment for symptomatic uterine prolapse has been a hysterectomy, which is usually performed vaginally in combination with an apical suspension procedure, and repair of coexisting defects.

Vaginal hysterectomy and repair

Several methods of vault suspension are used at the time of this surgery and include the following:

- Uterosacral suspension: the vault is suspended to the uterosacral ligaments with a delayed absorbable stitch.
- McCall culdoplasty: a delayed absorbable suture is inserted through the full thickness of the posterior vagina laterally. The suture is then passed through each uterosacral ligament and back out the posterior vaginal wall. The stitch on either side is tied, suspending the apex to the uterosacral ligaments.
- Abdominal sacrohysteropexy: suspension of the vagina or uterus to the sacral promontory with an intervening mesh depending if the woman wants to preserve the uterus or not.
- Manchester repair: this combines anterior vaginal wall repair with amputation of the cervix and uterosacral ligament suspension.
- Sacrospinous hysteropexy: involves fixation of the uterus to the sacrospinous ligament. Variations of this technique have been described:
  - If an abdominal hysterectomy is performed because a woman has an enlarged uterus which cannot be removed vaginally, additional intraperitoneal vault support procedures will be required including Moschowitz, Halban, and uterosacral plication.

Evidence base Surgical management

Women with uterine prolapse who have *no preference about preserving* their uterus[8] should be offered a choice of:

- Vaginal hysterectomy, with or without vaginal sacrospinous fixation with sutures
- Vaginal sacrospinous hysteropexy with sutures
- Manchester repair
- Abdominal sacrohysteropexy using mesh.

Women with uterine prolapse who *wish to preserve* their uterus may be offered any of the above-listed procedures except a hysterectomy.

When a mesh procedure is performed:

- Explain the type of mesh that will be used and whether or not it is permanent.
- Ensure that the details of the procedure and its subsequent short- and long-term outcomes are recorded in a national registry.
- Give written information about the implant (including its name, manufacturer, date of insertion, and the implanting surgeon's name and contact details).

Learning point Surgical management of posterior compartment prolapse

- Transvaginal approach: consists of either midline posterior colporrhaphy in a manner similar to that in the anterior compartment or a site-specific defect repair.
- Transanal approach: considered less effective than transvaginal repairs.
- Perineorrhaphy: reapproximation of torn dense perineal connective tissue including the bulbocavernosus and perineal muscles in an effort to restore the perineal body when deficient.

Learning point Surgical management of the vaginal vault

- Abdominal sacrocolpopexy: suspension of the vagina vault to the sacral promontory with an intervening mesh.

- Vaginal sacrospinous fixation: fixation of the vaginal vault to the sacrospinous ligament with the variations discussed previously.
- Other: transvaginal repairs include iliococcygeal suspensions, and high paravaginal suspensions of the apical vaginal fornices to the arcus tendineus at the level of the ischial spine or to the endopelvic fascia.
- Colpocleisis: operation which obliterates the lumen of the vagina. This is only an option for women who do not wish to maintain sexual activity.

Future directions Vaginal mesh

The use of mesh in anterior and posterior compartment surgery is associated with an increased risk of complications and lower effectiveness than native tissue repair.[18,19] At the time of writing this chapter, the use of vaginal mesh is paused in the UK awaiting implementation of recommendations made by the Independent Medicines and Medical Devices Safety Review.[20] The use of abdominal mesh is under high-vigilance scrutiny and should be used after careful discussion with the patient and at a multidisciplinary team meeting.

Evidence base Abdominal sacrocolpopexy versus vaginal sacrospinous fixation

A Cochrane review[16] included three randomized controlled trials that compared abdominal sacrocolpopexy versus vaginal sacrospinous fixation. Its meta-analysis showed that abdominal sacrocolpopexy was associated with significantly lower rates of recurrent vault prolapse, and less postoperative SUI and dyspareunia. There were no statistically significant differences in patient satisfaction, the number of women reporting prolapse symptoms, objective failure at any site, reoperation rates for SUI, and reoperation rates for prolapse. Sacrospinous fixation resulted in a reduction in operative time, it was less expensive to perform, and women had an earlier return to their daily activities.[17]

Future directions Recurrent prolapses

NHS England are commissioning units to undertake specialist work and management of recurrent prolapse will be undertaken in these specialist units.

Vaginal hysterectomy and anterior repair were performed uneventfully. The patient was well after surgery. Five years later, she went on to develop significant posterior compartment prolapse for which she underwent a posterior colporrhaphy and perineorrhaphy.

A final word from the expert

POP is very common and one in ten women will require surgery over their lifetime for this condition. It usually affects women after the menopause but can occur in younger women of childbearing age too. It almost always occurs in women who have had vaginal deliveries, but a caesarean is only protective if all deliveries are exclusively by caesarean section. Combined vaginal and caesarean births do not offer protection.

When it affects a woman before she has completed her family, women should be encouraged to avoid surgery and consider it after their family is complete. This avoids the need for unnecessary caesarean sections and risk of the prolapse returning due to further childbearing.

Symptoms can sometimes be minimal, and surgery should be undertaken when there are bothersome symptoms rather than purely because an asymptomatic POP has been diagnosed. Women should be advised to perform their pelvic floor exercises as this will treat minor grades of prolapse and will also prevent recurrence if they proceed with surgery.

In women opting for pessary control, regular follow-up is required and they should be kept under surveillance to detect any complications that can arise from long-term pessary use. Women opting for surgery should be given the range of options in accordance with the 2019 NICE guidelines (NG123).

Women opting for surgery should be forewarned of the risk of recurrence and the one in three lifetime risk of needing further prolapse and/or incontinence surgery and the one in ten risk of the same compartment prolapsing again.

Baseline assessment of pelvic floor symptoms including urinary, bowel, and sexual dysfunction should be undertaken prior to and after treatment particularly surgery. Women should be informed that treatment of the prolapse is not guaranteed to cure the other symptoms of pelvic floor dysfunction and some women may develop SUI following treatment of prolapse (occult incontinence) whereas others may develop dyspareunia due to the formation of scar tissue after surgery.

All complex cases should be discussed at a multidisciplinary team meeting and where facilities exist, all primary cases of prolapse scheduled for surgery should also be discussed. Recurrent prolapse surgery should be undertaken by adequately trained surgeons in units which are commissioned to undertake this work.

References

1. Haylen BT, Maher CF, Barber MD, et al. An International Urogynecological Association (IUGA)/International Continence Society (ICS) joint report on the terminology for female pelvic organ prolapse (POP). *Neurourol Urodyn.* 2016;35(2):137–168.
2. Samuelsson EC, Arne Victor FT, Tibblin G, et al. Signs of genital prolapse in a Swedish population of women 20 to 59 years of age and possible related factors. *Am J Obstet Gynecol.* 1999;180(2 Pt 1):299–305.
3. Beck RP. Pelvic relaxational prolapse. In: Kase NG, Weingold AB, eds. *Principles and Practice of Clinical Gynecology*. New York: John Wiley & Sons; 1983:677–685.
4. DeLancey JO. Anatomic aspects of vaginal eversion after hysterectomy. *Am J Obstet Gynecol.* 1992;166(6 Pt 1):1717–1724.
5. Bump RC, Mattiasson A, Bø K, Brubaker LP, DeLancey JO, Klarskov P. The standardization of terminology of female pelvic organ prolapse and pelvic floor dysfunction. *Am J Obstet Gynecol.* 1996;175(1):10–17.
6. Lowenstein L, FitzGerald MP, Kenton K, Dooley Y, Templehof M, Mueller ER. Patient-selected goals: the fourth dimension in assessment of pelvic floor disorders. *Int Urogynecol J Pelvic Floor Dysfunct.* 2008;19(1):81–84.
7. Laycock J. Pelvic muscle exercises: physiotherapy for the pelvic floor. *Urol Nurs.* 1994;14(3):136–40.
8. National Institute for Health and Care Excellence. Urinary incontinence and pelvic organ prolapse in women: management. NICE guideline [NG123]. National Institute for Health and Care Excellence. 2019. https://www.nice.org.uk/guidance/ng123
9. National Institute for Health and Care Excellence (NICE) guideline. Urinary incontinence and pelvic organ prolapse in women: management: tools and resources. NICE guideline [NG123]. National Institute for Health and Care Excellence. 2019. https://www.nice.org.uk/guidance/ng123/resources
10. Hagen S, Stark D, Glazener C, et al. Individualised pelvic floor muscle training in women with pelvic organ prolapse (POPPY): a multicentre randomised controlled trial. *Lancet.* 2014;383(9919):796–806.
11. Committee on Practice Bulletins-Gynecology, American College of Obstetricians and Gynecologists. ACOG Practice Bulletin No. 79: pelvic organ prolapse. *Obstet Gynecol.* 2007;109(2 Pt 1):461–473.
12. National Institute for Health and Care Excellence. Sacrocolpopexy using mesh for vaginal vault prolapse repair. Interventional procedures guidance [IPG583]. National Institute for Health and Care Excellence. 2009. https://www.nice.org.uk/guidance/ipg583
13. Hagen S, Stark D. Conservative prevention and management of pelvic organ prolapse in women. *Cochrane Database Syst Rev.* 2011;12:CD003882.
14. Hagen S, Stark D, Glazener C, Sinclair L, Ramsay I. A randomized controlled trial of pelvic floor muscle training for stages I and II pelvic organ prolapse. *Int Urogynecol J Pelvic Floor Dysfunct.* 2009;20(1):45–51.

15. Morse AN, O'Dell KK, Howard AE, Baker SP, Aronson MP, Young SB. Midline anterior repair alone vs anterior repair plus vaginal paravaginal repair: a comparison of anatomic and quality of life outcomes. *Int Urogynecol J Pelvic Floor Dysfunct.* 2007;18(3):245–9.
16. Maher C, Feiner B, Baessler K, Schmid C. Surgical management of pelvic organ prolapse in women. *Cochrane Database Syst Rev.* 2013;4(4):CD004014.
17. Royal College of Obstetricians and Gyanecologists, British Society of Urogynaecology. *Post-Hysterectomy Vaginal Vault Prolapse*. London: Royal College of Obstetricians and Gyanecologists; 2015.
18. Morling JR, McAllister DA, Agur W, Fischbacher CM, Glazener CM, Guerrero K. Adverse events after first, single, mesh and non-mesh surgical procedures for stress urinary incontinence and pelvic organ prolapse in Scotland, 1997–2016: a population-based cohort study. *Lancet.* 2017;389(10069):629–640.
19. Campbell P, Jha S, Cutner A. Vaginal mesh in prolapse surgery. *Obstet Gynecol.* 2018;20(1):49–56.
20. Independent Medicines and Medical Devices Safety Review. First Do No Harm—The report of the Independent Medicines and Medical Devices Safety Review 2020.

SECTION 10

Reconstruction

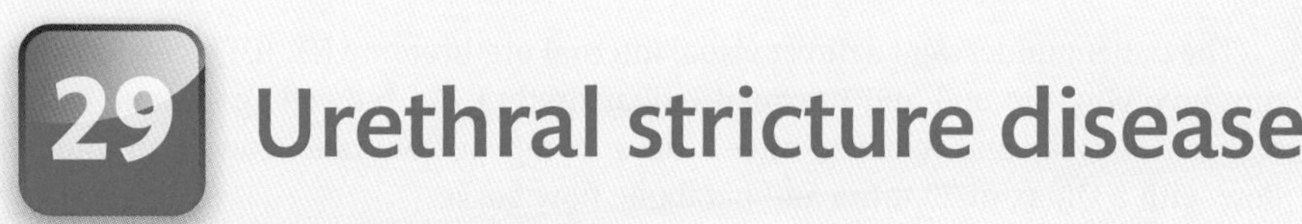

29 Urethral stricture disease

Jamie V. Krishnan and Nadir I. Osman

Expert commentary Christopher R. Chapple

Case history 1

A 19-year-old man was referred by his general practitioner (GP) with gradually worsening voiding lower urinary tract symptoms for 2 years. He was otherwise fit and well with no history of perineal trauma, urethral instrumentation, or sexually transmitted infection. No abnormalities were found on examination. Urinalysis showed a trace of blood. Urethral stricture, bladder neck dysfunction, and bladder underactivity were considered in the differential diagnoses.

Uroflowmetry, ultrasound scanning for post-void residual urine, retrograde urethrography, and a flexible cystourethroscopy were requested. Uroflowmetry showed reduced maximal flow rate (Qmax) of 5.5 mL/s and a prolonged plateau pattern (Figure 29.1a). There was no residual urine on the ultrasound scan. The urethrogram suggested a narrowing in the mid and proximal bulbar urethra and flexible cystoscopy demonstrated the distal end of the impassable stricture (Figure 29.1b,c).

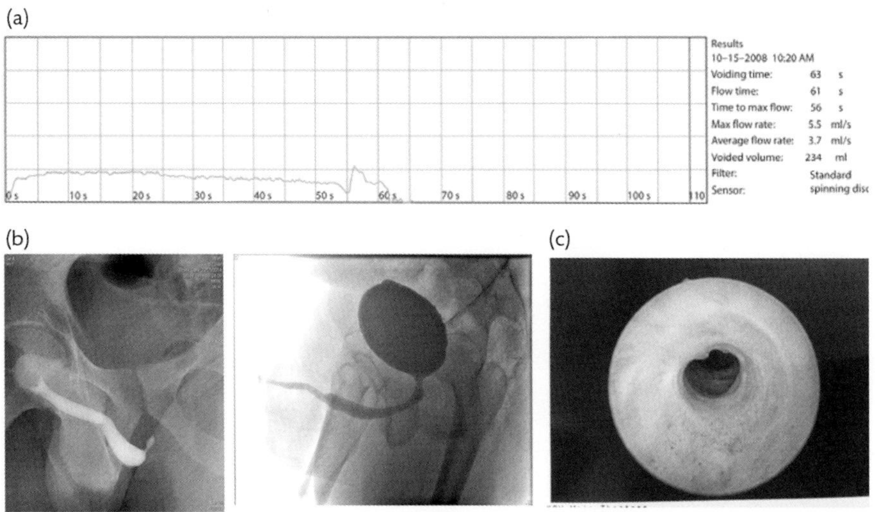

Figure 29.1 (a) Flow rate of patient with urethral stricture. (b) Retrograde urethrogram highlighting a bulbar stricture. (c) View of a bulbar stricture during attempted flexible cystoscopy.

The patient underwent a direct visual internal urethrotomy (DVIU) of a 1.5 cm stricture involving the mid and proximal bulbar urethra. An indwelling silicone catheter was left in place and removed after 2 days. A repeat flow rate showed an improved flow with a Qmax of 20 mL/s and parabolic flow curve.

The patient was subsequently followed up with uroflowmetry and post-void residual estimation every 4 months for a period of 1 year with no change in flow parameters and post-void residual before being discharged back to his GP.

Case history 2

The 19-year-old man in case history 1, who had undergone a DVIU, was re-referred by his GP several months following discharge with a resumption in voiding difficulties. He underwent repeat uroflowmetry which showed a further deterioration in Qmax and flexible urethroscopy confirmed an impassable urethral stricture. A urethrogram showed bulbar urethral narrowing.

He was counselled for the possible treatment options of (1) repeat DVIU followed by long-term intermittent self-dilatation (ISD) or (2) urethroplasty. He chose to have a urethroplasty.

Case history 3

A 72-year-old man had a transurethral resection of the prostate procedure 2 years before. His flow improved significantly after the operation but started deteriorating after a few months. He presented with a poor flow with a Qmax of 3 mL/s. Urethroscopy revealed an impassable submeatal narrowing. Urethrography confirmed a lengthy stricture of his penile urethra. He underwent urethral dilatation and was instructed to perform ISD postoperatively but found this difficult. He wanted to discuss other options. The options discussed with him included a permanent suprapubic catheter, substitution urethroplasty, or a perineal urethrostomy. He chose to have a perineal urethrostomy.

Clinical tip Flowchart illustrating the management of a urethral stricture

See Figure 29.2.

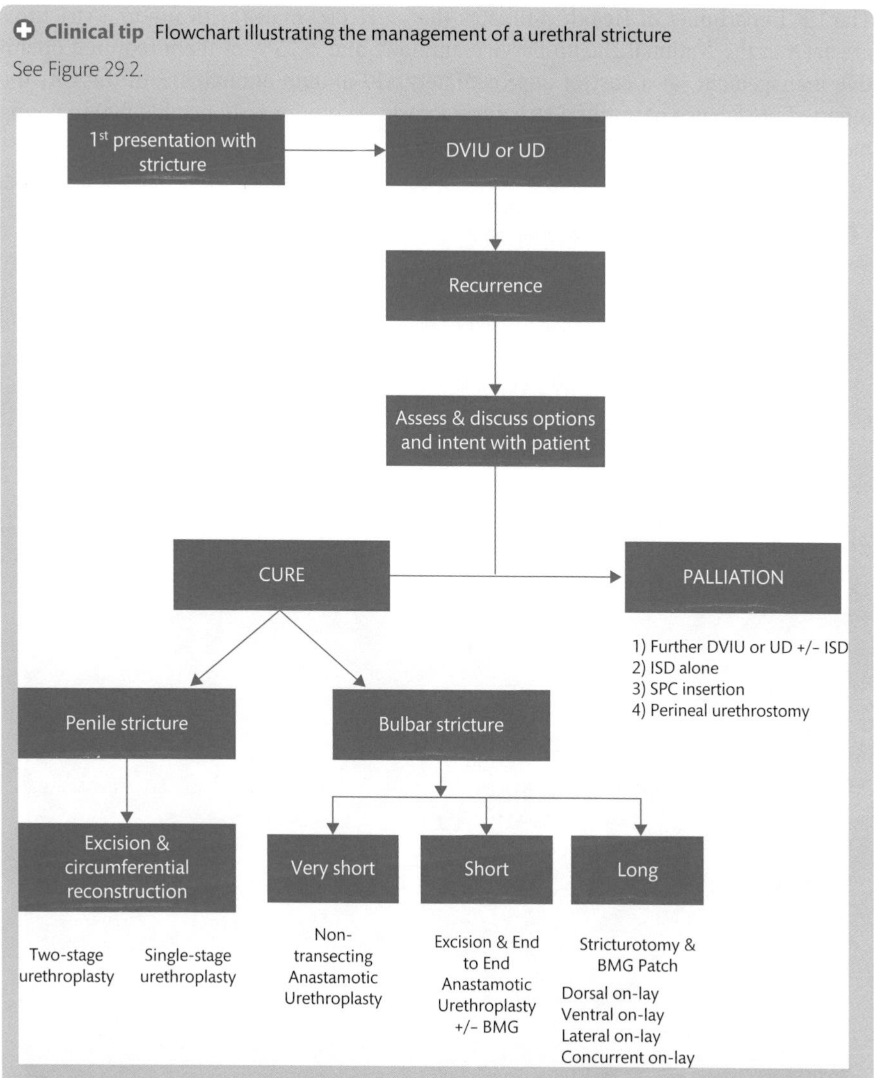

Figure 29.2 Algorithm demonstrating management options. BMG, buccal mucosal graft; DVIU, direct visual internal urethrotomy; ISD, intermittent self-dilatation; SPC, suprapubic catheter; UD, urethral dilation.

Introduction

Learning point Definition and pathology

A urethral stricture is defined as a constriction of the urethral lumen caused by concentric scarring, involving the epithelium, and extending to a variable depth into the corpus spongiosum. The underlying pathology is that of an ischaemic spongiofibrosis. This definition applies to the part of the urethra surrounded by spongiosal tissue, the anterior urethra. It is important to recognize that the configuration of the urethra does vary, being thickest ventrally in the bulbar urethra and uniformly narrowing in the penile urethra. Narrowings of the posterior urethra are conventionally termed stenoses and not considered as stricture.

The UK Department of Health estimates that > 16,000 males with urethral strictures are seen in the National Health Service annually and > 75% of them required operative management, at a cost of approximately £10 million annually.[1,2] In the UK, the reported prevalence of urethral strictures across age groups is 10 per 100,000 in young men and up to 100 per 100,000 in those > 65 years.[3]

Learning point Anatomical considerations

The urethra is 15–25 cm long, anatomically divided into anterior and posterior urethra. The anterior urethra consists of the meatus, navicular fossa, penile (or pendulous) urethra, and the bulbar urethra (extends from the penoscrotal junction to inferior perineal fascia). The penile urethra runs ventrally within the corpus spongiosum, which is a mass of spongy tissue, expanded posteriorly to form the urethral bulb which lies opposed to the urogenital diaphragm. The urethra enters the bulb near its superior aspect. Spongiosal tissue distal to the bulb sits in a groove on the under-surface of the conjoined corpora cavernosa and tapers along its length until it expands to form the glans penis distally. Figure 29.3 demonstrates this and the relative position of the urethra within the spongiosum in cross section.

The posterior urethra consists of the membranous urethra, prostatic urethra, and bladder neck. The membranous urethra contains the distal urethral sphincter in its wall and is surrounded by

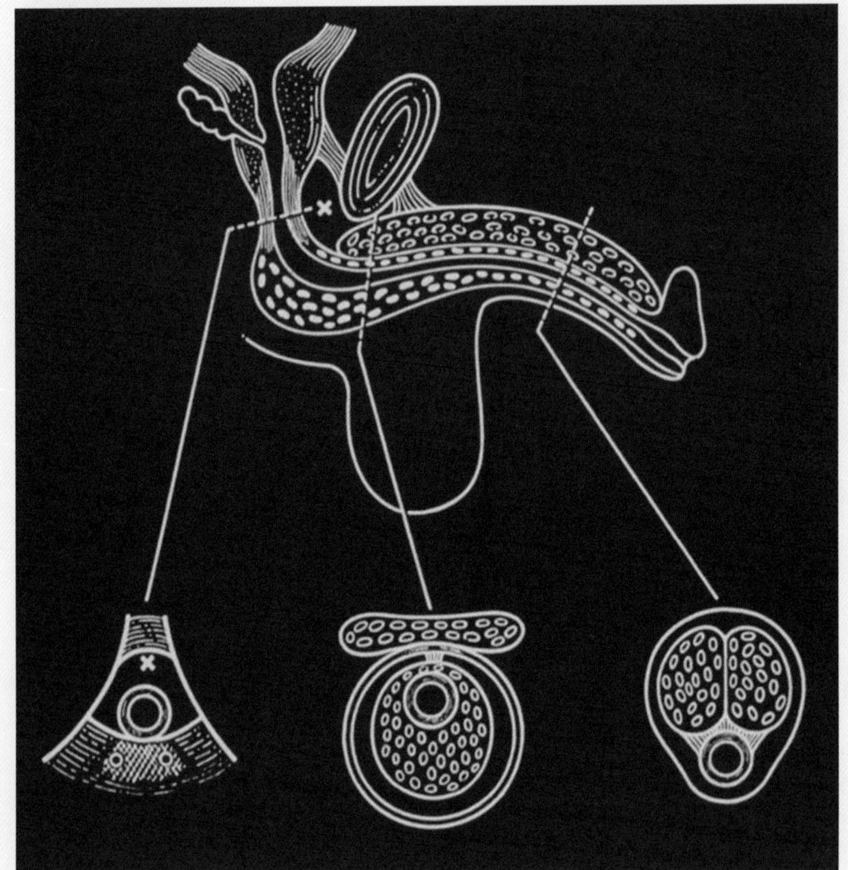

Figure 29.3 Illustration of the urethra and its relations within the corpus spongiosum.

the periurethral part of the pelvic diaphragm as it passes through it. The bladder neck consists of a prominent sphincter in males. Each section of urethra is lined by a different variation of epithelial cells: fossa navicularis by squamous epithelium, penile and bulbar urethra by pseudostratified columnar epithelium, and the membranous and prostatic urethra by transitional epithelium.[4]

The Scarpa's fascia of the lower abdominal wall continues down into the perineum where it is termed Colles' fascia. It extends on to the penile shaft where it is called the penile fascia or Gallaudet's fascia.

The blood supply to the urethra is segmental which means that it is possible to mobilize the urethra without ischaemic problems along its whole length, provided that the proximal and distal blood supply is intact. The inferior vesical, middle rectal, and pudendal arteries, arising from the anterior division of the internal iliac artery, provide the urethral blood supply. The internal pudendal artery gives three main branches: (1) the bulbourethral artery, which supplies the bulb of the penis, the membranous and penile urethra; (2) the dorsal artery, which runs dorsal to the corpora cavernosa within the Buck's fascia; and (3) paired cavernosal arteries, within the corpus cavernosum, which run along the length of the shaft.

Aetiology

Learning point Aetiology of urethral strictures

Strictures of the anterior urethra are broadly caused by lichen sclerosis in 30%, instrumentation (including catheterization, cystoscopy, hypospadias repair) in 30%, and are idiopathic in 30%. About 10% of urethral strictures are caused by direct trauma (fall astride injuries), where there is very limited spongiofibrosis and an anastomotic repair is usually successful in these cases. Conversely, ischaemia is the common underlying pathology in urethral strictures, but is rarely referred to as such.[5] The aetiology of strictures varies slightly between the bulbar and penile urethra as shown in Table 29.1.[6]

Posterior urethral stenoses, on the other hand, are usually caused by severe trauma and are often associated with pelvic fractures and involve a distraction injury or avulsion of the membranous urethra and are otherwise known as pelvic fracture urethral injury.[7] Much less common, but increasing in incidence, certain treatments for prostate cancer (high-intensity focused ultrasound, radiotherapy, brachytherapy; radical retropubic prostatectomy) can lead to prostatic urethral strictures and distraction injuries and fistulae. A complicating feature of these cases is the damage to blood supply resulting from radiotherapy.

Table 29.1 Aetiology of urethral strictures by site

	Idiopathic	Iatrogenic	Inflammatory	Trauma
Penile	15%	40%	40%	5%
Bulbar	40%	35%	10%	15%

Pathophysiology

Strictures occur as a result of a process termed ischaemic spongiofibrosis. Focal extravasation of urine occurs as a result of an insult (infective, inflammatory, iatrogenic) leading to subepithelial fibrosis within the corpus spongiosum, and as consequence the vascular supply is lost and fibrotic plaques form. If the fibrotic foci coalesce circumferentially around the urethra, then a stricture may form.[8]

Clinical features

Seventy per cent of patients present with voiding lower urinary tract symptoms (hesitancy, poor flow, terminal dribbling or a feeling of incomplete voiding).[9] Acute presentations include acute urinary retention, recurrent urinary tract infections, epididymo-orchitis, or periurethral abscesses[10]

Investigations

Clinical tip Considerations when planning treatment

A patient with poor dexterity may not be a suitable candidate for DVIU and ISD; equally, a patient with multiple comorbidities may not be an appropriate candidate for major reconstructive surgery.

Assessment of these patients includes history and the use of a patient-reported outcome questionnaire to ascertain symptom severity and bother (e.g. urethral stricture patient reported outcome measure and the Sexual Health Inventory for Men (SHIM)).[11,12] Clinical examination is typically unremarkable, note should be taken of lichen sclerosis and the location of the urethral meatus; occasionally periurethral fibrosis is palpable; and digital rectal examination is essential to assess prostate size and consistency in older men. Urinary flow rate shows a long slow protracted pattern with a plateau, as shown in Figure 29.1.[13] A post-void ultrasound may reveal large post-micturition residual volumes, which may necessitate more urgent management.

Expert comment Endoscopic treatment

In the case of a young and fit individual, often even if much older, treatment with curative intent is appropriate. The location and length of the stricture will determine the optimal form of treatment. Endoscopic treatment has most success in short bulbar stricture and least success in long penile strictures. There is no evidence to suggest DVIU is more efficacious than urethral dilatation; hence, both options are valid.[14]

Expert comment Assessment of urethral strictures

Symptoms and flow rates are poor measures of urethral calibre. There is no reduction in uroflow until the calibre of the urethra is <11 French gauge.[15] With a normally functioning bladder, a stricture does not usually become manifest until the stricture is very tight.

Retrograde urethrography is essential to delineate the full length of the urethra. It is not possible to comment on the status of the posterior urethra on a retrograde urethrogram. Only an antegrade or voiding urethrogram delineates the posterior urethra. Voiding cystourethrography can be performed as adjunct, distending the urethra proximal to the stricture.[9] This is clearly easier in patients with a suprapubic catheter *in situ*. In some situations, flexible cystoscopy is of value to visibly assess the state of the urethral wall in terms of diseases such as lichen sclerosis and it will also provide an impression rigidity of radiologically non-stenosed regions. This aids preoperative planning in terms of the likely need for grafting, the length of graft that may be required, and the surgical approach.

Follow-up with flexible cystourethroscopy after patients undergo a urethroplasty enables early identification of recurrence, morphologic characterization of the recurrence pattern, and, thus, determination of required intervention.[16]

Clinical tip Planning management

A number of factors need to be taken into account when planning management of patients with urethral strictures, including:

- Stricture characteristics: length, location, calibre, associated problems (e.g. balanitis xerotica obliterans, hypospadias)
- Patient characteristics: age, comorbidities, dexterity, severity of symptoms
- Patient choice: curative or palliative treatment, long-term catheter.

Generally, endoscopic treatment is performed as first line for short bulbar strictures; for those with longer strictures, particularly in the penile urethra, a primary urethroplasty may be more appropriate. If primary endoscopic treatment fails, further endoscopic intervention is considered highly likely to fail and hence is palliative in nature. In general, patients wishing to pursue a second endoscopic intervention should be instructed to perform clean ISD postoperatively to maintain urethral patency.

Reconstruction for bulbar strictures is almost always a single-stage urethroplasty. Short strictures may be treated with excision and end-to-end anastomosis or a non-transecting excision and anastomosis. Longer strictures require a stricturotomy and augmentation with buccal mucosal graft (BMG). The stricturotomy may be made on the dorsal, ventral, or lateral aspect of the urethra. The grafts are typically laid on to the stricturotomy.[17] A systematic review by Mangera et al. found no significant difference in average success rates between the various techniques for single-stage

Table 29.2 A comparison of buccal mucosal and skin grafts

Buccal mucosa	Skin
Full thickness—no contraction	Split thickness—contracts
Full thickness—good take	Full thickness—poor take
Abundant vessels between dermal and subdermal plexus	Fewer vessels between dermal and subdermal plexus
Hairless	Hairy
Used to being wet or dry	Not used to being wet
Limited supply	Limitless supply
Durable	Penile skin: 20 years; scrotal skin: 10 years

bulbar urethroplasties.[18] Penile strictures typically require a two-stage substitution urethroplasty usually using BMG. Single-stage urethroplasty can also be also performed although the recurrence rate is felt to be higher with the latter in penile urethra.

Historically, penile or scrotal skin flaps and grafts were used for augmentation procedures. Bladder mucosa grafts were also tried briefly, before being abandoned. BMG was originally described > 100 years ago but popularized in the contemporary era as the graft of choice following Burger's report in 1992.[19] Table 29.2 provides a comparison of skin and BMG for urethroplasties.[20]

Expert comment Qmax and symptoms

Patients with a Qmax >10 mL/s typically do not have troublesome symptoms and have a low likelihood of developing complications and as such may be suitable for a watch-and-wait approach. Those with a Qmax of 5–10 mL/s are more likely to develop a urinary tract infection and if this were the case, then intervention would be warranted. A Qmax <5 mL/s indicates troublesome symptoms and complications are common and as such should be treated.[9]

Learning point Graft uptake

Several factors negatively influence successful 'take' of a graft, these include an inadequately prepared graft (too thick, fatty) or bed, poor vascularity, and infection. Care must be taken to ensure the chance of 'take' is optimized.

There are three main stages of graft uptake:

1. Imbibition: first 48 hours. Where the graft receives nutrients from the plasma through direct contact.
2. Inosculation: day 2–3. Where there is an establishment of communication channels between adjacent blood vessels.
3. Vascularization: day 3–7. Exact mechanism unknown. Angiogenesis occurs with anastomosis between donor site and graft.

Evidence base Grafts versus flaps

A meta-analysis by Wessells and McAninch showed no difference in cure rate between the use of grafts and flaps. Thus, factors once believed to be less important (e.g. scarring, time taken to harvest, donor site morbidity) came to the forefront when deciding which to use, making grafts preferable.[21]

Prognosis

Success rates of urethroplasty are quoted at 85–90% for bulbar urethroplasties and around 80% for penile urethroplasties. With regard to bulbar strictures, dorsal and ventral onlay procedures carry similar success rates of 88.4% and 88.8% respectively.[22]

Future directions The OPEN study

The OPEN study is a randomized, open label, superiority trial of 'OPen urethroplasty versus ENdoscopic urethrotomy' for recurrent bulbar urethral strictures (after prior minimally invasive treatment). The long-anticipated results were recently published and while urethroplasty had a lower rate of reintervention (15%), the difference between it and urethrotomy (29%) was far lower than anticipated. The success of urethrotomy was much higher than anticipated. The question has to be posed as to the case selection for entry into this study and whether all patients who entered had a similar profile to that expected for a patient for whom urethroplasty is recommended (e.g. failed urethrotomy). Although this study raises some interesting questions, reconstruction in expert hands remains the best long-term solution for patients seeking the best chance of a cure.[23]

Clinical tip DVIU for initial presentations

In summary, a DVIU is indicated with curative intent at first presentation for short bulbar strictures. This carries around a 50% cure rate. If unsuccessful, the course of further treatment (cure vs palliation) should be determined by involving the patient. If cure is the aim, urethroplasty should be considered.

A final word from the expert

Urethral strictures have been recognized as a considerable source of morbidity for thousands of years. The classic paradigm has been to undertake minimally invasive treatment by way of urethral dilatation and latterly urethrotomy, followed by palliation with intermittent dilation in refractory cases. In the modern era, surgical reconstruction has become the accepted treatment option in refractory cases and was championed by pioneers such as Richard Turner-Warwick and John Blandy among others. In recent years, attempts have been made to better define the place of minimally invasive treatments and reconstruction in the treatment algorithm for anterior urethral stricture disease; however, this has been hampered by the lack of any high-level evidence.

References

1. Department of Health. NHS reference costs. http/www.dh.gov.uk/en/Publicationsandstatistics/Publications/PublicationsPolicyAndGuidance/DH_111591
2. Department of Health. NHS Hospital Episode Statistics. http://www.hesonline.nhs.uk
3. McMillan A, Pakianathan M, Mao NH, Macintyre CC. Urethral stricture and urethritis in men in Scotland. *Genitourin Med.* 1994;70(6):403–405.
4. Schenkman NS, Manger JP. Male urethra anatomy. Medscape. 2016. https://emedicine.medscape.com/article/1972482-overview#a2
5. Nacey JN. Urinary catheter toxicity. *NZ Med J.* 1991;104(918):355–356.
6. Lumen N, Hoebeke P, Willemsen P, De Troyer B, Pieters R, Oosterlinck W. Etiology of urethral stricture disease in the 21st century. *J Urol.* 2009;182(3):983–987.
7. Kulkarni SB, Barbagli G, Kulkarni JS, Romano G, Lazzeri M. Posterior urethral stricture after pelvic fracture urethral distraction defects in developing and developed countries, and choice of surgical technique. *J Urol.* 2010;183(3):1049–1054.
8. Chambers RM, Baitera B. The anatomy of urethral stricture. *Br J Urol.* 1977;49(6):545–551.
9. Mundy AR, Andrich DE. Urethral strictures. *BJU Int.* 2010;107(1):6–26.
10. Thompson H. *The Pathology and Treatment of Stricture of the Urethra Both in the Male and the Female*. London: John Churchill; 1865.
11. Kluth, LA, Dahlem R, Becker A. Validation of a patient-reported outcome measure (PROM) for urethral stricture surgery: a prospective study at a German tertiary care center. *Eur Urol Suppl.* 2015;14(2):e954a.
12. Benson CR, Hoang L, Clavell-Hernández J, Wang R. Sexual dysfunction in urethral reconstruction: a review of the literature. *Sexual Med Rev.* 2018;6(3):492–503.
13. Arya M, Shergill I, Fernando H, et al. *Viva Practice for the FRCS(Urol) and Postgraduate Urology Examinations*. 2nd ed. Masterpass. Boca Raton, FL: CRC Press; 2018.
14. Steenkamp JW, Heyns CF, Dr Kock ML. Internal urethrotomy vs dilatation as treatment for male urethral strictures: a prospective randomized comparison. *J Urol* 1997;157(1):98–101.
15. Smith J. Urethral resistance to micturition: British Association of Urological Surgeons Prize Essay. *BJU Int.* 1968;40(2):125–156.
16. Goonesinghe SK, Hillary CJ, Nicholson TR, Osman NI, Chapple CR. Flexible cystourethroscopy in the follow-up of post urethroplasty patients and characterisation of recurrences. *Eur Urol.* 2015;68(3):523–529.
17. Patterson JM, Chapple CR. Surgical techniques in substitution urethroplasty using buccal mucosa for the treatment of anterior urethral strictures. *Eur Urol.* 2008;53(6):1162–1171.
18. Mangera A, Patterson JM, Chapple CR. A systematic review of graft augmentation urethroplasty techniques for the treatment of anterior urethral strictures. *Eur Urol.* 2011;59(5):797–814.

19. Burger RA, Muller SC, el-Damanhoury H, et al. The buccal mucosal graft for urethral reconstruction: a preliminary report. *J Urol.* 1992;147(3):662–664.
20. Bryk DJ, Yamaguchi Y, Zhao LC. Tissue transfer techniques in reconstructive urology. *Korean J Urol.* 2015;56(7):478–486.
21. Wessells H, McAninch JW. Use of free grafts in urethral stricture reconstruction. *J Urol.* 1996;155(6):1912–1915.
22. Andrich DE, Leach CJ, Mundy AR. The Barbagli procedure gives the best results for patch urethroplasty of the bulbar urethra. *BJU Int.* 2001;88(4):385–389.
23. Goulao B, Carnell S, Shen J, et al. Surgical treatment for recurrent bulbar urethral stricture: a randomised open-label superiority trial of open urethroplasty versus endoscopic urethrotomy (the OPEN Trial). *Eur Urol.* 2020;78(4):572–580.

CASE

30 Urethral diverticulum

Anudini Ranasinghe and Tamsin Greenwell

Expert commentary Jeremy Ockrim

Case history

A 34-year-old woman was referred by her local urologist to our tertiary unit for excision of a complex recurrent urethral diverticulum (Figure 30.1a). She had undergone initial excision of the diverticulum and concomitant insertion of a rectus fascial sling for associated stress urinary incontinence (SUI) 5 years earlier.

She gave a 12-month history of recurrent urinary tract infections (UTIs), frequency of micturition, urge incontinence, and incomplete emptying requiring intermittent self-catheterizing eight times per day. She also complained of vaginal pain and dyspareunia, especially during attempts at penetrative sexual intercourse.

Learning point Histopathology of urethral diverticulum

Urethral diverticula are rare entities affecting between 0.02% and 6% of the female population,[1,2] although they are found in up to 40% of women undergoing investigation for unexplained lower urinary tract symptoms in specialist centres.[3]

First described by William Hey in 1805, they are localized, epithelium-lined urethral outpouchings.[4,5] Histologically, they are difficult to distinguish from paraurethral cysts. Their lining is composed of squamous epithelial cells in 42%, columnar epithelial cells in 32%, a combination of both squamous and columnar cells in 18%, and cuboidal cells in 14%. The majority of diverticula (77%) show signs of inflammation or ulceration.[6]

Learning point Causes of urethral diverticulum

Most urethral diverticula are acquired and presumed to arise from rupture of chronically obstructed and infected periurethral glands into the lumen of the urethra.[7,8] Risk factors for the development of urethral diverticula are vaginal birth trauma and previous vaginal or urethral surgery. In recent years, bladder outlet obstruction (BOO), particularly in the form of bulking agents, and mid-urethral tapes/slings have been implicated in the development of urethral diverticula.[9–12]

Learning point Signs and symptoms of urethral diverticulum

The classic description of symptoms from a urethral diverticulum have been described as dysuria, dyspareunia, and urinary dribbling. However, this triad is only present in approximately 25% of patients,[3] with the majority presenting with non-specific symptoms such as recurrent UTIs, anterior vaginal pain, swelling, discharge, or urgency lower urinary tract symptoms. Their non-specific clinical presentation combined with their relative rarity, means that the diagnosis is often delayed.[13] It has been reported that the average delay in diagnosis ranges from 11 to 72 months.[3,13] In addition to bothersome presenting symptoms, there is also a long-term risk of malignant transformation in urethral diverticula in up to 9%.[3]

Urethral diverticula can pose both a diagnostic and surgical challenge and so a high index of suspicion is required for timely and successful diagnosis and subsequent surgical treatment in experienced hands.

Awareness of this diagnosis is important, as many patients suffer symptoms for years before the diagnosis is made and referral made. Additionally, the risk of associated carcinoma arising in urethral diverticula is low but significant. Patients must be counselled of a 1–9% long-term risk if the diverticulum is left untreated and for most patients this is a compelling reason for surgical excision.

Expert comment Diagnosis of urethral diverticula

The clinical diagnosis of urethral diverticula is challenging. The diagnosis is found in direct proportion to 'the avidity with which it is sought'. While some patients have obvious periurethral swellings, in many cases the diagnosis is dependent on imaging. While ultrasound, voiding computed tomography urethrography, and video urodynamic studies (VUDS) have all been described, fine-slice magnetic resonance imaging (MRI) has now been established as the modality of choice with the greatest sensitivity and offering the greatest anatomical detail for subsequent surgical planning. We also perform VUDS as standard to assess preoperatively for bladder and outlet function. This enables us to counsel the patients on symptom cause and predict symptom resolution following intervention. We can quantify the risk of postoperative (stress) urinary incontinence dependent on the diverticulum size, position, and configuration (simple, partial, or complete horseshoe configurations) along with the preoperative VUDS findings.

The patient was investigated with an T2-weighted, small field of vision, post-void pelvic MRI (urethral diverticulum protocol) which showed a recurrent, dorsal, large horseshoe diverticulum surrounding the urethra for 300° from 3 o'clock to 5 o'clock position (Figure 30.1b) measuring 2.0 × 2.0 × 1.8 cm. The superior portion of a previous Martius fat pad was also demonstrated. She had VUDS, which demonstrated severe detrusor overactivity with peak pressures of 74 cmH_2O with leak. SUI was not shown but severe BOO with a Pdet Qmax of 70 cmH_2O for a Qmax of 6 mL/s (Solomon Greenwell BOO Index 58),[14] and a post-void residual of 200 mL (Figure 30.1c). MRI and VUDS are standard investigations in our unit for all patients with urethral diverticulum.

A transrectal ultrasound was also performed in an attempt to delineate the path of her rectus fascial sling behind the pubis and relationship to the diverticulum. Ultrasound did not identify the sling but did demonstrate the circumferential diverticulum surrounding the proximal to mid urethra.

Her case was discussed at the multidisciplinary team meeting. Her symptom complex was considered to be a consequence of her urethral diverticulum. It was possible that the diverticulum had recurred as a consequence of BOO from the rectus fascial sling, although it was impossible to exclude a persistent/recurrent urethral diverticulum as the primary cause. Detrusor overactivity was felt to be consequent to BOO.

The patient had extensive counselling regarding the options for managing her symptomatic recurrent complex urethral diverticulum. She was offered the options of the following:

1. Conservative management with observation and/or anticholinergic or beta-agonist; or botulinum toxin to treat her urgency incontinence symptoms. She would continue to be catheter dependent. Her urgency symptoms would be unlikely to completely resolve, and her pain/dyspareunia would persist. There is a risk of up to 9% of

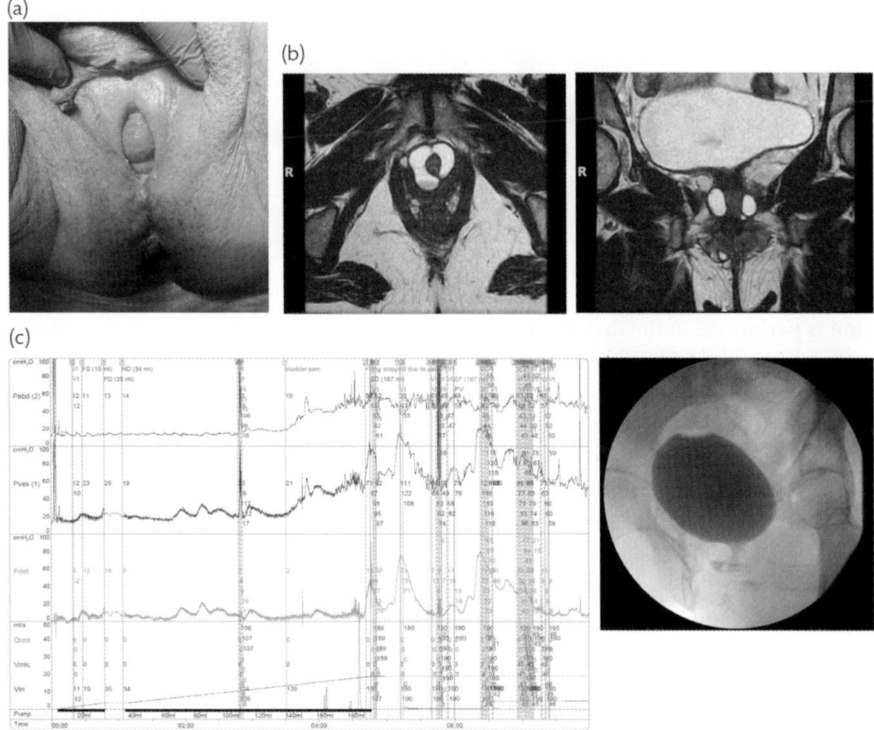

Figure 30.1 Clinical assessment and investigation of urethral diverticula. (a) A large urethral diverticulum seen bulging behind the urethral meatus. (b) MRI scan showing a recurrent, dorsal, large horseshoe diverticulum surrounding the urethra for 300° from 3 o'clock to 5 o'clock. (c) Video cystometrography showing detrusor overactivity and BOO.

malignant transformation with untreated urethral diverticula.[13] This would require annual follow-up with vaginal examination and MRI pelvis, although MRI surveillance for urethral carcinoma is unproven.

2. Marsupialization of the diverticulum—this may reduce the bulk and infections but risks creating a fistula between the urethra and the vagina and persistent leak. There would be no guarantee that her outflow obstruction and catheter dependency would resolve. The risk of malignant transformation would not change.[15]
3. Excision of the recurrent urethral diverticulum with urethrolysis and Martius labial fat pad interposition—considered the standard of management for urethral diverticula.[16]

Expert comment Risk of urethral diverticulum excision

There is a 98% chance that the diverticulum can be completely excised (2% chance that it may recur) and a 1–2% chance of the patient developing a new urethrovaginal fistula consequent to the excision.[16] She was informed of a 80–90% chance of being free of recurrent infections, >90% chance of resolution of her vaginal pain and dyspareunia, a 70–90% chance of being relieved of her outflow obstruction, and consequently a >50% chance of her detrusor overactivity, the cause of her urge incontinence, settling.[16]

The main risk of urethral diverticulum excision is *de novo* or worsening SUI in 10–30%. The risk of SUI is higher with larger and more extensive horseshoe diverticula and repeat surgery. The SUI improves and can be managed in the majority of patients with conservative measures. Due to the complexity of this lady's recurrent diverticulum including the horseshoe configuration with dorsal extension around the urethra, and the urethrolysis required to deal with the obstructive rectus fascia sling, the patient was advised her risk of significant postoperative SUI was 20–30%. She was told that she had a 10–15% risk of eventually requiring further salvage surgery for SUI at 12 months.[17]

The patient was informed that at our institution a Martius labial fat pad interposition is performed in the majority of urethral diverticula excisions to cover the urethral reconstruction and fill the defect. The risk of labial infection/abscess is <2%. Martius harvest can cause labial dissymmetry and discomfort. However, 80% of women find the cosmesis excellent or very good and <1% unsatisfactory. Labial discomfort generally settles with gentle massage of the wound, with persistence in <5%.[18,19] The patient was given the British Association of Urological Surgeons patient information sheets on excision of urethral diverticulum to complement the information provided in her clinic letter.

The patient opted for surgical excision of the recurrent urethral diverticulum, urethrolysis, and Martius fat pad interposition.

Clinical tip Surgical technique

In experienced hands, nearly all diverticula can be accessed and excised from a ventral approach through the anterior vaginal wall. Even those with circumferential configuration can be accessed from this incision, mobilizing the urethra as required, without the necessity for a dorsal approach to drop the urethra.

- The procedure is performed with the patient in steep lithotomy.
- A preliminary cystourethroscopy is performed to assess the urethra and bladder, which were unremarkable. Urethral diverticular os are not often identified and was not seen in this case. A CH16 urethral catheter was inserted.
- The anterior vaginal wall was infiltrated with 10 mL of 0.5% Xylocaine® with 1 in 200,000 adrenaline. A midline anterior vaginal wall incision was made, centred over the urethral diverticulum, and dissection of the periurethral tissue from the vaginal aspect of the diverticulum was performed. A large near-circumferential dorsal diverticulum was identified (Figure 30.2a).
- The plane between the urethra and the inner aspect of the diverticulum was then developed and the horseshoe diverticulum was completely dissected from dorsum to ventrum and excised in two halves (Figure 30.2b).
- The 5 o'clock opening into urethra was closed with a 5/0 Vicryl® in two layers (Figure 30.2c) and this was leak tested with Instillagel™ injected into the urethra using a 10 mL syringe attached to a 20-gauge Venflon™.
- A Martius labial fat pad was harvested on its inferolateral pedicle with the superior pedicle ligated. The Martius fat pad was tunnelled into the vaginal defect and secured around the urethra with 6 × 4/0 Vicryl® (Figure 30.3a,b).
- The fat pad donor site was closed in layers with 3/0 Vicryl® over a minivac drain. The vagina was closed with 3/0 Vicryl® (Figure 30.3c) and a Hibitane™-soaked vaginal pack was used to give vaginal compression for 48 hours.
- The procedure is covered by enoxaparin and three doses of perioperative antibiotics.
- The vaginal pack and labial drain were removed at 48 hours and the patient was discharged once comfortable on oral analgesia.
- A pericatheter urethrogram was organized 3 to 4 weeks postoperatively to ensure the urethra had healed and the catheter was removed.

Expert comment

Concomitant anti-incontinence procedures

We **do not** perform concomitant anti-incontinence procedures at the time of urethral diverticulum surgery, as the majority do not require further intervention, and the placement of a fascial sling or colposuspension sutures around a fragile (healing) urethra has potential risk. The morbidity of Martius fat pad harvest is low. In our series of >130 patients, significant clinical issues with labial dissymmetry or discomfort were much less than 5%.

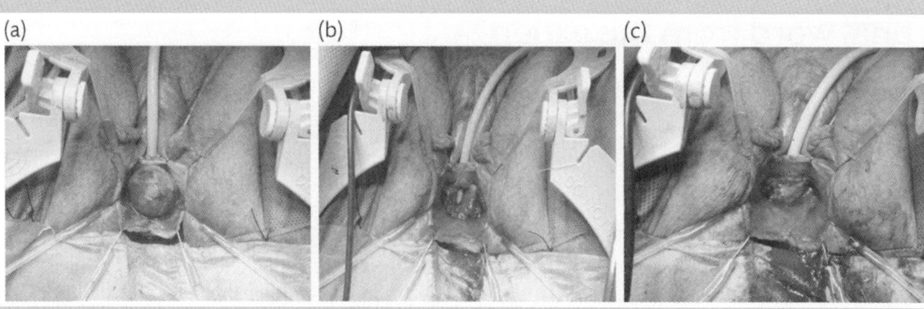

Figure 30.2 Exposure, dissection, and excision of the urethral diverticulum. (a) A large near-circumferential dorsal diverticulum. (b) Horseshoe diverticulum bivalved. The urethral opening (os) can be seen at 7 o'clock. (c) The 5 o'clock opening into urethra was closed with a 5/0 Vicryl® in two layers.

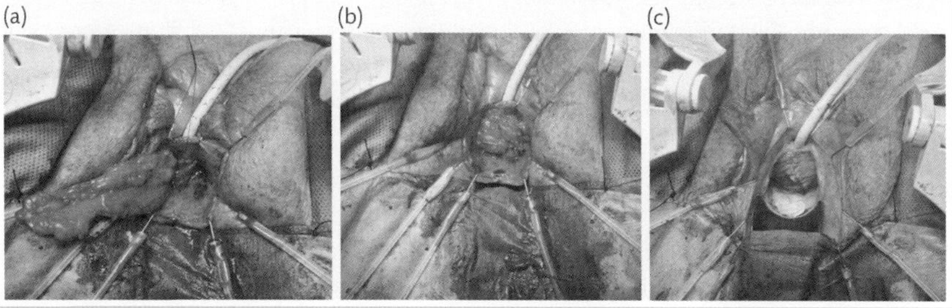

Figure 30.3 Martius labial fat pad interposition. (a) Martius labial fat pad was harvested on its inferolateral pedicle with the superior pedicle ligated and tunnelled into the vaginal defect. (b) Martius fat pad interposition and secured around the urethra with 6 × 4/0 Vicryl®. (c) Final appearance.

Expert comment Surgical excision and reconstruction

In the majority of cases, the dissection to remove the diverticulum leaves a urethral defect (differentiating a diverticulum from a paraurethral cyst), which can be primary repaired using fine-gauge Vicryl®. We test this repair to ensure that it is 'watertight' using Instillagel™ to retrograde fill the urethra using a CH20 Venflon™.

We are enthusiasts for the use of Martius fat pad interposition for much of our vaginal surgery including vesicovaginal fistulae and urethral diverticula. The fat pad is easy to harvest and interpose between the urethral repair and the vagina closure. The use of the Martius fat pad has reduced our failure (fistula) rate to <1%. In addition, the preservation of a distinct plane between the urethra and vagina allows much simpler access for salvage (incontinence) surgery. We have been able to salvage >90% of stress incontinent (10–20% of complex) patients with autologous slings or rarely an artificial urinary sphincter.

At 3 months, the patient was voiding well, and her preoperative vaginal pain had completely settled. She did complain of mild SUI (one pad). She was referred for pelvic floor exercises and her SUI improved over the next 9 months. At 12 months she was infection free, dry, and sexually active. She was delighted with the resolution of her symptoms.

Evidence base Management of urethral diverticulum

Between 1805 and 1954, only 17 cases of urethral diverticulum in women were described in the medical literature. Davis and Telinde published the defining series of 121 cases of urethral diverticula in 1958. Since that time, the literature and knowledge of this rare but important condition has blossomed. We would recommend recent reviews by O'Connor et al. (2018),[20] Bodner-Adler et al. (2016),[21] and Crescenze and Goldman (2015).[22]

Future directions Surgical options

About 150 new cases of urethral diverticula are diagnosed in the UK each year (Hospital Episode Statistics data 2016–2017). Further analysis is required to define which patients could be safely managed by excision and urethral reconstruction alone, and which patients would be best served by concomitant Martius fat pad interposition. It seems sensible that patients with a higher risk of SUI and thus secondary intervention would have Martius fat pads placed as the default position.

Expert comment Centralization of complex urethral diverticula

Most urethral diverticula are treated by surgeons (urologists and urogynaecologists) with limited experience of this delicate and often challenging surgery. There is general acceptance that rare and complex conditions should be centralized in expert centres and specialist commissioning is now developing along these lines.

A final word from the expert

Urethral diverticula are a rare diagnosis but cause substantive morbidity and distress. Many patients suffer debilitating lower urinary tract symptoms and pain for years before the diagnosis is thought of and diagnosed.

In expert hands, surgical excision and urethral reconstruction is successful in well over 90% of cases, with alleviation of the distressful symptom complex that this condition causes. The main risk of stress incontinence can be marginalized by the judicious use of the Martius fat pad interposition and subsequent salvage anti-incontinence procedures.

In the era in which the complications of interventions for SUI are becoming more apparent, long-term BOO from bulking agents, mesh tapes, and slings may be shown to be a significant contributory factor in the aetiology and development of urethral diverticula.

The centralization of complex female urology and concentration of surgical experience in specialist centres will lead to greater understanding and better functional outcomes for women with urethral diverticula.

References

1. Andersen MJ. The incidence of diverticula in the female urethra. *J Urol.* 1967;98(1):96–98.
2. El-Nasher SA, Bacon MM, Kim-Fine S, Weaver AL, Gebhart JB, Klingele CJ. Incidence of female urethral diverticulum: a population-based analysis and literature review. *Int Urogynecol J.* 2014;25(1):73–79.
3. Ockrim JL, Allen DJ, Shah PJ, Greenwell TJ. A tertiary experience of urethral diverticulectomy: diagnosis, imaging and surgical outcomes. *BJU Int.* 2009;103(11):1550–1554.
4. Hey W. Collection of pus in the vagina. In: *Practical Observations in Surgery*. Philadelphia, PA: James Humphreys; 1805:303–305.
5. Davis HJ, Telinde RW. Urethral diverticula: an assay of 121 cases. *J Urol.* 1958;80(1):34–39.
6. Tsivian M, Tsivian A, Schreiber L, Sidi AA, Koren R. Female urethral diverticulum: a pathological insight. *Int Urogynecol J Pelvic Floor Dysfunct.* 2009;20(8):957–960.
7. Routh A. Urethral diverticulum. *Br Med J.* 1890;8:360–365.
8. Cocco AE, MacLennan GT. Unusual female suburethral mass lesions. *J Urol.* 2005;174(3):1106.
9. Clemens JQ, Bushman W. Urethral diverticulum following collagen injection. *J Urol.* 2001;166(2):626.
10. Kumar D, Kaufman MR, Dmochowski RR. Case reports: periurethral bulking agents and presumed urethral diverticula. *Int Urogynecol J.* 2011;22(8):1039–1043.
11. Athanasopoulos A, McGuire EJ. Urethral diverticulum: a new complication associated with tension-free vaginal tape. *Urol Int.* 2008;81(4):480–482.
12. Hammad FT. TVT can also cause urethral diverticulum. *Int Urogynecol J Pelvic Floor Dysfunct.* 2007;18(4):467–469.
13. Greenwell TJ, Spilotros M. Urethral diverticula in women. *Nat Rev Urol.* 2015;12(12):671–680.
14. Solomon E, Yasmin H, Duffy M, Malde S, Ockrim J, Greenwell T. Concordance of urodynamic definitions of female bladder outlet obstruction. *Eur Urol Suppl.* 2017;16(3):e1965–e1966.
15. Spence HM, Duckett JW Jr. Diverticulum of the female urethra: clinical aspects and presentation of a simple operative technique for cure. *J Urol.* 1970;104(3):432–437.

16. Malde S, Sihra N, Naaser S, et al. Urethral diverticulectomy with Martius labial fat pad interposition improved symptom resolution and reduces recurrence. *BJU Int.* 2017;119(1):158–163.
17. Malde S, Naaseri S, Kavia R, et al. Preliminary report on the effect of urethral diverticulum magnetic resonance imaging configuration on the incidence of new onset urodynamic stress urinary incontinence following excision. *Urol Ann.* 2017;9(4):321–324.
18. Malde S, Pakzad M, Spilotros M, et al. The uses and outcomes of the Martius fat pad in urology. *World J Urol.* 2017;35(3):473–478.
19. Wilson A, Pillay S, Greenwell TJ. How and why to take a Martius labial interpositional flap in female urology. *TAU* 2017;6 (Supp 2):S81–S87.
20. O'Connor E, Iatropoulou D, Hashimoto S, Takahashi S, Ho DH, Greenwell T. Urethral diverticulum carcinoma in females—a case series and review of the English and Japanese literature. *Transl Androl Urol.* 2018;7(4):703–729.
21. Bodner-Adler B, Halpern K, Hanzal E. Surgical management of urethral diverticula in women: a systematic review. *Int Urogynecol J.* 2016;27(7):993–1001.
22. Crescenze IM, Goldman HB. Female urethral diverticulum: current diagnosis and management. *Curr Urol Rep.* 2015;16(10):71.

CASE

Management of ketamine-induced bilateral upper urinary tract injury

Ishtiakul G. Rizvi

Expert commentary Mohammed Belal

Case history

A 25-year-old male was admitted with signs of sepsis and acute kidney injury (AKI) on 26 October 2015. His vital signs were stable with one spike of temperature (38°C) on admission.

His blood parameters were reported as creatinine 517 μmol/L, estimated glomerular filtration rate (eGFR) 12 mL/min/1.73 m^2, C-reactive protein 298 mg/L, white blood cell count 15.5 × 10^9/L, and normal coagulation profile; however, an ultrasound scan (USS) of the urinary tract showed bilateral hydronephrosis. He underwent emergency bilateral nephrostomy insertion under general anaesthesia (GA) by the interventional radiology team because he was unable to tolerate the procedure under local anaesthesia or sedation.

His past medical history included mental behaviour disorder, ketamine-induced cystitis, and he is a known case of a chronic ketamine abuser. He has allergies to latex, tramadol, dust, and talcum powder and he is also known for having a very low pain threshold.

He underwent multiple endoscopic and percutaneous urological interventions including a complex reconstructive urological procedure (clam ileocystoplasty and Mitrofanoff procedure on 23 January 2015) due to ketamine-induced lower urinary tract injury.

Learning point Ketamine

Ketamine is an *N*-methyl-D-aspartate antagonist. It is metabolized in the liver to become an active form - norketamine, that is excreted in the urinary system. It has been used as an anaesthetic and analgesic agent since the 1960s.[1] It is also considered as a treatment option for major depression,[2] treatment-resistant depression,[3] bipolar affective disorder,[4] and pain. It has strong psychostimulant properties and its usage as a recreational drug was first reported in the 1970s.[5] Nowadays, ketamine is a common recreational street drug and its usage increased from 0.8% (in 2007–2008) to 2.1% (in 2010–2011) among young people in the UK aged between 16 and 24 years.[6]

The patient was initially referred in June 2009 for severe storage lower urinary tract symptoms with a history of chronic ketamine abuse. However, his renal function was normal and imaging showed no evidence of obstructive uropathy. Rigid cystoscopy under GA revealed inflamed bladder mucosa, ulceration, and bleeding on contact and bladder biopsy reported active inflammation. These findings were discussed with him in detail and he was offered bladder instillation therapy for symptom management.

He was strongly advised to stop using ketamine and was warned that progression of the disease would cause further bothersome urinary symptoms unless he stopped using ketamine. The potential consideration of bladder removal in case of failed medical management was mentioned. The patient refused to accept any forms of management (including medical management or bladder instillation) and was discharged back to community care.

In April 2013, the patient was re-referred to urology for the investigation of haematuria. A computed tomography scan revealed left hydronephrosis; his renal function was normal (eGFR >90 mL/min/1.73 m^2). However, a mercaptoacetyltriglycine (MAG3) renogram (May 2013) reported poor drainage of the left kidney and video urodynamics (July 2013) showed a small-capacity bladder, loss of compliance, with evidence of detrusor overactivity. Rigid cystoscopy with retrograde study (September 2013) demonstrated a small bladder capacity of 100 mL, petechial haemorrhage, and left hydronephrosis with left hydroureter. All of these findings were discussed in the local functional urology multidisciplinary team meeting.

The patient refused to accept simple cystectomy and urinary diversion with ileal conduit and its associated adverse effects on fertility and erectile function. Therefore, a clam ileocystoplasty with a Mitrofanoff was offered. Furthermore, he also declined to perform urethral self-catheterization but agreed to do self-catheterization via a Mitrofanoff. He was also strongly advised regarding stoppage or abstinence of ketamine for at least 6 months prior to the surgical intervention.

Expert comment Surveillance and compliance

The importance of regular surveillance from 2009 onwards could have been helpful in monitoring disease progression, avoid potential complication and making decision of early intervention. Therefore regular surveillance either by general practitioner or primary team, early social support, education about fatal consequence of ketamine abuse and take measures to abstinence from ketamine abuse are essential. It will be helpful not only to abstinence from ketamine abuse but also helpful to avoid disease progression and/or its serious consequences. However, compliance of the patient is an important issue.

Learning point Ketamine abuse

Ketamine abuse leads to serious urological conditions and the most common presentation is ketamine-associated ulcerative cystitis (severe lower urinary tract symptoms with dysuria, frequency, urgency, and haematuria).[7] However, a limited number of cases have been reported previously in the published literature regarding ketamine's effects throughout the urinary tract or upper tract involvement. Nevertheless, it is a complex and increasingly prevalent challenging clinical condition. The management of ketamine induced upper tract injury requires a holistic and multidisciplinary approach.

The patient developed AKI and sepsis in July 2014 prior to the planned surgical procedure (clam ileocystoplasty and Mitrofanoff) and imaging revealed worsening left hydronephrosis. His MAG3 renogram showed an obstructed left kidney and poor drainage of the right kidney. Therefore, he underwent emergency bilateral nephrostomy tube insertion under GA for the drainage of both kidneys.

Expert comment Monitoring of the abstinence of ketamine usage

Aggressive holistic management (including involvement of the general practitioner, the community nurse, psychiatric team and social support) is necessary for the regular monitoring of the abstinence of ketamine usage. It is also essential to educate the patient about the consequence of continuous ketamine abuse. It will be helpful not only to reduce the incidence of admission with deteriorating urinary symptoms or renal function and improvement of the patient's compliance but also to proceed on the further medical and surgical intervention within the expected time.

The patient underwent clam ileocystoplasty with ileal chimney and Mitrofanoff formation and bilateral ureteric reimplantation in January 2015 following abstinence of ketamine usage for >6 months while maintaining his bilateral nephrostomy tubes *in situ*. His bilateral nephrostogram in February 2015 reported no obvious obstruction on the left side but slow flow of contrast on the right side. He was discharged with bilateral nephrostomy tubes *in situ* but clamped for observation.

Clinical tip Ileal chimney

In this particular case, an ileal chimney was made along with the clam ileocystoplasty procedure in anticipation of future reconstructive procedures (if disease progressed to the upper urinary tract or renal pelvis), such as formation of ileal conduit. It is important and necessary to plan ahead about further or future reconstructive procedure in advance because sometimes patient require multiple surgical interventions when there is an evidence of disease progression or no improvement or worsening of symptoms. Therefore the necessity of thinking ahead in reconstructive functional urology procedure is essential.

The patient failed to perform self-catheterization via his Mitrofanoff due to stenosis of the Mitrofanoff channel within a few weeks of the procedure (March 2015). He needed an emergency rigid cystoscopy with suprapubic catheter insertion due to a failed trial of Mitrofanoff dilatation and failed retrograde bilateral ureteric stent reinsertion under GA. Subsequently, bilateral antegrade stent insertion was performed by the interventional radiology team to allow free drainage of both kidneys.

Bilateral ureteric stents were removed on 23 October 2015 (creatinine 136 µmol/L and eGFR 55 mL/min/1.73 m^2) following improvement of his renal function. However, he subsequently developed AKI and signs of sepsis on 26 October 2015 (creatinine 517 µmol/L, eGFR 12 mL/min/1.73 m^2, C-reactive protein 296 mg/L). His USS reported bilateral hydronephrosis and he required emergency bilateral nephrostomy tube insertion on 26 October 2015.

Expert comment Disease progression

Progression of the disease may occur despite cessation of ketamine usage and therefore necessity of keeping bilateral nephrostomy tube in situ with a plan of regular change until consideration of any major reconstructive procedure. This particular patient had bilateral ureteric stents including resonant (metallic) stent, however ureteric stents failed to drain both kidneys effectively which led to repeated hospital admissions with AKI or blocked nephrostomies, with signs of urosepsis requiring changes or re-insertion of nephrostomy tubes.

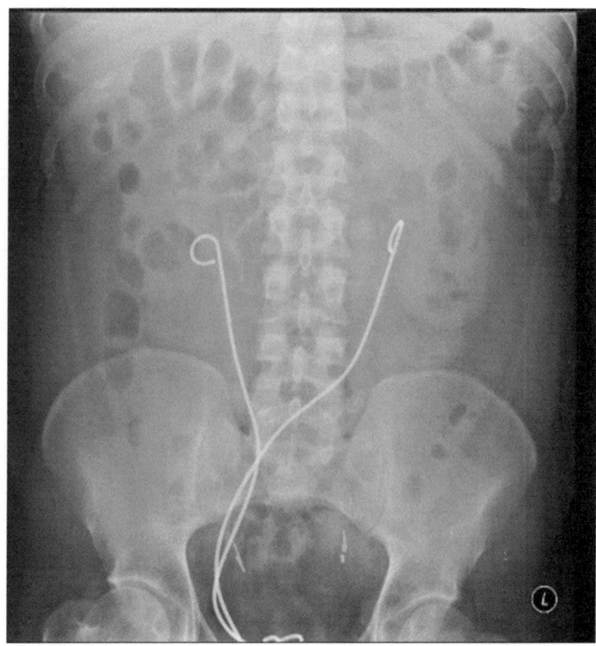

Figure 31.1 Bilateral resonant stents *in situ*.

Rigid cystoscopy and bilateral retrograde resonant (metallic) ureteric stents were inserted under GA in January 2016 due to bilateral pelviureteric junction obstruction reported on nephrostogram (Figure 31.1). He was discharged after removal of both nephrostomy tubes following the procedure with improved stable renal function (creatinine 146 μmol/L and eGFR 51 mL/min/1.73 m^2).

Expert comment Disease progression and further surgery

There is an evidence of disease progression because the patient developed bilateral hydronephrosis with AKI despite having bilateral resonant (metallic) ureteric stents *in situ*. It was proven that bilateral ureteric stent failed to ensure effective drainage of both kidneys and the patient required emergency nephrostomy tube insertion for the improvement of renal function and ensure effective drainage of the renal system. Therefore, the necessity of further reconstructive surgery was paramount.

The patient was readmitted with AKI (creatinine 317 μmol/L, eGFR 21 mL/min/1.73 m^2) and USS reported bilateral hydronephrosis (March 2016) despite having bilateral resonant ureteric stents. Subsequently, he had emergency bilateral nephrostomy insertion (March 2016) by the interventional radiology team (Figure 31.2).

The patient was discharged with bilateral nephrostomies (3-monthly changes) until a further planned reconstructive procedure was made. He had further admissions due to urosepsis and required changes of bilateral nephrostomies due to blockage or dislodgement.

Finally, the patient underwent ileal segmental anastomosis with a continuous isoperistaltic ileal segment running from the left renal pelvis to the right renal pelvis and an anastomosis to the end of the previous ileal chimney (Figure 31.3) in February 2017. It is similar to a roux-en-Y configuration and bilateral nephrostomies were left on free

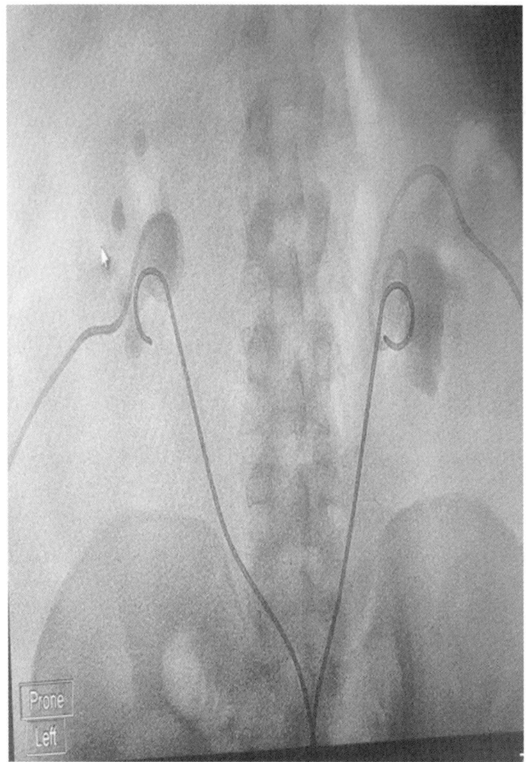

Figure 31.2 Bilateral nephrostogram showing evidence of obstruction at the pelviureteric junction bilaterally. There is visualization of the renal pelvis and no evidence of contrast passing into both ureters despite having bilateral resonant (metallic) ureteric stents.

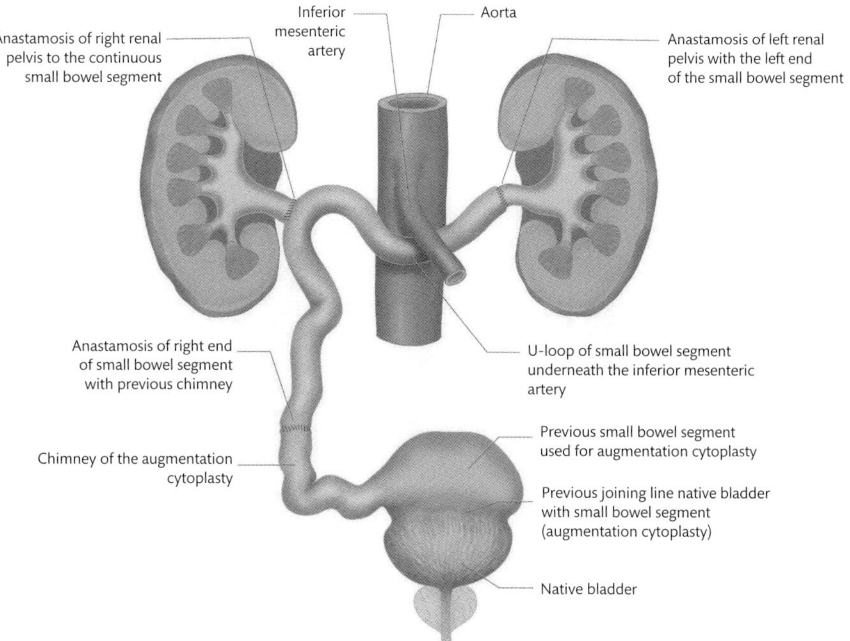

Figure 31.3 Schematic diagram of the complex reconstructive procedure.
Courtesy: University Hospitals Birmingham illustration department, Andrew Dakin.

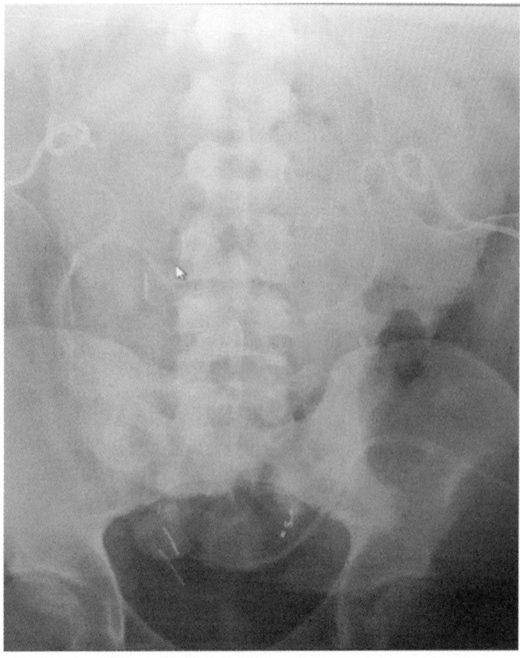

Figure 31.4 Post-reconstructive procedure X-ray of the kidneys, ureters, and bladder showing bilateral ureteric stents lying within the configuration of the anastomosis with bilateral nephrostomies *in situ*.

drainage with the bilateral ureteric stents *in situ* (Figure 31.4) as part of the reconstruction. His baseline creatinine level and eGFR were 147 µmol/L and 47 mL/min/1.73 m^2 respectively at the time of operation.

A bilateral nephrostogram was performed within 6 weeks of the reconstructive surgical procedure (March 2017) which showed no evidence of obstruction with free drainage of contrast (Figure 31.5). Both nephrostomies and ureteric stents were removed and renal function remained stable (creatinine 157 µmol/L and eGFR 42 mL/min/1.73 m^2).

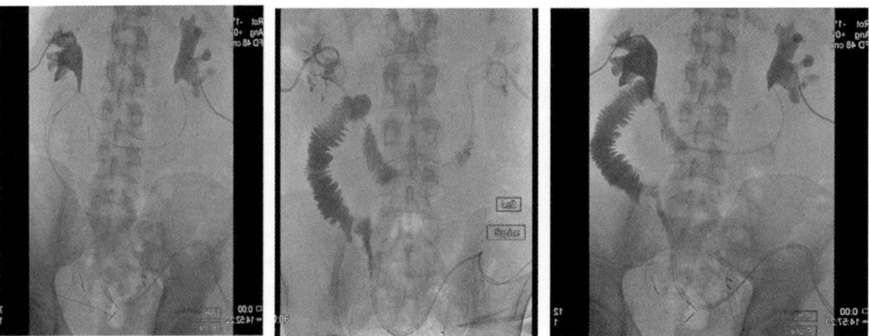

Figure 31.5 Post-reconstruction nephrostograms showing the configuration of procedure with bilateral stents and nephrostomies *in situ*. Visualization of the ileal segment from the left renal pelvis to the right renal pelvis and contrast moving down to the ileal chimney to the augmented bladder.

Clinical tip Anastomoses

The complications of anastomoses involving bowel and urinary tracts are well recognized and it has significant impact on the outcome of the procedure. The numbers of anastomoses are usually high in reconstructive procedures. Therefore, performing a minimum number of anastomoses while using small bowel (ileum) as a continuous segment joining the left renal pelvis, right renal pelvis, and with the previous ileal chimney (three anastomoses) reduces the chance of anastomotic-related complications. The importance of planning reconstructive surgical procedure (such as using of bowel segment and number of anastomotic sites) is crucial.

Clinical tip Mobilization of the ileal segment

The selected segment of the ileum needs to be mobilized under the inferior mesenteric artery following mobilization of both small bowel and large bowel, similar to a standard retroperitoneal lymph node dissection procedure. However the ileal segment can also be mobilized through a mesentery window, but in our case, it was done through the formal method to reduce the tension on the mesentery and also to make the ileal segment become isoperistaltic. It has significant relation to the early recovery of the post operative period, reduce morbidity and eventually the outcome of the procedure.

Clinical tip Metabolic complications

One of the common long term complications of reconstructive procedure is malabsorption syndrome due to using a significant length of bowel segment. It is necessary to monitor the serum biochemical level regularly to rule out any biochemical abnormalities such as serum bicarbonate, serum vitamin B12 and serum folate level. Low serum bicarbonate level is one of most common abnormalities and requires regular sodium bicarbonate supplementation. Therefore lifelong follow up after the reconstructive procedure is essential to monitor and treatment of the biochemical abnormalities.

Outcome and follow-up

The patient's baseline creatinine level (157–220 μmol/L) and eGFR (38–46 mL/min/ 1.73 m^2) remained stable at a follow-up of 34 months.

The MAG3 renogram in July 2017 showed sluggish flow on the left side (due to the surgical configuration) with no obvious obstruction in the right side and the USS in December 2017 demonstrated stable left hydronephrosis with mild fullness of the right renal pelvis.

He was under regular urology follow-up every 3 months for the first year and currently, every 6 months to monitor his renal function along with USS surveillance for hydronephrosis. Furthermore, he is now on regular sodium bicarbonate supplementation therapy for his low serum bicarbonate level.

In addition, he is under regular follow-up with the renal physician team for chronic kidney disease as part of a multidisciplinary and holistic management approach to manage this rare catastrophic clinical condition involving the entire urinary tract following chronic ketamine abuse.

Expert comment Multidisciplinary team involvement and education of the patient

Multidisciplinary team involvement is essential (such as renal medicine, urology, psychiatry, and social support) for the holistic management of the patient with chronic ketamine abuse. The importance of patient's education and appropriate information regarding potential disease progression or complication should be discussed in a specialized clinic. This group of patient should be under regular follow up and ensure about abstinence from ketamine abuse by providing adequate social and mental support. They also need lifelong follow up which will help to monitor the disease progression and involvement of multidisciplinary team earlier for planning of further management prior to the development of catastrophic consequence.

Discussion

The incidence of ketamine-associated urinary tract injury (cystitis and upper tract involvement) is a complex and challenging syndrome.

It needs a patient-centred approach including consideration of the patient's psychosocial issues and co-morbidities, and long-term abstinence of ketamine is essential for treatment to be successful.[8]

There are various treatment modalities and the use of intravesical agents such as dimethylsulfoxide and hyaluronic acid (Cystistat®) is also common. But no medical management shows any significant success if there is evidence of continued ketamine abuse.[8]

Medical management relies on symptomatic control with combinations of anticholinergic, antibiotic, steroid, and non-steroidal anti-inflammatory drugs.[9]

Disease progression or failed medical management leads to consideration of surgical management such as hydrodistension, urinary diversion, augmentation cystoplasty,[10,11] autotransplantation, and pyelovesicostomy.[12]

It has been reported that ureteric transmural inflammation and ulceration leads to stricture and hydronephrosis.[13] Ureteric stenting is the most common form of management of obstructive uropathy prior to extensive surgical intervention.

Small bowel interposition is commonly used for ureteric reconstruction in case of extensive ureteric injuries and the common complications of small bowel interposition as part of reconstruction are metabolic abnormalities, mucus production, and renal dysfunction. Furthermore, the risk of small bowel syndrome with formation of renal stones, dehydration, and malabsorption syndrome is higher if the patient has had prior small bowel resection.

Evidence base Ketamine abuse and hydronephrosis

Ketamine induced cystitis (frequency, urgency, nocturia, dysuria and suprapubic pain) is the most common urological presentation due to direct toxic effects of ketamine and its metabolites. However, toxic effects of ketamine in the upper urinary tract are becoming a well-recognized clinical condition leading to development of hydronephrosis or obstructive uropathy. Chu et al. reported 30 out of 59 patients (51%) presenting with lower urinary tract symptoms due to ketamine abuse had unilateral or bilateral hydronephrosis on renal USS.[9] However. Tam et al. reported 8.1% had hydronephrosis in a cohort of 160 patients.[14]

Evidence base Risk factors for hydronephrosis

Most of these patients in Chu et al.[9] case series were found to have hydronephrosis and hyroureter down to the level of vesico-ureteric junctions on intravenous urogram implying upper tract involvement was due to long term decrease in bladder compliance however in Yee et al. series ureteric obstruction was found in some patient and level of obstruction varied from vesicoureteric junction to the pelvic-ureteric junction. Yee et al. reported that age, full blood count, serum creatinine level, and abnormal serum liver enzyme profile were associated with the risk of hydronephrosis. The resolution of hydronephrosis was noted in some patients following abstinence of ketamine usage but require further study to confirm. However, permanent toxicity to the upper urinary tract is still of concern with long-term ketamine abuse.[15]

Learning point Pathological changes

Gross pathological changes of the urinary tract include contracted bladder, thickening of the bladder wall, adhesion to the peritoneum, dilatation of ureters, and thickening of the ureteric wall.

Endoscopic pathological changes are erythematous bladder mucosa (bleeds easily), ulceration of bladder mucosa and laceration on hydrodistension, swelling, and oedematous mucosa of the ureter.

Microscopic pathological changes are denuded urothelium, formation of granulation tissue with infiltration by mast cells, eosinophils, lymphocytes, and plasma cells, fibrinoid necrosis of arterioles, focal calcification, muscle hypertrophy, collagen accumulation, thickening of ureteric wall, and ureteric mucosal infiltration by inflammatory cells and eosinophils.[16–19]

Here, we report our case of ketamine-induced complete bilateral upper urinary tract obstruction / uropathy involving both renal pelvises managed with ileal segmental anastomoses. The ileal segment passes from the left renal pelvis to the right renal pelvis and was anastomosed to the previous ileal chimney (roux-en-Y configuration). It ensures normal flow of urine following failed augmentation cystoplasty and medical management. This case highlights the multidisciplinary management of renal dysfunction and biochemical abnormalities and demonstrates the challenging surgical treatment following devastating effects of bilateral upper urinary tract involvement due to chronic ketamine usage that developed following augmentation cystoplasty. It also helps us to develop awareness regarding ketamine effects throughout the entire urinary tract (lower and upper urinary tract). In this case, we report 34 months of surgical outcome of the complex surgical management of ketamine-induced bilateral upper urinary tract obstruction and the necessity of involvement of a multidisciplinary team (renal medicine, urology) for lifelong follow-up.

Conclusion

The surgical management of ketamine-induced bilateral upper urinary tract injury is complex and needs a holistic approach for lifelong follow-up. However, surgical intervention is based on local expertise and tailed to the individual patient. To the best of our knowledge, this is the first case reported using iso-peristaltic ileal segmental anastomosis involving both renal pelvis with continuation of the ileal segment to the previous ileal chimney of the clam ileocystoplasty procedure with 34 months of follow-up.

A final word from the expert

Ketamine-induced urinary tract injury is increasing because of its popularity as a common recreational street drug among the younger generation. It has catastrophic consequences due to its devastating effects on the urinary tract and it needs lifelong multidisciplinary team management. Abstinence of using ketamine is the most important step of reducing the progression of the disease; however, permanent toxicity still remains high in chronic ketamine abuse.

The management of the ketamine-induced lower urinary tract injury includes management of symptoms (medical management) and surgical intervention (failed medical management). However, upper urinary tract injury needs surgical intervention such as ureteric stenting and ileal interposition of the ureter if hydronephrosis develops due to benign ureteric stricture following chronic ketamine abuse.

The maintenance of potency is important during consideration of extensive surgical management of the younger patient; therefore, the option of cystectomy may not be popular among this group of patients. The importance of increasing bladder capacity to improve the bladder compliance is essential in case of a small non-compliant bladder. However, extensive upper urinary tract damage may occur despite cessation of using ketamine and ultimately leads to a bespoke solution to be formulated.

There are currently no guidelines available regarding management of ketamine-induced upper urinary tract injury. Therefore, careful patient selection, planning of surgical intervention, discussion in a multidisciplinary team meeting, holistic approach including the patient's education of the disease process with their involvement in the management plan, involvement of other specialities (such as renal medicine), and lifelong follow-up are essential for the optimal management of ketamine-induced upper urinary tract injury.

References

1. Lankenau SE, Sanders B. Patterns of ketamine use among young injection drug users. *J Psychoactive Drugs.* 2007;39(1):21–29.
2. Walter M, Li S, Demenescu LR. Multistage drug effects of ketamine in the treatment of major depression. *Eur Arch Psychiatry Clin Neurosci.* 2014;264(Suppl 1):S55–65.
3. Wan LB, Levitch CF, Perez AM, et al. Ketamine safety and tolerability in clinical trials for treatment-resistant depression. *J Clin Psychiatry.* 2015;76(3):247–252.
4. Best SR. Combined ketamine/transcranial magnetic stimulation treatment of severe depression in bipolar I disorder. *J ECT.* 2014;30(4):e50–e51.
5. Kalsi SS, Wood DM, Dargan PI. The epidemiology and patterns of acute and chronic toxicity associated with recreational ketamine use. *Emerg Health Threats J.* 2011;4:7107.
6. Forster JA, Harrison SC. Ketamine uropathy: rising to the challenges of a new condition. *BJU Int.* 2012;109(9):1277–1278.
7. Shahani R, Streutker C, Dickson B. Ketamine-associated ulcerative cystitis a new clinical entity. *Urology.* 2007;69(5):810–812.
8. Lai Y, Wu S, Ni L. Ketamine-associated urinary tract dysfunction: an under recognized clinical entity. *Urol Int.* 2012;89(1):93–96.
9. Chu PSK, Ma WK, Wong SCW. The destruction of the lower urinary tract by ketamine abuse: a new syndrome? *BJU Int.* 2008;102(11):1616–1622.
10. Ng CF, Chiu PKF, Li ML. Clinical outcomes of augmentation cystoplasty in patients suffering from ketamine-related bladder contractures. *Int Urol Nephrol.* 2013;45(5):1245–1251.
11. Misra S, Chetwood A, Coker C. Ketamine cystitis: practical considerations in management. *Scand J Urol.* 2014;48(5):482–488.
12. Raison NT, O'Brien T, Game D, Olsburgh J. Autotransplantation for the management of ketamine ureteritis. *BMJ Case Rep.* 2015;2015:bcr2014207652.
13. Hopcroft SA, Cottrell AM, Mason K, et al. Ureteric intestinal metaplasia in association with chronic recreational ketamine abuse. *J Clin Pathol.* 2011;64(6):551–552.

14. Tam YH, Ng CF, Pang KK, et al. One stop clinic for ketamine-associated uropathy: report on service delivery model, patients' characteristics and non-invasive investigations at baseline by a cross-sectional study in a prospective cohort of 318 teenagers and young adults. *BJU Int.* 2014;114(5):754–760.
15. Yee CH, Teoh JY, Lai PT, et al. The risk of upper urinary tract involvement in patients with ketamine associated uropathy. *Int Neurourol J.* 2017;21(2):128–132.
16. Jhang JF, Hsu YH, Kuo HC. Possible pathophysiology of ketamine-related cystitis and associated treatment strategies. *Int J Urol.* 2015;22(9):816–825.
17. Chung SD, Wang CC, Kuo HC. Augmentation enterocystoplasty is effective in relieving refractory ketamine-related bladder. *Neurourol Urodyn.* 2014;33(8):1207–1211.
18. Chu PS, Kwok SC, Lam KM, et al. 'Street ketamine'-associated bladder dysfunction: a report of ten cases. *Hong Kong Med J.* 2007;3(4):311–313.
19. Huang LK, Wang JH, Shen SH, Lin AT, Chang CY. Evaluation of the extent of ketamine-induced uropathy: the role of CT urography. *Postgrad Med J.* 2014;90(1062):185–190.

CASE

32 Vesicovaginal fistula

Sachin Malde

Expert commentary Arun Sahai

Case history

A 48-year-old lady was referred to our centre with a history of vaginal leak 2 months post laparoscopic total hysterectomy and bilateral salpingo-oophorectomy. The gynaecological surgery was performed for potential malignancy based on blood tests and imaging but her final histology was benign. The patient reported urinary leak from the vagina day 1 post surgery. She was managed with a urinary catheter at the referring hospital. Despite this she continued to have a vaginal leak. The local urology team were asked to review the patient and a cystoscopy and bilateral retrograde studies were performed, which revealed evidence of some suture material in the bladder above the trigone, and above and medial to the left ureteric orifice with no evidence of ureteric injury. The suture material was removed endoscopically and a catheter was left for a further 2 weeks. A cystogram performed at that time suggested a vesicovaginal fistula (VVF) and the patient was referred to our centre.

On review in our clinic, the patient was noted to have a background of mixed connective tissue disorder, autoimmune arthritis requiring steroids, type 1 diabetes, coeliac disease, depression, and had two previous Caesarean sections. The patient reported worsening of urinary incontinence and vaginal leak despite the indwelling urethral catheter and so this was removed just prior to our first review.

Prior to the hysterectomy the patient did not complain of bothersome lower urinary tract symptoms or incontinence. She was clearly distressed with her symptoms and a number of investigations were organized including midstream specimen of urine, urea and electrolytes, cystoscopy plus examination under anaesthetic/methylene blue test/retrograde studies, and an up-to-date computed tomography intravenous urogram. At cystoscopy, a clear VVF was demonstrated (Figure 32.1). This was assessed both intravesically with the cystoscope and vaginally. A well-formed 1 cm × 0.5 cm fistula was seen approximately 1 cm above and medial to the left ureteric orifice. Bilateral retrograde studies were performed which were normal and she was noted to have a good capacity bladder. The rest of her bladder was unremarkable. The computed tomography intravenous urogram revealed normal upper tracts and no evidence of pelvic collection. The midstream specimen of urine was clear and her renal function normal.

Expert comment Urgent referrals

If a VVF is suspected early, urgent referral to a specialist is required for diagnosis, as early repair is feasible if identified typically within the first week. After this time, oedema, inflammation, potential tissue necrosis, and infection make successful repair of the VVF challenging. Expert opinion would suggest that if a VVF is identified later than this time, the optimal time for repair would be after 3 months and some may argue at 6 months.

Learning point Aetiology of VVF

- Obstetric trauma, for example, prolonged labour (commonest in low-resourced/underdeveloped world).
- Other obstetric causes include Caesarean section, forceps delivery, and uterine rupture.
- Pelvic surgery, for example, hysterectomy (commonest in developed/well-resourced world); others include benign and malignant colorectal, gynaecological, and urological surgery.
- Pelvic radiation.
- Advanced pelvic malignancy.
- Foreign body.
- Trauma—pelvic fracture, sexual.
- Congenital.

Clinical tip Removing urethral catheters prior to surgical repair

The catheter will cause an inflammatory reaction on the posterior wall of the bladder and often will involve the bladder base, which is often the site of the VVF. In our view, removing the catheter in advance of the planned repair will allow the catheter reaction to settle, optimizing the chances of a successful repair. Furthermore, the patient will often find the catheter uncomfortable and, as in this case, it usually does not prevent vaginal leak.

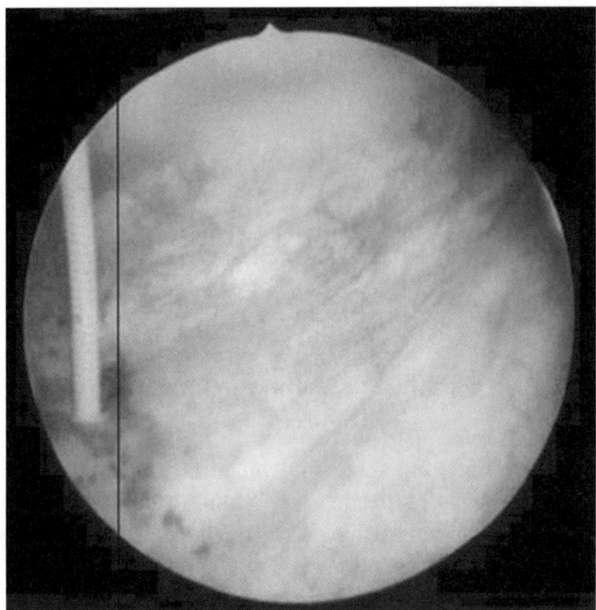

Figure 32.1 Cystoscopic view of a VVF with sensor guidewire placed through it.

Clinical tip Cystoscopy and examination under anaesthetic

Always perform your own evaluation of the urinary incontinence. At cystoscopy and examination under anaesthetic, it is important to assess the location and size of the fistula and the quality of the tissue planned for repair. There may be more than one VVF! Retrograde studies should be performed routinely to assess for ureteric involvement and ureterovaginal fistula or ureteric injury. Furthermore, one must decide whether the VVF can be repaired through the vaginal or abdominal route or in select cases where the tissue quality is so poor a further delay and re-evaluation or urinary diversion may be required. In cases of uncertainty, attempt to place a small catheter or Fogarty balloon catheter through the VVF with the tubing exiting through the vagina. Then place gentle traction onto the tubing to see if this helps with bringing the VVF into the field of view to allow vaginal repair. In our opinion, the vaginal route of repair is preferable and will allow a quicker postoperative recovery. In cases where the VVF cannot be easily identified and doubt remains about the diagnosis, a methylene blue test should be performed.

Learning point Methylene blue test

This involves placing three appropriately sized swabs into the vagina sequentially to fill the upper, mid, and lower (closest to the introitus) portions of the vaginal length. Ensure the vagina is dry prior to inserting the three swabs. Methylene blue is then instilled into the bladder via a catheter (at least 200 mL) and the catheter removed. The dye is left in the bladder for at least 15 minutes. The swabs can then be removed. Blue staining on the upper swab indicates a VVF. Blue staining on the lower swab indicates either a urethrovaginal fistula or contamination of the dye from urethral leak into the introitus (careful removal of the catheter is required and also caution to not over-distend the bladder with dye). Finally, a wet upper swab that has no dye suggests a ureterovaginal fistula. If all swabs are dry with no staining there is unlikely to be a VVF.

Learning point Abdominal route for VVF repair

The abdominal route for VVF repair is required if the VVF is thought to be inaccessible per vagina, the ureter is involved or at risk of compromise from vaginal repair, or simultaneous augmentation cystoplasty is required. In such cases, the abdominal route is preferred. Ureteric reimplantation can be performed at the same time if required or planned. In abdominal cases of repair, typically the posterior bladder is bivalved to the fistula site and using sharp dissection the plane between the bladder and vagina separated and developed. The vagina is then closed and the greater omentum or peritoneum mobilized and used as an interposition graft over the repair site before closing the bladder.

Expert comment Advanced pelvic malignancy and radiotherapy

In cases of advanced pelvic malignancy and/or as a result of cancer treatment such as radiotherapy as a cause of VVF, repair may not be possible if the tissue quality is too poor. In a wide radiotherapy field, there may be concomitant problems such as ureteric stricture(s), enteritis/proctitis, and the environment may be too hostile to allow healing and repair. In selected cases where oncologically it is appropriate, a urinary diversion procedure should be considered, such as an ileal conduit.

A week later the patient underwent elective vaginal repair of the fistula with Martius fat pad interposition. In brief, she was positioned in a supine Trendelenburg position with her legs in lithotomy. A 6-French (Fr) ureteric catheter was fed up the left ureter in order to help protect and identify any ureteric injury during VVF repair and was secured to a 14 Fr urethral catheter draining the bladder. A lone star retractor was set up to help facilitate retraction of tissues. An 8 Fr catheter was utilized to catheterize the fistula with the tubing being exteriorized through the vagina. This helped to bring the VVF into the surgical field and be more accessible. In addition, 2/0 Vicryl® stay sutures were utilized either side of the VVF and tacked to the lone star retractor to bring the VVF into the field of view. The fistula was sharply circumscribed and a plane developed between the bladder and vaginal walls. Stay sutures were again employed to facilitate retraction of the dissected edge of the vaginal tissue. The bladder defect was exposed with a 0.5 cm margin all around and was closed with interrupted 3/0 polydioxanone sutures and was leak tested to be watertight. As there was a distinct lack of good-quality pubocervical fascia to close over the bladder as a second layer, a Martius fat pad was harvested from the right on its inferior pedicle and tunnelled into the fistula repair site with the use of a Statinsky clamp. The fat pad was laid over the repair and fixed to the fascia with three 2/0 Vicryl® sutures beyond the repair site. A suction drain was placed in a dependent position in the labial wound and the subcutaneous tissue closed with 2/0 Vicryl®. The labial skin was then closed with 3/0 Vicryl® Rapide and vaginal skin with 3/0 Vicryl®. A vaginal pack was left *in situ* overnight. She went on to make an unremarkable recovery and was discharged on postoperative day 3 with her catheter *in situ*. She then had a cystogram 3 weeks later, which showed no demonstrable leak from the bladder. Her catheter was removed. She had follow-up at 3 and 12 months and was discharged with no evidence of any vaginal leak.

Clinical tip Martius fat pad

Have a low threshold for the use of a Martius fat pad. It is important when repairing a VVF that there is a three-layer closure with non-overlying suture lines. Typically, the bladder, pubocervical fascia, and vaginal skin can make up the three layers and are closed at differing levels, for example, horizontal closure of the bladder and vertical closure of the pubocervical fascia and then lateral closure of the vaginal skin to prevent overlying suture lines (a risk for a recurrent VVF). However, often the pubocervical fascia cannot be well preserved during the dissection or the fistula is complex (i.e. large defect, radiotherapy) or the surgeon feels the tissue quality is poor, and so an interposition fat pad should be used. In our hands the Martius fat pad is an excellent choice.

Expert comment Martius fad pad

The Martius fat pad is the most suitable interposition pad to use for vaginal VVF repair. It receives its blood supply through two pedicles, superior based on external pudendal and inferior based on the internal pudendal artery. One pedicle is sacrificed, typically the superior one, and the labial fat pad is then swung into the vaginal field after dissection of the space between the labia and the sidewall of the vagina (Figure 32.2).

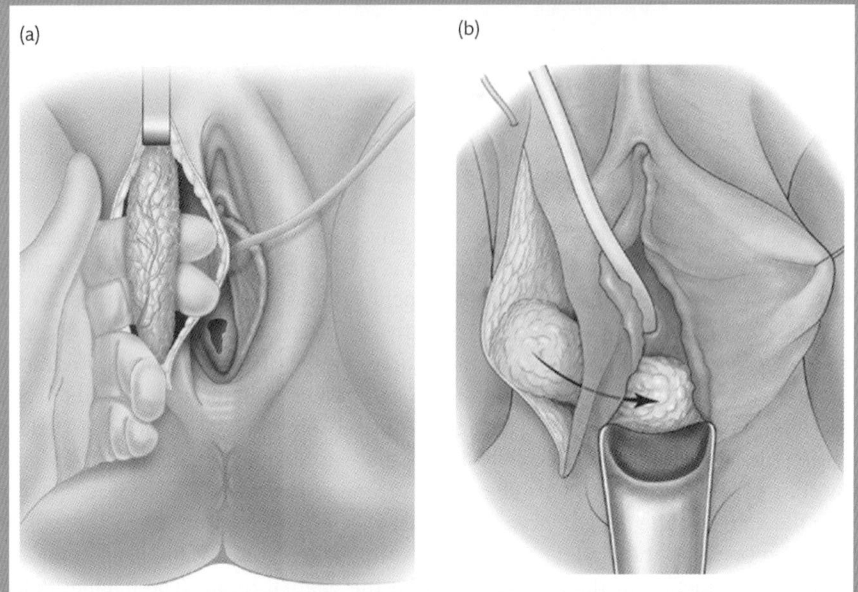

Figure 32.2 (a) Exposure of labial fat pad.[1] (b) Martius fat pad swung into the vaginal surgical field through a lateral vaginal wall tunnel. The graft is based on its inferior pedicle blood supply in this case.[1]

Discussion

The World Health Organization (WHO) has estimated that 2 million women from sub-Saharan Africa and Asia have fistulae and approximately 50,000–100,000 new women are affected each year.[2] Adler et al., in their systematic review and meta-analysis, were able to provide more robust estimates on prevalence, suggesting 1.60 (95% confidence interval (CI) 1.16–2.10) per 1000 women of reproductive age in sub-Saharan Africa and 1.20 (95% CI 0.10–3.54) per 1000 in South Asia regions.[2] The commonest cause in this population is obstructed labour. In the developing world, there is a distinct lack of services, poor obstetric care, as well as a lack of health-seeking behaviour. However, in the industrialized world, gynaecological or pelvic surgery are the main causes of VVF.

Expert comment Classification of VVF

Several classifications systems exist and the commonest utilized are those related to obstetric VVF such as Waaldijk's and Goh's classifications.[3,4] However, for iatrogenic fistula, the International Consultation on Incontinence has suggested using the WHO classification from 2006.

In general, there is a lack of high-quality studies in this field. According to the European Association of Urology guidelines on the management of non-obstetric urinary fistula, the majority of evidence is level 3 and recommendations are grade C, suggesting a need for better quality studies.[5]

Evidence base Systematic review: aetiology, treatment, and outcomes of urogenital fistulae in low- and well-resourced countries

In a systematic review[6] over a 35-year period, 49 articles were identified and suggested that in well-resourced countries, 83% of fistulae occurred following surgery, whereas in low-resourced countries, 95% were associated with childbirth. Conservative approaches, such as catheter drainage, are more likely to be successful for non-radiotherapy fistulae. The median overall closure rate was 95% and 87%, in high- and low-resourced countries, respectively. Closure was significantly more likely using a transvaginal rather than a transabdominal technique (91% vs 84% success).

Evidence base UK series of urogenital fistulae

Hilton reported on his own tertiary referral experience over 25 years from the UK.[7] Hospital episode statistics had suggested in the UK between 2000 and 2010 approximately 105 urogenital fistulae cases were surgically treated per year in the UK, suggesting it is a relatively uncommon procedure. Approximately three-quarters of the 348 women in his series were related to VVF. Of all urogenital fistulae, the commonest cause was surgical (two-thirds of the entire cohort) and mostly due to hysterectomy. Obstetrics aetiology was seen in 11% and radiotherapy cases were responsible for 10%. Spontaneous closure occurred in 7% of women who were managed with no treatment, indwelling catheter, or ureteric stenting. The anatomical closure rate at the first operation was 96%, although 2% reported residual urinary incontinence. Success was higher in patients who were undergoing surgical repair for the first time. The author suggested the need for centralization of urogenital fistulae as the volume was generally low in the UK and it was clear that previous failed repair had a negative influence on the chance of subsequent successful repair.

Learning point WHO classification of fistula (2006)

Simple fistula with good prognosis

- Single fistula <4 cm.
- VVF.
- Bladder neck not involved.
- No circumferential defect.
- Minimal tissue loss.
- No ureteric involvement.
- First attempt at repair.

Complex fistula with uncertain prognosis

- Fistula >4 cm.
- Multiple fistula.
- Mixed fistula (e.g. cervical, rectal).
- Bladder neck involvement.
- Scarring.
- Circumferential defect.
- Extensive tissue loss.
- Radiation.
- Intravaginal ureters.
- Previous failed repair.

Expert comment The 6th International Consultation on Incontinence

The management of VVF is summarized in the 6th International Consultation on Incontinence document and is summarized in Figure 32.3.[8]

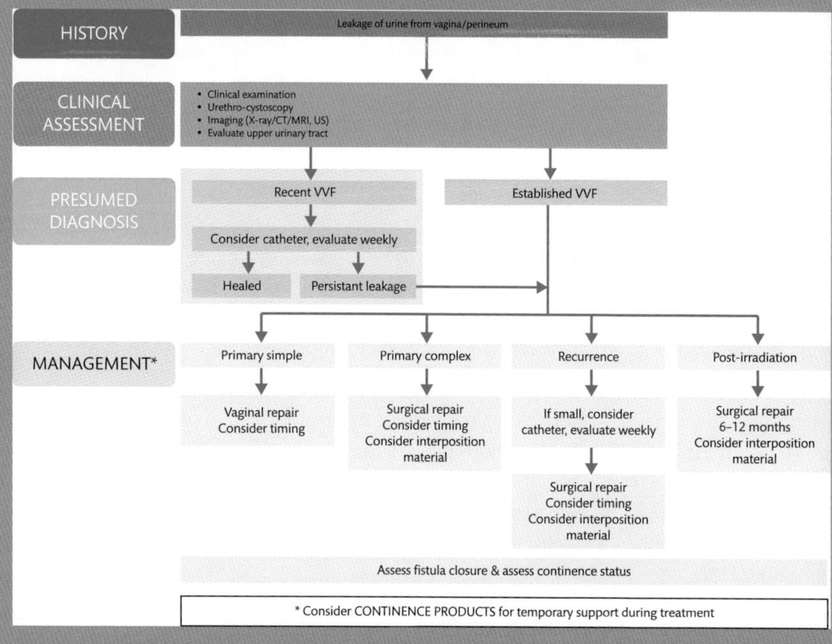

Figure 32.3 Algorithm for management of VVF.

Future directions Minimally invasive VVF repair

Minimally invasive VVF repair has been performed using laparoscopic techniques,[9] combined vesicoscopic, laparoscopic, and vaginal approach,[10] and with a robotic-assisted laparoscopic approach.[11] The robotic-assisted technique appears attractive as this approach has three-dimensional vision and magnification, and suturing in the pelvis is technically easier compared to the laparoscopic approach. In 2017, Bora et al. reported on 30 such cases, with a 93% successful outcome.[12] At the time of writing, this is the largest series to date. A four-port transperitoneal technique was employed and the same principles of the open abdominal approach were adhered to. Packing of the vagina is required with roller gauze to prevent leak of the pneumoperitoneum. Ninety per cent of the cases were subsequent to hysterectomy. Mean fistula size was 10.4 mm (range 5–30 mm). Eighteen patients had an interposition flap consisting of omentum, peritoneum, or sigmoid colon epiploicae. Mean duration of surgery was 133 minutes with a mean blood loss of 50 mL. Median duration of stay was 7.5 days. The authors comment that patients in general were ready for discharge on postoperative day 4 but due to the nature of their tertiary referral practice patients, they preferred to stay a little longer for reassurance due to them living at very remote sites. Two early recurrences were seen, after 2 days post catheter removal and at 3 months.

The outcomes of this approach are encouraging but it is clear that larger, comparator studies are required before understanding if this approach is beneficial. Furthermore, this approach is more costly and effectiveness in this regard will need to be studied carefully.

A final word from the expert

VVF is a devastating complication with considerable physical and psychosocial effects. Obstetric trauma due to lack of obstetric healthcare resources is a major global health issue and the majority of VVFs worldwide are preventable; in well-resourced countries VVF is a relatively rare consequence of pelvic surgery or radiotherapy. Due to its considerable impact on quality of life, as well as potential associated medicolegal consequences, it is important that patients are referred early to specialist surgeons with expertise in VVF repair. The best chance for successful VVF closure is the first chance, with any successive surgery converting a potentially 'simple' fistula into a challenging 'complex' fistula with lower rates of successful closure. Therefore, detailed surgical planning is essential.

Evaluation of a patient with VVF fundamentally involves three key decisions:

1. When should the fistula be repaired?
2. How should it be repaired (abdominal or vaginal approach)?
3. Should an interposition graft be used (and if so, which)?

If recognized in the immediate postoperative period then early repair is recommended, even up to 2 weeks following the initial surgery as long as the patient is clinically well (e.g. not overtly septic or other factors that may compromise surgical repair). Otherwise, repair should be delayed until 3 months to allow local tissue quality to improve, increasing the likelihood of successful closure.

The decision of whether to perform a vaginal or abdominal approach depends upon patient factors (body mass index, extent of previous pelvic surgery/radiotherapy, vaginal access and tissue quality, patient's wishes), fistula factors (size, location, presence of any associated ureteric injury), and expertise of the surgeon. These factors should be assessed with a thorough evaluation consisting of cross-sectional imaging, cystoscopy, and examination under anaesthetic in order to determine the optimal approach.

The principles of achieving a successful surgical outcome are adequate exposure of the fistula, excision of avascular tissue, ensuring a tension-free, layered closure with non-overlapping suture lines, and catheter drainage of the bladder for 2–3 weeks (depending upon complexity of the fistula and local tissue quality). The use of a pedicled interposition flap between the suture lines can aid successful outcome, especially in complex fistula with poor local tissue vascularity (e.g. following pelvic irradiation). Omental or labial fat pad flaps are most readily available depending upon the surgical approach.

Finally, prevention is better than cure and improving obstetric care in low-resourced countries will prevent most cases of VVF worldwide. Awareness of the surgical anatomy of the lower urinary tract, and careful surgical technique, may prevent iatrogenic cases. The development of specialist fistula centres in areas of high VVF prevalence would allow timely access and treatment for patients with VVF, and in well-resourced countries early referral to a specialist VVF surgeon is essential. Ultimately, abiding by the basic principles of reconstructive surgery will ensure a successful outcome.

References

1. Malde S, Spilotros M, Wilson A, et al. The uses and outcomes of the Martius fat pad in female urology. *World J Urol.* 2017;35(3):473–478.
2. Adler AJ, Ronsmans C, Calvert C, Filippi V. Estimating the prevalence of obstetric fistula: a systematic review and meta-analysis. *BMC Pregnancy Childbirth.* 2013;13:246.
3. Goh JT. A new classification for female genital tract fistula. *Aust N Z J Obstet Gynaecol.* 2004;44(6):502–504.
4. Waaldijk K. Surgical classification of obstetric fistulas. *Int J Oynaecol Obstetr.* 1995;49(2):161–163.
5. Burkhard FC, Bosch JLHR, Cruz F, et al. EAU guidelines on urinary incontinence in adults. European Association of Urology. 2018. https://uroweb.org/wp-content/uploads/EAU-Guidelines-on-Urinary-Incontinence-2018-large-text.pdf
6. Hillary CJ, Osman NI, Hilton P, Chapple CR. The aetiology, treatment, and outcome of urogenital fistulae managed in well- and low-resourced countries: a systematic review. *Eur Urol.* 2016;70(3):478–492.
7. Hilton P. Urogenital fistula in the UK: a personal case series managed over 25 years. *BJU Int.* 2012;110(1):102–110.
8. De Ridder D, Browning A, Mourad S, et al. In: Abrams P, Cardozo L, Wagg A, Wein A, eds. *Incontinence*, Vol. 2. 6th ed. Bristol: International Continence Society; 2016:2145–2202.
9. Shah SJ. Laparoscopic transabdominal transvesical vesicovaginal fistula repair. *J Endourol.* 2009;23(7):1135–1137.
10. Grange P, Giarenis I, Rouse P, Kouriefs C, Robinson D, Cardozo L. Combined vaginal and vesicoscopic collaborative repair of complex vesicovaginal fistulae. *Urology.* 2014;84(4):950–954.
11. Sundaram BM, Kalidasan G, Hemal AK. Robotic repair of vesicovaginal fistula: case series of five patients. *Urology.* 2006;67(5):970–973.
12. Bora GS, Singh S, Mavuduru RS, et al. Robot-assisted vesicovaginal fistula repair: a safe and feasible technique. *Int Urogynecol J.* 2017;28(6):957–962.

SECTION 11

Male infertility and sexual dysfunction

Male factor infertility: management of the azoospermic patient

Matthew Young

Expert commentary Oliver Kayes

Case history

A 31-year-old male is referred to the reproductive medicine clinic with an 18-month history of failure to conceive. He is otherwise fit and well with no history of urogenital infection, previous inguinoscrotal surgery, or cryptorchidism. He has no history of erectile or ejaculatory dysfunction. He does not recall any significant family history. His partner (age 32 years) has a child from a previous relationship for which she did not require any fertility investigations or treatments. Clinical examination reveals a phenotypical male with a body mass index (BMI) of 26 kg/m^2. There is no evidence of gynaecomastia. Both testes are small (approximate volume 4 cc) but have a normal consistency. No other abnormality is detected on regional examination.

Expert comment Causes of male factor infertility

Approximately half of involuntarily childless couples involve male infertility-associated factors, usually with abnormal semen parameters. For this reason, all male patients should undergo preliminary testing and if diagnosed with subfertility then referred for further medical evaluation by a urologist trained in male reproduction as part of a multidisciplinary assessment of infertility. Up to 30% of cases may identify no identifiable cause which is historically termed idiopathic male infertility. Other recognized causes of male infertility are highlighted in Table 33.1.

Table 33.1 **Recognized cause of male factor infertility**

Diagnosis	Unselected patients with male factor infertility (%)	Azoospermic patients (%)
All	100	11.2
Infertility of known (possible) cause	42.6	42.6
Undescended testes	8.4	17.2
Varicocele	14.8	10.9
Sperm autoantibodies	3.9	-
Testicular tumour	1.2	2.8
Other	5.0	1.2
Idiopathic infertility	30.0	13.3
Hypogonadism	10.1	16.4
Klinefelter syndrome (47,XXY)	2.6	13.7
XX male	0.1	0.6
Primary hypogonadism of unknown cause	2.3	0.8

Learning point Definition of infertility

Infertility is defined as the inability to achieve a spontaneous pregnancy within 12 months with regular (every 2–3 days) and unprotected sexual intercourse. Primary infertility refers to couples who have never had a child and cannot achieve a pregnancy. Secondary infertility refers to individuals who have been able to conceive at least once previously. Ideally, all newly referred couples who are struggling to conceive should be assessed simultaneously with a detailed clinical history and examination.

Table 33.1 **Continued**

Diagnosis	Unselected patients with male factor infertility (%)	Azoospermic patients (%)
Secondary hypogonadism	1.6	1.9
Kallmann syndrome	0.3	0.5
Idiopathic hypogonadotropic hypogonadism	0.4	0.4
Residual after pituitary surgery	<0.1	0.3
Late onset hypogonadism	2.2	–
Constitutional delay of puberty	1.4	–
Other	0.8	0.8
Systemic disease	2.2	0.5
Cryopreservation due to malignancy	7.8	12.5
Disturbance of erection/ejaculation	2.4	–
Obstruction	2.2	10.3
Vasectomy	0.9	5.3
Cystic fibrosis	0.5	3.0
Others	0.8	1.9

Re-formatted from Nieschlag E, Behre HM and Nieschlag S (eds). *Andrology: Male Reproductive Health and Dysfunction*. 2010, Springer Verlag: Berlin.

Clinical tip Clinical history

The following should be evaluated in the clinical history:

- Duration of failure to conceive (months).
- Primary (no history of children) or secondary (children from a previous relationship).
- History of cryptorchidism.
- History of infections—urogenital (e.g. mumps orchitis, tuberculosis) or sexually transmitted.
- Regional surgery (e.g. orchidopexy, hernia repair, vasectomy).
- History of trauma or testicular torsion.
- Previous malignancy.
- Age of puberty.
- Lifestyle—smoking/alcohol/anabolic steroid use/recreational drugs (e.g. cannabis, cocaine).
- Family history (genetic abnormalities/congenital abnormalities/infertility history).
- Occupational exposure to radiation/chemicals.
- Gonadotoxic treatments (e.g. chemotherapy, radiotherapy, immunotherapy).
- Sexual dysfunction—erectile dysfunction/premature ejaculation.

Mandatory first-line testing includes a semen fluid analysis in an accredited andrology laboratory and microbiological sampling, primarily to exclude any sexually transmitted infections. If the semen fluid analysis is abnormal, then a repeat sample is compulsory. Careful interpretation of the semen fluid analysis results should aim to identify men with normal or abnormal parameters based on published WHO criteria and establish (1) degree subfertility (mild, moderate, or severe); and (2) evidence of obstruction, infection, or inflammation. Men with severe subfertility (total sperm count < 5 million) should go on to have further laboratory testing. Our patient's results can be seen in Table 33.2.

Clinical tip Clinical examination

Clinical examination should include the following:

- Body composition—height/weight/BMI/gynaecomastia.
- Evidence of inguinoscrotal surgery.
- Regional lymphadenopathy.
- Penile abnormalities—deformity/hypospadias/meatal stenosis/phimosis.
- Testes—volume/consistency/scrotal position/mass or swelling.
- Epididymis—dilatation/defects/induration/cysts.
- Spermatic cord—varicocele/Valsalva manoeuvre.
- Vas deferens abnormalities.

Table 33.2 Semen analysis parameters for case study patient with WHO lower reference limits

Parameter	Case study patient values	Lower reference limit (WHO criteria)
Semen volume (mL)	**4.5**	1.5 (1.4–1.7)
Total sperm number (million/ejaculate)	**0**	39 (33–46)
Sperm concentration (million/mL)	**0**	15 (12–16)
Total motility (progressive, non-progressive, %)	**0**	40 (38–42)
Progressive motility (PR, %)	**0**	32 (31–34)
Vitality (live spermatozoa, %)	**0**	58 (55–63)
Sperm morphology (normal form, %)	**0**	4 (3–4)
pH	**7.4**	≥7.2

Expert comment Semen analysis

Ejaculate analysis has been standardized (Table 33.3), with consensus that modern semen analysis must follow these guidelines. However, it has become evident that more complex investigations beyond simple semen analysis may be required. Such cases may include recurrent pregnancy loss (i.e. miscarriage) following natural or assisted conception and men with unexplained male infertility. In these patients there is evidence that the sperm DNA may be damaged, resulting in pregnancy failure.

Table 33.3 WHO standardized values for semen analysis

Parameter	Lower reference limit (range)
Semen volume (mL)	1.5 (1.4–1.7)
Total sperm number (10^6/ejaculate)	39 (33–46)
Sperm concentration (10^6/mL)	15 (12–16)
Total motility	40 (38–42)
Progressive motility (PR, %)	32 (31–34)
Vitality (live spermatozoa, %)	58 (55–63)
Sperm morphology (normal forms, %)	4 (3–4)
Other consensus threshold values	
pH	>7.2
Peroxidase-positive leukocytes (10^6/mL)	<1.0

Re-formatted from WHO, *WHO Laboratory Manual for the Examination and Processing of Human Semen*, 5th edn. 2010.

Learning point Male urogenital infections

Male urogenital infections are a potentially reversible cause of male factor infertility. Men with confirmed sexually transmitted infections have not been conclusively shown to be at increased risk of infertility; however, such infections (e.g. *Chlamydia*) ae likely to pose a potential risk to the female urogenital tract rather than a direct effect on male reproduction. The presence of bacteria in the urogenital tract may lead to chronic inflammation of the prostate and epididymis which may cause obstruction and lead to oligospermia and/or reduced seminal volume. The role of the microbiome and effects on sperm function requires further elucidation.

Clinical tip Semen analysis interpretation

It is important to distinguish between the following conditions:

- Oligospermia: <15 million spermatozoa/mL.
- Asthenozoospermia: <32% motile spermatozoa.
- Teratozoospermia: <4% normal forms.

All three phenomenon occurring simultaneously represent oligoasthenoteratospermia (OAT) syndrome.

Clinical tip Laboratory investigations

Laboratory investigations include the following:

- Semen analysis.
- Microbiology analysis—sexually transmitted diseases (*Chlamydia trachomatis/Neisseria gonorrhoeae*), urinary tract infection (coliforms, *Klebsiella, Pseudomonas*), tuberculosis.
- Reproductive hormone levels:
  - Follicle-stimulating hormone (FSH).
  - Luteinizing hormone (LH).
  - Total testosterone.
  - Prolactin.
- Leucocytospermia.
- Genetic screening.
- Sperm DNA damage or fragmentation (e.g. COMET test; sperm chromatin structure assay).

Learning point Genetic abnormalities

- Genetic abnormalities, such as numerical and structural chromosomal abnormalities, are found more frequently in men with unexplained oligozoospermia/azoospermia. These findings can be as high as 13.7% in men with non-obstructive azoospermia (NOA) and 4.6% in oligozoospermia.
- A higher frequency of cytogenetic abnormalities and Y chromosome deletions are observed with increasing severity of testicular dysfunction.
- Klinefelter syndrome (KS) is the most common chromosomal aneuploidy found in azoospermic men.
- *CFTR* gene mutations (i.e. cystic fibrosis-associated genes) are the most common finding in infertile couples. In MFI, it is often associated with congenital vas deferens abnormalities and obstruction.
- Y-chromosome microdeletions are rarer but confer important diagnostic and prognostic information. Y-chromosome deletions are inherited and will cause infertility in biological male offspring.
- Structural and numeric chromosomal anomalies can result in spontaneous abortions and multiple congenital defects in the offspring.

This patient is diagnosed with **azoospermia** so it is important to perform further investigations. The endocrinological tests required at this stage are FSH, LH, and testosterone levels. Our patient's results can be seen in Table 33.4. A comprehensive understanding of the normal functioning hypothalamic–pituitary–gonadal axis is important when interpreting these results (Figure 33.1).

Expert comment Spermatozoa of infertile men

The spermatozoa of infertile men show an increased rate of aneuploidy, structural chromosomal abnormalities, and DNA damage, carrying the risk of passing genetic abnormalities on to the next generation. Positive testing will require a formal referral for genetic counselling and possibly pre-implantation genetic diagnosis.

Learning point Hypogonadism

Differentiating between hypergonadotropic hypogonadism (high FSH/LH) and hypogonadotropic hypogonadism (low FSH/LH) is important.

Primary hypogonadism (aka hypergonadotropic hypogonadism) causes include testicular insufficiency, disturbed spermatogenesis, KS, cryptorchidism, anorchia, testicular dysgenesis, history of orchitis or testicular torsion, previous chemo/radiotherapy, and testicular tumour.

Secondary hypogonadism (aka hypogonadotropic hypogonadism) causes include: hypothalamic-pituitary dysfunction, Kallmann syndrome, idiopathic, pituitary tumours, anabolic steroid abuse, obesity. Patients with hypogonadotropic hypogonadism require cranial imaging (computed tomography or magnetic resonance imaging).

Differentiation can be made between NOA and obstructive azoospermia (OA) by reference to the serum FSH levels. An elevated FSH level indicates an increased probability of diagnosing NOA.

Our patient suffers from hypergonadotropic hypogonadism, suggesting the primary pathology lies at the testicular level. He has primary testicular deficiency. Our patient undergoes a scrotal ultrasound scan which does not reveal any significant pathology and despite there being no clinical evidence of OA, he also undergoes a screening transrectal ultrasound scan. This was also normal.

Table 33.4 Serum hormone levels for our patient

Parameter	Patient's results	Reference range
FSH	**40**	1.5–12.4 IU/L
LH	**18**	1–9 IU/L
Testosterone	**6.8**	8–30 nmol/L

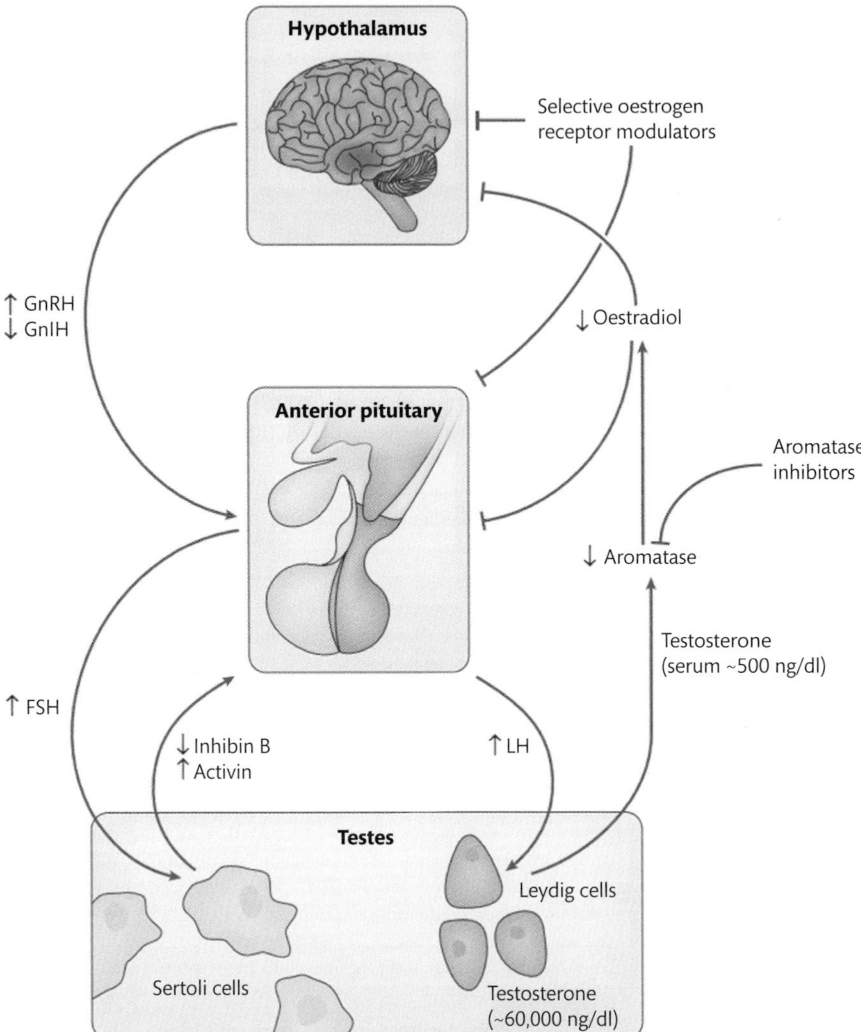

Figure 33.1 The hypothalamic–pituitary–gonadal axis. Secretion of the anterior pituitary luteinizing hormone (LH) and follicle-stimulating hormone (FSH) are stimulated by the pulsatile release of gonadotropin-releasing hormone (GnRH) and inhibited by the release of gonadotropin-inhibiting hormone (GnIH) from the hypothalamus. Selective oestrogen receptor modulators (SERMs) competitively inhibit hypothalamic oestrogen receptors, which leads to increased anterior pituitary gonadotropin release and subsequent endogenous testosterone production. Inhibin B is secreted by the testicular germinal epithelium (primarily Sertoli cells) in response to FSH and subsequently acts on the anterior pituitary in a negative-feedback loop, inhibiting FSH production. Activin has an agonistic effect on the pituitary secretion of FSH and its release is inhibited by inhibin B. Aromatase inhibitors are used to correct a diminished testosterone:oestrogen ratio.

Reused with permission from Springer Nature. Kathrins M and Niederberger C. *Nat Rev Urol.* 2016;13(6):309–23 (Figure 1).

Expert comment Hypergonadotropic hypogonadism

In men with testicular deficiency, hypergonadotropic hypogonadism (also called primary hypogonadism) typically presents with higher levels of FSH and LH. Low testosterone levels may or may not be observed. FSH levels often negatively correlate with the number of spermatogonia.

FSH levels are often elevated with absent or diminished spermatogonia. Occasionally it is possible to observe normal FSH readings associated with a normal number of spermatogonia but no mature spermatozoa are identified. This process is termed 'maturation arrest' with failure of spermatogenesis at the spermatocyte/spermatid level. Importantly, for patients undergoing sperm extraction, FSH levels do not accurately predict the presence of spermatogenesis, as men with maturation arrest on histology may have both normal FSH levels and testis volume. Furthermore, men with NOA and high levels of FSH may still harbour focal areas of spermatogenesis which can be targeted using microsurgical sperm extraction surgery.

The results of our patient's genetic screening return 6 weeks after his initial assessment. His chromosome analysis revealed 47,XXY—consistent with KS. Often patients with this diagnosis are asymptomatic and go unrecognized until they try to conceive. This is a common cause of NOA with one in eight azoospermic men (cf. 1 in 500 general population) diagnosed with classic meiotic disjunction on genetic testing.

Learning point Sex chromosome abnormalities (KS and variants (47,XXY; 46,XY/47,XXY mosaicism))

KS is the most common sex chromosome abnormality. Adult males with KS often have small but firm testes, along with features of primary hypogonadism. The overall phenotype of a patient is the final result of genetic, hormonal, and age-related factors. The phenotype ranges from the characteristics of a normally virilized male to the stigmata of androgen deficiency. In the majority of KS cases, infertility and reduced testis volume are the only detectable clinical features.

Men with KS frequently have impaired Leydig cell function. This has a direct impact on testosterone production, leading to testosterone deficiency when compared to the general population. More obvious features of hypogonadism are infrequently displayed, along with cardiovascular and renal problems. Sperm production and the presence of germ cells are variable in males with KS, being more often observed in mosaicism, 46,XY/47,XXY. The production of 24,XY sperm has been reported in 0.9–7.0% of men with KS and in up to 25% of men with somatic karyotype 47,XXY. In patients with azoospermia, open testicular sperm extraction (TESE) or microdissection testicular sperm extraction (mTESE) are established therapeutic options, with spermatozoa being recovered in up to 50% of cases. Some data suggest improved outcomes with sperm extraction performed at a younger age; however, TESE in the peripubertal and prepubertal KS patient is still considered experimental.

There is limited published information regarding the prevalence of aneuploidies in children of KS fathers being conceived by intracytoplasmic sperm injection (ICSI) versus the general population. However, contemporary European guidelines support the role of in-depth counselling regarding potential genetic abnormalities in any biological offspring. The role of pre-implantation genetic diagnosis remains unclear. Close follow-up of men with KS is advocated, with androgen replacement to be considered if levels are found to be hypogonadal. Men with KS are at greater risk of cardiovascular disease and metabolic syndrome.

The final investigation in the patient pathway is a testicular biopsy. This should also be considered a therapeutic procedure in nearly all cases, as sperm may be harvested for *in vitro* fertilization. European Association of Urology guidelines support the role of testicular biopsy in unexplained NOA. A truly diagnostic testicular biopsy is reserved for confirmation of patients with OA in patients with normal sized testes and normal gonadotropin levels.

Learning point Testicular biopsy

Approximately 50% of men with NOA will have spermatozoa that can be used for ICSI identified within focally, active testicular tissue. A good correlation exists between histology at biopsy and the likelihood of finding mature sperm cells at sperm retrieval and ICSI. Currently there is no role for testicular fine-needle aspirate mapping outside of a research setting. However, the greater the number of testicular biopsies performed, the higher the chance of a successful retrieval. Microsurgical techniques allow identification of focal areas of potential spermatogenesis by targeting fuller and dilated tubules at × 200 magnification. Currently, ICSI outcomes appear to be poorer for patients with NOA versus OA (live birth rates 19% vs 28%, respectively).

Our patient undergoes a combined procedure for testicular biopsy and sperm harvesting for ICSI. The procedure of choice in this situation is mTESE. This procedure offers a 50–54% success rate of harvesting testicular sperm, with reported 61% fertilization rates and a cumulative pregnancy rate of nearly 30% per ICSI cycle. Success rates in KS are likely to be much lower but published figures suggest that performing TESE/mTESE in subjects with KS results in sperm retrieval rates of close to 50%, with pregnancy rates and live birth rates approaching 50%, with the results being independent of any clinical or biochemical parameters tested.

Our patient went on to have spermatozoa successfully harvested by mTESE but unfortunately the subsequent treatment cycle of ICSI was unsuccessful. Further sperm retrieval and ICSI are planned. Pre-implant genetic diagnosis could be offered, following appropriate counselling, to this patient to avoid the risk of implanting an embryo with a known severe genetic disorder that may end in an unsuccessful pregnancy.

Expert comment mTESE

Unadjusted sperm retrieval rate after mTESE are reported to be 52% in a pooled data analysis of studies comparing conventional TESE with mTESE. mTESE appears to offer a 1.5 × improvement in sperm retrieval versus TESE. Salvage mTESE after failed TESE/TESA has also resulted in 46.5% published successful sperm retrieval rate. mTESE is associated with a lower complication rate in relation to haematoma and fibrosis formation. Equivalence is observed on recovery to baseline testosterone level during long-term follow-up.

Clinical tip Role of adjuvant therapies to improve sperm retrieval in NOA

No randomized controlled trials exist supporting the role of endocrine therapies to potentiate spermatogenesis in NOA. However, studies evaluating their empirical use appear to demonstrate improved sperm quality and output. Endogenous FSH and testosterone levels, both of which are required for spermatogenesis, have been shown to be increased by human chorionic gonadotropin, human menopausal gonadotropin, and clomiphene citrate. Evidence has shown that these treatments prior to mTESE increased the sperm in ejaculate, thus obviating the need for surgical sperm retrieval and a greater likelihood of a successful sperm retrieval in persistently azoospermic men (57% vs 33.6%) when compared to a control group.

Summary

The causes of MFI are varied and in part poorly understood. Our case highlights the optimal assessment of male patients who have been unable to conceive after 12 months of regular, unprotected intercourse. This case focuses on the implications of genetic abnormalities (specifically KS) but other factors should always be considered, including testicular insufficiency, hypogonadotropic hypogonadism, anatomical obstructions of the seminal tract, urogenital infections, ejaculatory dysfunction, and idiopathic male infertility (30–40% of MFI cases).

Patients should always be assessed simultaneously alongside their partner in a dedicated fertility clinic setting as part of a specialist multidisciplinary team approach.

Future directions

Men with infertility are vulnerable to being under-investigated and inappropriately counselled regarding their chances and options for becoming a father. An expanding portfolio of diagnostic testing is opening the door for men who suffer permanent infertility following chemotherapy, radiation, and other medical treatments. Currently, sperm freezing is the standard of care method to preserve male fertility. Testicular tissue freezing is an experimental option to preserve the fertility of prepubertal boys and others who cannot produce sperm. Testicular tissues contain spermatogonial stem cells (SCC) and new SCC-based techniques currently in the research pipeline may be available in the male fertility clinic of the future. Alongside a better understanding of the role of oxidative stress and improved molecular prognostic biomarkers, these scientific advances will hopefully translate to better patient selection and novel targeting for innovative therapeutics in the future.

A final word from the expert

MFI affects up to 50% of infertile couples and management is dependent on careful assessment and understanding of the primary reproductive abnormality. Men with azoospermia represent approximately 10–15% of men referred for fertility investigations. Men with OA benefit from microsurgical reconstruction, endoscopic treatment, or advanced sperm retrieval and ICSI techniques. Conversely, men with NOA represent a greater diagnostic and therapeutic challenge. The advent of improved *in vitro* fertilization methods has allowed a larger proportion of these men to father their own biological offspring using modern assisted conception procedures rather than being confined to donor insemination programmes. Multidisciplinary teams involving a urologist with a specialist MFI interest are strongly recommended.

Further reading

Ashraf CM, Dharmaraj P, Sankalp S, et al. Microdissection testicular sperm extraction (micro-TESE): results of a large series from India. *Andrology.* 2014;3:113.

Baazeem A, Belzile E, Ciampi A, et al. Varicocele and male factor infertility treatment: a new meta-analysis and review of the role of varicocele repair. *Eur Urol.* 2011;60(4):796–808.

Corona G, Pizzocaro A, Lanfranco F, et al. Sperm recovery and ICSI outcomes in Klinefelter syndrome: a systematic review and meta-analysis. *Hum Reprod Update.* 2017;23(3):265–275.

De Braekleer M, Ferec C. Mutations in the cystic fibrosis gene in men with congenital bilateral absence of the vas deferens. *Mol Hum Reprod.* 1996;2(9):669–677.

Dohle GR. Inflammatory-associated obstructions of the male reproductive tract. *Andrologia.* 2003;35(5):321–324.

Hamdy FC, Eardley I. Section 7. In: *Oxford Textbook of Urological Surgery*. 1st ed. Oxford: Oxford University Press; 2017:839–942.

Hussein A, Ozgok Y, Ross L, Niederberger C. Clomiphene administration for cases of non-obstructive azoospermia: a multicenter study. *J Androl.* 2005;26(6):787–791.

Junwirth A, Diemer T, Kopa Z, Krausz C, Minhas S, Tournaye H. European Association of Urology guidelines on male infertility. European Association of Urology. 2019. https://uroweb.org/wp-content/uploads/EAU-Guidelines-on-Male-Infertility-2019.pdf

Lamfranco F, Kamischke A, Zitzmann M, et al. Klinefelter's syndrome. *Lancet* 2004;364(9430):273–283.

Nieschlag E, Behre HM, Nieschlag S, eds. *Andrology: Male Reproductive Health and Dysfunction*. Berlin: Springer Verlag; 2010.

Pierik FH, Dohle GR, van Muiswinkel JM, Vreeburg JT, Weber RFA. Is routine scrotal ultrasound in infertile men advantageous? *J Urol.* 1999;162(5):1618–1620.

Rowe, T. Fertility and a woman's age. *J Reprod Med.* 2006;51:157.
van Assche E, Bonduelle M, Tournaye H, et al. Cytogenetics of infertile men. *Hum Reprod.* 1996;11(Suppl 4):1–24.
World Health Organization. *WHO Laboratory Manual for the Examination of Human Semen and Sperm-Cervical Mucus Interaction.* 5th ed. Cambridge: Cambridge University Press; 2010.
World Health Organization. *WHO Manual for the Standardized Investigation and Diagnosis of the Infertile Couple.* Cambridge: Cambridge University Press; 2000.
Weidner W, Krause W, Ludwig M. Relevance of male accessory gland infection for subsequent fertility with special focus on prostatitis. *Hum Reprod Update.* 1999;5(5):421–432.

CASE

34 Erectile dysfunction

James Tracey and Majid Shabbir

Expert commentary Majid Shabbir

Case history

A 46-year-old male was referred for a 6-month history of erectile dysfunction (ED). His primary issue is maintaining a firm erection long enough for sexual intercourse. Previously, erections were satisfactory. He has a stable, supportive partner but now lacks confidence and is avoiding intercourse. He does not have morning erections anymore, has smoked daily since the age of 18 years, and has a family history of coronary artery disease (CAD).

Clinical tip History

- The goal in the history is to discover the 4 Cs: **Causes**, **Comorbidities**, **Complicating factors**, and **Contraindications** to treatment.
- Identifying potential **causes** helps determine if the ED is psychogenic, organic, or mixed. Ask about duration of onset, situational ED, morning or night erections, genital trauma, penile curvature, and priapism events.
- Important **comorbidities** include CAD, hypertension, hyperlipidaemia, diabetes, peripheral vascular disease, prostate diseases, pelvic floor pain, pelvic surgery, psychiatric health, and smoking. It is important to ask about medications and, specifically, recreational drug use as the patient rarely offers this information without prompting.
- **Complicating factors** include lack of desire, premature or anejaculation, anorgasmia, pain with intercourse, sexual orientation issues, psychosocial stresses, partner age, and health. All may lead to significant changes in sexual function that can cause or contribute to ED and should be clearly defined to obtain the best result from treatment. Including partners in the consultation can impact decisions in up to 58% of cases.[5]
- **Contraindications** can include use of oral nitrates or alpha blockers and fitness for intercourse.

The patient's ED is not situational. He has no penile curvature or history of priapism. He denies any lower urinary tract symptoms (LUTS), pelvic discomfort, or any past medical history. He takes no medications and does not use recreational drugs. He has never had concerns of a lack of desire, ejaculation, orgasm, or pain with intercourse. He has minimal stress but leads a sedentary lifestyle. He can walk up two flights of stairs briskly; his partner is 39 years old and healthy. On examination he has normal external genitalia, a small, non-tender prostate and palpable lower extremity pulses. His blood pressure is 128/84 mmHg. His body mass index (BMI) is 32 kg/m^2. His sexual health index for men score is 17/25. Initial testing sent includes a urinalysis, full blood count, basic metabolic panel, morning total testosterone, fasting blood glucose, glycated haemoglobin (HbA1c), and lipid profile. All testing returned

Learning point
Epidemiology of ED

- ED prevalence is as high as 52% in men 40–70 years old with 10% exhibiting severe ED.[1]
- ED increases progressively after the age of 40 years.[2]
- The degree of bother is inversely related to age.[3]
- The rate of progression, remission, and stability is near equivalent.[4]

within normal limits except an elevated glucose and HbA1c of 75 mmol/mol indicating a type 2 diabetes mellitus (DM) diagnosis.

Expert comment Metabolic equivalents of the task

Intercourse is equivalent to mild to moderate non-sexual activity or 3–4 metabolic equivalents of the task (METS) at orgasm. This is equivalent to walking 1 mile on level ground in 20 minutes, briskly climbing two flights of steps in 10 seconds, or being able to golf (4–5 METs). However, this generalization does not cover all situations as intercourse in the older, the less fit, an extramarital setting with an unfamiliar person and location, or after excessive alcohol intake may raise the METS requirement. Completing 4 minutes on a standard treadmill stress test without concerns is more indicative of a safe level (5–6 METS).[6]

Evidence base Risk factors that predict ED

The risk factors that predict ED are shown in Table 34.1.[7–9] Odd ratios are displayed with diabetes being the prominent risk factor.

Table 34.1 Risk factors for ED

Risk factor	Odds ratio
Diabetes mellitus (DM)	4.1
Prostate disease	2.9
Peripheral vascular disease	2.6
Cardiac disease	1.8
Hyperlipidaemia	1.7
Hypertension (HTN)	1.6
Major depressive disorder	1.7
Smoking	1.5

Learning point ED and CAD risk

- ED occurs in up to 71% of DM.[10]
- CAD and ED are both commonly caused by endothelial dysfunction.
- **ED is an independent risk factor and early marker for the development of CAD with a lead-time of 2–5 years prior to a coronary event**. This has been established across continents and held true over time.[11–13] **It is imperative to assess a new ED patient's cardiac risk**.
- Both the Princeton Consensus Panel and UK Guidelines identify three risk levels:
  1. **Low-risk patients can be cleared for treatment** and include asymptomatic CAD and fewer than three risk factors (excluding sex) of CAD. Risk factors are controlled HTN, DM, smoking, hyperlipidaemia, sedentary lifestyle, family history or early CAD, mild, stable angina, previous revascularization, uncomplicated past myocardial infarction (MI), mild valvular disease, or chronic heart failure New York Heart Association (CHF NYHA) class I/left ventricular dysfunction.
  2. **Intermediate risk requires further evaluation** with a stress test prior to treatment to reclassify as high or low risk.
  3. **High-risk patients should not receive treatment for ED** and include unstable/refractory angina, uncontrolled HTN, CHF NYHA class III/IV, MI or cerebrovascular accident within 2 weeks, high-risk arrhythmias, hypertrophic obstructive cardiomyopathy, and moderate–severe valve disease.[14–16]

With his new diagnosis of ED and diabetes, he has more than three risk factors for CAD (DM, family history of CAD, smoking, sedentary lifestyle) and so is classified as 'intermediate' risk. He was referred for a stress test which reclassified him as low risk. He was started on metformin, an exercise and weight loss regimen, and a smoking cessation programme. Evidence has shown modification of lifestyle risk factors can improve sexual function.[18] He was offered sildenafil and sexual health counselling. He declined the latter. At 3-month follow-up he did not feel the sildenafil was helping enough and was experiencing mild gastric reflux and flushing during use.

Expert comment Intercourse and risk of MI

There is a >2 relative risk of non-fatal MI in the 2 hours after intercourse, with an absolute risk of roughly 20 events per million.[17]

Learning point Physiology of erections

Erection begins with sexual stimulation (thoughts or physical contact) causing the parasympathetic nervous system to release nitric oxide (NO) from sinusoidal endothelium. NO causes the activation of guanylyl cyclase, thus converting guanosine triphosphate guanosine triphosphate (GTP) to cyclic guanosine monophosphate (cGMP) in smooth muscle cells. cGMP accumulation activates K^+ and Ca^{2+} channels causing a decrease in intracellular calcium thereby allowing smooth muscle fibres to relax. The helicine arteries then dilate increasing blood flow to the corpus cavernosa. Phosphodiesterase type 5 (PDE5) breaks down cGMP (into 5′-GMP) and inhibitors (PDE5is) of this enzyme bolster erections by blocking cGMP degradation. The first PDE5i was sildenafil citrate, which was originally synthesized in England, and while studied for hypertension and angina was found to have extensive erectogenic properties.[19]

Learning point Comparison of PDE5is

See Table 34.2.

- There are no randomized-controlled trials comparing the efficacy of PDE5i directly. However, rates of successful erections were relatively similar for each when compared to placebo.
- PDE5i are affected by meals (fatty) with tadalafil being minimally affected.
- All are contraindicated with organic nitrates for 24 hours except tadalafil for 48 hours.[20,21]
- Vardenafil is contraindicated with alpha blockers, the remaining can be administered with caution with a 6-hour window of separation recommended.
- All have side effects of facial flushing (4–12%), nasal congestion (1–10%), headache (13–16%), and dyspepsia (4–12%).[22–24]

Table 34.2 Comparison of PDE5 inhibitors

Drug	Dosage	Half-life ($T_{1/2}$)	Peak plasma conc.	Cross-reactivity	Side effects
Sildenafil	25–100 mg	4 h	60 min	PDE6	Blue-green visual change
Vardenafil	5–20 mg	4 h	60 min	PDE6	Visual changes and QT prolongation
Tadalafil	10–20 mg on demand or 2.5–5 mg daily	17.5 h	120 min	PDE11	Muscle aches
Avanafil	50–200 mg	5 h	30 min	Limited PDE6	Visual change

Clinical tip How to assess for sildenafil failure

- Ask what dose was tried, how it was taken, was there sexual stimulation after, did they have side effects, and how many attempts were tried?
- Sildenafil dosages are 25–100 mg. Only two of three patients met success in completing intercourse on the starting dose.[22]
- It should be taken on an empty stomach. High-fat meals cause a reduction in plasma concentration while alcohol delays gastric emptying and absorption. If food or alcohol has been had, the patient should wait 2–3 hours before taking the dose.
- PDE5is require sexual stimulation to have an effect.
- On average, it can take up to six attempts to get everything right.
- Prior to second-line therapy being initiated, one should determine whether the trial was adequate, re-educate, and ensure dose titration was performed.
- Consider switching to a different PDE5i if side effects are an issue, a partial response is obtained, or one medication offers a lifestyle advantage over another.

The patient was taking the 100 mg dose but usually just after a meal with wine. Otherwise, he had appropriate sexual stimulation within 1–4 hours and tried the medication several times. He was re-educated but due to side effects was switched to tadalafil.

Learning point Use of PDE5Is

- PDE5is are not associated with MI, stroke, or mortality in patients with stable angina, CAD, HTN, DM, or heart failure.[25]
- Though more common, side effects cause discontinuation in <5% of patients.[26]
- There is little to no harm in starting at the highest dose and decreasing if need be.
- PDE5is have been shown to increase not only penile rigidity but improve orgasmic function, patient and partner satisfaction, quality of life, and even depressive symptoms.[27,28]
- Given the ease of use they should be offered as first-line therapy.

The patient returns 7 years later to our clinic with worsening ED, occasional nocturia, urgency, slow stream, and decreased libido despite utilizing 20 mg on-demand tadalafil. He has since been diagnosed with HTN and hyperlipidaemia and is on lisinopril and simvastatin. Repeat blood work reveals an early-morning total testosterone level of 8.3 nmol/L, prostate-specific antigen level of 1.7 ng/mL, and appropriate control of his diabetes and lipids.

Evidence base Hypogonadism

- Testosterone therapy in hypogonadal men with ED can improve certain sexual characteristics, possibly including ED; PDE5is may have improved efficacy in a eugonadal state.[29]
- It is important to check testosterone on a morning fasted sample, along with sex hormone-binding globulin to obtain an accurate reading of free and total testosterone and avoid over-diagnosing hypogonadism. An early-morning fasted sample can be 20% higher than an improper sample.
- Treatment of hypogonadism has secondary benefits of improved lethargy, depression, limits osteoporosis, and helps build lean muscle mass.[30]
- Tadalafil has been shown to decrease LUTS and improve ED in men when taken as a 5 mg daily dose.[31]

The patient was switched to tadalafil 5 mg daily and started on testosterone gel. One month later his early-morning testosterone level was 19.5 nmol/L. He noticed an improvement in his erection quality, energy, sexual desire, and LUTS. Six months later his DRE, prostate-specific antigen, haemoglobin, cholesterol, liver function test profile, and total testosterone remained in the normal range.

Four years later, the patient returns with worsening ED despite tadalafil and testosterone. He has started two additional medications to keep his blood sugars controlled. A penile Doppler is performed revealing a peak systolic velocity (PSV) of 25 mL/s and retrograde flow in diastole after a second 10 mcg injection of alprostadil was given due to the initial dose not producing an adequate erection.

Expert comment
Testosterone replacement

Testosterone replacement is not felt to be associated with cardiac risk. However, side effects include increased haematocrit, concerning for an elevated risk of deep vein thrombosis; mild fluid retention, which can worsen heart failure; worsening sleep apnoea; breast enlargement; and LUTS. Haemoglobin, cholesterol, prostate-specific antigen, and testosterone levels; liver function; and digital rectal examination require intermittent monitoring while on therapy.

Expert comment Specific investigations

More specific evaluations are reserved for non-responders to oral medications, candidates for penile implant, Peyronie's disease, post priapism or traumatic ED, lifelong ED, concern for psychogenic ED, and medicolegal situations.

A penile Doppler with intracavernosal alprostadil is the most useful functional test. A PSV >30 cm/s is normal. A PSV of ≤25cm/s is indicative of arteriogenic ED. A reversal of flow in diastole is expected and the end-diastolic velocity should be <3 cm/s. A reading of >5 cm/s is indicative of a continued outflow from the cavernosal space and is sometimes referred to as a 'venous leak' phenomenon. However, the results must be correlated with the clinical picture. High stress during the test can lead to an artificially poor erection during the test. One cannot diagnose venous leak if an inadequate erection is achieved. Always ask the patient if the erection they achieved during the ultrasound scan was representative of their normal state. If they achieved a better erection when back in the changing room after the test was completed, this can be indicative of an anxiety related suppression of the effect of alprostadil during the test, and puts the poor vascular dynamics readings into the correct perspective.

Additional tests can be used in this situation and include nocturnal penile tumescence testing if psychogenic ED is suspected. Other specialised tests used to investigate ED include a magnetic resonance imaging if there has been significant trauma, priapism, or anatomical abnormality and angiography in cases of pelvic trauma. Dynamic infusion cavernosometry and cavernosography are very rarely indicated.

After being counselled on further treatment options, the patient chose intracavernosal injections with alprostadil and was started at a 10 mcg dose after a test dose of 5mcg was performed and taught in clinic. He given instructions for dose escalation at home.

Learning point Second-line treatments

Alprostadil is a prostaglandin-E1 analogue that induces cyclic adenosine monophosphate (cAMP) signalling thereby decreasing intracellular calcium to bolster erections.

Intraurethral alprostadil deposits come in pellets (Medicated Urethral System for Erection, MUSE) or cream (Vitaros).

- Pellet dosages are 250–1000 mcg with 43% total efficacy and 65% in those who responded to an office trial. Penile pain and erythema were reported in 32%.[32]
- Cream dosages are 200–300 mcg showing significant improvement of ED.[33]
- Other side effects occur in 2–5% and include dizziness, hypotension-induced syncope, sweating, priapism, and urethral bleeding.[34]

Intracavernosal injection (ICI) of alprostadil monotherapy at dosages of 5–40 mcg has an efficacy of >70%.[35,36] Other formulations of ICI include bimix (papaverine + phentolamine), trimix (papaverine + alprostadil + phentolamine), or quadmix (which includes atropine) but require a compounding pharmacy.

- ICI carries the highest risk of priapism of all ED treatments at 0.3–7% with alprostadil ICI monotherapy carrying the least risk.
- Other complications include varying levels of pain in 7–34% that often decreases over time, 1–12% develop nodules or fibrosis, and haematoma in 6–25%.[35,36]

Vacuum erection devices are a non-pharmacological therapy that can be highly effective, safe, and less expensive in the long term.

- These devices use negative pressure to draw blood into the corporal sinusoids and are made of three components: a cylinder that is placed around the penis, a pump to draw air out of cylinder, and a compression ring to limit venous outflow.
- Although 92% of patients achieve erections firm enough for intercourse,[37–39] long term satisfaction of the vacuum devices range from 35% to 70%.
- The most common side effects are discomfort, petechiae, ejaculatory difficulty due to the compression ring, penile coldness, and numbness.[40]

Clinical tip Use of second-line therapies

Intraurethral alprostadil is used after micturition, 15–30 minutes before sexual activity:

- To place, lift the penis straight up and place the pellet applicator 3 cm into urethra, depress the button, and move the applicator from side to side to separate the pellet before removing the applicator, and 'rolling the urethra' to aid absorption. The cream is squeezed into the opened urethra without needing to insert an applicator, and any excess cream is rubbed over the glans to allow it to absorb. An initial trial in clinic should be done to assess for syncope and need for dose escalation.[41]

Intracavernosal injection produces on-demand erections within 5–10 minutes:

- A ½ inch 27- or 30-gauge needle is placed into the corporal space lateral to the dorsal nerve complex. An initial dose should be administered in clinic to assess the technique and response. Dose titration can occur at home.
- Special 'dual chamber' applicators are available for alprostadil monotherapy.
- Injections may be given by patients or their partner.
- The site of injection should be massaged for 30 seconds unless the patient is anticoagulated. Then pressure should be placed for 5–10 minutes.
- Patients need to be made aware of the risk of priapism and be provided with a treatment algorithm for it. Terbutaline and pseudoephedrine have been studied to facilitate detumescence in ICI-induced priapism.[42,43]

- If in 3–4 hours there is no detumescence, an emergency room visit is required for immediate attention to prevent lasting and irreversible damage to the cavernosal tissue.

Vacuum erection devices produce on-demand, immediate erections:

- Patients should be instructed about a learning curve with vacuum erection devices.
- The open end of the cylinder is placed over the penis against the pubis to create an airtight seal with lubricant used to facilitate the seal. Devices come with single-hand operation attached to the end of the cylinder. The constriction ring should be placed over the cylinder before beginning so it can be rolled onto the base of the penis immediately after negative pressure is released and before removal of the cylinder.
- A constriction band should not be left on for >30 minutes as this may lead to ischaemia.

After 5 years, the patient returns to our clinic for further refractory ED despite 40 mcg alprostadil ICI. One year ago, cardiac ischaemic changes were found on a stress test. Angiography revealed two-vessel CAD and he had drug-eluting stents placed with a good outcome. He continues on aspirin and has initiated insulin. On a follow-up stress test, he completed a 4-minute protocol without any changes. Over the last 9 months, he tried using a vacuum erection device but was unsatisfied. He wants to know if there is anything else that can be done.

Clinical tip Counselling for penile implants

- Penile prosthesis has the highest level of patient satisfaction (up to 90%) for severe ED.[44–46]
- On-demand erections are achieved with preserved sensation and ejaculation.
- Placement irreversibly inhibits the ability to have or stimulate a natural erection.
- Devices change the feel of the flaccid penis.
- The erection does not replicate a natural erection and lacks glans engorgement. These factors can lead to a perception of decreased size.
- Glans engorgement can be improved with co-use of PDE5is or topical alprostadil.[47]
- There are semi-rigid, two- and three-piece inflatable devices.
- Infection rate has been reported as 1% in virgin and 2–3% with revision cases.[48,49] The risk is increased in patients with poor diabetic control or extensive fibrosis post priapism.
- If infection occurs, a hastened explant of the infected device must be performed.
- Prothesis salvage for infection was reported by Mulcahy et al. as 80–90% successful after explant, thorough washout, and immediate reimplantation of a new device. This is not appropriate in the setting of a severe local infection, sepsis, or a resistant organism.[50]
- Other complications include erosion (1–6%), mechanical failure rates (approximately 10% at 5 years, 20% at 10 years, 30% at 15 years), pump or reservoir displacement (1–2%), auto-inflation (1%), scrotal swelling and bruising, chronic pain, new or worsening curvature, transient difficulty with ejaculation or retention, phimosis, sensory change, cylinder aneurysm, inguinal hernia, and supersonic transporter (SST) deformity (i.e. glans tilt or droop) which can cause difficulty with penetration.
- Reoperation rates range from 5% to 15% at 5 years.[51,52]
- Predictors of satisfaction include realistic expectations, BMI <30 kg/m^2, and no Peyronie's disease or history of prostatectomy.
- Predictors of dissatisfaction are perceived loss of length, decreased glanular engorgement, altered sensation, and partner dissatisfaction.[53]

Learning point Types of devices

- Two main vendors: Coloplast and Boston Scientific.
- Three main prosthesis options: malleable/semi-rigid, two-piece or three-piece inflatable.
- **Boston Scientific** three-piece inflatable devices include the AMS 700™ CX, CXR, and LGX. The 700™ CX is considered the base standard and expands in girth. The 700™ CXR does not expand as

greatly and thus is used for scarred corporal bodies or small penis size. The 700™ LGX expands in girth (18 mm) and length (15%).

- Boston Scientific's three-piece inflatable device is coated with an antibacterial coating known as InhibiZone™ that consists of rifampicin and minocycline, has the Momentary Squeeze™ pump, and the reservoir is called the Conceal™.
- Boston Scientific has a two-piece inflatable device (Ambicor™) that is used when reservoir placement places a patient at undo risk (e.g. renal transplant/neobladder/bilateral mesh hernia repairs), but the patient declines a malleable device. This device does not come coated in InhibiZone™.
- Boston Scientific also has the Spectra™ malleable device. It is non-antibiotic coated and comes in girths of 9.5, 11, and 13 mm.
- **Coloplast's** three-piece device is the Titan® Touch. It has a narrow base and standard cylinders that expand in girth to 21 mm.
- Coloplast devices have hydrophilic coating allowing for tailored antibiotic solution to be impregnated into device, have the one-touch release pump, and the reservoir is the CL (Cloverleaf) design.
- Coloplast's malleable device is the Genesis® which also has a hydrophilic coating, and comes in 9.5, 11, and 13 mm girths.
- Both companies' three-piece devices have lock-out valves limiting auto-inflation.
- Both pumps allow detumescence without the need to hold the deflate button while compressing the penis/cylinders to empty.

Expert comment Which device to recommend

The most important thing when deciding on an implant is to involve the patient and ideally their partner. They should have the opportunity to see the devices in person, learn how the mechanism works, watch videos about the devices, and ideally speak to a patient who has had one before. This should be done over more than one consultation to allow the patient to make a considered and informed choice. With all the information on board, the patient should choose the device that suits them best. This will lead to better satisfaction. Except in cases where there may be a particular medical reason why one type of implant may not be suitable, all should be considered. Implant counselling is often best done by a specialist nurse to allow more time for an unbiased consultation.

Clinical tip Preoperative considerations

- No device should be placed in the presence of a systemic, cutaneous, or urinary infection. Untreated voiding dysfunction due to either bladder outlet obstruction or neurogenic bladder is a contraindication.
- Good diabetic control is important. A recent correlation between HbA1c and infection rate was published revealing an infection rate of 1.3% with HbA1c level of <6.5%, 1.5% for 6.5–7.5%, 6.5% for 7.6–8.5%, 14.7% for 8.6–9.5%, and 22.4% for >9.5% ($p < 0.001$). A HbA1c threshold level of 8.5% predicted infection with sensitivity of 80% and specificity of 65%.[54]
- Intravenous anti-Gram positive and negative coverage is required for preoperative induction and recommended for 24 hours postoperatively. Regimens include an aminoglycoside + vancomycin or first- or second-generation cephalosporin.
- Shaving should be done immediately prior to incision so small cuts do not become infected ahead of time. Patients should be instructed to not shave themselves prior to surgery.
- Chlorhexidine decreases skin flora compared to povidone-iodine.[55]

Clinical tip Operative considerations

- A no-touch technique has been advocated by some experts.[56]
- Incision options include subcoronal, infrapubic, and penoscrotal, each with their own benefits and limitations.
- A ventral scrotoplasty after placement may improve perceived length.[57]

- There is a 4.5% risk of proximal perforation, which is more common than lateral and distal perforations and is often caused by smaller dilators.
- Risk of proximal perforation increases in revision surgery but can be readily repaired at the time of surgery with a rear tip extender sling anchored to the corporal body.
- If perforation is not recognized and repaired an extrusion can occur.[58,59]
- Use a clank test to assess for crossover.
- If a crossover does occur, place a large dilator into the receiving side of the crossover and re-dilate the side that caused the septum perforation.
- Urethral injury most commonly occurs during distal dilation, scrotal dissection, or penile modelling.
- If a distal urethral injury occurs during dilating, the urethra should be repaired via a distal counter incision and the case delayed for 3 months. However, if the opposite cylinder is in position already, it can be left in place.
- A Foley catheter is used to drain the bladder to avoid injury during reservoir placement.[60]
- If the space of Retzius is obliterated, as in a post-prostatectomy setting, ectopic placement of the reservoir is an established option.
- A Gibson-type counter-incision can be made to ensure safe placement of the reservoir.
- If a bladder injury is identified, as by blood in the catheter, make a counter incision, explore, and close the bladder, then place the reservoir on the opposite side.
- Lastly, when modelling for curvature, ensure extra support to the distal corpora to minimize risk of distal perforation.

Clinical tip Postoperative considerations

- Perform a wound check at 2 weeks post surgery.
- Patients can then be taught to cycle the device from 3 weeks.
- Patients should perform daily cycling to expand the capsule during its maturation.
- Intercourse should be delayed for 6 weeks.
- Distal erosion is more common in those with impaired sensation and can be repaired using a fibrous capsule cap or graft cap through a distal incision and re-dilating the distal space through the medial wall of the capsule.
- Twenty per cent of patients rarely or never use their device, but despite this the satisfaction rate approaches 90%.

The patient elected to have a three-piece inflatable device placed. His HbA1c level was checked preoperatively and was elevated at 92 mmol/mol (10.6%). His procedure was postponed until he optimized his glycaemic control and his HbA1c dropped to 56 mmol/mol (7.3%). The device was then placed without complication. At 3 months after surgery, he was satisfied with the quality of his erection and happy he could initiate a more routine sexual relationship with his partner again.

A final word from the expert

ED is common problem. The key steps are to differentiate psychogenic from organic ED, to identify any potentially reversible causes, and to identify any coexisting pathological risk factors. Given the common aetiological factors for atherosclerosis and endothelial dysfunction leading to both ED and CAD, development of the former is often a warning sign of future cardiovascular disease, and gives an opportunity to change the course of the individual's future health and outcome. The management of ED has been transformed by PDE5is, which have become more accessible as the post-patent costs have dropped significantly. For those who fail to respond to this first line, a stepwise approach to management as outlined here moving through injectable agents and vacuum devices and leading up to penile prosthesis can effectively manage ED, an important element of a man's life and psychological well-being.

References

1. Feldman, HA, Goldstein I, Hatzichristou DG, Krane RJ, McKinlay JB. Impotence and its medical and psychosocial correlates: results of the Massachusetts Male Aging Study. *J Urol.* 1994;151(1):54–61.
2. Lindau ST, Schumm LP, Laumann EO, Levinson W, O'Muircheartaigh CA, Waite LJ. A study of sexuality and health among older adults in the U.S. *NEJM.* 2007;357(8):762–764.
3. Holden CA, McLachlan RI, Pitts M, et al. Men in Australia Telephone Survey (MATeS): a national survey of the reproductive health and concerns of middle-aged and older Australian men. *Lancet.* 2005;366(9481):218–224.
4. Travison TG, Shabshigh R, Kupelian V, O'Donnell AB, McKinlay JB. The natural progression and remission of erectile dysfunction: results from the Massachusetts Male Aging Study. *J Urol.* 2007;177(1):241–246.
5. Tiefer L, Schuetz-Mueller D. Psychological issues in diagnosis and treatment of erectile disorders. *Urol Clin North Am.* 1995;22(4):767–773.
6. Nehra A, Jackson G, Miner M, et al. The Princeton III Consensus Recommendations for the Management of Erectile Dysfunction and Cardiovascular Disease. *Mayo Clin Proc.* 2012;87(8):766–778.
7. Laumann EO, Kang JH, Glasser DB, Rosen RC, Carson CC. Lower urinary tract symptoms are associated with depressive symptoms in white, black and Hispanic men in the United States. *J Urol* 2008;180(1):233–240.
8. Cao S, Yin X, Wang Y, Zhou H, Song F, Lu Z. Smoking and risk of erectile dysfunction: systematic review of observational studies with meta-analysis. *PLoS One.* 2013;8(4):e60443.
9. Martin-Morales A, Sanchez-Cruz JJ, Saenz de Tejada I, et al. Prevalence and independent risk factors for erectile dysfunction in Spain: results of the Epidemiologia de la Disfuncion Erectil Masculina Study. *J Urol.* 2001;166(2):569–574.
10. Guiliano FA, Leriche A, Jaudinot EO, de Gendre AS. Prevalence of erectile dysfunction among 7689 patients with diabetes or hypertension, or both. *Urology.* 2004;64(6):1196–1201.
11. Hodges LD, Kirby M, Solanki J, O'Donnell J, Brodie DA. The temporal relationship between erectile dysfunction and cardiovascular disease. *Int J Clin Pract.* 2007;61(12):2019–2025.
12. Montorsi P, Ravagnani PM, Galli S, et al. Association between erectile dysfunction and coronary artery disease. Role of coronary clinical presentation and extent of coronary vessels involvement: the COBRA Trial. *Eur Heart J.* 2006;27(22):2632–2639.
13. Chew KK, Finn J. Erectile dysfunction as a predictor for subsequent atherosclerotic cardiovascular events: finds from a linked-data study. *J Sex Med.* 2010;7(1):192–202.
14. DeBusk R, Drory Y, Goldstein I, et al. Management of sexual dysfunction in patients with cardiovascular disease: recommendations of the Princeton Consensus Panel. *Am J Cardiol.* 2000;86(2):62F–68F.
15. Kostis JB, Jackson G, Rosen R, et al. Sexual dysfunction and cardiac risk (the Second Princeton Consensus Conference). *AM J Cardiol.* 2005;96(12):85M–93M.
16. Jackson G, Betteridge J, Dean J, et al. A systematic approach to erectile dysfunction in the cardiovascular patient: a consensus statement—update 2002. *Int J Clin Pract.* 2002;56(9):663–671.
17. Muller JE. Triggering of cardiac events by sexual activity: findings from a case crossover analysis. *Am J Cardiol.* 2000;86(2):14F–118F.

18. Gupta BP, Murad MH, Clifton MM, Prokop L, Nehra A, Kopecky SL. The effect of lifestyle modification and cardiovascular risk factor reduction on erectile dysfunction: a systematic review and meta-analysis. *Arch Intern Med.* 2011;171(20):1797–1803.
19. Boolell M, Allen MJ, Ballard SA, et al. Sildenafil: an orally active type 5 cyclic GMP-specific phosphodiesterase inhibitor for the treatment of penile erectile dysfunction. *Int J Impot Res.* 1996;8(2):47–52.
20. Cheitlin MD, Hutter AM Jr, Brindis RG, et al. Use of sildenafil (Viagra) in patients with cardiovascular disease. Technology and Practice Executive Committee. *Circulation.* 1999;99(1):168–177.
21. Kloner RA, Mitchell M, Emmick JT. Cardiovascular effects of tadalafil. *Am J Cardiol.* 2003 92(9):37–46.
22. Padma-Nathan H, Steers WD, Wicker PA. Efficacy and safety of oral sildenafil in the treatment of erectile dysfunction: a double blind, placebo-controlled study of 329 patients. Sildenafil Study Group. *Int J Clin Pract.* 1998;52(6):375–379.
23. Brock GB, McMahon CG, Chen KK, et al. Efficacy and safety of tadalafil for the treatment of erectile dysfunction: results of integrated analysis. *J Urol.* 2002;168(4):1332–1336.
24. Martin Morales A, Mirone V, Dean J, Costa P. Vardenafil for the treatment of erectile dysfunction: an overview of the clinical evidence. *Clin Interv Aging.* 2009;4:463–472.
25. Kloner RA. Cardiovascular effects of the 3 phosphodiesterase-5 inhibitors approved for the treatment of erectile dysfunction. *Circulation.* 2004;110(19):3149–3155.
26. Morales A, Gingell C, Collins M, Wicker PA, Osterloh IH. Clinical Safety or oral sildenafil citrate (VIAGRA) in the treatment of erectile dysfunction. *Int J Impot Res.* 1998;10(2):69–73.
27. Hatzichristou D, Cuzin B, Martin-Morales A, et al. Vardenafil improves satisfaction rates, depressive symptomatology, and self-confidence in a broad population of men with erectile dysfunction. *J Sex Med.* 2005;2(1):109–116.
28. Montorsi F, Althof SE. Partner responses to sildenafil citrate (Viagra) treatment of erectile dysfunction. *Urology.* 2004;63(4):762–767.
29. Isidori AM Buvat J, Corona G, et al. A critical analysis of the role of T in erectile function. *Euro Urol* 2014;65(1):99–112.
30. Basaria S, Dobs AS. Testosterone making an entry into the cardiometabolic world. *Circulation.* 2007;116(23):2658–2661.
31. Porst H, Reohrborn CG, Secrest RJ, Esler A, Viktrup L. Effects of tadalafil on lower urinary tract symptoms secondary to benign prostatic hyperplasia and on erectile dysfunction in sexually active men with both conditions: analysis of pooled data from four randomized, placebo-controlled tadalafil clinical studies. *J Sex Med.* 2013;10(8):2044–2052.
32. Padma-Nathan H, Hellstrom WJ, Kaiser FE, et al. Treatment of men with erectile dysfunction with transurethral alprostadil. Medicated Urethral System for Erection (MUSE) Study Group. *N Engl J Med.* 1997;336(1):1–7.
33. Padma-Nathan H, Yeager JL. An integrated analysis of alprostadil topical cream for the treatment of erectile dysfunction in 1732 patients. *Urology.* 2006;68(2):386–391.
34. Hellstroum WJ, Bennett AH, Gesundheit N, et al. A double-blind, placebo-controlled evaluation of the erectile response to transurethral alprostadil. *Urology.* 1996;48(6):851–856.
35. Porst H, Buvat J, Meuleman E, Michal V, Wagner G. Intracavernous Alprostadil Alfadex—an effective and well tolerated treatment for erectile dysfunction. Results of a long-term European study. *Int J Impot Res.* 1998;10(4):225–231.
36. Lue TF. Erectile dysfunction. *N Engl J Med.* 2000;342:1802–1813.
37. Nadig PW, Ware JC, Blumoff R. Non-invasive device to produce and maintain an erection-like state. *Urology.* 1986;27(2):126–131.
38. Sidi AA, Decher EF, Zhang G, Lewis JH. Patient acceptance of and satisfaction with an external negative pressure device for impotence. *J Urol.* 1990;144(5):1154–1156.
39. Dutta TC, Eid JF. Vacuum constriction devices for erectile dysfunction: a long-term, prospective study of patients with mild, moderate, and severe dysfunction. *Urology.* 1999;54(5):891–893.

40. Levine LA, Dimitriou RJ. Vacuum constriction and external erection devices in erectile dysfunction. *Urol Clin North Am.* 2001;28(2):335–342.
41. Cai T, Palumbo F, Liguori G, et al. The intra-meatal application of alprostadil cream (Vitaros®) improves drug efficacy and patient's satisfaction: results from a randomized, two-administration route, cross-over clinical trial. *Int J Impot Res.* 2019;31(2):119–125.
42. Lowe FC, Jarow JP. Placebo-controlled study of oral terbutaline and pseudoephedrine in management of prostaglandin E1-induced prolonged erections. *Urology.* 1993;42(1):51–53.
43. Priyadarshi S. Oral terbutaline in the management of pharmacologically induced prolonged erection. *Int J Impot Res.* 2004;16(5):424–426.
44. Brinkman MJ, Henry GD, Wilson SK, et al. A survey of patients with IPP for satisfaction. *J Urol.* 2005;174(1):253–257.
45. Montorsi F, Rigatti P, Carmignani G, et al. AMS three-piece inflatable implants for erectile dysfunction: a long-term multi-institutional study in 200 consecutive patients. *Eur Urol.* 2000;37(1):50–55.
46. Bernal RM, Henry GD. Contemporary patient satisfaction rates for three-piece inflatable penile prosthesis. *Adv Urol.* 2012;2012:707321.
47. Mulhall JP, Jahoda A, Aviv N, Valenzuela R, Parker M. The impact of sildenafil citrate on sexual satisfaction profiles in men with a penile prosthesis in situ. *BJU Int.* 2004;93(1):97–99.
48. Carson CC. Efficacy of antibiotic impregnation of inflatable penile prosthesis in decreasing infection in original implants. *J Urol.* 2004;171(4):1611–1614.
49. Nehra A, Carson CC, Chapin AK, Ginkel AM. Long-term infection outcomes of 3-piece antibiotic impregnated penile prosthesis used in replacement implant surgery. *J Urol.* 2012;188(3):899–903.
50. Mulcahy JJ, Brant MD, Ludlow JK. Management of infected penile implants. *Tech Urol.* 1995;1(3):115–119.
51. Deuk Choi Y, Jin Choi Y, Hwan Kim J, Ki Choi H. Mechanical reliability of the AMS 700CXM inflatable penile prosthesis for the treatment of male erectile dysfunction. *J Urol.* 2001;165(3):822–824.
52. Wilson SK, Delk JR, Salem EA, Cleves MA. Long-term survival of inflatable penile prosthesis: single surgical group experience with 2,384 first time implants spanning two decades. *J Sex Med.* 2007;4(4):1074–1079.
53. Trost LW, Baum N, Hellstrom WJ. Managing the difficult penile prosthesis patient. *J Sex Med.* 2013;10(4):893–906.
54. Habous M, Tal R, Tealab A, et al. Defining a glycated haemoglobin (HbA1c) level that predicts increased risk of penile implant infection. *BJU Int.* 2018;121(2):293–300.
55. Yeung LL, Grewal S, Bullock A, Lai HH, Brandes SB. A comparison of chlorhexidine-alcohol vs povidone-iodine for eliminating skin flora before genitourinary prosthetic surgery: a randomized controlled trial. *J Urol.* 2013;189(1):136–140.
56. Eid JF, Wilson SK, Cleves M, Salem EA. Coated implants and 'no touch' surgical technique decreases risk of infection in IPP implantation to 0.46%. *Urology.* 2012;79(6):1310–1315.
57. Miranda-Sousa A, Keating M, Moreira S, Baker M, Carrion R. Concomitant ventral phalloplasty during penile implant surgery: a novel procedure that optimizes patient satisfaction and their perception of phallic length after penile implant surgery. *J Sex Med.* 2007;4(5):1494–1499.
58. Szotok MJ, DelPizzo JJ, Sklar GN. The plug and patch: a new technique for repair of corporal perforations during placement of penile prosthesis. *J Urol.* 2000;163(4):1203–1205.
59. Wilson SK. Rear tip extender sling: a quick and easy repair of crural perforation. *J Sex Med.* 2010;7(3):1052–1055.
60. Henry G, Hsiao W, Karpman E, et al. A guide for inflatable penile prosthesis reservoir placement: pertinent anatomical measurements of the retropubic space. *J Sex Med.* 2014;11(1):273–278.

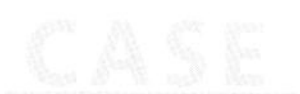

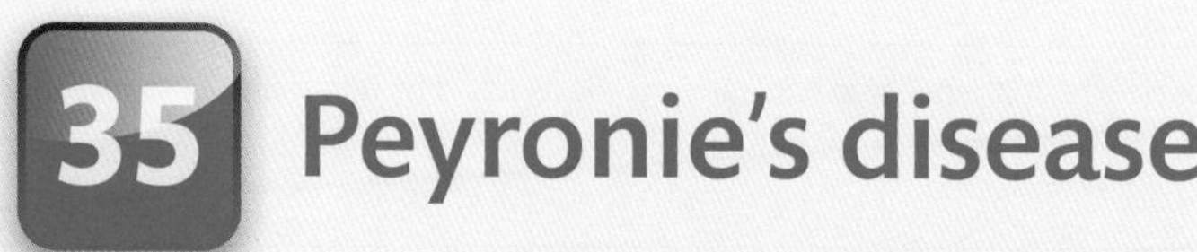

35 Peyronie's disease

Sarah Prattley

Expert commentary Rowland Rees

Case history

A 51-year-old gentleman was referred to the andrology clinic with a 2-year history of penile curvature. The curvature had been stable for approximately 18 months and no longer caused painful erections. This resulted in him being unable to have sexual intercourse; however, his erectile function was not impaired.

Questioning and photographic evidence revealed a marked dorsal curvature of 70°. His erectile function was satisfactory, without the need for adjunctive therapy. The patient had recently started a new relationship, but had been unable to achieve penetrative intercourse due to the curvature. This was affecting his psychosexual health which subsequently led to mild depression. The patient had a past medical history of asthma, and took a combination budesonide and formoterol 160/4.5 mcg inhaler. He was also a smoker with a 20 pack-year history. He had no evidence of Dupuytren's contracture or Ledderhose disease.

On examination and self-taken photograph depicting degree of curvature, the patient was found to have a 70° dorsal curvature at tumescence with associated waist deformity, with a stretched penile length of 11 cm. There was palpable plaque disease on the dorsal aspect of the penis which was non-tender.

Learning point Phases of Peyronie's disease

There are two distinct phases of Peyronie's disease (PD), and it is important to identify which phase the patient is in as this will help guide management, advice, and monitoring.

Active disease

This is characterized by active symptoms that are dynamic and changing. Pain related to inflammation can be experienced along the active area of disease in the tunica albuginea. Deformity at this stage may not be fully developed and may change over the subsequent months. The natural history of PD is that plaque-related pain improves or resolves in approximately 90% of patients in the first 12–18 months. However, improvement in curvature is limited to 3–13%, with predictors of progression versus resolution unclear.[1,2] Stabilization of plaque disease and curvature occurs in 47–67% of patients and worsens in 30–50%.[2,3] Erectile function during this stage may be compromised by pain or deformity but can be intact. During this stage, conservative and medical therapy can be considered to attempt to limit symptoms and progression.

Stable disease

Stable disease is characterized by a lack of symptom change or progression for >3 months, and is typically 1 year following the onset of symptoms.[4] Pain may still be present but is less common. There is often a plaque palpable which can become hard, and can be assessed by ultrasound.[5] However, the size and magnitude of the plaque bears no influence on the degree of deformity.[6] It is at this stage that surgical intervention can be considered.

Learning point Psychosexual impact

It is essential that the psychosexual impact of PD on patients is assessed and managed appropriately. Approximately 48% of men with PD are affected by depression, with 26% moderately and 22% severely affected, and 81% reporting emotional distress associated with PD.[7,8] Four core domains have been identified as being important to men with PD: physical appearance and self-image; sexual function and performance; PD-related pain and discomfort; and social stigmatization and isolation.[9]

Depression has been associated with a twofold increase in sexual problems, namely reduction in sexual desire, libido, erectile dysfunction (ED), and orgasm. Antidepressants can cause treatment-emergent sexual dysfunction, further affecting overall problems.[10] This can result in exacerbation of ED symptoms in PD.

Expert comment The presence of ED

It is essential to establish if ED is present as this will impact intervention. A trial of phosphodiesterase type 5 inhibitors can be given to see if ED can be improved.

Patients need to be counselled appropriately as performing surgical intervention in patients with refractory ED will render any repair useless. Such patients can be considered for penile prosthesis.

Expert comment Evaluation of PD

There is currently no internationally accepted standard of evaluation for PD. Current recommendations in the examination for PD include degree of curvature and stretched penile length, which is equivalent to erect length.[11] This can be with self-photograph, vacuum-assisted erection test, or pharmacological-induced erection. The International Index of Erectile Function may be useful but has not been validated in PD.[12] Peyronie's Disease Questionnaire may be helpful in establishing baseline scores and in determining change over time (level of evidence 2a).[13]

Ultrasound scan measurement of plaque size is user dependent and inaccurate, and is not recommended in everyday clinical practice (level of evidence 3).[6] Doppler ultrasound scanning can be used in those with ED, for vascular assessment (level of evidence 2a).[14]

Clinical tip Erection test

When performing the artificial erection test, it is best to compress the base of the penis against the pubic bone, so as not to miss any proximal element to the curvature. A tourniquet can then be used if proximal disease is excluded.

Clinical tip Mobilization of the neurovascular bundle

Great care needs to be taken when mobilizing the neurovascular bundle in order to avoid neurovascular complications such as glans ischaemia. It can be performed laterally to medially, or medially to laterally after excising the dorsal vein.

Given the degree of curvature and waist deformity of the penis, a Nesbit or its alternative penile-shortening procedures was ill-advised due to the degree of penile length loss, therefore the patient was counselled regarding a Lue procedure, and advised to stop smoking and continue with his exercise programme while awaiting intervention. The management of stable PD depends on whether ED is present and penile length (Figure 35.1).

The operation involved initial circumcision, followed by degloving of the penis down to the level of Buck's fascia. Two butterfly needles were inserted from the glans into the corpora cavernosa. An erection test was then performed with normal saline and a tourniquet around the base of the penis to further characterize site, plane, and degree of curvature (Figure 35.2a).

As the site of the curvature and plaque disease was on the dorsal aspect of the penis at the level of the midshaft, the neurovasculature was mobilized with Buck's fascia. This allowed for direct access to the affected tunica albuginea. A modified H incision was made into the point of maximum curvature of the tunica thereby creating a window for grafting with bovine collagen Permacol® (Figure 35.2b).

Finally, a repeat erection test was completed after closure of Buck's fascia to determine if any further corrections were required, with an accepted residual curvature of up to 10° (Figure 35.2c). The skin was then replaced and sutured closed.

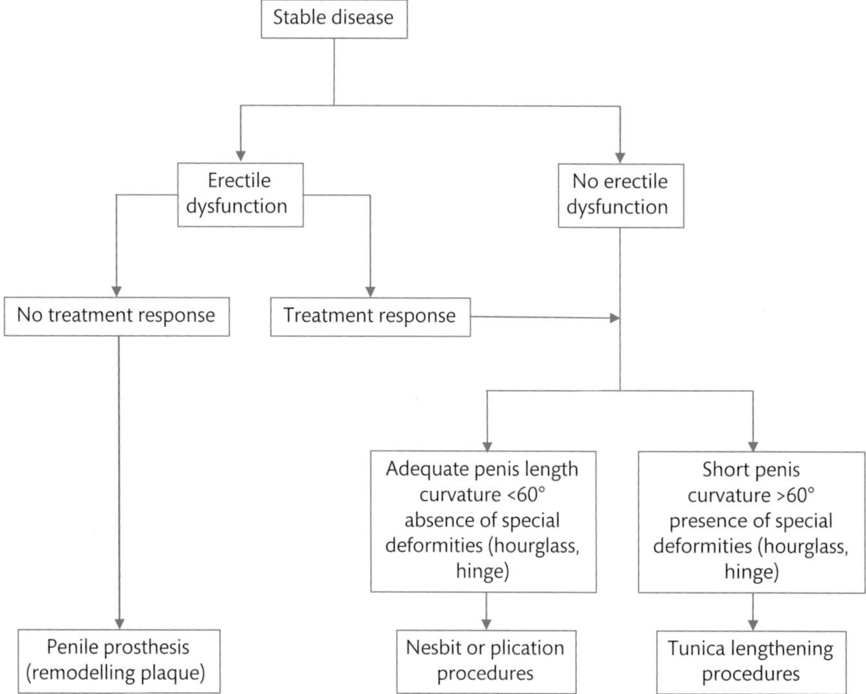

Figure 35.1 Surgical algorithm for PD.[4]

Expert comment Congenital penile curvature

Penile curvature can either be congenital or acquired. Congenital penile curvature is rare with an incidence of <1% and results from disproportionate development of the tunica albuginea of the corporal bodies, with the most common curvature being ventrally.[15] Any intervention is deferred until after puberty and intervention shares the same principles as PD.

Congenital penile curvature typically affects the entirety of the tunica rather than an affected site with PD. Surgical correction therefore should take place in specialized centres only with clinicians used to dealing with challenging cases.

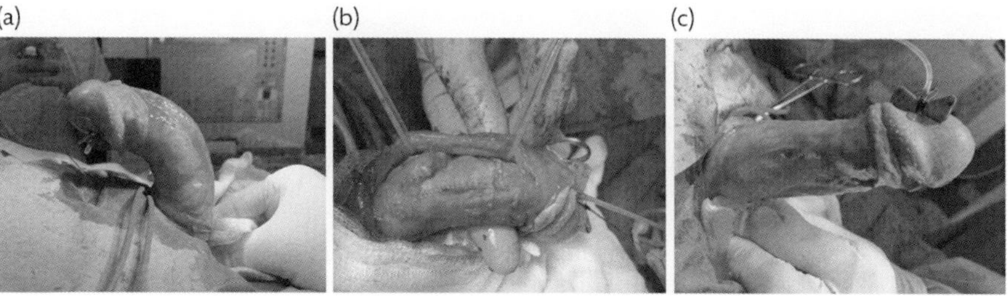

Figure 35.2 Intraoperative images of penile straightening surgery (Lue's). (a) Erection test to characterize site, plane, and degree of curvature. (b) Modified H incision. (c) Final erection test following closure of Buck's fascia.

Learning point Prevalence and aetiology of PD

PD is a fibrotic disease of the tunica albuginea which results in a focal loss of elasticity at the involved site of plaque formation. During erection, non-uniform expansion results in curvature at the site due to loss of longitudinal stretch.[16]

The aetiology of PD is unclear; however, the most widely accepted hypothesis is that of a localized response to endogenous factors from repetitive microvascular injury or trauma within the bilayer of the tunica albuginea in genetically susceptible individuals.[17,18] This results in a prolonged inflammatory process, characterized by remodelling of connective tissue into a dense fibrotic plaque.[19]

The prevalence of PD is 0.4–9%[3,20]; this figure may be higher in specific high-risk subgroups, with a typical age at presentation being 55–60 years. Risk factors include trauma, genetic susceptibility, diabetes, hypertension, lipid abnormalities, ischaemic cardiomyopathy, ED, smoking, and alcohol excess.[21]

Learning point Non-surgical management of PD

Conservative therapy is predominantly focused towards patients in the early stages of the disease, when the plaque has not densely fibrosed or calcified. However, the efficacy in distinct patient populations is yet to be demonstrated.[4]

There are a multitude of treatment options for PD; however, due to the incomplete aetiological understanding there is a lack of efficacious treatment, and large multicentre series or randomized controlled trials are lacking.[21] Non-surgical treatment modalities have focused on disrupting or reducing the acute phase process. Options include oral, mechanical, topical, and intralesional therapies (Table 35.1).

While other therapies may have potential benefit in differing stages of PD including potassium para-aminobenzoate, intralesional and topical verapamil, intralesional interferon, and iontophoresis, they have not shown sufficient evidence to be recommended.[4] Other therapies have shown little or no benefit such as vitamin E, tamoxifen, colchicine, acetyl esters of carnitine, pentoxifylline, extracorporeal shockwave lithotripsy, and intralesional steroids and are currently not recommended by the European Association of Urology.[4]

Table 35.1 Non-surgical management of PD

Oral	Topical	Mechanical
Vitamin E	Verapamil	Iontophoresis
Potassium para-aminobenzoate	H-100 gel	Extracorporeal shockwave lithotripsy
Tamoxifen		Traction device
Colchicine		Vacuum device
Acetyl esters of carnitine		
Pentoxifylline		

Evidence base Intralesional collagenase *Clostridium histolyticum*

Intralesional collagenase *Clostridium histolyticum* (CCH) is the only medical therapy approved by the US Food and Drug Administration and European Medicines Agency for the treatment of PD with dorsal or lateral curvature >30°. Two large, randomized, placebo-controlled, double-blind trials (IMPRESS I and II) have confirmed its efficacy[22] with improvement in curvature of 34% versus 18.2% in placebo. Peyronie's Disease Questionnaire and International Index of Erectile Function scores improved and overall satisfaction rates were also higher.[22,23] Significant adverse events related to this included three corporeal ruptures, all requiring surgical repair, and three haematomas.

The International Consortium on Sexual Medicine guidelines recommend the use of intralesional CCH should be limited to stable curvature between 30° and 90°, with normal erectile function, and no underlying hour-glass deformity, plaque calcification, or proximally located plaque at the base of the penis, level of evidence 2. Clinical trials have not yet established CCH use in ventral curves, or complex PD effect in these groups.[21] Its use during the acute phase is currently under investigation.[24]

Evidence base Traction device

A recent non-randomized controlled trial into the use of traction device in the acute phase of PD found that there was a mean improvement curvature of the penis of 20° in 55 patients, compared to 41 patients in the non-intervention group. There was also improved sexual function, reported pain level, and a reduction in the need for surgical intervention.[25] However, in order to attain these results, it requires commitment from a patient perspective. The traction device needs to be worn for a minimum of 6 hours a day for 6 months. In practice, this is difficult to achieve, and therefore vacuum devices are more commonly used despite lack of high-level evidence.[4]

Future directions Developments in non-surgical management of PD

Recent development in non-surgical management have included the use of hyaluronic acid, plasma-rich platelets, H-100 gel, and combination therapy. Further larger-scale studies are required to assess their efficacy.[26]

There is also increasing evidence for the role of mesenchymal stem cell therapy. This may result in beneficial effects of local growth and repair, leading to regeneration of tissue. Studies involving rat models injected with adipose tissue-derived stem cells into tunica albuginea and corpus cavernosum showed statistically significant results in the improvement of erectile function through prevention of fibrosis during the acute phase.[27] It has also been used in conjunction with interferon and has shown promising results.[28] Very few human studies have been performed to date and with small numbers but results show that it may be beneficial.[29]

Learning point Penile shortening surgery

There have been developments of penile shortening surgery throughout the years, since the Nesbit procedure was first documented in 1965.[30] There are three techniques in current use for the management of penile curvature. All procedures involve techniques performed on the convex side of the penis, opposite to the site of plaque formation, in order to achieve penile straightening.

- **Nesbit procedure**: excision of a 5–10 mm elliptical section of the tunica albuginea or approximately 1 mm for every 10° of curvature.
- **Plication Heineke–Mikulicz principle (Yachia or Lemberger)**: after exposure, single or multiple longitudinal incisions to the convex side of the penis, with a vertical incision and a horizontal closure to the tunica, thus applying the Heineke–Mikulicz principle.
- **'Sixteen-dot' Lue procedure**: parallel plication of the tunica albuginea with non-absorbable suture under minimal tension. The central point of curvature needs to be established, then 16 (two pairs) or 24 dots (three pairs) are marked at 0.5 cm distance from each other and plicated.

Satisfaction rates in those with normal erectile function preoperatively are 74–94% for Nesbit corporoplasty and 52–98% for plication procedures in patients with PD, while success rates for penile straightening ranges from 57–100% to 73–96% respectively.[31] Degrees of complications and risks vary between the different methods but include penile shortening, ED, change in sensation, recurrent curvature, palpable sutures, and the potential need for circumcision at the time of operation.[32]

Learning point Penile lengthening procedures

Penile lengthening procedures, as described in the case of our patient, are performed on the concave side of the penis, and require a graft. While the aim of the procedure is to preserve length, 17–40% of patients still experience a degree of shortening over time.[33]

A Lue procedure as described, involves either a 'H' or double-'Y' incision into the tunica albuginea, creating a defect on the affected concave side which is grafted. In a recent review of plaque incision and grafting, successful straightening was reported in 80–96.4% of patients; however, ED rates were

Expert comment The aim of surgical management

The aim of surgical intervention is to correct the curvature of the penis in a patient with stable disease, allowing for sexual intercourse and improvement in quality of life. It is usually recommended to wait a year from the onset of symptoms before performing any surgical intervention. There are three types of surgical strategies available for patients with PD or congenital curvature: a penile shortening procedure, a penile lengthening procedure, or prosthesis.

Learning point Penile prosthesis

This is typically reserved for patients with severe PD, usually in combination with ED with or without complex deformity such as a hinge deformity, particularly if non-responsive to phosphodiesterase type 5 inhibitors. Penile prostheses are often used in conjunction with grafting or plication techniques in order to achieve sufficient correction, where intraoperative modelling of the penis through manually bending in the opposite direction to the curvature is not sufficient.[4,33]

higher than for penile shortening procedures. The percentage of patients requiring adjunctive therapy was between 4.6% and 67.4% postoperatively, and 0–11.8% were unable to achieve erection.[34] Factors that are associated with increased rates of ED are excision of plaque, the use of larger grafts, preoperative ED, age >60 years, and ventral curvature.[35]

Future directions Penile volume-loss deformity

Penile volume-loss deformity is often overlooked, it is reported to be present in 65% of men with PD curvature and 10–13% of those with <10° curvature. This can result in global penile length loss, hourglass deformity, unilateral indentation, distal tapering, or proximal or distal girth loss. These changes alone can result in axial instability, psychological distress, and decreased sexual activity. Volume loss deformities are often difficult to quantify and are typically not reported in outcome measurements. Further quantitative investigation is required for the development of volume-restoring therapies.[36]

A final word from the expert

PD is a poorly recognized but fairly common condition primarily affecting the ageing male, with a peak age of incidence in the early 50s. The pathophysiology has yet to be fully clarified, but there is an association with vascular risk factors such as diabetes and other fibrotic conditions such as Dupuytren's contracture.

It typically has an acute inflammatory phase followed by a chronic and stable phase which usually plateaus within a year of symptom onset, resulting in fibrosis of the tunica albuginea. It can present in a similar way to those with a clear history of penile injury.

Symptoms include a palpable lump in the penis, penile pain (in the acute phase), penile shortening, or ED, but the commonest reason to seek medical attention is a penile curvature during erection, prohibiting sexual intercourse.

Patient assessment includes taking a clear history of the symptoms, defining the patient's main concerns, examining the penis, and a reliable assessment of the degree of curvature or deformity—either by good photographic evidence or a pharmacologically induced erection in the clinic. If left alone in the acute phase, there is a 3–13% chance of improvement of the curvature and a 30–50% chance of further progression.

Treatment choices should be directed at the patient's concerns and priorities. There is no effective medical therapy that can reverse the fibrosis of PD, and realistic options lie between mechanical stretching therapy, intratunical injections, or surgery. The evidence for mechanical stretching therapy such as the vacuum erection device or penile stretchers is low level, and the success rates low, but the risks are minimal. Rather than just wait, patients may opt to do this in the early phase of the disease when it is too early to consider surgery.

More recently, level 1 evidence has emerged for the benefits, though modest, of intratunical injections of CCH (Xiapex®) as an option for those not ready for or not wanting to consider surgery. On average, a 34% improvement in curvature can be achieved, and the results are better in the milder curvatures.

Surgery remains a mainstay of treatment for stable disease (>1 year). Curvatures of <60° can be corrected by shortening the convex side (corporoplasty) by a number of methods such as excision, plication, or the Heineke–Mikulicz principle. This will cause a geometric and proportional shortening of the erect penis, and is therefore not advised in curvatures of >60°. For more severe curvatures, an incision and grafting procedure is advised which aims to lengthen the shortened concave side, though this is associated with a significant complication profile including ED and recurrent curvature. For this reason, a penile prosthesis is recommended as the best option where there is a combination of severe curvature and pre-existing ED.

Severe PD/penile fibrosis can be a challenging problem to treat, impossible to reverse, and often associated with psychological morbidity, so it is vital to manage patient expectations and counsel patients appropriately from the start.

References

1. Berookhim BM, Choi J, Alex B, Mulhall JP. Deformity stabilisation and improvement in men with untreated Peyronie's disease. *BJU Int.* 2014;113(1):133–136.
2. Grasso M, Lania C, Blanco S, Limonta G. The natural history of Peyronie's disease. *Arch Esp Urol.* 2007;60(3):326–331.
3. Mulhall JP, Creech SD, Boorjian SA, et al. Subjective and objective analysis of the prevalence of Peyronie's disease in a population of men presenting for prostate cancer screening. *J Urol.* 2004;171(6):2350–2353.
4. Katzimouratidis K, Eardley I, Giuliano F, Moncada I, Salonia A. Guidelines on penile curvature. European Association of Urology. 2015. https://uroweb.org/wp-content/uploads/EAU-Guidelines-Penile-Curvature-2015.pdf
5. Nehra A, Alterowitz R, Culkin DJ, et al. Peyronie's disease: AUA guidelines. American Urological Association. 2015. https://www.auanet.org/documents/education/clinical-guidance/Peyronies-Disease.pdf
6. Porst H, Vardi Y, Akkus E, et al. Standards for clinical trials in male sexual dysfunction. *J Sex Med.* 2010;7(2):414–444.
7. Farrell MR, Corder CJ, Levine LA. Peyronie's disease among men who have sex with men: characteristics, treatment, and psychosocial factors. *J Sex Med.* 2008;5(9):2179–2184.
8. Cavallini G. Psychological aspects of Peyronie's disease. In: Cavallini G, Paulis G, eds. *Peyronie's disease.* Cham: Springer; 2015:71–72.
9. Nelson CJ, Mulhall JP. Psychological impact of Peyronie's disease: a review. *J Sex Med.* 2013;10(3):653–660.
10. Kennedy SH, Rizvi S. Sexual dysfunction, depression, and the impact of antidepressants. *J Clin Psychopharmacol.* 2009;29(2):157–164.
11. Wessells H, Lue T, McAninch J. Penile length in the flaccid and erect states: guidelines for penile augmentation. *J Urol.* 1996;156(3):995–997.
12. Rosen RC, Riley A, Wagner G, Osterloh IH, Kirkpatrick J, Mishra A. The international index of erectile function (IIEF): a multidimensional scale for assessment of erectile dysfunction. *Urology.* 1997;49(6):822–830.
13. Hellstrom WJ, Feldman R, Rosen RC, Smith T, Kaufman G, Tursi J. Bother and distress associated with Peyronie's disease: validation of the Peyronie's disease questionnaire. *J Urol.* 2013;190(2):627–634.
14. Hellstrom WJ, Bivalacqua TJ. Peyronie's disease: etiology, medical, and surgical therapy. *J Androl.* 2000;21(3):347–354.
15. Yachia D, Beyar M, Aridogan IA, Dascalu S. The incidence of congenital penile curvature. *J Urol.* 1993;150(5):1478–1479.
16. Bella AJ, Perelman MA, Brant WO, et al. Peyronie's disease (CME). *J Sex Med.* 2007;4(6):1527–1538.
17. Brock G, Hsu GL, Nunes L, von Heyden B, Lue TF. The anatomy of the tunica albuginea in the normal penis and Peyronie's disease. *J Urol.* 1997;157(1):276–281.
18. Gonzalez-Cadavid NF. Mechanism of penile fibrosis. *J Sex Med.* 2009;6(3):353–362.
19. Kumar B, Narang T, Gupta S, Gulati M. A clinic-aetiological and ultrasonographic study of Peyronie's disease. *Sex Health.* 2006;3(2):113–118.

20. Schwarzer U, Sommer F, Klotz T, et al. The prevalence of Peyronie's disease: results of a large scale survey. *BJU Int.* 2001;88(7):727–730.
21. Chung E, Ralph D, Kagiolu A, et al. Evidence-based management of Peyronie's disease. *J Sex Med.* 2016;13(6):905–923.
22. Gelbard M, Goldstein I, Hellstrom WJ, et al. Clinical efficacy, safety and tolerability of collagenase clostridium histolyticum for the treatment of Peyronie disease in 2 large double-blind, randomized, placebo controlled phase 3 studies. *J Urol.* 2013;190(1):199–207.
23. Gelbrand M, Lipshultz LI, Tursi J, et al. Phase 2b study of the clinical efficacy and safety of collagenase Clostridium histolyticum in patients with Peyronie disease. *J Urol.* 2012;187(6):2268–2274.
24. Yang KK, Bennett N. Peyronie's disease and injectable collagenase Clostridium histolyticum: safety, efficacy, and improvements in subjective symptoms. *Urology.* 2016;94:143–147.
25. Martinez-Salamanca JI, Egui A, Moncada I, et al. Acute phase Peyronie's disease management with traction device: a non-randomised prospective controlled trial with ultrasound correlation. *J Sex Med.* 2014;11(2):506–515.
26. Randhawa K, Shukla CJ. Non-invasive treatment in management of Peyronie's disease. *Ther Adv Urol.* 2019;11:1–13.
27. Castiglione F, Hedlund P, Van der Aa F, et al. Intratunical injection of human adipose tissue-derived stem cells prevents fibrosis and is associated with improved erectile function in a rat model of Peyronie's disease. *Eur Urol.* 2013;63(3):551–560.
28. Gocke A, Abd Elmageed ZY, Lasker GF, et al. Intratunical injection of genetically modified adipose tissue-derived stem cells with human interferon α-2b for treatment of erectile dysfunction in a rat model of tunica albugineal fibrosis. *J Sex Med.* 2015;12(7):1533–1544.
29. Levy JA, Marchand M, Iorio L, Zribi G, Zahalsky MP. Effects of stem cell treatment in human patients with Peyronie disease. *J Am Osteopath Assoc.* 2015;115(10):e8–e13.
30. Nesbit RM. Congenital curvature of the phallus: report of three cases with description of corrective operation. *J Urol.* 1965;93:230–232.
31. Çayan S, Aşcı R, Efesoy O, et al. Comparison of patient's satisfaction and long-term results of two penile plication techniques: lessons learned from 387 patients with penile curvature. *Urol.* 2019;129:106–112.
32. Ralph D, Gonzalez-Cadavid N, Mirone V, et al. The management of Peyronie's disease: evidence-based 2010 guidelines. *J Sex Med.* 2010;7(7):2359–2374.
33. Gaffney CD, Pagano MJ, Weinberg AC, et al. Lengthening strategies for Peyronie's disease. *Transl Androl Urol.* 2016;5(3):351–362.
34. Rice P, Somani BK, Rees RW. Twenty years of plaque incision and grafting for Peyronie's disease: a review of literature. *Sex Med.* 2019;7(2):115–128.
35. Mulhall J, Anderson M, Parker M. A surgical algorithm for men with combined Peyronie's disease and erectile dysfunction: functional and satisfaction outcomes. *J Sex Med.* 2005;2(1):132–138.
36. Margolin EJ, Pagano MJ, Aisen CM, Onyeji IC, Stahl PJ. Beyond curvature: prevalence and characteristics of penile volume-loss deformities in men with Peyronie's disease. *Sex Med.* 2018;6(4):306–315.

36 Ejaculatory orgasmic disorders

Maria Satchi

Expert commentary David Ralph

Case history

A 50-year-old Afro-Caribbean male was referred to a tertiary urology service for investigation and management of an 18-month history of delayed and absent ejaculation and difficulty reaching orgasm. He felt the time to reach orgasm was prolonged and this was followed by small volume of ejaculate or more often, a 'dry ejaculate'. He was able to achieve a spontaneous erection; however, he felt this was not as rigid as it had once been. He was most troubled by the reduction or on occasion, absence of the ejaculate and said that in only one in 20 episodes he would note a small volume expelled, the rest remained 'dry'. On the occasion he was able to reach orgasm, he felt the urine was cloudy.

Expert comment Ejaculation versus orgasm

Ejaculation and orgasm, although linked, are two separate neurophysiological processes that occur during peak sexual arousal. In the absence of an underlying neurological disorder, ejaculation typically promotes a state of orgasm. However, ejaculation can occur without orgasm and vice versa. It is therefore important to view ejaculatory disorders and orgasmic disorders separately with an understanding of the underlying physiology. During the history taking process ascertain if the symptoms have been lifelong or acquired, present during masturbation and sexual intercourse and if situational or consistent. This will help to explore an organic versus psychological cause.

Learning point Physiology of ejaculation

Ejaculation is under control of the autonomic nervous system, predominantly the sympathetic nervous system, and has been described in two phases: emission and expulsion.

The **emission phase** can be stimulated by tactile stimulation of the glans penis or by visual or physical stimulation which is under cerebral control. On activation, sensory information is sent via the dorsal penile nerve and pudendal nerve which enter the spinal cord at S2–S4 to relay information to the thalamus and sensory cortex. Central coordination of afferent sensory information is mainly in the medial preoptic area, paraventricular nucleus, and periaqueductal grey and this plays an important role in sexual function.

Sympathetic efferent nerve fibres from T10–L2 via the hypogastric nerves reach the pelvic plexus and stimulate smooth muscle contraction of the epididymis and vas deferens to propel sperm to reach the prostatic urethra via the ejaculatory ducts along with the glandular secretions from the seminal vesicles, bulbourethral glands, and prostate to form seminal fluid. Contraction of the internal urethral sphincter with simultaneous relaxation of the external urethral sphincter prevents retrograde ejaculation (RE) into the bladder and promotes forward antegrade ejaculation.

During the **expulsion phase**, somatosensory information reaches S2–S4 of the spinal cord via the dorsal penile and pudendal nerves. Onuf's nucleus in S2–S4 of the spinal cord sends out efferent somatomotor signals to stimulate rhythmic contraction of the ischiocavernosus and bulbocavernosus muscle which are under control of the somatic nerves. To achieve antegrade ejaculation, the bladder neck remains closed.[1]

Prior to this, the patient had no concerns regarding his ability to orgasm or ejaculate. He was unable to identify any specific triggers or new medications that coincided with the onset of his symptoms. On review of his past medical history, he was a human immunodeficiency virus (HIV)-positive male, diagnosed 18 years ago with a consistently undetectable viral load and a CD4 count of 700 cells/mm^3. He had no prior history of abdominal or pelvic surgery. His only medication was his long-term antiretroviral medications aciclovir and Eviplera®, a combination of emtricitabine, rilpivirine, and tenofovir. He was in a stable, loving relationship and could not identify any psychological stressors or triggers.

Expert comment HIV-positive men

Ejaculatory and orgasmic disorders in HIV-positive men on highly active antiretroviral therapy have been reported in various studies ranging in prevalence between 24% and 49%. Similarly, other studies have not found a significant positive association. The evidence regarding an association between HIV-positive patients and ejaculatory disorders is not robust enough to draw definite conclusions. Patients with HIV, similar to non-infected individuals, may have other comorbidities and psychosexual issues that impact sexual function. They should be investigated and managed in the same way.[2] This differentiation can help with diagnosis and streamline management.

Learning point Classification of ejaculatory disorders

Ejaculatory disorders should be classified as lifelong where it is noted from the patients first sexual experiences and lasts throughout, or acquired, where the current problem was preceded by normal experiences. It should be differentiated from situational or consistent, and if the symptom is present during masturbation and sexual intercourse. The impact on sexual activity and quality of life should be noted and this can be done via patient questionnaires to assess the problem objectively.

Ejaculatory disorders can be classified as follows:

- **Premature ejaculation** (PE): according to the International Society of Sexual Medicine, PE is the inability to delay ejaculation in the majority of cases of vaginal penetration causing personal distress. It can be defined as intravaginal ejaculatory latency time of ≤1 minute (in lifelong PE) or a bothersome reduction in intravaginal ejaculatory latency time to ≤3 minutes (in acquired PE).
- **Delayed ejaculation** (DE): marked delay or inability to achieve ejaculation where a prolonged period of stimulation may be required and causes personal distress. There is no defined time period.[3].
- **Retrograde ejaculation** (RE): absence of antegrade ejaculation and can be partial or complete. Partial RE refers to sperm identified in the post-orgasmic urinalysis associated with an antegrade ejaculate as well.
- **Anejaculation**: complete absence of antegrade ejaculation or RE.

Orgasmic disorders can be primary (lifelong) or secondary (acquired). They can be classified as follows:

- **Delayed orgasmia** (DO): World Health Organization 2nd Consultation on Sexual Dysfunction defines DO as persistent or recurrent difficulty, delay in, or absence of attaining orgasm after sufficient sexual stimulation, which causes personal distress.
- **Anorgasmia** (AO): The International Consultation on Sexual Medicine defines anorgasmia as the perceived absence of orgasm, independent of the presence of ejaculation.

Learning point Drug history

A review of drug history is vital as pharmacotherapies can affect sexual function. Antipsychotic medication that acts to block dopamine receptors in the brain can affect ejaculation causing DE or RE. Out of the atypical antipsychotics, clozapine, has also been reported to cause RE. Methyldopa can cause DE. Monoamine oxidase inhibitors and selective serotonin reuptake inhibitors (SSRIs) that increase serotonin levels, can delay ejaculation and orgasm.[4] Alpha-1-adrenoceptor blockers can affect ejaculatory volume with tamsulosin having the greatest effect compared to others such as alfuzosin.[5]

Learning point SSRIs

Serotonin (5HT) is thought to inhibit ejaculation. Consequently, SSRIs which inhibit the reuptake of 5HT in the central nervous system can delay ejaculation and be used in the treatment of PE.[6] Dapoxetine is a short-acting SSRI licensed for the use in PE. Other SSRIs such as paroxetine and fluoxetine and tricyclic antidepressants such as clomipramine have been used; however, these are unlicensed. These medications should not be used in young patients with bipolar disorder and should be prescribed with caution in those with depression as there is an increased risk of suicide attempts or thoughts. It should also not be offered to those trying to conceive as may have unfavourable effects on sperm parameters. In patients already on an SSRI with DE/AO, alternatives should be considered if possible and advice sought from the lead physician.

On review of his social history, the patient had been an ex-smoker for 20 years, denied any recreational drug use, and consumed 10 units of alcohol per week. Examination of the external genitalia was normal.

Prior to his referral to the urology department, his general practitioner had organized a thyroid function test, full blood count, renal profile, lipid profile, and testosterone, fasting glucose, and glycated haemoglobin (HbA1c) tests. All blood counts were within normal limits.

Learning point Hormonal regulation of ejaculation

Hormones can influence the regulation of ejaculation and therefore should be assessed.

- **Testosterone**: Elevated testosterone has been associated with PE, and low testosterone with DE and reduced ejaculate volume. It is thought to play a role through its action on androgen receptors on the medial preoptic area and pelvic floor muscles.[3,7]
- **Thyroid hormones**: hyperthyroidism has been associated with PE, and hypothyroidism with DE.[8]
- **Prolactin**: hyperprolactinaemia has been associated with anorgasmia and DE, and low levels of prolactin with PE.[3] Hyperprolactinaemia also inhibits gonadotropin-releasing hormone resulting in decreased testosterone via the hypothalamic-pituitary-gonadal axis.
- **Oxytocin**: significance is unclear; however, an increase in level is noted after orgasm, reaching baseline approximately 10 minutes later.[7]

Expert comment Systemic examination for hormonal dysfunction

Examination of this patient should not only focus on the external genitalia but also look for systemic signs and symptoms of endocrine disturbance. On examination, a loss of muscle mass, central obesity, loss of body hair, small testes may be suggestive of low testosterone. Gynaecomastia may be seen in both hypogonadism and hyperprolactinaemia. Patients with hyperthyroidism may have a visible tremor, sweating and unexplained weight loss whilst those with hypothyroidism may have a history of weight gain.

A large study of men with sexual dysfunction identified that patients reporting PE had higher testosterone levels compared to those with DE. Patients with DE had a higher prevalence of hypogonadism compared to those with PE suggesting testosterone influenced the ejaculatory pathway.[9] It is therefore important to consider endocrine disorders as an underlying cause, as correction of these conditions may reverse the ejaculatory or orgasmic dysfunction.

Expert comment Psychosexual elements

At this stage, further questions should be directed at investigating a psychosexual cause that would benefit from counselling. If the DE/DO is situational as opposed to consistent, occurring only during sexual intercourse with a certain partner and not during masturbation or with other partners, this is more likely to suggest a psychosexual element. A patient's masturbatory techniques or practices or psychosexual triggers can be embarrassing to openly discuss but must be explored. Hyperstimulation from excessive masturbation has been linked to DO and increased frequency of masturbation linked to decline in penile sensitivity.[10] Asking these questions can identify patients who would benefit from psychosexual counselling.

To investigate his concerns further, a transrectal ultrasound (TRUS) scan was organized to look for an obstructive cause of his anejaculation/reduced ejaculatory volume. A post-void orgasmic urine was requested looking for the presence of sperm to suggest RE as the underlying pathology. For his concerns of suboptimal erectile function, sildenafil, an oral phosphodiesterase type 5 inhibitor was prescribed to help improve his erectile function. Psychosexual counselling was offered, but the patient declined.

At his follow-up appointment, the TRUS scan showed a closed bladder neck, and no evidence of ejaculatory duct obstruction. A post-orgasmic urine analysis of 28 mL of urine showed sperm at a concentration of 0.4×10^6 million/mL suggesting RE.

Learning point Causes and diagnosis of RE

Out of the ejaculatory disorders, RE is typically organic and results from failure of the bladder neck to close, causing retrograde passage of seminal fluid into the bladder. The diagnosis can be made in patients with absent or low ejaculatory semen volume (defined as <1.5 mL by the World Health Organization) with a post-orgasmic urine sample indicating the presence of sperm. No clear sperm concentration has been defined. It can be partial or complete, where sperm is seen in both the antegrade ejaculate and post-ejaculatory urine sample in partial retrograde ejaculation and only in the post-ejaculatory urine sample with absent antegrade ejaculation when complete (Table 36.1).[4,11]

Table 36.1 Causes of RE

Neurological	Spinal cord injury/shock
	Retroperitoneal lymph node dissection
	Pelvic surgery—radical prostatectomy, cystectomy, abdominoperineal resection
	Diabetes mellitus
	Multiple sclerosis
	Cerebrovascular accident
Anatomical	Bladder outflow obstruction
Medication	Alpha-adrenergic blockers
	Typical antipsychotics
	Clozapine (atypical antipsychotic)
Congenital	Incompetent bladder neck (lifelong RE)
Idiopathic	

Data from: Hendry. Disorders of ejaculation: congenital, acquired and functional. *Br J Urol.* 82, 331–341 (1998). Segraves, R. T. Effects of psychotropic drugs on human erection and ejaculation. *Arch Gen Psychiatry.* 46, 275–284 (1989).

The trial of sildenafil made an improvement to his erectile function only. He still remained bothered by delayed orgasm with predominantly dry ejaculates. He was given a trial of yohimbine to be titrated from 5 mg up to a maximum of 40 mg once daily. He was also given pseudoephedrine 60 mg titrated from once a day to three times a day, to start the day before anticipated sexual activity. This was prescribed to manage his delayed orgasm and ejaculatory dysfunction.

Learning point Management of RE

In this case, the focus was on treating a bothersome symptom rather than achieving sperm for conception. Around 2% of patients presenting to fertility clinics are as a result of RE. Alpha-adrenergic agonists, such as pseudoephedrine, can be used to increase bladder neck tone and promote antegrade ejaculation; however, there is no established treatment protocol.[12] It is the author's practice to start on 60 mg pseudoephedrine the day before intended sexual activity. This can be increased up to 60 mg three times a day. Imipramine, a serotonin and noradrenaline reuptake inhibitor with anticholinergic activity, can also be used at 25–75 mg taken approximately 3 hours before sexual intercourse. Urinary sperm retrieval can also be attempted from a post ejaculatory urine specimen, usually after alkalization or dilution or urine with fluids, and the retrieved sperm is then used for assisted reproductive technology (ART).[13] Penile vibratory stimulation or electroejaculation can achieve an antegrade ejaculate in patients with a neurogenic cause such as diabetes or spinal injury. Samples obtained through these methods can then be used for ART in the form of intravaginal insemination, intrauterine insemination, in vitro fertilisation (IVF) or intracytoplasmic sperm injection (ICSI). Surgical techniques to bring about bladder neck closure are rarely performed but have been reported with successful outcomes of achieving antegrade ejaculation[14] (Table 36.2).

Table 36.2 Medical and surgical options for treatment of RE

Alpha-adrenergic agonist	Pseudoephedrine hydrochloride Midodrine
Anticholinergics	Imipramine (tricyclic antidepressant)
Surgical	Bladder neck collagen injection V-Y plasty bladder neck reconstruction Young–Dees bladder reconstruction

Data from: Jefferys, A., Siassakos, D. & Wardle, P. The management of retrograde ejaculation: a systematic review and update. *Fertil Steril*. 97, 306–312.e6 (2012). Mehta, A. & Sigman, M. Management of the dry ejaculate: a systematic review of aspermia and retrograde ejaculation. *Fertil Steril*. 104, 1074–1081 (2015).

Learning point Causes and treatment of orgasmic disorders

Orgasm occurs as a consequence of physical and mental sexual stimulation and arousal. The onset is usually triggered by ejaculation and stimulated by the increase in pressure within the prostatic urethra that occurs with closure of the bladder neck and expulsion of the seminal fluid.[10] A man's ability to orgasm after every sexual encounter has been reported to decrease with age. This can be as a result of comorbidities such as diabetes or hypothyroidism, decreased stamina of both the patient and partner to reach completion, and age-related changes in penile sensitivity.[10,15] In patients reporting loss of penile sensation, neurophysiological investigations such as biothesiometry or pudendal somatosensory evoked potentials can be done to assess the sensory vibratory perception threshold and afferent signals from the dorsal nerve of penis respectively[10] (Table 36.3).

Often a definite cause cannot be found, and empirical treatment with oral medication can be trailed. There are no large randomized controlled studies in the empirical treatment of AO/DO. At the author's institution, yohimbine is used. Yohimbine is titrated up from 5 mg to a maximum of 40 mg daily dosing. Obtained from the *Pausinystalia johimbe* tree, it is an alpha-2-adrenergic receptor blocker and $5HT_{1a}$ receptor agonist. It can be used to achieve orgasm and can be used in patients on SSRIs experiencing symptoms of sexual dysfunction. A small study of 29 patients demonstrated 19 out of 29 were able to achieve orgasm with or without the assistance of penile vibratory stimulation.[16]

Other drugs that have been trialled in small studies include bupropion, amantadine, cyproheptadine, and oxytocin.[17]

Table 36.3 Causes and treatment of delayed orgasm/anorgasmia

	Cause	Treatment
Endocrine	Hypogonadism Hyperprolactinaemia Hypothyroidism	Treat underlying disorder; aim to normalize hormone levels
Pharmacological	Antipsychotics Antidepressants, SSRIs Opioids	Liaise with lead physician to assess if change to alternative is appropriate
Decreased penile sensation	Age related Diabetes Lifelong	Optimize HbA1c Neurology referral in cases of abnormal neurophysiological investigations
Penile hyperstimulation	Excessive masturbation Personalized masturbatory techniques	Psychosexual counselling for masturbation retraining
Psychosexual		Psychosexual counselling

Data from: Jenkins, L. C. & Mulhall, J. P. Delayed orgasm and anorgasmia. *Fertil Steril.* 104, 1082–1088 (2015).

At his next follow-up visit, the patient had not noticed an improvement in the ability to orgasm with daily yohimbine and had therefore stopped it after 1 month. He felt the pseudoephedrine had made some improvement when taken at a dose of 60 mg twice daily started the day before intended sexual activity. He had come to terms with his ejaculatory dysfunction as he was not aiming to ejaculate to conceive, but rather to 'feel like a man'. He wanted to continue with the pseudoephedrine on an as-required basis. He admitted that he was under a lot of pressure recently and therefore these issues were currently not at the forefront. Finding time to test the effect of the medications was difficult. A further follow-up appointment was organized in 6 months and the option of psychosexual counselling re-visited again, which the patient said he would consider for the next appointment.

Discussion

In both ejaculatory and orgasmic disorders there can be an overlap in the neurotransmitters and hormones identified in association with these disorders at each end of the spectrum.

DE or AO has been associated with hypothyroidism and hypogonadism, whereas PE has been associated with hyperthyroidism and high levels of testosterone. Treatment of the hormonal imbalances have also demonstrated an element of reversibility. Assessment of the patient should be systemic, focusing not only not only on the genital examination but also looking for signs of endocrine disorders during the examination. Laboratory tests should be performed for prolactin, testosterone and thyroid hormones. This should be performed in the morning between 8-11am and fasted to capture peak levels of testosterone which has a circadian variation.

A review of a patient's medication history is important as antipsychotics and antidepressants, mainly SSRIs, that increase serotonin levels have been found to inhibit or delay the ejaculatory pathway. If this is identified, we suggest liaising with the patient's lead physician or psychiatrist to discuss an alternative that may not elevate serotonin levels in the brain.

Similarly, in patients with PE, the same principle can be applied in an attempt to delay ejaculation. Dapoxetine is the only licensed SSRI for use in PE and should be used with caution in young patients and avoided in patients with a significant psychiatric history. For Pharmacological management should not be a first-line management in PE, however, and treatment should start with psychosexual therapy with a focus on behavioural strategies to delay ejaculation. The **stop–start technique** and the **squeeze technique** are often taught in an attempt to maintain a level of sexual excitement below the threshold for ejaculation.[18] Topical anaesthetics such as eutectic mixture of local anaesthetics (EMLA) cream or lidocaine/prilocaine cream or spray or lidocaine only spray have been found to be effective in increasing intravaginal ejaculatory latency time.[19] Tramadol, a serotonin and norepinephrine reuptake inhibitor and opioid receptor agonist, has also been used as off-label treatment for PE. There is, however, limited long-term data and further information is needed regarding its potential for addiction and side effects.[20] In patients reporting lifelong PE, behavioural management and psychosexual counselling should be offered in combination with pharmacological treatment.

In patients who experience organic ejaculatory dysfunction secondary to pelvic surgery or retroperitoneal lymph node dissection, spinal cord injury, or diabetes, explore the patient's wishes regarding fertility. This will help guide management towards sperm retrieval should the use of sympathomimetics fail to achieve antegrade ejaculation. Various techniques such as electroejaculation or surgical sperm retrieval can be employed to retrieve sperm subsequently used in ART such as IVF or ICSI. Anejaculation should be differentiated from RE with a post-orgasmic urine test looking for the presence of sperm. If sperm is identified in the urine, the sperm can be extracted and used in ART. A TRUS or multiparametric magnetic resonance imaging (MRI) of the prostate will also be useful to for look for an obstructive cause with consequent ejaculatory duct obstruction causing reduced ejaculatory volume or anejaculation.

Explore an underlying psychological cause and offer psychosexual counselling for those presenting with orgasmic or ejaculatory disorders or both. Patients can adopt techniques to focus on improving their current problem either to delay or hasten ejaculation and orgasm. Where appropriate, it is often helpful to offer treatment to the couple to focus on issues together.

A final word from the expert

Managing patients with orgasmic and ejaculatory disorders can be challenging and it is important to manage patient expectations from the start. Often, they can be multiple and cause the patient embarrassment and distress when trying to vocalize their concerns. I find it useful to tease out their most problematic symptom and focus on the time of onset, triggers such as life events or new medications that may have been started simultaneously, and if it is situational or consistent. This line of questioning prioritizes symptom management and helps to identify a psychosexual issue.

My next focus is to identify the reason the patient has sought help. This is to assess if the symptoms are causing personal distress only or if fertility is also an issue. This will help focus the line of treatment options if fertility is the priority.

Asking personal questions about masturbation techniques or excessive masturbation can be challenging but this may indicate hyperstimulation as a cause and unless these questions are asked, patients may not be aware or accept this as an issue. Therefore, if psychosexual counselling is simply offered without a cause, patients may decline in the belief that there is purely a pathological cause for their symptoms. Access to a psychosexual counsellor is important to offer to patients with an ejaculatory or orgasmic disorder. For example, masturbation retraining, cognitive therapy, and psychosexual counselling are not within the armamentarium of the general urologist and such patients should have access to specialists who are able to offer this.

During follow-up visits when assessing the efficacy of medications, revisit the timing and dose of administration. On occasion, patients may not have done this correctly and is worth revisiting prior to marking them as unresponsive to the medication.

References

1. Wein AJ, Kavoussi LR, Campbell MF, eds. *Campbell-Walsh Urology*. 10th ed. Philadelphia, PA: Elsevier Saunders; 2012.
2. Collazos J. Sexual dysfunction in the highly active antiretroviral therapy era. *AIDS Rev.* 2007;9(4):237–245.
3. Di Sante S, Mollaioli D, Gravina GL, et al. Epidemiology of delayed ejaculation. *Transl Androl Urol.* 2016;5(4):541–548.
4. Hendry WF. Disorders of ejaculation: congenital, acquired and functional. *Br J Urol.* 1998;82(3):331–341.
5. Giuliano F. Impact of medical treatments for benign prostatic hyperplasia on sexual function. *BJU Int.* 2006;97(Suppl 2):34–38.
6. Waldinger MD, Olivier B. Utility of selective serotonin reuptake inhibitors in premature ejaculation. *Curr Opin Investig Drugs.* 2004;5(7):743–747.
7. Alwaal A, Breyer BN, Lue TF. Normal male sexual function: emphasis on orgasm and ejaculation. *Fertil Steril.* 2015;104(5):1051–1060.
8. Carani C, Isidori AM, Granata A, et al. Multicenter study on the prevalence of sexual symptoms in male hypo- and hyperthyroid patients. *J Clin Endocrinol Metab.* 2005;90(12):6472–6479.
9. Corona G, Jannini EA, Mannucci E, et al. Different testosterone levels are associated with ejaculatory dysfunction. *J Sex Med.* 2008;5(8):1991–1998.
10. Jenkins LC, Mulhall JP. Delayed orgasm and anorgasmia. *Fertil Steril.* 2015;104(5):1082–1088.
11. Segraves RT. Effects of psychotropic drugs on human erection and ejaculation. *Arch Gen Psychiatry.* 1989;46(3):275–284.
12. Shoshany O, Abhyankar N, Elyaguov J, Niederberger C. Efficacy of treatment with pseudoephedrine in men with retrograde ejaculation. *Andrology.* 2017;5(4):744–748.
13. Jefferys A, Siassakos D, Wardle P. The management of retrograde ejaculation: a systematic review and update. *Fertil Steril.* 2012;97(2):306–312.
14. Mehta A, Sigman M. Management of the dry ejaculate: a systematic review of aspermia and retrograde ejaculation. *Fertil Steril.* 2015;104(5):1074–1081.
15. Rowland DL. Penile sensitivity in men: a composite of recent findings. *Urology.* 1998;52(6):1101–1105.

16. Adeniyi AA, Brindley GS, Pryor JP, Ralph DJ. Yohimbine in the treatment of orgasmic dysfunction. *Asian J Androl.* 2007;9(3):403–407.
17. Abdel-Hamid IA, Elsaied MA, Mostafa T. The drug treatment of delayed ejaculation. *Transl Androl Urol.* 2016;5(4):576–591.
18. Jannini EA, Ciocca G, Limoncin E, et al. Premature ejaculation: old story, new insights. *Fertil Steril.* 2015;104(5):1061–1073.
19. Martyn-St James M, Cooper K, Ren K, et al. Topical anaesthetics for premature ejaculation: a systematic review and meta-analysis. *Sex Health.* 2016;13(2):114–123.
20. Martyn-St James M, Cooper K, Kaltenthaler E, et al. Tramadol for premature ejaculation: a systematic review and meta-analysis. *BMC Urol.* 2015;15:6.

SECTION 12

Emergency urology and trauma

CASE

37 Testicular torsion controversies

Lona Vyas and Mohamed Noureldin

Expert commentary Suks Minhas

Case history

A 19-year-old male presented to the accident and emergency department at 4 pm with right-sided scrotal pain. He was a student and was taking regular antidepressants. He previously had a left inguinal hernia repair and left orchiopexy, for undescended testis during childhood. He had developed sudden onset of pain, 11 hours previously at 5 am, which was severe enough to wake him up from his sleep. He took paracetamol tablets but this did not improve his pain. He denied having any history of trauma related to his testis. He had noticed some frequency in passing urine on the day of presentation.

Learning point Incidence

The two main peaks of age of torsion are perinatally and prepubertally. The annual incidence of testicular torsion (TT) is 4.5 in 100,000 males between 1 and 25 years of age. It is more common in the age group between 16 and 24 years, with an incidence of 2.8 per 100,000 males per year. According to Mansbach and his colleagues' database registry, approximately 86% of torsions occur above the age of 10 years. Moreover, about one-third of all the cases will result in orchidectomy.[1,2] However, torsion cannot be reliably excluded in adults of any age.

Learning point Aetiology

The mechanism of TT remains an enigma. There are a number of theories to explain this.

Extravaginal torsion

This occurs in perinatal life as the testes are descending into the scrotum, the tunica vaginalis (TV) has not fully developed and therefore is not fixed to the inner layer of the scrotum. This congenital defect may allow the spermatic cord to twist proximal to the TV leading to torsion. A reported association with extravaginal torsion is a long mesorchium together with cryptorchidism, which can present as an incarcerated inguinal hernia.[3,4]

Intravaginal torsion and the bell clapper deformity

In the bell clapper deformity (BCD), the epididymis and testis lie intravaginally leaving them hanging freely within the vaginal sac and risks subsequent twisting of the cord. The evidence, however, is contentious. Reports suggest that 12% of the male population have the defect, though far fewer boys have TT related to this.[5] However, Scorer and Farrington reported about 80% of patients who had torsion also had a BCD.[5] Another interesting association is that 78% of boys with a BCD have the same deformity on the contralateral side. Therefore, this places the other testis at an increased risk of torsion in the future.

Traumatic events

Between 4% and 8% of males can present with TT and acute scrotum secondary to trauma. However, it is often difficult to differentiate this from a scrotal haematoma.[6]

Genetic factors

The role of genetic factors as a cause of TT are unclear as some animal models have not translated to human studies. However, more recently INSL3 and its receptor RXLF2 have been shown to be associated with TT.[7,8]

Learning point Pathophysiology

The twisting of the spermatic cord as the testis torts results in ischaemia secondary to reduced blood flow. This initiates a cascade of biochemical and cellular pathways resulting in tissue necrosis. There is no predisposition to laterality. A small study reported that TT was right sided in 48% compared to 52% on the left.[9] The reported range of the degree of torsion are 180° to 1080°, with a median of 360° in the salvage group compared to 540° in the orchidectomy group.[9,10]

On examination, the patient looked well with stable vital signs. On focused clinical examination, the right hemi-scrotum looked swollen in comparison to the left side, with associated erythema of the right hemi-scrotal skin. The right testis was also tender to touch. The right testis was higher than the left in position, with absence of the cremasteric reflex. Urine dipstick test came back as negative.

Clinical tip Diagnosis

The time to diagnosis is critical in TT. The three main phases can be categorized as acute (within 24 hours), subacute (1–10 days), and the chronic phase (>10 days). Ideally, a diagnosis should be made within 4 hours; however, delayed presentation may delay surgical intervention.

The diagnosis of torsion is based on history, symptoms, and physical signs.

Adolescents with TT can present with sudden onset of unilateral scrotal symptoms including pain, swelling, erythema, as well as signs of nausea, vomiting, and occasionally fever. Other non-specific symptoms include abdominal pain and urinary dysfunction.[11–14]

Classic findings on clinical examination can include:

- Positive Prehn's sign (elevation of the scrotum does not improve pain symptoms)[14]
- Brunzel's sign (high-riding testis with horizontal lie)[15]
- Ger's sign (retraction of scrotal skin associated with BCD)[16]
- Absence of the cremasteric reflex.

Expert comment Diagnosis and predictive models

The diagnosis of TT using clinical examination alone can be challenging. Predictive models have been described to assist the clinician in diagnosis. These have included scoring systems[17] or specific factors including absence of ipsilateral cremasteric reflex, nausea and vomiting, and scrotal skin changes which have been described as predictive factors. Other factors include time to presentation,[18,19] heterogeneity on ultrasound images, and high position of the testis.

Studies have reported a 'high lie' in only 33–55% of cases.[20] The absence of the cremasteric reflex can be associated with other conditions and has a specificity of only 66%.[21,22] The diagnosis of torsion can be misleading and includes several other differential diagnoses (Table 37.1).

Urine analysis

Diagnostic yield is often improved with the use of dipstick urine analysis to eliminate infective causes.[23]

Table 37.1 Suggestive sign for common differentials of testicular torsion

Testicular torsion	Torsion of appendix	Epididymo-orchitis
Nausea Severe pain No history of trauma Lower abdominal pain	Blue dot associated with necrosis of the appendix Isolated tenderness of upper pole of testis Earlier age History of trauma	Fever Tenderness secondary to inflammation Often sexually active Puberty and older males Epididymal tenderness

The radiographer performed an urgent scrotal ultrasound, which revealed enlargement of the right testis, a small hydrocele, and a marked reduction in vascularity of the right testis in comparison to the left.

Learning point Imaging

Unilateral testicular pain, swelling, and high lie are non-specific, and therefore make a clinical diagnosis difficult. Imaging techniques can be used as an adjunct to assist in the diagnosis, particularly in cases of delayed torsion (>24 hours).

Colour Doppler ultrasound is the most utilized imaging modality with a specificity of 97–100% and sensitivity of 63–99%.[14,23–25] Other useful signs are the identification of the whirlpool sign which is associated with the twisted spermatic cord.[26]

A novel method of ultrasound scanning is contrast enhanced ultrasonography which has been reported to improve visualization of the vasculature compared to standard colour Doppler for smaller testes such as neonates and early TT. This has a sensitivity of 96% and specificity of 100%.[25,27] Interestingly, SonoVue®, the agent used for contrast ultrasound, is not licensed for use in children in Europe. It is used in a few centres in the UK.

Both scintigraphy and dynamic contrast-enhanced subtraction magnetic resonance imaging have comparable sensitivity and specificity to ultrasonography.[28–31] The advantages include a higher sensitivity and ability to differentiate between TT and other acute scrotal pathology. However, it is expensive, not widely available, with little expertise, and is dye dependent. It also would lead to a delay in diagnosis and therefore has an academic use rather than utility in routine clinical practice.[32]

Scrotal scintigraphy requires the use of intravenous 99mTc-pertechnetate radionuclide dye to identify cold spots which highlight absence of the microcirculation. Late hyperperfusion in delayed presentation of TT can give a false-positive signal and therefore this test is more sensitive in the early stages of torsion. However, again delayed diagnosis, cost, and radiation exposure reduce the availability of this modality.[5,33]

However, ultrasonography does not accurately recognize the early phase of torsion.[34] Associated signs are scrotal wall swelling, abnormal positioning of the testis or epididymis, enlargement of the testis, as well as the presence of a reactive hydrocele.[15,35]

Evidence base Guidelines on imaging

The National Institute for Health and Care Excellence guidelines in the UK do not recommend the use of any imaging studies in managing of the acute scrotum if torsion is clinically suspected as this may delay management and increase the risk of testicular infarction and orchidectomy.[36] However, the European Association of Urology guidelines (paediatric), recommend Doppler ultrasonography due to its high sensitivity ranging from 63% to 100% with the aim to minimize the number of cases requiring surgical exploration. It is stated clearly that this should not delay the surgical management[37] (Table 37.2).[38]

Evidence base Colour Doppler versus high-resolution ultrasonography

In a multicentre study in 2007, colour Doppler was compared to high-resolution ultrasonography in surgically verified cases of torsion. The colour Doppler was inferior at identifying reduced flow; 76% compared to 96% of cases of twisted spermatic cords on high-resolution ultrasound scanning.

Table 37.2 Summary of different guidelines

European Association of Urology[37]	Doppler ultrasound is an effective imaging tool to evaluate the acute scrotum and comparable to scintigraphy and dynamic contrast-enhanced subtraction magnetic resonance imaging. This should not delay the intervention
National Institute for Health and Care Excellence[36]	In patients with a history and physical examination suggestive of torsion, imaging studies should **not** be performed as they may delay treatment, therefore prolonging the ischaemic time. Negative surgical exploration is preferable to a missed diagnosis as all imaging studies have a false-negative rate
American Urological Association[38]	If the diagnosis is questionable, scrotal ultrasonography is readily available; this test is the single most useful adjunct to the history and physical examination in the diagnosis of torsion

Data from Thakkar HS, Yardley I, Kufeji D. Management of paediatric testicular torsion—are we adhering to Royal College of Surgeons (RCS) recommendations. *Ann R Coll Surg Engl*. 2018; Dogan HS, Stein R, 't Hoen LA, Bogaert G, Nijman RJM, Tekgul S, et al. Do EAU/ESPU guidelines recommendations fit to patients? Results of a survey on awareness of spina bifida patients. *Eur Urol Suppl*. 2019; Kurtz MP. Evaluation of the pediatric patient with a non-traumatic acute scrotum. *AUA Update Ser*. 2015.

Due to the delay in ultrasound, the decision was made to take the patient directly to theatre for urgent scrotal exploration. The patient was consented carefully for infection, bleeding, infertility, as well as the possibility of right orchidectomy and contralateral fixation. Under general anaesthesia, a midline scrotal incision was performed, and the right testis was delivered. On opening the TV, the testis was found to be dark blue in colour (Figure 37.1) and the cord was untwisted. Warm swabs were wrapped around the testis for 10 minutes, but the testicular colour did not improve and orchidectomy was performed. A three-point fixation of the contralateral testis was performed with non-absorbable sutures. The patient was discharged the following morning after review.

Clinical tip Management

Testicular torsion is a surgical emergency that requires prompt surgical exploration and detorsion. The testis may be excised if unsalvageable or fixed if viable.

Learning point Testicular fixation

Fixation of the testis to the inner scrotal wall prevents re-torsion. If torsion is diagnosed, contralateral fixation must be performed as the BCD is usually present on both sides. The literature describes several techniques for testicular fixation.[12–14,39,40]

A popular method involves stitching a non-absorbable suture from the tunica albuginea (TA) to the median septum or scrotal wall.[41,42] Another technique is to fenestrate the TV to produce strong adhesions between the TA and inner scrotal wall.[43] To reduce the risk of recurrence post fixation, the technique of axial fixation at four points compared to three has been described.[42]

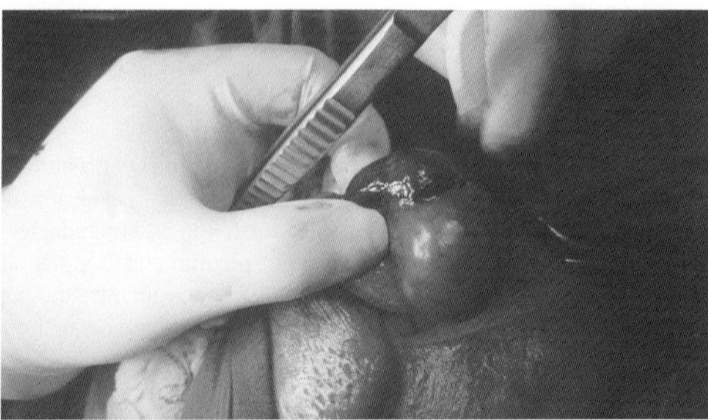

Figure 37.1 Dark blue testis during exploration for testicular torsion from ASUH, Cairo, Egypt 2017.

The main criticism of suturing of the TA is a breach of the blood–testis barrier, which may lead to impaired spermatogenesis.[44] Animal studies have also suggested a higher level of anti-sperm antibodies after orchidopexy.[45,46] Therefore, often paediatric surgeons use a subcutaneous dartos pouch, to avoid suturing of the TA. The testis is fixed in an extravaginal position.[47,48]

Other non-breaching techniques include a Jaboulay's repair and reliance of adhesions between testicular integuments[49] as well as fixation of the TV to the dartos fascia.[45]

Expert comment Contralateral testicular fixation

Catastrophic bilateral testicular loss has impelled recommendations for fixation of the contralateral healthy testis, particularly in boys with BCD.[50,51] Some urologists have adopted similar practice with other pathological causes, which may increase the risk of bilateral complications.[52] Current guidance from the American Urological Association recommends further research into the area as the long-term outcome data are lacking.[53] In the absence of evidence-based guidelines, the decision for contralateral testicular fixation should be based on experience and non-comparative retrospective studies. Therefore, patients and their parents must be thoroughly counselled on both the advantages and disadvantages of each option together with the possible implications prior to surgery.[54]

Learning point Timing of testicular fixation

Door to detorsion time is an important and independent factor affecting testicular preservation and survival. The literature demonstrates that fixing the torted testis within the first 6 hours has the highest probability of salvage rates. This rate decreases with the length of delay in exploration and detorsion of the testis (Figure 37.2).[55] Another important factor includes prehospital delay. Fast efficient hospital management improves the former and education may improve the latter.[56]

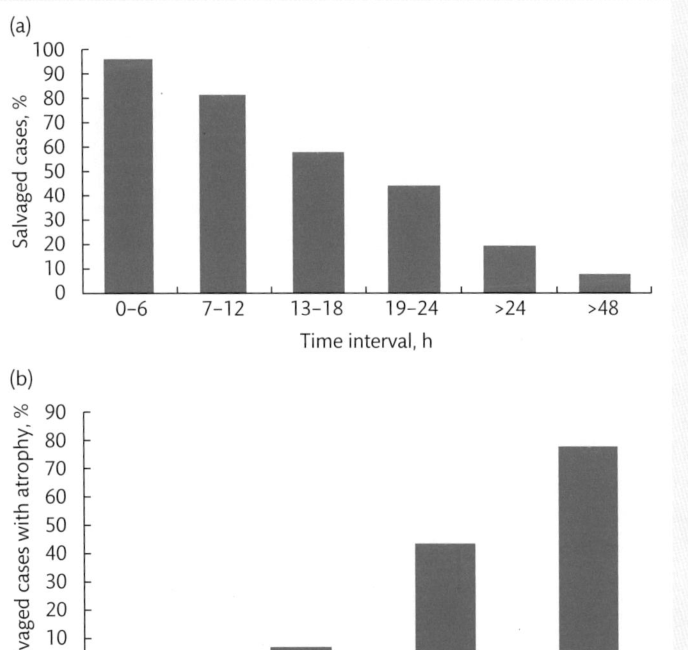

Figure 37.2 Immediate (early) surgical salvage rate after torsion (a) and subsequent atrophy rate of surgically salvaged testes (b) after torsion of various time intervals.
From Visser and Heynes (2003).[55]

Evidence base Testicular fixation

Case studies have advocated fixation of testis despite the clinical appearance of ischaemia in a case of a solitary testis.[57] Often postoperatively normal testicular blood flow can be detected on subsequent ultrasonography, testosterone levels normalize, and cryopreserved semen 50 hours later can also be normal. Therefore, there is a chance of salvage despite the testis appearing completely ischaemic.

A small study (n = 3) describing a technique to decrease ischaemia caused by localized compartment syndrome by making a small window in the TA has been described.[58] The team reported that the intercompartmental pressure decreased dramatically and the colour improved. One case developed this further by adding a TV flap for coverage and found the risk of orchidectomy was less than fasciotomy alone (35.9% vs 15%).[59]

Clinical tip Orchidectomy

Orchidectomy is the final surgical option and a delay in diagnosis will potentially lead to a necrotic unsalvageable testis at exploration. Orchidectomy may be performed in up to 42% of surgically explored cases.[60,61] In all cases detorsion should be performed and only when all attempts to reperfuse the testis have failed and the testis remains unsalvageable. In this case, the surgeon should proceed to orchidectomy.[57,62]

It is extremely important to consent the patient carefully prior to surgery discussing all possible findings, procedures, and complications of surgery.

Expert comment Testicular prosthesis

Post orchidectomy, a urologist must consider both the late effects of the surgery as well as the patient's body image. Insertion of a testicular prosthesis may help to restore patient self-esteem. Around a quarter of testicular prosthesis insertions are performed post TT orchidectomy. Between 68% and 91% of men were satisfied with their prosthesis and body image postoperatively.[63] Historical teaching recommends a delay in prosthesis insertion after torsion to avoid the risk of infection. However, experience from breast surgeons who often insert silicone breasts after mastectomy has changed the current concept of prosthesis timing.[64] A recent study demonstrated that simultaneous insertion of prosthesis with orchidectomy after torsion does not increase complication rates.[65] Moreover, the evidence supporting the concept of delayed insertion is low level.[66]

A final word from the expert

Although TT is one of the most frequent urological emergencies, there are still several controversial areas in management as this chapter has highlighted. There is emerging evidence of an association between TT and genetic disorders as well as an increased incidence in families.[62,67] Environmental causes remain unclear. No single symptom is solely pathognomonic of the disease[20] nor is there an effective imaging technique, which can differentiate diagnosis of TT with a high degree of sensitivity and specificity.[24,32,33,68,69]

Discrepancies in surgical technique, non-invasive manual detorsion, and surgical fixation still rely on surgical experience and surgeon preference.[12,70] Minimizing long-term risk is paramount; however, there is still no consensus on a superior suturing technique, three-point or four-point fixation, and a TA protective approach.[14,46]

Several medical therapies have been used in animal models but very few reliably translate to humans.[71–81] For clinicians to streamline management of this common condition worldwide and ensure uniformity of clinical practice, well-designed multicentre studies are required. Increasing litigation[62] and more access to patients for information necessitates doctors to participate and collaborate in studies to improve evidence-based practice for TT.

References

1. Mansbach JM, Forbes P, Peters C. Testicular torsion and risk factors for orchiectomy. *Arch Pediatr Adolesc Med.* 2005;159(12):1167–1171.
2. Williamson RCN. Torsion of the testis and allied conditions. *Br J Surg.* 1976;63(6):465–476.
3. Zilberman D, Inbar Y, Heyman Z, et al. Torsion of the cryptorchid testis—can it be salvaged? *J Urol.* 2006;175(6):2287–2289.
4. Weiss AP, Van Heukelom J. Torsion of an undescended testis located in the inguinal canal. *J Emerg Med.* 2012;42(5):538–539.
5. Johansen TEB. Anatomy of the testis and epididymis in cryptorchidism. *Andrologia.* 1987;19(5):565–569.
6. Seng YJ, Moissinac K. Trauma induced testicular torsion: a reminder for the unwary. *J Accid Emerg Med.* 2000;17(5):381–382.
7. Sozubir S, Barber T, Wang Y, et al. Loss of Insl3: a potential predisposing factor for testicular torsion. *J Urol.* 2010;183(6):2373–2379.
8. Dajusta DG, Granberg CF, Villanueva C, Baker LA. Contemporary review of testicular torsion: new concepts, emerging technologies and potential therapeutics. *J Pediatr Urol.* 2013;9(6 Pt A):723–730.
9. Sessions AE, Rabinowitz R, Hulbert WC, Goldstein MM, Mevorach RA. Testicular torsion: direction, degree, duration and disinformation. *J Urol.* 2003;169(2):663–665.
10. Hayn MH, Herz DB, Bellinger MF, Schneck FX. Intermittent torsion of the spermatic cord portends an increased risk of acute testicular infarction. *J Urol.* 2008;180(4 Suppl):1729–1732.
11. Yang C, Song B, Tan J, Liu X, Wei GH. Testicular torsion in children: a 20-year retrospective study in a single institution. *ScientificWorldJournal.* 2011;11:362–368.
12. Drlík M, Kočvara R. Torsion of spermatic cord in children: a review. *J Pediatr Urol.* 2013;9(3):259–266.
13. Gatti JM, Patrick Murphy J. Current management of the acute scrotum. *Semin Pediatr Surg.* 2007;16(1):58–63.
14. Sharp VJ, Kieran K, Arlen AM. Testicular torsion: diagnosis, evaluation, and management. *Am Fam Physician.* 2013;88(12):835–840.
15. Prando D. Torsion of the spermatic cord: the main gray-scale and doppler sonographic signs. *Abdom Imaging.* 2009;34(5):648–661.
16. Corriere JN. Horizontal lie of the testicle: a diagnostic sign in torsion of the testis. *J Urol.* 1972;107(4):616–617.
17. Boettcher M, Krebs T, Bergholz R, Wenke K, Aronson D, Reinshagen K. Clinical and sonographic features predict testicular torsion in children: a prospective study. *BJU Int.* 2013;112(8):1201–1206.
18. Castañeda-Sánchez I, Tully B, Shipman M, Hoeft A, Hamby T, Palmer BW. Testicular torsion: a retrospective investigation of predictors of surgical outcomes and of remaining controversies. *J Pediatr Urol.* 2017;13(5):516–516.
19. Srinivasan A, Cinman N, Feber KM, Gitlin J, Palmer LS. History and physical examination findings predictive of testicular torsion: an attempt to promote clinical diagnosis by house staff. *J Pediatr Urol.* 2011;7(4):470–474.
20. Mellick LB. Torsion of the testicle: it is time to stop tossing the dice. *Pediatric Emergency Care.* 2012;28(1):80–86.
21. Hughes ME, Currier SJ, Della-Giustina D. Normal cremasteric reflex in a case of testicular torsion. *Am J Emerg Med.* 2001;19(3):241–242.

22. Murphy FL, Fletcher L, Pease P. Early scrotal exploration in all cases is the investigation and intervention of choice in the acute paediatric scrotum. *Pediatr Surg Int.* 2006;22(5):413–416.
23. Kadish HA, Bolte RG. A retrospective review of pediatric patients with epididymitis, testicular torsion, and torsion of testicular appendages. *Pediatrics.* 1998;102(1 Pt 1):73–76.
24. Kaye JD, Shapiro EY, Levitt SB, et al. Parenchymal echo texture predicts testicular salvage after torsion: potential impact on the need for emergent exploration. *J Urol.* 2008;180(4 Suppl):1733–1736.
25. Yusuf GT, Sidhu PS. A review of ultrasound imaging in scrotal emergencies. *J Ultrasound.* 2013;16(4):171–178.
26. Vijayaraghavan SB. Sonographic differential diagnosis of acute scrotum: real-time whirlpool sign, a key sign of torsion. *J Ultrasound Med.* 2006;25(5):563–574.
27. Coley BD, Frush DP, Babcock DS, et al. Acute testicular torsion: comparison of unenhanced and contrast-enhanced power Doppler US, color Doppler US, and radionuclide imaging. *Radiology.* 1996;199(2):441–446.
28. Blask ARN, Bulas D, Shalaby-Rana E, Rushton G, Shao C, Majd M. Color Doppler sonography and scintigraphy of the testis: a prospective, comparative analysis in children with acute scrotal pain. *Pediatr Emerg Care.* 2002;18(2):67–71.
29. Paltiel HJ, Connolly LP, Atala A, Paltiel AD, Zurakowski D, Treves ST. Acute scrotal symptoms in boys with an indeterminate clinical presentation: comparison of color Doppler sonography and scintigraphy. *Radiology.* 1998;207(1):223–231.
30. Terai A, Yoshimura K, Ichioka K, et al. Dynamic contrast-enhanced subtraction magnetic resonance imaging in diagnostics of testicular torsion. *Urology.* 2006;67(6):1278–1282.
31. Yuan Z, Luo Q, Chen L, Zhu J, Zhu R. Clinical study of scrotum scintigraphy in 49 patients with acute scrotal pain: a comparison with ultrasonography. *Ann Nucl Med.* 2001;15(3):225–229.
32. Terai A, Yoshimura K, Ichioka K, et al. Dynamic contrast-enhanced subtraction magnetic resonance imaging in diagnostics of testicular torsion. *Urology.* 2006;67(6):1278–1282.
33. Amini B, Patel CB, Lewin MR, Kim T, Fisher RE. Diagnostic nuclear medicine in the ED. *Am J Emergy Med.* 2011;29(1):91–101.
34. Burks DD, Markey BJ, Burkhard TK, Balsara ZN, Haluszka MM, Canning DA. Suspected testicular torsion and ischemia: evaluation with color Doppler sonography. *Radiology.* 1990;175(3):815–821.
35. Cokkinos DD, Antypa E, Tserotas P, et al. Emergency ultrasound of the scrotum: a review of the commonest pathologic conditions. *Curr Probl Diagn Radiol.* 2011;40(1):1–14.
36. Thakkar HS, Yardley I, Kufeji D. Management of paediatric testicular torsion—are we adhering to Royal College of Surgeons (RCS) recommendations. *Ann R Coll Surg Engl.* 2018;100(5):397–400.
37. Dogan HS, Stein R, 't Hoen LA, et al. Do EAU/ESPU guidelines recommendations fit to patients? Results of a survey on awareness of spina bifida patients. *Eur Urol Suppl.* 2019;38(6):1625–1631.
38. Kurtz MP. Evaluation of the pediatric patient with a non-traumatic acute scrotum. *AUA Updat Ser.* 2015;34:7.
39. Caesar RE, Kaplan GW. Incidence of the bell-clapper deformity in an autopsy series. *Urology.* 1994;44(1):114–116.
40. Bolln C, Driver CP, Youngson GG. Operative management of testicular torsion: current practice within the UK and Ireland. *J Pediatr Urol.* 2006;2(3):190–193.
41. Hamdy FC, Hastie KJ, Pagano F. Torsion of the testis: a new technique for fixation. *Eur Urol.* 1994;25(4):338–339.
42. Antao B, MacKinnon AE. Axial fixation of testes for prevention of recurrent testicular torsion. *Surgeon.* 2006;4(1):20–21.
43. Morse TS, Hollabaugh RS. The 'window' orchidopexy for prevention of testicular torsion. *J Pediatr Surg.* 1977;12(2):237–240.

44. Coughlin MT, Bellinger MF, LaPorte RE, Lee PA. Testicular suture: a significant risk factor for infertility among formerly cryptorchid men. *J Pediatr Surg.* 1998;33(12):1790–1793.
45. Mazaris E, Tadtayev S, Shah T, Boustead G. Surgery illustrated Focus on details a novel method of scrotal orchidopexy: description of the technique and short-term outcomes. *BJU Int.* 2012;110(11):1838–1842.
46. Cerasaro TS, Nachtsheim DA, Otero F, Parsons CL. The effect of testicular torsion on contralateral testis and the production of antisperm antibodies in rabbits. *J Urol.* 1984;132(3):577–579.
47. Redman JF, Barthold JS. Technique for atraumatic scrotal pouch orchiopexy in management of testicular torsion. *J Urol.* 1995;154(4):1511–1512.
48. Shanbhogue LKR, Miller SS. Subcutaneous dartos pouch fixation for testicular torsion. *Br J Surg.* 1987;74(6):510.
49. Lent V, Stephani A, Kaplan GW, Winslow BH. Eversion of the tunica vaginalis for prophylaxis of testicular torsion recurrences. *J Urol.* 1993;150(5 Pt 1):1419–1421.
50. Favorito LA, Cavalcante AG, Costa WS. Anatomic aspects of epididymis and tunica vaginalis in patients with testicular torsion. *Int Braz J Urol.* 2004;30(5):420–424.
51. Martin AD, Rushton HG. The prevalence of bell clapper anomaly in the solitary testis in cases of prior perinatal torsion. *J Urol.* 2014;191(5 Suppl):1573–1577.
52. Arnbjornsson E, Kullendorff CM. Testicular torsion in children—bilateral or unilateral operation. *Acta Chir Scand.* 1985;151(5):425–427.
53. Kolon TF, Herndon CDA, Baker LA, et al. Evaluation and treatment of cryptorchidism: AUA guideline. *J Urol.* 2014;192(2):337–345.
54. Abdelhalim A, Chamberlin JD, McAleer IM. A survey of the current practice patterns of contralateral testis fixation in unilateral testicular conditions. *Urology.* 2018;116:156–160.
55. Visser AJ, Heyns CF. Testicular function after torsion of the spermatic cord. *BJU Int.* 2003;92(3):200–203.
56. Gold DD, Lorber A, Levine H, et al. Door to detorsion time determines testicular survival. *Urology.* 2019;133:211–215.
57. Woodruff DY, Horwitz G, Weigel J, Nangia AK. Fertility preservation following torsion and severe ischemic injury of a solitary testis. *Fertil Steril.* 2010;94(1):352–352.
58. Kutikov A, Casale P, White MA, et al. Testicular compartment syndrome: a new approach to conceptualizing and managing testicular torsion. *Urology.* 2008;72(4):786–789.
59. Figueroa V, Pippi Salle JL, et al. Comparative analysis of detorsion alone versus detorsion and tunica albuginea decompression (Fasciotomy) with tunica vaginalis flap coverage in the surgical management of prolonged testicular ischemia. *J Urol.* 2012;188(4 Suppl):1417–1422.
60. Zhao LC, Lautz TB, Meeks JJ, Maizels M. Pediatric testicular torsion epidemiology using a national database: incidence, risk of orchiectomy and possible measures toward improving the quality of care. *J Urol.* 2011;186(5):2009–2013.
61. Cost NG, Bush NC, Barber TD, Huang R, Baker LA. Pediatric testicular torsion: demographics of national orchiopexy versus orchiectomy rates. *J Urology.* 2011;185(6 Suppl):2459–2463.
62. DaJusta DG, Granberg CF, Villanueva C, Baker LA. Contemporary review of testicular torsion: new concepts, emerging technologies and potential therapeutics. *J Pediatr Urol.* 2013;9(6):723–730.
63. Bodiwala D, Summerton DJ, Terry TR. Testicular prostheses: development and modern usage. *Ann R Coll Surg Engl.* 2007;89(4):349–353.
64. Jarrett JR, Cutler RG, Teal DF. Subcutaneous mastectomy in small, large, or ptotic breasts with immediate submuscular placement of implants. *Plast Reconstr Surg.* 1978;62(5):702–705.
65. Bush NC, Bagrodia A. Initial results for combined orchiectomy and prosthesis exchange for unsalvageable testicular torsion in adolescents: description of intravaginal prosthesis placement at orchiectomy. *J Urol.* 2012;188(4 Suppl):1424–1428.

66. Marshall S. Potential problems with testicular prostheses. *Urology.* 1986;28(5):388–390.
67. Shteynshlyuger A, Freyle J. Familial testicular torsion in three consecutive generations of first-degree relatives. *J Pediatr Urol.* 2011;7(1):86–91.
68. Pepe P, Panella P, Pennisi M, Aragona F. Does color Doppler sonography improve the clinical assessment of patients with acute scrotum? *Eur J Radiol.* 2006;60(1):120–124.
69. Yusuf GT, Sidhu PS. A review of ultrasound imaging in scrotal emergencies. *J Ultrasound.* 2013;16(4):171–178.
70. Cornel EB, Karthaus HFM. Manual derotation of the twisted spermatic cord. *BJU Int.* 1999;83(6):672–674.
71. Bajory Z, Varga R, Janovszky Á, Pajor L, Szabó A. Microcirculatory effects of selective endothelin—a receptor antagonism in testicular torsion. *J Urol.* 2014;192(6):1871–1877.
72. Ozbek O, Altintas R, Polat A, et al. The protective effect of apocynin on testicular ischemia-reperfusion injury. *J Urol.* 2015;193(4):1417–1422.
73. Acar O, Esen T, Colakoglu B, Camli MF, Cakmak YO. Improving testicular blood flow with electroacupuncture-like percutaneous nerve stimulation in an experimental rat model of testicular torsion. *Neuromodulation.* 2015;18(4):324–328.
74. Meštrović J, Drmić-Hofman I, Pogorelić Z, et al. Beneficial effect of nifedipine on testicular torsion-detorsion injury in rats. *Urology.* 2014;84(5):1194–1198.
75. Akgül T, Karagüzel E, Sürer H, et al. Ginkgo biloba (EGB 761) affects apoptosis and nitric-oxide synthases in testicular torsion: an experimental study. *Int Urol Nephrol.* 2009;41(3):531–536.
76. Erol B, Bozlu M, Hanci V, Tokgoz H, Bektas S, Mungan G. Coenzyme Q10 treatment reduces lipid peroxidation, inducible and endothelial nitric oxide synthases, and germ cell-specific apoptosis in a rat model of testicular ischemia/reperfusion injury. *Fertil Steril.* 2010;93(1):280–282.
77. Hekimoglu A, Kurcer Z, Aral F, Baba F, Sahna E, Atessahin A. Lycopene, an antioxidant carotenoid, attenuates testicular injury caused by ischemia/reperfusion in rats. *Tohoku J Exp Med.* 2009;218(2):141–147.
78. Karakaya E, Ateş O, Akgür FM, Olguner M. Rosuvastatin protects tissue perfusion in the experimental testicular torsion model. *Int Urol Nephrol.* 2010;2(2):357–360.
79. Karaguzel E, Sivrikaya A, Mentese A, et al. Investigation of tyrphostin AG 556 for testicular torsion-induced ischemia reperfusion injury in rat. *J Pediatr Urol.* 2014;10(2):223–229.
80. Zhang Y, Lv Y, Liu YJ, et al. Hyperbaric oxygen therapy in rats attenuates ischemia-reperfusion testicular injury through blockade of oxidative stress, suppression of inflammation, and reduction of nitric oxide formation. *Urology.* 2013;82(2):489–489.
81. Haj M, Shasha SM, Loberant N, Farhadian H. Effect of external scrotal cooling on the viability of the testis with torsion in rats. *Eur Surg Res.* 2007;39(3):160–169.

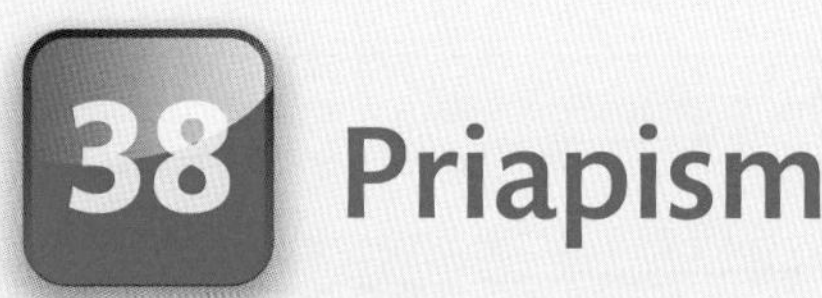

Priapism

Thomas Ellul and Nicholas Bullock

Expert commentary Ayman Younis

Case history

A 37-year-old gentleman presented acutely to the emergency department with a prolonged, painful erection. He had taken cocaine earlier in the day and subsequently developed an erection that had not subsided for 8 hours despite ejaculation. This was his first presentation with any urological complaint. Despite receiving analgesia in the emergency department, he was in significant discomfort. The urologist on call attended and following an examination, made a diagnosis of acute priapism.

Learning point Definition, classification, and epidemiology of priapism

Priapism is defined as complete or partial penile tumescence that persists for >4 hours in the absence of sexual stimulation, or after ejaculation.[1-3] Incidence rates of priapism vary, dependent on the population being studied. This distinction is most relevant for populations with a high prevalence of sickle cell disease (SCD) (a major risk factor for the development of priapism). Overall incidence of priapism is estimated to be 1.5 per 100,000 and can occur in any age group. Typically, there is a bimodal peak of incidence, between 5 and 10 years in children and 20 and 50 years in adults.[4] Priapism is divided into three main subtypes: ischaemic, non-ischaemic, and stuttering priapism. The aetiologies of these are summarized in Table 38.1.

Ischaemic or 'low-flow' priapism

This is a persistent erection marked by rigidity of the corpora cavernosa and by little or no cavernous arterial inflow.[1] The patient typically complains of penile pain and examination reveals a rigid erection of the corpora with relative flaccidity of the glans. The ischaemic subtype accounts for 95% of presentations with priapism. It is marked by rigidity of the corpora cavernosa with little arterial inflow

Table 38.1 Summary of aetiological factors for ischaemic and non-ischaemic priapism

Ischaemic priapism	Non-ischaemic priapism
Idiopathic	Blunt perineal or penile trauma
Haematological disorders (SCD, thalassaemia, leukaemia, multiple myeloma)	Metastatic malignancy to the penis
Infections (rabies, malaria, scorpion sting)	Acute spinal cord injury
Metabolic disorders (amyloidosis, gout, homocystinuria)	Following intracavernosal injections or aspiration
Neurogenic disorders (syphilis, spinal cord injury, cerebrovascular accident)	
Neoplasms (pelvic/perineal infiltration or metastases)	
Medications (erectile dysfunction medications, antipsychotics, recreational drugs)	

Adapted from Johnson et al. (2019).[6]

and thus is a compartment syndrome of the penis. This results in venous stasis within the corpora cavernosa due to obstruction and subsequently leads to intracavernosal acidosis, anoxia, hypercarbia, and glucopaenia.[5]

Non-ischaemic or high-flow priapism

This is a persistent erection caused by unregulated inflow of the cavernosal arteries.[1] The patient typically reports a non-painful, partial erection. Non-ischaemic priapism is most commonly caused following perineal trauma whereby fistulation occurs between the cavernosal artery and the sinusoidal tissue. This unregulated arterial inflow leads to incomplete tumescence as the veno-occlusive mechanisms created by smooth muscle relaxation are not activated. Therefore, the corporal tissues remain well oxygenated and thus are not at high risk of becoming ischaemic.

Stuttering priapism

This refers to a condition whereby patients experience frequent, recurrent episodes of priapism, which typically presents in a similar fashion to ischaemic priapism but tends to be self-limiting. Tumescence tends to last for <3 hours and is most commonly seen in patients with SCD. Although most presentations of stuttering priapism are self-limiting, a small proportion of patients may develop a prolonged, ischaemic priapism which requires urgent intervention and management as with any ischaemic priapism presentation.

Learning point Ischaemic priapism in SCD

Patients with SCD are an important subgroup of those presenting with priapism and their underlying condition often warrants additional management considerations. While a comprehensive overview of the genetics and pathophysiology of SCD is beyond the scope of this case, in brief, this comprises a group of autosomal recessive inherited disorders caused by mutations in the *HBB* gene, which encodes the beta-globin protein. Beta-globin, together with alpha-globin, makes up HbA, the most common form of haemoglobin in adults. HbA containing two mutant beta-globin subunits, known as HbS, is able to polymerize when under conditions of deoxygenation, leading to the formation of fibrous precipitates that distort the shape of erythrocytes (known as sickling) which in turn reduces their elasticity and renders them susceptible to haemolysis.[7]

One of the hallmark complications in patients with SCD is vaso-occlusive crisis in which a complex interplay between a number of mechanisms results in the obstruction of blood vessels by sickled erythrocytes, leading to ischaemia, pain, haemolytic anaemia, and organ injury.[8] The clinical manifestations, severity, and duration of vaso-occlusive crises vary significantly and depend on the organ system involved. Occlusion of venous outflow from the corpora cavernosum leads to ischaemic priapism, which constitutes >95% of priapism presentations in patients with SCD.[9] However, contemporary research has shown that mechanical obstruction of flow is only one component of the pathophysiology of priapism in SCD, with studies suggesting that defects in erectile regulatory pathways, such as aberrant nitric oxide signalling, also play an important role.[10]

The prevalence of priapism in men with SCD is in the order of 35%, with episodes usually beginning after onset of puberty.[11] Although the majority present as ischaemic events, a small proportion experience stuttering priapism, with recurrent transient and self-limiting episodes. Erections do not typically occur in the setting of another vaso-occlusive illness, although other sites of pain are often present. While precipitating factors include those common to other complications of SCD, such as infection and dehydration, episodes may also occur upon waking or following sexual intercourse.[11]

Clinical tip Ischaemic priapism in SCD

As well as the standard clinical assessment, it is important to identify any precipitating factors or other complications of vaso-occlusive crises. Many episodes of priapism are brief and resolve with conservative measures such as hydration, exercise, and masturbation with ejaculation. If the erection persists >4 hours, patients should present to the emergency department and be managed in the manner outlined in Figure 38.1. Additionally, dehydration should be corrected with intravenous fluids, oxygen supplementation if hypoxic, and treatment of any underlying precipitating illness. Pain should

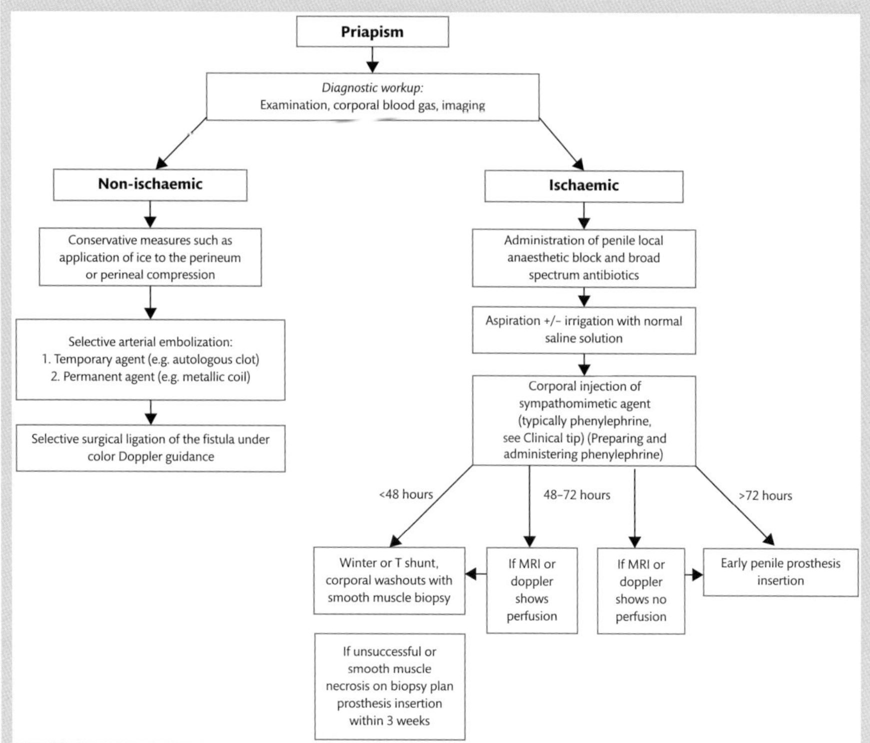

Figure 38.1 Management of ischaemic and non-ischaemic priapism.
Adapted from the BAUS Section of Andrology and Genitourethral Surgery (2018),[14] Salonia et al. (2014),[15] and Zacharakis et al. (2014)[17].

be controlled adequately and early involvement of a haematologist is fundamental, with patients ideally being managed jointly in a specialist unit with expertise in SCD.

Over 20% of patients with SCD will go on to develop ED and therefore early education and prompt management are fundamental.[11] Conservative approaches such as avoidance of known precipitants should be employed. There is limited evidence to support the use of medical prophylaxis, with some small series describing improved outcomes with use of hydroxyurea, pseudoephedrine, sildenafil, and leuprolide.[12]

A local anaesthetic penile ring block was performed, using 10 mL 1% lidocaine. This improved the pain and allowed for lateral puncture of the right corpus cavernosum to be performed using a 19-gauge 'butterfly' needle. The first blood aspirated was sent for blood gas analysis. This demonstrated hypoxia, acidosis, and hypercarbia (pH of 6.8, PO_2 of 0.7 kPa, PCO_2 of 7.5 kPa, and lactate of 7.1 mmol/L) in keeping with an ischaemic priapism. Recurrent aspirations and irrigation with saline solution were attempted. However, due to the significant ischaemic change, very little blood could be withdrawn and therefore this procedure was unsuccessful in achieving detumescence.

Expert comment SCD

In patients with SCD, priapism can be part of a sickle cell crisis, hence systemic management should include supportive measures such as fluid resuscitation, oxygen administration, and potentially blood exchange transfusion. This is in addition to managing the actual priapism as in idiopathic type.

Learning point Investigations

All patients presenting with a priapism of any type must undergo full blood count analysis and, in selected cases, a blood film should be performed to ensure haematological disorders are identified as a potential underlying cause. As an initial test to elucidate the nature of the priapism, corporal blood gas analysis must be performed for estimation of PO_2, pH, and glucose using a standard blood gas analyser. The presence of hypoxia, acidosis, and glucopenia confirms a diagnosis of ischaemic priapism. Normoxia correlated with the clinical history indicates that this is a non-ischaemic priapism; however, this should be confirmed with penile Doppler studies.

Clinical tip Aspiration and blood gas analysis

Prior to aspiration of blood, a penile block should be administered. The most prevalent agent in the authors' practice is 1% lidocaine (which must not contain adrenaline) and can be administered as a ring block or dorsal penile nerve block. Subsequently, a 19-gauge needle or butterfly must be inserted into the corpus cavernosum, either through the lateral penile shaft (towards the base of the penis) or through the glans penis into the tip of the corpus cavernosum, followed by aspiration of blood from the corpora. The first blood aspirated should be sent for blood gas analysis. It is advisable to use a 10 mL syringe for aspiration, as larger-volume syringes may create too high a pressure and thus prevent straightforward aspiration. If the aspirated blood is highly viscous and dark, this indicates ongoing hypoxia of the corporal tissues and ideally aspiration should continue until bright red arterial blood is present. If aspiration is not possible, or failing to achieve tumescence, this should be abandoned and instillation of sympathomimetic agent should be trialled.

The patient was placed on cardiac monitoring and intracorporal instillation of phenylephrine was performed in 200 mcg aliquots at 5-minute intervals. Detumescence was achieved after injection of 400 mcg of phenylephrine. The patient did not require further intervention for re-tumescence and was discharged on a course of co-amoxiclav.

Clinical tip Preparing and administering phenylephrine

Administration of a sympathomimetic agent is a fundamental step in the management of ischaemic priapism. Phenylephrine is the usual drug of choice, owing to its high selectivity for the alpha-1-adrenergic receptor with minimal beta-adrenergic receptor-mediated adrenergic or chronotropic effects.[13] Given the potential for potentially life-threatening adverse effects it is fundamental that the drug is prepared and administered correctly, with provision for appropriate patient monitoring. A practical guide, as adapted from the British Association of Urological Surgeons consensus document for the management of priapism[14] and European Association of Urology guidelines,[15] is given below:

1. Phenylephrine ampules are usually available as 10 mg in 1 mL. Dilute this in 49 mL of normal saline using a 50 mL syringe, giving a final concentration of 200 mcg/mL.
2. Establish the baseline heart rate and blood pressure prior to giving the initial injection and repeat these measurements at a minimum of every 15 minutes. Exercise particular vigilance in those with pre-existing cardiovascular disease.
3. Administer a 1 mL (200 mcg) aliquot directly into the corpus cavernosum at the 3 or 9 o'clock position towards the base of the penis, thereby avoiding the urethra and the course of the dorsal neurovascular bundle.
4. Give further aliquots every 3–5 minutes up to a maximum dosage of 1000 mcg for no more than 1 hour.
5. If the priapism persists despite the above, then proceed to the next step in the management pathway, as outlined in Figure 38.1.

Expert comment Monitoring during phenylephrine instillation

It is not always possible to perform phenylephrine instillation in a bed equipped with cardiac monitoring equipment. If this is the case, it is advisable to utilize an automatic observation machine which can regularly monitor blood pressure and heart rate via pulse oximetry and, if possible, apply defibrillator pads (on a monitoring setting) which allow for continuous heart tracing to ensure no arrhythmias are caused.

Unfortunately, the patient continued to use cocaine and therefore represented 2 weeks later. Similarly, blood gas analysis demonstrated ischaemic priapism which required phenylephrine to achieve detumescence. On subsequent outpatient assessment, the patient reported that he had erectile dysfunction (ED) despite use of over-the-counter sildenafil. He was trialled on regular phosphodiesterase type 5 inhibitors unsuccessfully.

A magnetic resonance imaging (MRI) scan was performed which demonstrated bilateral corporal fibrosis, as shown in Figure 38.2. The patient subsequently underwent implantation of an inflatable penile prosthesis.

Learning point Imaging

In unclear or refractory cases, penile Doppler studies may note a paradoxically increased systolic velocity in the proximal penile shaft. This is especially relevant if aspiration or shunt surgery has already been attempted or when there is fibrosis starting to develop in the distal corpus cavernosum.

If no underlying cause if clearly identified, it is imperative that abdominal and pelvic imaging using computed tomography or MRI is performed in order to ensure that underlying pelvic or abdominal malignancy is not overlooked (Table 38.1).

Penile MRI, as demonstrated in Figure 38.2, may provide useful information regarding the viability of the corporal tissue in refractory cases as well as aiding in the decision to proceed with penile prosthesis surgery.

Learning point Management of ischaemic priapism

Ischaemic priapism constitutes a compartment syndrome and therefore warrants prompt emergency intervention. The aim of treatment is to alleviate pain and achieve detumescence while ameliorating hypoxia, acidosis, and glucopenia within the corpora and thus prevent progression to smooth muscle necrosis with subsequent fibrosis and ED. Following confirmation of the diagnosis, treatment should follow a stepwise approach, as outlined in Figure 38.1. Given that the prognosis is directly related to the duration of priapism, contemporary guidelines suggest categorizing patients into three groups: <48 hours, 48–72 hours, and >72 hours.[14] In patients presenting after 48 hours it is unlikely that aspiration or sympathomimetic agent instillation will be effective. Therefore, in such

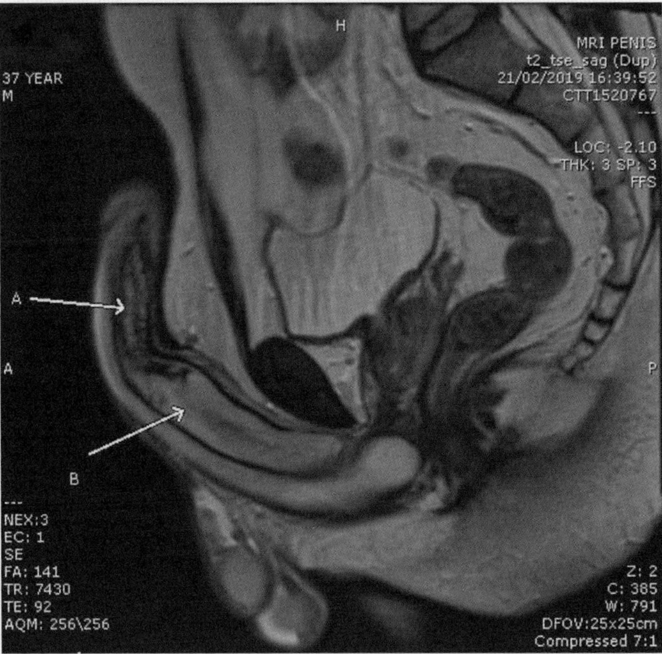

Figure 38.2 MRI scan demonstrating corporal fibrosis (arrow A) and healthy corporal tissue (arrow B).

patients a 'shunt' procedure is often required. The commonest, and most straightforward approach is a 'T-shunt'. This involves using a No. 10 blade scalpel and making a stab incision through the glans penis into the corporal head and then rotating the blade 90° laterally. This procedure creates a fistula between the cavernosal blood and the corpus spongiosum, thus allowing venous drainage and detumescence. In those patients for whom this is ineffective, or those presenting after 72 hours, it is likely there is little or no viable smooth muscle within the corpus cavernosum and so long-term ED is almost inevitable.[16] Some authors therefore advocate early insertion of a penile prosthesis in this patient group as this not only treats the inevitable ED and prevents shortening, but is also easier to perform and associated with fewer complications than a delayed procedure due to the absence of corporal fibrosis.[15,17–19]

Expert comment Penile prosthesis

Immediate insertion of malleable penile prosthesis should be considered in prolonged priapism (>48 hours) and in those refractory to intracavernosal vasoactive treatment and/or failed shunting. Penile prosthesis is mainly to avoid penile shortening that ensues due to cavernosal fibrosis because of prolonged ischaemia.

Learning point Management of non-ischaemic priapism

In non-ischaemic priapism, the blood within the corpus cavernosum is well oxygenated and therefore the risk of smooth muscle necrosis with progression to fibrosis is low. This form of priapism is therefore not considered a urological emergency and hence there is time for appropriate evaluation and patient counselling prior to instigating definitive management.

As with ischaemic priapism, treatment generally follows a stepwise approach, as demonstrated in Figure 38.1. Although conservative approaches are successful in 60–70% of cases, ED has been reported in up to 30% and so referral to a specialist andrology unit for selective arterial embolization is usually the modality of choice for those that fail to respond.[20] A number of different embolization materials have been described and are generally classified as either temporary, such as autologous blood clot,[21,22] or permanent, such as metallic coils or acrylic glue.[22,23] Although no randomized trials have been conducted, small series report success rates of up to 89%, with restoration of potency in around 80% of cases.[15,24] Surgical management involves selective ligation of the fistula but is associated with a number of risks and is therefore reserved for those unsuitable for or have failed embolization.

Expert comment Recurrent ischaemic priapism

In stuttering priapism, each acute episode should be managed as ischaemic type. Recurrent presentations with ischaemic priapism and subsequent numerous cavernosal aspirations may lead to the conversion of the priapism type from ischaemic to non-ischaemic.

Learning point Management of stuttering priapism

Stuttering priapism represents a rare subset and hence there is a paucity of published literature concerning management. Emergency management is required for acute episodes while longer-term treatment is aimed at preventing future episodes. The principal approach in patients with idiopathic stuttering priapism is the reduction of circulating androgens using gonadotropin-releasing hormone agonists/antagonists or antiandrogens such as bicalutamide, although these should be reserved for those who have reached full sexual maturation.[25,26] A range of other agents have also been described, including 5-alpha-reductase inhibitors, alpha-adrenergic agonists, phosphodiesterase type 5 inhibitors, and intracavernosal injections of sympathomimetic agents.[2,15,27] The management of stuttering priapism in patients with SCD warrants additional considerations.

Evidence base Management of priapism

Priapism is a rare condition, with an estimated incidence of 5.34 per 100,000 men per year in the US.[28] This, combined with the fact that ischaemic priapism is a urological emergency that mandates urgent detumescence, renders the design and execution of high-quality randomized studies challenging. Consequentially the evidence surrounding the management of priapism is of generally low level, with current guidelines based largely on small retrospective series and expert consensus.[2,14,15]

A final word from the expert

Priapism (among genital emergencies) is a relatively rare condition and clinicians are often unfamiliar with it. It can occur in all ages and requires prompt assessment and management. Due to the rarity of this condition, there are no unified guidelines and therefore treatment recommendations of priapism are an outcome of clinical studies and level 4 evidence at most. Recent recommendations and consensus statements have been published by the British Association of Urological Surgeons Section of Andrology and Genito-Urethral Surgery.[14]

The management of priapism is mainly to resolve the consequential pain in the short term and to restore erectile function in the long term. Clinical assessment of priapism starts from taking a careful history, exploring its onset, precipitating factors, and paying special attention to possible systemic causes such as illicit drugs, medications, pelvic malignancy, haematological disorders, and genital trauma. Clinical assessment should include abdominal, rectal, and penile examination.

Treatment of priapism depends on its onset and type. Simple measures such as physical exercise or a cold shower may suffice in simple cases. The treatment algorithm for each type is detailed in the main body of this article. Awareness of the basic management of priapism and early discussion with a specialist centre is vital to minimize the risk of irreversible consequences (such as cavernosal fibrosis) that may result from a delay in treatment.

References

1. Broderick GA, Kadioglu A, Bivalacqua TJ, Ghanem H, Nehra A, Shamloul R. Priapism: pathogenesis, epidemiology, and management. *J Sex Med.* 2010;7(1 Pt 2):476–500.
2. Montague DK, Jarow J, Broderick GA, et al. American Urological Association guideline on the management of priapism. *J Urol.* 2003;170(4 Pt 1):1318–1324.
3. Burnett AL, Bivalacqua TJ. Priapism: new concepts in medical and surgical management. *Urol Clin North Am.* 2011;38(2):185–194.
4. Cherian J, Rao A, Thwaini A, Kapasi F, Shergill I, Samman R. Medical and surgical management of priapism. *Postgrad Med J.* 2006;82(964):89–94.
5. Muneer A, Minhas S, Freeman A, Kumar P, Ralph DJ. Investigating the effects of high-dose phenylephrine in the management of prolonged ischaemic priapism. *J Sex Med.* 2008;5(9):2152–2159.
6. Johnson MJ, Hallerstrom M, Alnajjar HM, et al. Which patients with ischaemic priapism require further investigation for malignancy? *Int J Impot Res.* 2020;32(2):195–200.
7. Kato GJ, Piel FB, Reid CD, et al. Sickle cell disease. *Nat Rev Dis Primers.* 2018;4:18010.
8. Manwani D, Frenette PS. Vaso-occlusion in sickle cell disease: pathophysiology and novel targeted therapies. *Blood.* 2013;122(24):3892–3898.
9. Broderick GA. Priapism and sickle-cell anemia: diagnosis and nonsurgical therapy. *J Sex Med.* 2012;9(1):88–103.
10. Bivalacqua TJ, Musicki B, Kutlu O, Burnett AL. New insights into the pathophysiology of sickle cell disease-associated priapism. *J Sex Med.* 2012;9(1):79–87.
11. Adeyoju A, Olujohungbe A, Morris J, et al. Priapism in sickle-cell disease; incidence, risk factors and complications—an international multicentre study. *BJU Int.* 2002;90(9):898–902.
12. Kato GJ. Priapism in sickle-cell disease: a hematologist's perspective. *J Sex Med.* 2012;9(1):70–78.
13. Lee M, Cannon B, Sharifi R. Chart for preparation of dilutions of alpha-adrenergic agonists for intracavernous use in treatment of priapism. *J Urol.* 1995;153(4):1182–1183.
14. British Association of Urological Surgeons Section of Andrology and Genito-Urethral Surgery, Muneer A, Brown G, et al. BAUS consensus document for the management of male genital emergencies: priapism. *BJU Int.* 2018;121(6):835–839.
15. Salonia A, Eardley I, Giuliano F, et al. European Association of Urology guidelines on priapism. *Eur Urol.* 2014;65(2):480–489.
16. Spycher M, Hauri D. The ultrastructure of the erectile tissue in priapism. *J Urol.* 1986;135(1):142–147.
17. Zacharakis E, Garaffa G, Raheem AA, Christopher AN, Muneer A, Ralph DJ. Penile prosthesis insertion in patients with refractory ischaemic priapism: early vs delayed implantation. *BJU Int.* 2014;114(4):576–581.
18. Rees R, Kalsi J, Minhas S, Peters J, Kell P, Ralph D. The management of low-flow priapism with the immediate insertion of a penile prosthesis. *BJU Int.* 2002;90(9):893–897.
19. Sedigh O, Rolle L, Negro C, et al. Early insertion of inflatable prosthesis for intractable ischemic priapism: our experience and review of the literature. *Int J Impot Res.* 2011;23(4):158–164.

20. Shigehara K, Namiki M. Clinical management of priapism: a review. *World J Mens Health.* 2016;34(1):1–8.
21. Numan F, Cantasdemir M, Ozbayrak M, et al. Posttraumatic nonischemic priapism treated with autologous blood clot embolization. *J Sex Med.* 2008;5(1):173–179.
22. Kim KR, Shin JH, Song HY, et al. Treatment of high-flow priapism with superselective transcatheter embolization in 27 patients: a multicenter study. *J Vasc Interv Radiol.* 2007;18(10):1222–1226.
23. Liu BX, Xin ZC, Zou YH, et al. High-flow priapism: superselective cavernous artery embolization with microcoils. *Urology.* 2008;72(3):571–573.
24. Muneer A, Ralph D. Guideline of guidelines: priapism. *BJU Int.* 2017;119(2):204–208.
25. Muneer A, Garaffa G, Minhas S, Ralph D. The management of stuttering priapism within a specialist unit—a 25-year experience. *Br J Med Surg Urol.* 2009;2(1):11–16.
26. Muneer A, Minhas S, Arya M, Ralph D. Stuttering priapism—a review of the therapeutic options. *Int J Clin Pract.* 2008;62(8):1265–1270.
27. Yuan J, DeSouza R, Westney OL, Wang R. Insights of priapism mechanism and rationale treatment for recurrent priapism. *Asian J Androl.* 2008;10(1):88–101.
28. Roghmann F, Becker A, Sammon JD, et al. Incidence of priapism in emergency departments in the United States. *J Urol.* 2013;190(4):1275–1280.

CASE

Renal trauma

Hack Jae Lee

Expert commentary Christopher Anderson and Davendra M. Sharma

Case history

An otherwise fit and well 16-year-old male was found to be stabbed twice to his left flank on the street. He was air-lifted to the hospital as a trauma call. He complained of pain to his abdomen. He was given 1 g of tranexamic acid and was fluid resuscitated on his way to the hospital. He was examined as per Advanced Trauma Life Support® (ATLS®) protocol and was found with two stab wounds, both to his left flank with evisceration of large bowel. His observations were PO_2 100% on 15 L, respiratory rate of 20 breaths per minute, blood pressure of 110/85 mmHg, and heart rate of 110 beats per minute. Bloods showed a haemoglobin level of 90 g/dL, white cell count of 3.8×10^9/L, platelet count of 109×10^9/L, creatinine level of 130 µmol/L, and international normalized ratio of 1.5. His chest X-ray was normal and did not reveal any pneumoperitoneum.

He was stable enough to have a trauma computed tomography (CT) scan (Figure 39.1). The report revealed:

1. 'Laceration of the left kidney extending through the renal pelvis. There were active contrast extravasation and large volume retroperitoneal and intraperitoneal haematoma. Underlying vascular injury could not be excluded. Collecting system injury was felt high likely.'
2. 'Extruded loops of descending colon through abdominal wall defect. There was an abnormally thickened loop of bowel at the splenic flexure which was poorly enhancing concerning for ischaemic compromise. The remainder of the bowel were within normal limits.'
3. 'There were no thoracic injuries.'

Learning point American Association for the Surgery of Trauma renal injury scale

Renal injury can be subclassified depending on the severity of the injury using the American Association for the Surgery of Trauma (AAST) renal injury scale.[1]

- **Grade 1:** subcapsular, non-expanding haematoma without parenchymal laceration.
- **Grade 2**: superficial laceration ≤1 cm parenchymal depth without urinary extravasation. Non-expanding perirenal haematoma.
- **Grade 3:** laceration >1 cm parenchymal depth not involving the collecting system. Vascular injury or active bleeding confined within the perirenal fascia.
- **Grade 4:** laceration involving the collecting system with urinary extravasation. Laceration of the renal pelvis and/or complete ureteropelvic disruption. Main renal artery or vein injury with contained haemorrhage.
- **Grade 5:** shattered kidney with loss of identifiable parenchymal renal anatomy. Avulsion of renal hilum which devascularizes the kidney.

Expert comment AAST renal injury scale

The AAST renal injury scale is a useful tool to classify renal injury in order of severity. It is used worldwide and useful to predict clinical outcome. It correlates with the need for intervention and mortality. Its most recent revised version was in 2018.[1]

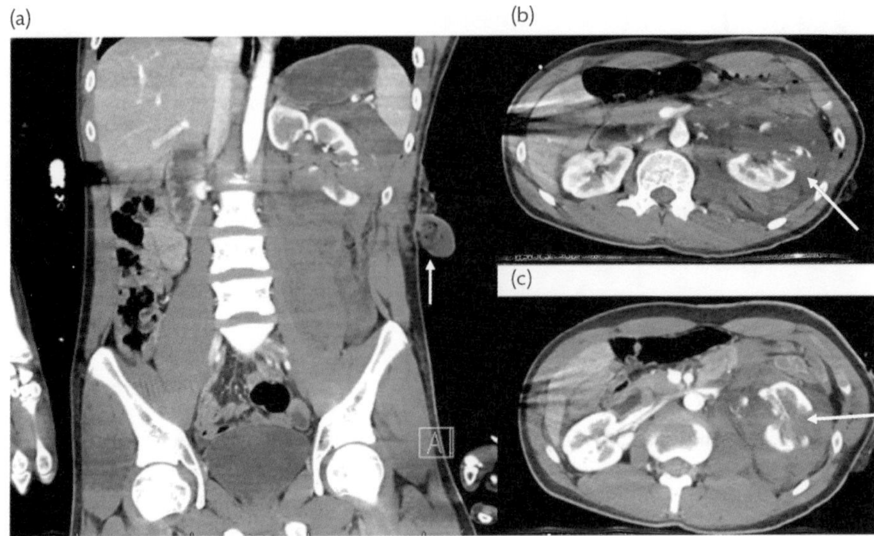

Figure 39.1 CT abdomen and pelvis with contrast following penetrating injury to left flank. (a) Extruded loops of descending colon can be seen through abdominal wall defect. (b) Large volume of retroperitoneal haematoma. (c) Complete laceration of the left kidney extending to the renal pelvis.

The patient's care involved various specialists including general surgeons, urologists, vascular surgeons, and interventional radiologists. Initial thought was to take the patient to theatre for damage control, washout of the abdomen, wound packing, and to re-look a few days later. Interventional radiology planned to embolize the kidney if the patient became unstable. However, after a multidisciplinary team discussion, the decision made was to take the patient to theatre for explorative laparotomy given his high-risk of bowel injury.

Expert comment
Multidisciplinary approach to polytrauma patients

Patients with renal trauma often have injuries to other visceral organs. It is important to discuss these patients with other specialities and adopt a multidisciplinary approach in management as in this case to give the patient the best optimal care. Note how the management of this patient changed after a multidisciplinary team discussion.

Learning point Management of major trauma

Penetrative trauma is becoming increasingly common with around 1600 major trauma cases a year in London (UK) alone.[2] When approaching a patient with suspected renal injury, taking a history and clinical examination is important. Patients will often have other significant injuries and is important to intervene as required. However, a definitive diagnosis will be achieved either by explorative laparotomy in haemodynamically unstable patients or with diagnostic imaging in those who are clinically stable. Explorative laparotomy and damage control have been the traditional teaching when managing penetrative abdominal injuries. Peritonitis, haemodynamic instability, and hollow viscus injury are all absolute indications for laparotomy.[3] There were concerns about bowel laceration and the patient became more haemodynamically unstable, therefore laparotomy was warranted.

Better understanding of potential organ injury with improved radiographic imaging has shifted managing abdominal injuries towards non-operative management in selective cases.[4] Demetriades et al. showed that out of 152 patients with penetrating injuries to abdominal solid viscera, 45 were stabbed. Out of the 45 patients with isolated organ injuries (liver 73%, kidney 30.3%, spleen 30.3%), 41 were managed without laparotomy and had a significantly shorter hospital stay than patients treated operatively.[5] However, this study did not include bowel injuries and this type of injury should almost always be explored.

On table, there was a through and through injury to the splenic flexure of the colon and lower pole of the left kidney. The patient also had a very large retroperitoneal haematoma. The patient had the injured part of the bowel resected and stapled off. As the hilum and the upper pole of the kidney appeared intact, a partial nephrectomy was carried out. The partial nephrectomy was performed by whole clamping of the renal artery and vein. The inferior pole was cut via the line of laceration. The collecting system was repaired with 2/0 Vicryl®, followed by two-layer renorrhaphy with V-Loc™ and sliding Hem-o-Lok® clip. Warm ischaemic time was 13 minutes. The patient had a re-look laparotomy 48 hours after. During the re-look, the patient had a washout and colic-colic anastomosis.

Expert comment Sliding-clip renorrhaphy

Renorrhaphy when performing partial nephrectomy has been a challenging part of the operation for the surgeon. Using sliding-clip renorrhaphy, which is performed by the use of Weck® Hem-o-Lok® clips that are slid into place, has shown to significantly shorten the overall procedure time and warm ischaemic time compared to traditional tied suture.[6]

Learning point Management of renal trauma

Renal trauma can cause injury to the renal parenchyma, hilum, and/or the collecting system. It accounts for approximately 1–5% of all trauma cases. The vast majority are blunt trauma but penetrating renal injury accounts for 20% in urban areas.[7] Management of these injuries has evolved over time with non-surgical management becoming increasingly common where possible. This has been possible because of improved patient selection using CT imaging and advancement of arterial embolization. The aim is to preserve as much renal parenchyma as possible and recurrent bleeding post embolization can be well managed with repeated embolization.[8] Expectant management for blunt renal trauma is fast becoming the standard of care worldwide. Non-operative management for penetrating renal injury is also becoming slowly accepted. However, patients with major blood loss, major renal parenchymal injury, renal vascular injury, and associated intra-abdominal injury should be considered for explorative laparotomy.[9]

The management of renal trauma is summarized in Figure 39.2.

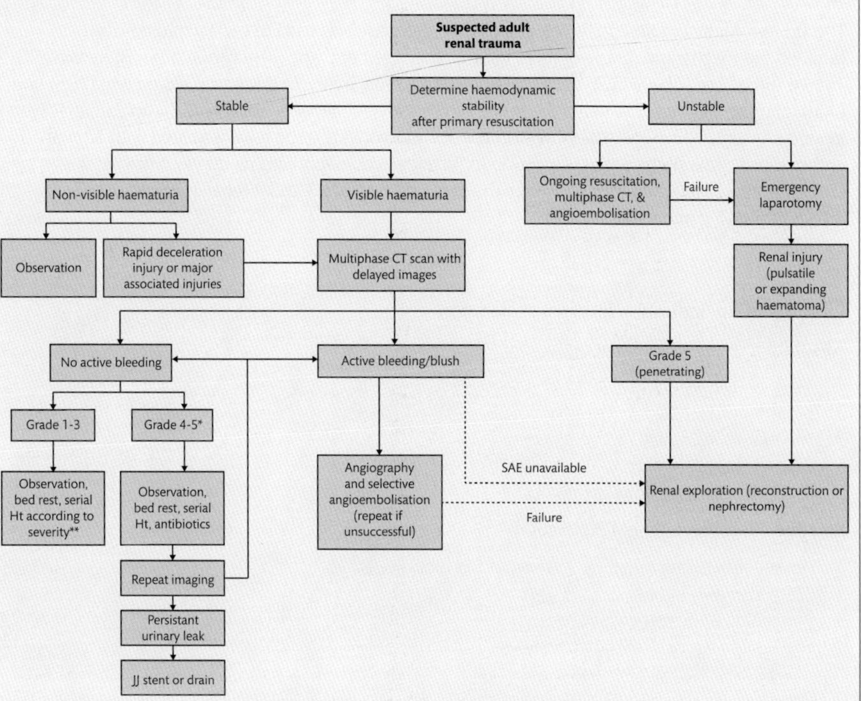

Figure 39.2 Management of renal trauma. Ht, haematocrit; SAE, selective angioembolization. * Excluding grade 5 penetrating injuries. ** Antibiotics should be administered for all penetrating injuries. --- If haemodynamically unstable.
Adapted from EAU guidelines on urological trauma (2020).

Learning point Conservative versus trauma nephrectomy

This practice of non-operative management was introduced in the early 2000s when clinicians recognized that most explorative laparotomies resulted in iatrogenic nephrectomies.[10] The role of selective renal artery embolization is becoming increasingly popular as an alternative to laparotomy in those patients who do not require surgery. There have been many studies which report good success rates (94% in one study) in achieving successful haemostasis in both penetrating and blunt grade 4 renal injuries. Embolization in those patients with renovascular injury was also highly successful for salvaging the kidney.[11,12]

Conservative management following penetrating renal injury is controversial and is less common as this group of patients are likely to have concomitant bowel injury and will require immediate explorative laparotomy. However, a large study with isolated, penetrative renal injury secondary to gunshot wounds revealed that the total number of patients requiring nephrectomy was 30 out of 206, with all grade 1–3 renal injuries managed conservatively.[13] The overall nephrectomy rate was 27% for penetrating renal injures and 7% for blunt renal trauma.[14]

Those patients selected for conservative management should be monitored in the intensive care unit setting where patients' physiological parameters can be monitored closely. Regular blood tests and examination should be undertaken especially during the early stages after injury. It is recommended to repeat the CT scan 36–72 hours after grade 3–5 renal injury or when patients show clinical signs of deterioration. Patients should be managed expectantly and have low threshold for intervention such as embolization to prevent morbidity and mortality. Given the unlikely need for any further intervention in minor renal injuries, routine CT is unlikely to add any value.[15]

Evidence base The Trauma Audit and Research Network database

The Trauma Audit and Research Network (TARN) database was used to review trauma cases. It outlined the mechanism, grade of renal trauma, management, and 30-day outcome. There were 1856 trauma cases of which 36 patients (1.9%) had a renal injury. In this group, 28 patient (78%) had blunt injury and eight (22%) had penetrating renal injury. All patients with grade 1 and 2 injuries were treated conservatively. One patient with grade 3, and two with grade 4 were treated with arterial embolization. One of the patients went on to have delayed nephrectomy due to unsuccessful embolization. Of the patients managed conservatively in grade 3 and 4 renal injury, all survived to 30 days following injury.[16]

Evidence base Predictors for embolization

There have been many studies to identify which patients are likely to require embolization. One study showed that of the 81 patients with high-grade injury (renal injury grade ≥3) who were haemodynamically stable and were treated conservatively, the predicting factors for subsequent embolization were[17]:

1. Intravascular contrast extravasation
2. Large perirenal haematoma distance of >25 mm
3. Extent of haematoma.

Clinical tip Indication for renal exploration

Absolute indications for renal exploration[19]:

1. Massive haemorrhage.
2. Expanding/pulsatile haematoma.
3. Penetrative injury with active bleeding.
4. Grade 5 vascular injury.
5. Associated intra-abdominal injuries.

Relative indication for renal exploration[19]:

1. Persistent bleeding requiring >3 units of red blood cells.
2. Bilateral kidney injury.
3. Worsening urine extravasation.
4. High-grade injury to solitary kidney.

Evidence base Percentage of cases requiring a nephrectomy

In a large study with 2467 patients, only 3% of grade 3 and 9% of grade 4 renal injuries required nephrectomies,[18] although it did go up as high as 85% for grade 5 renal injuries. This highlighted that many of these apparent severe renal injuries can be managed conservatively.

Expert comment Surgical approach

Despite best efforts to manage the patient non-operatively, it is inevitable to explore surgically in certain situations. The most common approach would be transperitoneal with the aim to identify and gain control of the renal hilum before renal exploration. Renal salvage can be improved by a consistent approach to evaluation, specific indications for retroperitoneal exploration, and vascular control before opening the retroperitoneum. This method reduces nephrectomy rates from 56% to 18%.[20] An expanding, central haematoma suggests injury to major vessels and should be surgically explored but a stable haematoma should not be opened.

During the operation, the feasibility of renal reconstruction should be considered. Isolated upper/lower pole injury, parenchymal defects, and isolated injuries to the renal pelvis are indications for nephron-sparing surgery. Renorrhaphy or partial nephrectomy requires good exposure of the kidney, debridement of non-viable tissue, control of bleeding by sutures, and tight closure of the collecting system and the parenchyma.[20] Repairing large vascular injuries is rarely effective and repair should be reserved for patients with solitary kidney or bilateral renal injuries.[21]

The patient had an uneventful recovery and was discharged after a few days.

Expert comment Follow-up imaging

Follow-up imaging is not routinely done for low-grade renal injuries. However, routine dimercaptosuccinic acid scintigraphy can be useful way to assess renal function in those patients with grade 3–5 renal injuries that have been salvaged a few months after the initial injury. They should also have their renal function and blood pressure monitored in the community.[22]

Learning point Complications of renal injury

Complications of renal trauma can be divided into either early, which occur within 1 month, or late complications. The most common complication following renal trauma is urinary extravasation. This accounts for 1–7% of cases and is seen as a collection of urine around the kidney that can be encapsulated or as free fluid in the retroperitoneum.[23] Urinomas are identified with urographic phase CT imaging. Small urinomas are usually reabsorbed spontaneously but can be complicated if they become infected, form a perinephric abscess, or increase in size. In such cases it may be necessary to insert a ureteric stent or image-guided percutaneous drainage. If there is progression of the urinoma despite this, then exploration should be considered.

Secondary haemorrhage is often seen in patients with grade 4 and 5 injuries usually between 7 and 14 days after the injury. This is frequently due to a ruptured arteriovenous fistula or pseudo-aneurysm.[24] Patients will develop new-onset flank pain, gross haematuria, and/or signs of haemorrhagic shock. Selective angio-embolization is the recommended treatment in these patients.[25]

Postrenal injury hypertension is a recognized complication following renal trauma which can happen at any time following the injury. It is thought to occur by increased renin secretion secondary to ischaemia from the renal trauma and subcapsular haematoma leading to chronic renal compression (known as Page kidney). This chronic renal compression also results in increased renin secretion that increases systemic blood pressure.[26,27] The incidence of postrenal injury hypertension differs in the literature but is thought to be between 1% and 5%.[28]

Other delayed complications include hydronephrosis, calculus formation, and chronic pyelonephritis and these should be treated expectantly.[25]

A final word from the expert

The kidney is the most commonly injured genitourinary organ and is becoming more common, especially in urban settings. Renal injury is suspected by the mechanism of injury such as blunt/penetrating injury to the flank, haemodynamic instability, and haematuria. It is important to understand that the degree of haematuria does not correlate with the severity of the renal injury.

The way we manage renal trauma has changed such that the conservative approach is favoured when possible. The aim is to conserve as much kidney function as possible and prevent iatrogenic nephrectomies. It is important to establish the diagnosis, rule out any other organ injury, and identify the degree of renal injury with a urographic phase CT in haemodynamically stable patients. Conservative management can be adopted in patients with blunt injury who are stable in all renal injury grades. This can also be applied to patients who are haemodynamically stable with penetrating low-grade renal injuries. These patients will require good supportive care in intensive therapy unit setting and should be managed expectantly with embolization or urinary drainage procedures if required.

Persistent bleeding despite embolization can be managed by re-embolization but there should be a low threshold to take these patients for explorative laparotomy for control of bleeding points. Every effort should be made to salvage the kidney by renorrhaphy or partial nephrectomy.

It is important to note that there are no set guidelines on how to manage patients with renal trauma. All patients should be managed individually and the management should be decided by a multidisciplinary team.

References

1. Moore EE, Shackford SR, Pachter HL, et al. Organ injury scaling: spleen, liver and kidney. *J Trauma.* 1989;29:(12):1664–1666.
2. Demetriades D, Hadjizacharia P, Constantinou C, et al. Selective nonoperative management of penetrating abdominal solid organ injuries. *Ann Surg.* 2006;244(4):620–628.
3. Butt M, Zacharias N, Velmahos G. Penetrating abdominal injuries: management controversies. *Scand J Trauma Resusc Emerg Med.* 2009;17:19.
4. McPhee M, Arumainayagam N, Clark M, Burfitt N, DasGupta R. Renal injury management in an urban trauma centre and implications for urological training. *Ann R Coll Surg Engl.* 2014;97(3):194–197.
5. Metcalfe D, Bouamra O, Parsons NR, et al. Effect of regional trauma centralization on volume, injury severity and outcomes of injured patients admitted to trauma centres. *Br J Surg.* 2014;101(8):959–964.
6. Benway BM, Wang AJ, Cabello JM, Bhayani SB. Robotic partial nephrectomy with sliding-clip renorrhaphy: technique and outcomes. *Eur Urol.* 2009;55(3):592–599.
7. Santucci RA, Fischer MB. The literature increasingly supports expectant (conservative)management of renal trauma—a systematic review. *J Trauma.* 2005;59(2):493–503.
8. Lin WC, Lin CH, Chen JH, et al. Computed tomographic imaging in determining the need of embolisation for high-grade blunt renal injury. *J Trauma Acute Care Surg.* 2013;74(1):230–235.
9. Wessels H, Suh D, Porter JR, et al. Renal injury and operative management in the United States: results of a population based study. *J Trauma.* 2003;54(3):423–430.
10. Breyer BN, Mcaninch JW, Elliott SP, Master VA. Minimally invasive endovascular techniques to treat acute renal haemorrhage. *J Urol.* 2008;179(6):2248–2252.
11. Chow SJ, Thompson KJ, Hartman JF, Wright ML. A 10-year review of blunt renal artery injuries at an urban level I trauma centre. *Injury.* 2009;40(8):844–850.
12. Voelzke BB, Mcaninch JW. Renal gunshot wounds: clinical management and outcome. *J Trauma.* 2009;66(3):593–600.
13. Keihani S, Xu Y, Presson AP, et al. Contemporary management of high-grade renal trauma: results from the American Association for the Surgery of Trauma Genitourinary Trauma Study. *J Trauma Acute Care Surg.* 2018;84(3):418–425.
14. Hotaling JM, Sorensen MD, Smith TG, Rivara FP, Wessells H, Voelzke BB. Analysis of diagnostic angiography and angioembolisation in the acute management of renal trauma using a national data set. *J Urol.* 2011;185(4):1316–1320.
15. Mcaninch JW, Carroll PR. Renal trauma: kidney preservation through improved vascular control—a refined approach. *J Trauma.* 1982;22(4):285–290.
16. McPhee M, Arumainayagam N, Clark M, Burfitt N, DasGupta R. Renal injury management in an urban trauma centre and implication for urological training. *Ann R Coll Surg Engl.* 2015;97(3):194–197.

17. David P, Bultitude MF, Koukounaras J, Royce PL, Corcoran NM. Assessing the usefulness of delated imaging in routine follow up for renal trauma. *J Urol.* 2010;184:973–977.
18. Santucci RA, McAninch JW, Safir M, Mario LA, Service S, Segal MR. Validation of the American Association for the Surgery of Trauma organ injury severity scale for the kidney. *J Trauma* 2001;50(2):195–200.
19. Erlich T, Kitrey N. Renal trauma: the best current practice. *Ther Adv Urol.* 2018;10(10):295–303.
20. Summerton DJ, Djakovic N, Kitrey ND, et al. EAU guidelines on urological trauma. European Association of Urology. 2014. https://uroweb.org/wp-content/uploads/24-Urological-Trauma_LR.pdf
21. Tillou A, Romero J, Asensio JA, et al. Renal vascular injuries. *Surg Clin North Am.* 2001;81(6):1417–1430.
22. Keller MS, Green MC. Comparison of short- and long-term functional outcome of nonoperatively managed renal injuries in children. *J Paediatr Surg.* 2009;44(1):144–147.
23. Titton RL, Gervais DA, Hahn PF, Harisinghani MG, Arellano RS, Mueller PR. Urine leaks and urinomas: diagnosis and imaging-guided intervention. *Radiographics.* 2003;23(5):1133–1147.
24. Mavili E, Dönmez H, Ozcan N, Sipahioğlu M, Demirtaş A. Transarterial embolisation for renal arterial bleeding. *Diagn Interv Radiol.* 2009;15(2):143–147.
25. Dinkel HP, Danuser H, Triller J. Blunt renal trauma: minimally invasive management with microcatheter embolisation experience in nine patients. *Radiology.* 2002;223(3):723–730.
26. Page IH. The production of persistent arterial hypertension by cellophane perinephritis. *JAMA.* 1939;113(23):2046–2048.
27. Goldblatt H, Lynch J, Hanzal RF, Summerville WW. Studies on experimental hypertension: I. The production of persistent elevation of systolic blood pressure by means of renal ischemia. *J Exp Med.* 1934;59:347–379.
28. Chedid A, Le Coz S, Rossignol P, Bobrie G, Herpin D, Plouin PF. Blunt renal trauma-induced hypertension: prevalence, presentation and outcome. *Am J Hypertens.* 2006;19(5):500–504.

CASE

40 Bladder and ureteric trauma

Guglielmo Mantica and Pieter V. Spies

Expert commentary André Van der Merwe

Case history

A 37-year-old male patient presented to the trauma unit with a gunshot wound to the forearm and a single gunshot wound to the pelvis. The patient was the victim of a firearm incident, but the circumstances of the event were not known. He presented to our trauma unit with a history of visible haematuria since the incident, which happened about 2 hours previously. On primary trauma survey, the patient was haemodynamically stable, fully conscious, and had a haemoglobin concentration of 12.5 g/dL. His vital signs were all within the normal ranges. He had completed treatment for pulmonary tuberculosis about 2 years ago. His medical history did not include surgical interventions or other chronic diseases.

The physical examination showed an entrance and an exit wound on the left forearm. Pulses were intact, but a fracture of the radius was suspected. The patient had clinical signs of an acute abdomen (guarding, rebound tenderness, rigid abdomen) and it was possible to identify an entrance wound in the right buttock without an exit wound. The digital rectal examination did not show lesions or clear signs of injury, but afterwards there were spots of blood on the glove.

A transurethral catheter (TUC) was inserted and frank blood was drained from the bladder.

Expert comment Initial assessment

Initial assessment may seem obvious, but it is not: the correct classification of any trauma patient starts by obtaining a detailed history and clinical examination, as per Advanced Trauma Life Support® (ATLS®) principles.[1] This allows the doctor to immediately decide on possible further investigations and therapies in an emergency setting, thereby saving precious time.

Clinical tip Haematuria and catheterization

In a trauma setting, haematuria may be the sign of an injury at any site in the urinary tract.[2] Therefore, if it is not possible to exclude a urethral injury with certainty from the clinical data, a trial of gentle TUC insertion must be performed with an atraumatic catheter. If any difficulty is experienced with the catheter insertion, a suprapubic catheter (SPC) or flexible cystoscopy-guided catheter insertion should be performed.

Subsequently, the patient underwent a multiphase contrast-enhanced abdominal and pelvic computed tomography (CT) intravenous urogram and cystography. These imaging tests showed penetrating trauma with fracture of the innominate bone, possible external iliac vein injury, and extraperitoneal bladder injury at the vesical ureteric junction with associated ureteric injury (Figure 40.1). Features were also highly concerning for rectal injuries. A penetrating trauma with a comminuted mid-radius fracture and radial and ulnar artery injuries were present.

The patient underwent urgent blood tests and arterial blood gas analysis (pH 7.31; PO_2 19.31 kPa; PCO_2 6.0 kPa; haemoglobin 8 g/dL; lactate: 2.1 mmol/L; HCO_3: 22.3 mmol/L; base excess: −3.4 mmol/L; oxygen saturation 99%). He was hydrated with 2 L of intravenous crystalloids and antibiotic coverage with intravenous amoxicillin/clavulanic acid (co-amoxiclav). Subsequently, the patient was taken for an urgent trauma laparotomy performed by trauma surgeons and urologists. The orthopaedic surgeons were pre-alerted to join in theatre in order to evaluate the innominate bone and radius injuries.

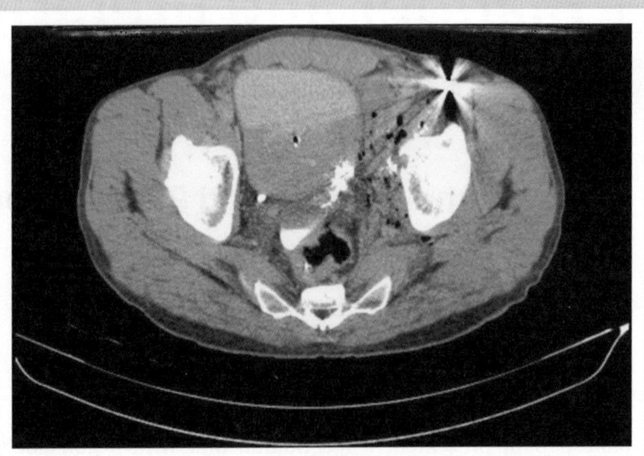

Figure 40.1 CT intravenous urogram showing left ureteric and bladder injuries due to gunshot wounds.

Learning point American Association for the Surgery of Trauma classification of bladder and ureteric injuries

Bladder injuries may be classified using the American Association for the Surgery of Trauma (AAST) scale which is based on radiological findings (Table 40.1).[3] This classification is periodically updated by the AAST and published in *The Journal of Trauma and Acute Care Surgery*. Similarly, ureteric injuries have an AAST classification with five different grades (Table 40.2).

Table 40.1 Bladder injuries classified using the AAST scale

Grade	Injury type	Description of injury
I	Haematoma	Contusion, intramural haematoma
II	Laceration	Partial thickness
III	Laceration	Extraperitoneal (>2 cm) or intraperitoneal (<2 cm) bladder wall laceration
IV	Laceration	Intraperitoneal bladder wall laceration >2 cm
V	Laceration	Intraperitoneal or extraperitoneal bladder wall laceration extending into the bladder neck or ureteral orifice (trigone)

Table 40.2 Ureteric injuries classified using the AAST scale

Grade	Injury type	Description of injury
I	Haematoma	Contusion or haematoma without devascularization
II	Laceration	<50% transection
III	Laceration	>50% transection
IV	Laceration	Complete transection with <2 cm devascularization
V	Laceration	Avulsion with >2 cm devascularization

Intraoperative findings revealed an extraperitoneal rectal injury which was repaired primarily with a covering loop colostomy. The left external iliac vein was injured and repaired with suture ligation. The bladder was bivalved surgically. A defect was found in the trigone of the bladder and repaired with dissolvable sutures.

Expert comment Surgical suction device and dyes

Do not use the surgical suction device directly on the bladder mucosa in order to avoid erythema, oedema, and bleeding that can make it difficult to correctly identify small injuries and the ureteric orifices. In a similar fashion, haemostatic swabs should also be used with gentle pressure as they can also cause swelling and erythema of the mucosa. The administration of intravenous methylene blue may be useful to identify the ureteric orifices if they are not clearly visible.[4] The utmost care should be used not to confuse methylene blue with Bonney's blue solution consisting of a high concentration of ethanol which is for external use only.

Both distal ureters were also dissected out and revealed a defect in the left distal ureter. The distal left ureter was tied off flush with the detrusor and the ureter was reimplanted into the left dome of the bladder, over a ureteric stent. A simple pop-in technique was used to minimize surgery time.

Learning point Ureteric injuries and repair

Even small ureteric injuries may heal with stricture formation, or persistent leaks may occur causing morbidity. The ureters have a delicate vascular supply and therefore surgical handling must be performed very gently and carefully in order to avoid microvascular injuries that may lead to necrosis.

General principles of ureteric repair are that the adventitia must be spared, the ureter should be debrided until the edges bleed, and a tension-free anastomosis should be performed.

In case of mid-upper ureteric injury, an uretero-ureterostomy can be attempted. The repair must be done over a double J stent, using a 4/0–5/0 absorbable monofilament for a waterproof, spatulated anastomosis. The peritoneum should be closed over the repaired ureter and a retroperitoneal drain inserted. In complex cases, omental wrapping of the repaired ureter may be considered.

In case of loss of a large part of the ureter, a more difficult approach such as renal autotransplantation or bowel interposition may be considered. However, they can be delayed to a better hospital setting and reconstructive expert supervision. In the emergency setting, the ureter can be tied off and a nephrostomy tube inserted as soon as the kidney becomes hydronephrotic. Alternatively, an intubated tube ureterostomy may be performed using the largest feeding tube that will enter the ureter with minimal friction, therefore allowing easy drainage but no risk of ureter necrosis.

Lower ureteric injuries are managed with ureteroneocystostomy. An extravesical approach can be utilized if no bladder injury is present, whereas the combined approach is favoured in cases where a bladder injury is suspected. The creation of a submucosal tunnel for a non-refluxing ureteric repair may be attempted keeping in mind the 5 (length):1 (width) principle. A watertight anastomosis of the spatulated ureter to the bladder mucosa is done using a 4/0–5/0 absorbable suture and should be performed after a double J stent insertion. During the extravesical approach, the detrusor layer may be closed over the anastomosis with an absorbable 3/0 suture to complete the ureter tunnelling. Tension should be avoided at all costs. If needed, further approaches such as a Boari flap or unilateral bladder mobilization with a psoas hitch can be performed in order to obtain a tension-free anastomosis.
In adults, a non-refluxing approach may not be essential and may be sacrificed in order to create a tension-free anastomosis.

Ureteric contusions without lacerations may be managed with the positioning of a double J stent only.

Expert comment Delaying ureteric repair

In a damage-control surgery setting ureteric repair may be delayed. It is, however, very important to exteriorize leaking urine, as an internal collection of urine in a critically ill patient might have morbid effects on acid-base balance and electrolytes. Infection usually follows a urine collection very swiftly. In these cases, there are a few options that you may consider[6]: insert a double J stent, ureteric exteriorization,[7,8] tie the ureter, and place a nephrostomy.[9] A nephrectomy has also been considered by some authors.[10]

Expert comment Bivalving the bladder

The bladder should be held in moderate tension with two to four stay sutures before being bivalved. These sutures must be retained as it will guide the closure of the bladder and should be full thickness. Afterwards, a bladder retractor (i.e. Marshall or Mason-Judd retractors) may be used. It is mandatory to bivalve the bladder in almost all bladder trauma to ensure adequate exposure for inspection and to identify the ureteric orifices.

Clinical tip Assessing ureteric injury

A careful intraoperative inspection of the retroperitoneum is of paramount importance in order to not miss any ureteric injuries.
In case of penetrating trauma, the entrance and exit wounds as well as the trajectory must be considered in detail. The ureteric peristalsis and palpation techniques are useful, but not able to completely exclude ureteric injury.

Evidence base Missed ureteric injury

A large meta-analysis of 429 ureteric injuries found an 11% missed ureteric injury rate.[5] This review demonstrated that a delayed diagnosis at laparotomy exploration leads to prolonged hospital stay and statistically increased rates of nephrectomy.

Evidence base Refluxing anastomoses

A refluxing anastomosis can be considered if ureteric length is insufficient for tunnelling. Refluxing anastomoses show no increase in complications related to urine reflux in some studies.[11,12]

The right ureter was canalized with an 8-French feeding tube and the defect in the trigone was repaired in two layers with 2/0 absorbable sutures. After the trigone was repaired, the feeding tube was removed from the right ureter.

The omentum was mobilized and pexied between the rectal and bladder injury repair lines. The bladder was closed with continuous 2/0 polyglactin sutures in a single layer, a SPC was also placed.

Expert comment Using feeding tubes

Feeding tubes may be very useful to identify and prevent inadvertent ligation of the ureteric meatus or intramural ureter during the suture of the bladder trigone. They can be easily removed after the repair is complete.

Evidence base Bladder drainage post repair

The European Association of Urology guidelines[2] highlight the importance of bladder drainage and the maintenance of the catheter, for at least 1 week, followed by its removal only after follow-up cystography. In contrast, The American Urological Association guidelines[15] state that a TUC should be preferred and that double drainage with a SPC is not necessary. A few studies have focused on this topic with the evidence of similar outcomes and complication rates for patients treated with SPC + TUC versus TUC only.[16–20]

Expert comment Bladder closure

The bladder can be closed in single or in double layers with absorbable 2/0 sutures as long as it is watertight and the bladder mucosa edges are approximated. There is no evidence to support the superiority of one of these two suturing techniques.[12,14]

The surgical repair of the left radius was done at a second operation. The TUC was removed as soon as the visible haematuria cleared, while the SPC was kept for 10 days postoperatively and was removed after a high-pressure cystogram showed no residual extravasation of contrast (Figure 40.2). The ureteric stent was removed 6 weeks after surgery and the patient had follow-up sonography 1 month later. Closing of the loop colostomy was done 6 months later after a loopogram showed no rectal extravasation.

Evidence base Cystography

Most authors advise to perform cystography before the removal of the TUC.[2,4,15,21,22] The cystography is usually performed between 7 and 14 days after repair. The time of the removal of the JJ stent is about 6 weeks.[2,4,15,23,24]

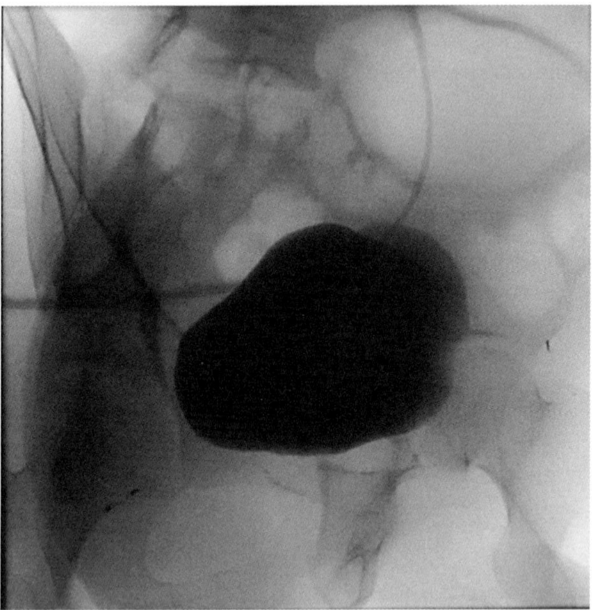

Figure 40.2 Lateral view cystogram performed 10 days after the surgical repair showing no contrast leak.

A final word from the expert

Ureteric injuries can be difficult to diagnose. They often occur concomitantly with other major injuries. The diagnosis is facilitated by protocol perfect trauma CT scans of the abdomen, with delayed phase images demonstrating the ureteric injury. Inadequate imaging with no delayed films is a major source of misdiagnosing ureteric injuries in trauma patients. It can be very challenging to diagnose ureteric injuries intraoperatively. Due to fluid shifts and possible acute tubular necrosis, urine output intraoperatively might be minimal making it challenging to diagnose small injuries. As the ureter resides inside a vascular adventitial sheath, it might also be difficult to diagnose complete transection of the ureter intraoperatively as the ureter might retract and the sheath around the ureter may obscure the injury. In a standard trauma operating room, once the patient is positioned for trauma surgery of the concomitant injuries, it is difficult and hazardous to move the patient into a position to perform cystoscopy and retrograde pyelograms or to do an on-table intravenous pyelogram with 10-minute films as often suggested in trauma literature. It is best to perform the correct type of CT imaging preoperatively and make a definitive diagnosis.

Lengthy reconstructive procedures in a critically injured patient should not be attempted, because increasing the length of surgery unnecessarily can potentiate the risk of breakdown of the repaired tissue when sutured in an inadequately perfused state. Exteriorization, as discussed above, must be performed to bridge the critically ill period after which reconstruction should be carefully planned and performed with the best expertise available.

Ureters should be handled with non-traumatic forceps such as DeBakey or fine fenestrated vascular surgery forceps. The use of loupe magnification is helpful to see small blood vessels supplying the ureter. While the usual teaching holds that the blood supply of the ureter enters above the pelvis from medial and inside the pelvis from lateral arteries, this must under no circumstances be followed dogmatically. Variation in blood supply is common. It is important to retain as much of the vascularity around the ureter as possible. Many of these will originate from branches of the renal artery.

Ureteric repairs in traumatically injured ureters should be drained internally by a ureteric stent and drained externally by a non-suction type drain in all cases. A persistent leak of urine may cause a stricture of the ureter. Similarly, undrained urine in tissue is toxic and can lead to urinoma and infection.

The key to the successful management of ureteric injuries is early diagnosis and management that takes the level of illness of the patient into account. In the critically ill patient, temporizing measures must prevail until reconstruction can be performed by a urologist experienced in reconstructive urology.

Similar to ureteric injuries, bladder injuries are diagnosed with an adequately performed, high-pressure cystogram. A CT cystogram is not an adequate test to rule out a bladder injury due to the low pressures in the bladder during this investigation. Accurate and early diagnosis of bladder trauma allows for correct classification and appropriate management.

Acknowledgement

We sincerely thank Dr Heidi Van Deventer for the English editing of this case.

References

1. Galvagno SM Jr, Nahmias JT, Young DA. Advanced Trauma Life Support(®) Update 2019: management and applications for adults and special populations. *Anesthesiol Clin.* 2019;37(1):13–32.
2. Kitrey ND, Djakovic N, Hallscheidt P, et al. EAU guidelines on urological trauma. European Association of Urology. 2020. https://uroweb.org/wp-content/uploads/EAU-Guidelines-on-Urological-Trauma-2020.pdf
3. Moore EE, Moore FA. American Association for the Surgery of Trauma Organ Injury Scaling: 50th anniversary review article of the Journal of Trauma. *J Trauma.* 2010;69(6):1600–1601.
4. Santucci RA, Doumanian LR. Upper urinary tract trauma. In: Wein AJ, Kavoussi LR, Campbell MF, eds. *Campbell-Walsh Urology*. 10th ed. Philadelphia, PA: Elsevier Saunders; 2012:1169–1189.
5. Kunkle DA, Kansas BT, Pathak A, et al. Delayed diagnosis of traumatic ureteral injuries. *J Urol.* 2006;176(6 Pt 1):2503–2507.
6. Cass AS. Blunt renal pelvic and ureteral injury in multiple-injured patients. *Urology.* 1983;22(3):268–270.
7. Ball CG, Kirkpatrick AW, Laupland KB, et al. Incidence, risk factors, and outcomes for occult pneumothoraces in victims of major trauma. *J Trauma.* 2005;59(4):917–924.
8. Gill IS, McRoberts JW. New directions in the management of GU trauma. *Mediguide Urol.* 1992;5:1–8.
9. Hirshberg A, Wall MJ Jr, Mattox KL. Planned reoperation for trauma: a two year experience with 124 consecutive patients. *J Trauma* 1994;37(3):365–369.
10. Velmahos GC, Degiannis E, Wells M, Souter I. Penetrating ureteral injuries: the impact of associated injuries on management. *Am Surg* 1996;62(6):461–468.
11. Wiesner C, Thuroff JW. Techniques for uretero-intestinal reimplantation. *Curr Opin Urol.* 2004;14(6):351–355.
12. Minervini A, Boni G, Salinitri G, et al. Evaluation of renal function and upper urinary tract morphology in the ileal orthotopic neobladder with no antireflux mechanism. *J Urol.* 2005;173(1):144–147.
13. Matlock KA, Tyroch AH, Kronfol ZN, McLean SF, Pirela-Cruz MA. Blunt traumatic bladder rupture: a 10-year perspective. *Am Surg.* 2013;79(6):589–593.
14. Urry RJ, Clarke DL, Bruce JL, Laing GL. The incidence, spectrum and outcomes of traumatic bladder injuries within the Pietermaritzburg Metropolitan Trauma Service. *Injury.* 2016;47(5):1057–1063.
15. Morey AF, Brandes S, Dugi DD 3rd, et al. Urotrauma: AUA guideline. *J Urol.* 2014;192(2):327–335.
16. Alli MO, Singh B, Moodley J, et al. Prospective evaluation of combined suprapubic and urethral catheterization to urethral drainage alone for intraperitoneal bladder injuries. *J Trauma.* 2003;55(6):1152–1156.
17. Volpe MA, Pachter EM, Scalea TM, et al. Is there a difference in outcome when treating traumatic intraperitoneal bladder rupture with or without a suprapubic tube? *J Urol.* 1999;161(4):1103-1105.
18. Thomae KR, Kilambi NK, Poole GV. Method of urinary diversion in nonurethral traumatic bladder injuries: retrospective analysis of 70 cases. *Am Surg.* 1998;64(1):77–80.
19. Parry NG, Rozycki GS, Feliciano DV, et al. Traumatic rupture of the urinary bladder: is the suprapubic tube necessary? *J Trauma.* 2003;54(3):431–436.
20. Margolin DJ, Gonzalez RP. Retrospective analysis of traumatic bladder injury: does suprapubic catheterization alter outcome of healing? *Am Surg.* 2004;70(12):1057–1060.
21. Inaba K, McKenney M, Munera F, et al. Cystogram follow-up in the management of traumatic bladder disruption. *J Trauma.* 2006;60(1):23–28.

22. Kim B, Roberts M. Laparoscopic repair of traumatic intraperitoneal bladder rupture: case report and review of the literature. *Can Urol Assoc J.* 2012;6(6):E270–E273.
23. Burks FN, Santucci RA. Management of iatrogenic ureteral injury. *Ther Adv Urol.* 2014;6(3):115–124.
24. Engelsgjerd JS, LaGrange CA. Ureteral injury. Treasure Island, FL: StatPearls Publishing; 2019. https://www.ncbi.nlm.nih.gov/books/NBK507817/

Penile fracture

Huw Garrod, Sacha Moore, and Iqbal Shergill

Expert commentary Christian Seipp

Case history

A 47-year-old male presented to the emergency department with a vague history of falling out of bed, in the middle of the night. He had a grossly swollen, bruised penis. He denied any haematuria. He stated the injury occurred approximately 8 hours previously, possibly when he had an early morning erection, but would not elaborate any further on the mechanism of injury.

He had no significant past medical history and took no regular medication.

He underwent an exploration within 24 hours via a circumferential penile incision and degloving which allowed evacuation of an extensive haematoma and repair of a defect in the corpora. No urethral injury was identified and he was discharged the following day.

Expert comment Exploration technique

Since the site of the injury was unknown in this patient, a degloving incision allowing thorough inspection was appropriate. When the site of injury is identified preoperatively, a more limited penoscrotal incision could be considered.

Learning point Epidemiology

In Western series, >90% of cases of penile fracture have been attributed to sexual intercourse. A 2014 Brazilian analysis of 30 cases of penile fracture confirmed that 'female on top' was the position most commonly associated with penile fracture. It has also been reported to occur during masturbation. In the Middle East, a practice called Taghaandan, the deliberate bending of the erect penis to achieve rapid detumescence, is associated with presentation of penile fracture. However, recent reports suggest a trend towards intercourse-related incidents as seen in the West.

Learning point Clinical presentation

Penile fracture is a rare urological emergency with an incidence of approximately 1 in 175,000. It is defined as a rupture of the tunica albuginea in one or both corpora cavernosa and is associated with urethral injury in 10–22% of cases.[1] Sexual intercourse is the most common precipitating factor where the penis slips out of the vagina and strikes the symphysis pubis or perineum.

Presentation

Penile fracture presents with a very characteristic set of symptoms and is generally considered a clinical diagnosis. Symptoms include:

- Sudden penile pain and swelling ('aubergine/eggplant' sign; Figure 41.1)
- Rapid detumescence
- Cracking or popping sound
- Haematuria (indicating possible urethral injury).

When these features are not present, the clinician should consider alternative diagnoses such as penile contusion, suspensory ligament rupture, and superficial vein rupture.

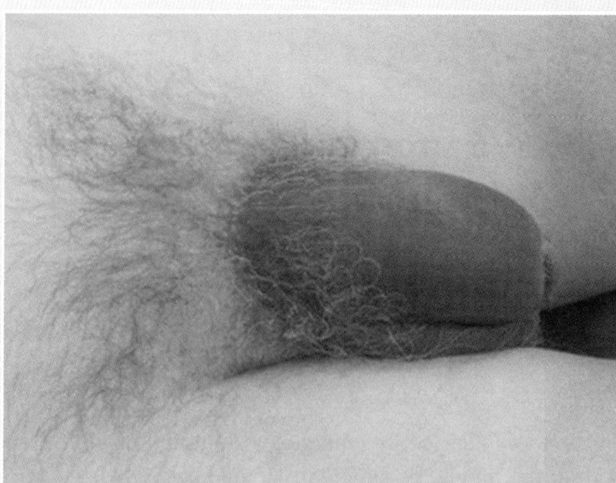

Figure 41.1 'Aubergine'-looking penis suggestive of penile fracture.

Examination

Alongside the features described previously described, there may be a tender palpable defect overlying the site of the defect in the tunica albuginea. If Buck's fascia is intact then the bruising will be confined to the penis. Rupture of Buck's fascia is associated with more extensive bleeding into the scrotum, perineum, and lower abdominal wall. Urethral injury may present as blood at the meatus, frank haematuria, painful voiding, or urinary retention.

Clinical tip Importance of clinical history

Penile fracture is a clinical diagnosis with a very characteristic history of a cracking or popping sound, severe pain, swelling, and immediate detumescence. Reports of haematuria should raise suspicion of a urethral injury.

Evidence base Fracture aetiology

A systematic review and meta-analysis by Amer et al. in 2016 assessed the aetiology of penile fracture in 1948 patients from 38 studies.[2] Bending and buckling of the penis during sexual intercourse was the most common single aetiology of penile fracture; this is typically caused by the blunt trauma of the penis hitting the perineum. Other more common causes include:

- Pressure during masturbation
- Forced flexion
- Rolling over onto the erect penis.

More uncommon causes reported in the literature include electrocution, firearm trauma, and utilization of a vacuum cleaner for the purposes of masturbation.

Additionally, meta-analysis of five studies assessing the effect of sexual position on likelihood of penile fracture demonstrated no significant impact on relative risk for any single position ($n = 76$; $p = 0.53$; $I^2 = 42\%$).

Learning point Pathophysiology

The thickness of the tunica albuginea reduces to 2 mm during tumescence making it more vulnerable to traumatic injury—for this reason true penile fractures only occur with an erect penis. Tears to the tunica albuginea are possible in a flaccid penis but are considered separate from penile fracture. Injuries most commonly occur on the ventrolateral area of the tunica where it is thinnest. Urethral injury is associated with penile fracture in between 20% and 50% of cases.

Learning point Investigation

Penile ultrasound is highly sensitive for detecting a defect in the tunica albuginea but is largely reserved as a 'rule out' procedure in cases where the history or clinical findings are not in keeping with a penile fracture. When an injury is identified, the sonographer should mark the site to help with surgical planning.

Penile magnetic resonance imaging (MRI) (Figure 41.2) has been advocated by recent guidelines when there is diagnostic doubt. It can identify smaller defects in the tunica than ultrasound and it can identify urethral injuries. It does however, remain a specialist investigation and will not be available in all centres.

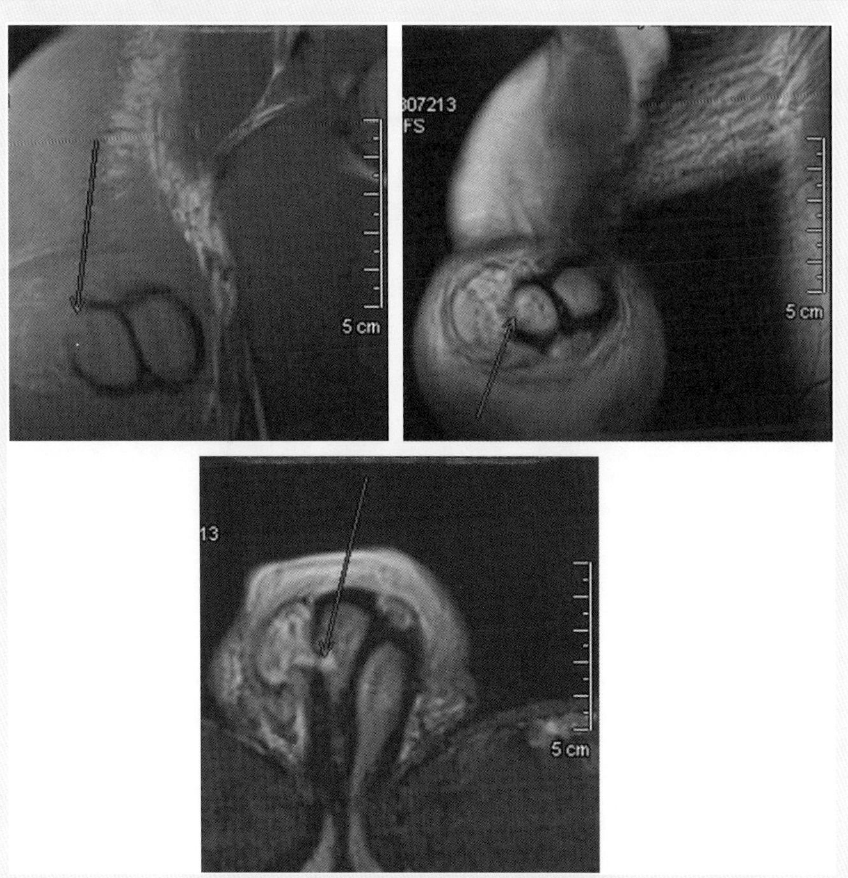

Figure 41.2 MRI demonstrating a penile fracture. There is a penile fracture half way down the penis, towards the dorsal surface of the right corpus cavernosum. There is a 11 mm defect in the tunica albuginea with a 24 × 16 mm haematoma in the subcutaneous tissue.

Despite the high risk, formal evaluation of the urethra is underutilized. To assess for a urethral injury, the urologist can perform a flexible cystoscopic examination at the time of surgery or a retrograde urethrogram preoperatively or on table.

Expert comment Flexible cystoscopy

Since almost all patients will be proceeding to surgery, a flexible cystoscopy on the table is easily performed and widely available. It has the additional benefit of allowing guidewire insertion for catheterization if a urethral injury is identified.

Expert comment Surgical repair

Once a diagnosis of penile fracture has been made, surgical repair should be carried out within 24 hours, or sooner if a urethral injury is suspected. Broad-spectrum antibiotics should be given preoperatively. The traditional approach is a circumferential subcoronal incision allowing complete degloving of the penis, exposing the injury and enabling identification of any associated injuries. This degloving approach is favoured when the site of injury is unknown or in the distal shaft (Figure 41.3a).

An alternative technique is a penoscrotal incision over the suspected injury, particularly in centres that have access to sensitive preoperative imaging such as MRI. Once localized, the injury should be repaired with a 0 or 2/0 absorbable suture such as PDS®, taking care to bury the knots (Figure 41.3b). A Foley catheter should be inserted postoperatively, particularly as there may be persistent significant penile swelling.

Clinical tip Conservative management

Conservative management of penile fracture is not considered best practice due to the high incidence of long-term sequelae. Impotence will be present in up to 60% of men and fibrosis and abnormal curvature in 35%. The only scenario where conservative management may be considered is when the patient has presented after an extended period of time and the acute injury has already settled.

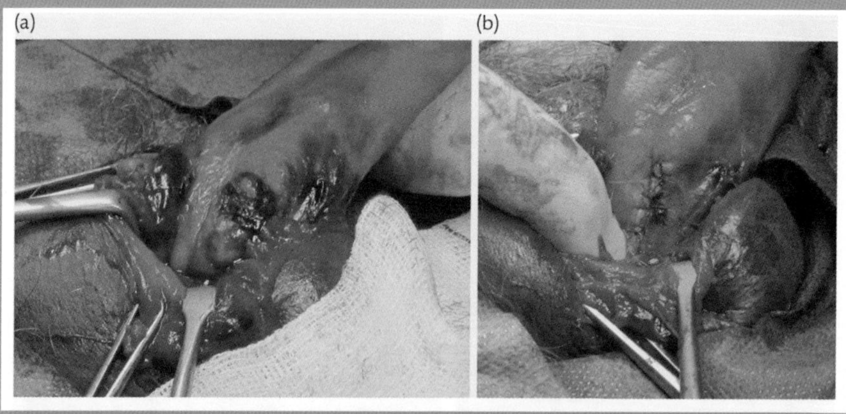

Figure 41.3 Penile fracture exploration and repair. (a) Degloving of the penis revealing the fracture site. (b) Repair of the defect using PDS®.

When a urethral repair is required, the edges should be exposed and closed with fine interrupted sutures such as 5/0 Polyglactin. A Foley catheter should be left in place for 2 weeks and a urethrogram performed before trial without catheter to ensure the urethra has fully healed.

Learning point Long-term complications

Complications of penile fracture include the formation of plaques or nodules, penile curvature, erectile dysfunction, and painful erections. There is conflicting evidence regarding the overall incidence of each of these, but prompt surgical management has been demonstrated to significantly reduce short- to medium-term erectile dysfunction and penile curvature.

Clinical tip Postoperative advice for patients

The British Association of Urological Surgeons 2018 consensus statement[3] recommends the following postoperative management plan for penile fracture patients:

- Patients should refrain from sexual activity for 6 weeks.
- Patients should be followed up in clinic 2 weeks after discharge.
- Patients with penile curvature or erectile dysfunction post fracture should be managed using the standard management pathways for these conditions.
- Emergency referral to a specialist unit is indicated where there is severe urethral disruption.

A final word from the expert

Penile fracture is the traumatic disruption of the tunica albuginea and enclosed corpus cavernosum as the result of blunt trauma to the erect penis. It is a rare yet easily recognized urological emergency characterized by the typical set of symptoms of popping sound, immediate detumescence, and rapid development of an increasing haematoma ('eggplant deformity'). Clinical presentation and physical examination are usually sufficient to establish the diagnosis. Depending on the size of the haematoma, it may not always be possible to palpate the ruptured tunica. Imaging such as ultrasound, penile MRI, or cavernosography can help in identifying the underlying defect, but are rarely necessary in general clinical practice—particularly as it may defer surgical exploration and management. Conservative management carries a high risk of complications such as infected haematoma, abscess, erectile dysfunction, penile curvature, and arteriovenous fistula. Once a patient is suspected of having sustained a penile fracture, early surgical management—as opposed to delayed therapy—provides the best possible outcome: degloving of the penile shaft through a circumferential subcoronal incision allows adequate evacuation of the penile haematoma and provides unparalleled access to both corpora and the urethra. The site of the fracture can be felt and it often shows large adherent clots. Once these have been removed, the tunical edges can be freshened and closed with interrupted polydioxanone sutures.

It is important to remember that penile fractures are often associated with concomitant urethral injuries. Haematuria or blood at the external urethral meatus are highly suggestive of a potential urethral injury and should prompt an on-table flexible cystoscopy. Routine catheterization at the time of surgery aids dissection and facilitates easy urethral repair in the event of a urethral tear.

Postoperative medication to suppress erections has not proven to be beneficial. It is sensible to prohibit sexual activities during the first 6 weeks of recovery.

In summary, rapid diagnosis through history and clinical examination combined with swift surgical intervention is the key for reconstruction with minimal long-term complications.

References

1. Lynch TH, Martínez-Piñeiro L, Plas E, et al. EAU guidelines on urological trauma. *Eur Urol.* 2005;47(1):1–15.
2. Amer T, Wilson R, Chlosta P, et al. Penile fracture: a meta-analysis. *Urol Int.* 2016;96(3):315–329.
3. Rees RW, Brown G, Dorkin T, et al. British Association of Urological Surgeons (BAUS) consensus document for the management of male genital emergencies - penile fracture. *BJU Int.* 2018;122(1):26–28.

SECTION 13

Renal transplantation

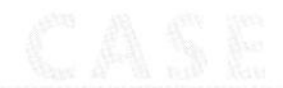

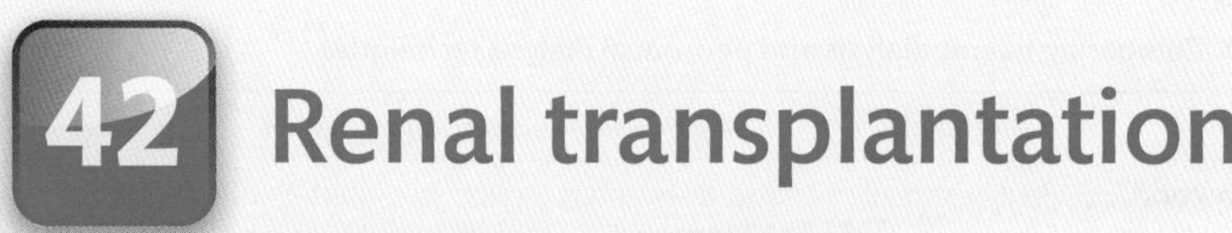

42 Renal transplantation

John M. O'Callaghan

Expert commentary James A. Gilbert

Case history

A 60-year-old male patient with type 2 diabetes is referred to the transplant service by his nephrologist due to a sustained fall in his estimated glomerular filtration rate (eGFR). He has been under their management for 2 years having been closely monitored by his general practitioner in the community.

Learning point Definition of chronic kidney disease

A patient is said to have chronic kidney disease (CKD) if they have abnormalities of kidney function or structure present for >3 months. The definition of CKD includes all individuals with markers of kidney damage or those with an eGFR of <60 mL/min/1.73m^2 on at least two occasions, 90 days apart (with or without markers of kidney damage). CKD is classified based on eGFR and the level of proteinuria, and helps to risk stratify patients. Patients are classified as G1–G5, based on the eGFR, and A1–A3 based on the albumin:creatinine ratio.

Expert comment Causes of CKD

The incidence of diseases that cause CKD changes with age; in childhood, CKD is often associated with congenital abnormalities, such as posterior urethral valves, vesicoureteric reflux, and Alport syndrome. In older patients, renovascular disease, diabetic nephropathy, and hypertensive nephropathy are the most common causes. Other recognized causes include autoimmune immunoglobulin A nephropathy and adult polycystic kidney disease. Some of these causes, such as immunoglobulin A disease, focal segmental glomerulosclerosis, and haemolytic uraemic syndrome can recur in the transplanted kidney. It is therefore important for the transplanting team to be aware of the primary cause of renal failure.

Renal replacement therapy

Some patients with CKD will opt to manage their renal failure conservatively, accepting that they will not survive the progressive accumulation of nitrogen waste products. Renal replacement therapy (RRT) includes various forms of dialysis such as haemodialysis, haemodiafiltration, and peritoneal dialysis (Table 42.1). These therapies are targeted at maintaining homeostasis of electrolytes, acid–base balance, nitrogen metabolites, and volume load. The dialysis options available are all incomplete solutions for CKD stage 5 and the expected 5-year survival of a patient on dialysis in the UK is 45%. Management is directed at the complications of kidney disease, namely acidosis, anaemia, hypervolaemia, and renal bone disease.

Table 42.1 Comparing haemodialysis and peritoneal dialysis techniques

	Haemodialysis	Peritoneal dialysis
Delivery method	Requires creation of an arteriovenous fistula or insertion of a central line	Requires insertion of a peritoneal catheter: radiologically or surgically
Burden	Usually 3 sessions of approximately 4 hours in hospital Can be done at home with adequate space, training, and facilities	Usually done every day at home Requires adequate space for storage of fluids and/or machine and patient capable of connecting fluid bags safely
Complications	Hypotension Line infection Line-associated central stenosis Cardiac failure Graft/fistula thrombosis Aneurysm formation Steal syndrome	Peritonitis Exit site infection Migrated/blocked tube Encapsulating peritoneal sclerosis (rare: 3% at 5 years) Loss of ultrafiltration
Contraindications	Poor cardiac function	Active inflammatory bowel disease or diverticular disease Abdominal hernia Severe peritoneal adhesions Abdominal stoma

During haemodialysis, water-soluble compounds small enough to pass across a semipermeable membrane diffuse down a concentration gradient and the application of pressure causes ultrafiltration of water and water loss. Options for haemodialysis access include temporary central lines (vascath), tunnelled central lines, autogenous arteriovenous fistulas, and synthetic arteriovenous grafts. The key to successful vascular access for haemodialysis is adequate planning. This starts with renal patients and their medical staff preserving veins by avoiding central lines where possible and limiting venepuncture in the cubital fossa or at the wrist. Arteriovenous fistulae using native venous conduits are associated with the highest long-term patency and lowest risk of infection; they should therefore be the vascular access of choice given enough time to plan and mature, which can take at least 6 weeks. Synthetic grafts have lower rates of primary failure and can be used earlier (in some cases immediately) but have higher complication rates; infection and thrombosis, for example. The UK Renal Association recommends that 60% of all incident patients with established end-stage kidney disease commencing planned haemodialysis should receive dialysis via a functioning arteriovenous fistula or graft, and 80% of all prevalent long-term dialysis patients should receive dialysis treatment via definitive access: arteriovenous graft, fistula, or Tenckhoff catheter.

Expert comment Initiation of RRT

The UK Renal Association makes key recommendations regarding the initiation of RRT: most patients with CKD stage 4–5, or with CKD stage 3 and rapidly declining function, should be under the care of a nephrologist. Patients should enter low-clearance programmes when the eGFR is <20 mL/min/1.73 m^2 and ideally should be referred to access surgeons at least 6 months before they are anticipated to require RRT to allow adequate time for planning. Patients should start RRT in a controlled manner, without the need for hospital admission and using an established access, and all patients should be encouraged to perform home dialysis therapy where possible.

Peritoneal dialysis involves a closed system in which an indwelling peritoneal catheter is used to instil hypertonic glucose-rich or amino acid-rich fluid to the peritoneal cavity. The fluid is then drained out completely after a dwell period. Peritoneal catheters can be inserted via a variety of techniques: open insertion via a small lower midline incision, laparoscopic insertion, or percutaneous/radiological.

The challenge for nephrologists is to provide the most appropriate RRT for the patient, each with its own benefits, risks, and individual considerations. Life expectancy and quality of life are greatly improved by renal transplantation though, and this should be considered for all patients who are likely to benefit.

Organ donation

The best first option is a pre-emptive transplant from a living donor, which have much better early graft function and long-term graft survival than kidneys from deceased donors (Figure 42.1). Live donation allows transplantation to take place on an elective basis and ideally before dialysis has commenced. Deceased donor allocation in the UK is determined by a complex mathematical process, which gives priority based on several factors, each of which are given points.

Deceased donors fall into two broad categories: donation after brain death (DBD) or donation after circulatory death (DCD). It should be noted that not all donor types are accepted in all countries and each has its own individual legislation. In the UK, only DBD and type III DCD are accepted; the Maastricht Classification of DCD defines class III as 'Planned withdrawal of life-sustaining therapy, expected cardiac arrest'. This is distinct from classes I, II, and IV, which include patients with sudden cardiac arrest out of hospital, with or without medical team resuscitation.

Following catastrophic brain injury, brainstem death is established through a number of bedside tests. The legal and ethical origin for this is the Harvard Committee of 1968, with modern criteria developed over subsequent years.

Learning point Kidney offering and matching criteria in the UK

- Blood group compatibility.
- Length of time on the waiting list: one point for every day waiting.
- Human leukocyte antigen (HLA) match between donor and recipient: more points for a better match.
- Difficult-to-match patients are awarded more points in order not to miss the rare chance of a transplant.
- Presence of antibodies in the recipient: these reduce the likelihood of a match (sensitization)—highly sensitized patients get more points.
- Paediatric recipients get more priority.

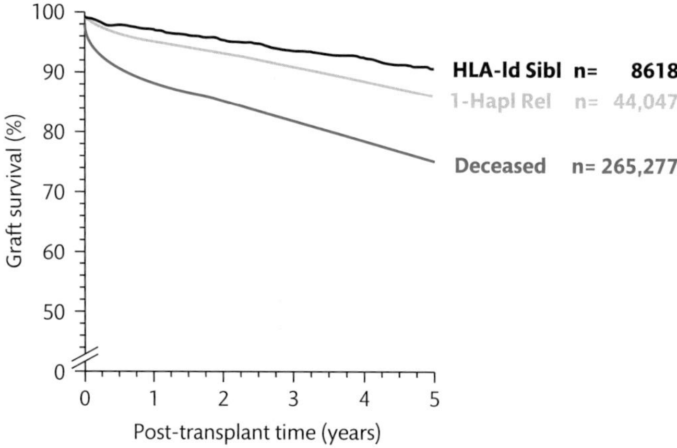

Figure 42.1 Graft survival for first kidney transplants in Europe (1990–2019), comparing different donor types. HLA-Id Sibl, live donor identical human leukocyte antigen-type sibling; 1-Hapl Rel, live donor haplotype relative; and deceased donors.

Collaborative Transplant Study, Heidelberg University.

Expert comment Brain death examination

Before brain death examination can begin, there needs to be evidence of a catastrophic brain injury and complicating or confounding medical problems must have been resolved. The testing must be undertaken by two doctors qualified for >5 years and the tests are done twice. The patient is assessed for the response to painful stimuli and the brainstem reflexes are tested: pupillary, oculocephalic, vestibulo-ocular (caloric), corneal, and gag reflexes. Lastly, the apnoea test is conducted: following pre-oxygenation, the ventilator is disconnected and the PCO_2 is allowed to climb. If it reaches 60 mmHg the test is positive, and the patient is brain dead.

Cerebral injury and brain death are associated with inflammatory processes that can directly injure organs and lead to further damage at reperfusion. Organs from DCD also undergo a period of warm ischaemia before retrieval. The simplest method of dealing with the harmful cellular processes after donor death has been to cool kidneys and flush out the donor blood with a chilled preservation fluid. Despite this, there is ongoing damage in cold-preserved organs, and hence the critical importance of limiting the cold ischaemic time (Figure 42.2). In current clinical practice, several preservation fluids are now used to flush the donor vessels *in situ* and on the workbench. In the UK, these include University of Wisconsin solution and Marshall's solution (hyper-osmolar citrate). The kidney is then packed in a sterile bag of this fluid and kept on ice in a cool box. Another well-described method of preservation is hypothermic machine perfusion (Figure 42.3): the renal artery is cannulated by one end of a system of tubing, and a pump generates a pulsatile or continuous flow of preservation solution through the renal vessels. Hypothermic machine perfusion has been associated with improved early graft function, particularly of DCD kidneys compared to static cold storage.

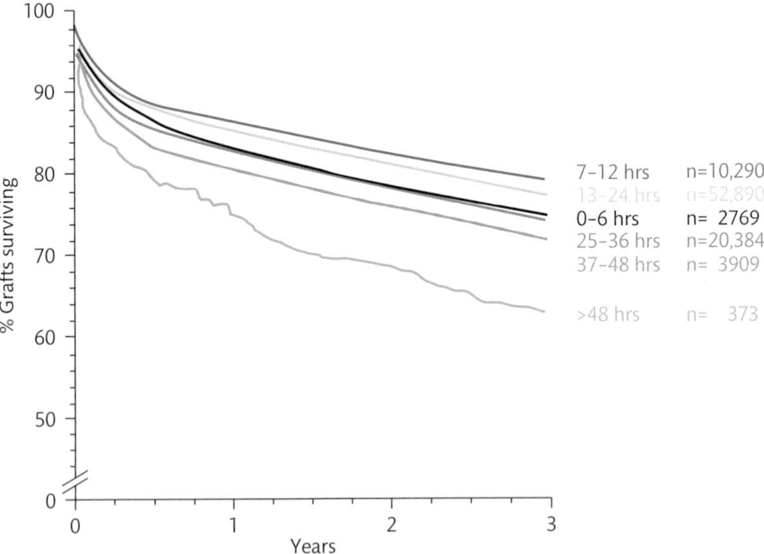

Figure 42.2 Graft survival of first cadaver kidneys showing the detrimental impact of longer cold ischaemic time (1990–2000).
Collaborative Transplant Study, Heidelberg University.

(a) (b)

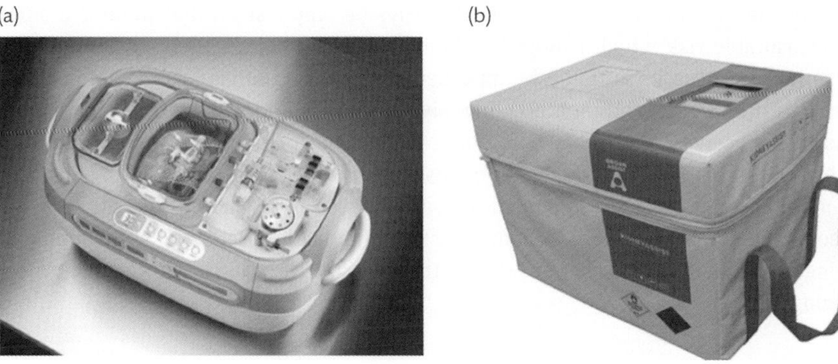

Figure 42.3 The Lifeport® from Organ Recovery Systems (a) and the Kidney Assist® from Organ Assist (b) are two of the commercially available, portable hypothermic machine perfusion systems. They pump chilled preservation fluid through the installed kidney via the renal artery and collect perfusion dynamic data.

Expert comment Techniques for live donor nephrectomy

Traditionally, live donor nephrectomy was undertaken using an open technique with a loin incision to access the kidney. In recent years it has become commonplace to use less invasive techniques, such as hand-assisted laparoscopic, or fully laparoscopic nephrectomy, both of which can be transperitoneal or retroperitoneal in approach. This has seen a significant improvement in postoperative pain experienced by patients, and a much more rapid recovery and return to full activities.

A relative comes forward as a potential live donor for our recipient and so he is not put on the waiting list for a deceased donor kidney, pending the outcome of the live donor's workup.

Live donor and recipient assessment

An overall assessment of the recipient must be made to assess fitness to undergo surgery, and to manage and withstand the necessary immunosuppression. An assessment of compliance is also important to pre-empt any problems with engagement for intensive follow-up, necessary blood tests, and monitoring of a scarce resource to get best outcomes. Patients with renal failure, especially in the setting of diabetes, have a high prevalence of ischaemic heart disease and so a careful evaluation of cardiac fitness is paramount. There is an absolute requirement for a suitable recipient artery for anastomosis, and therefore clinical, and in some cases sonographic assessment, of lower limb vasculature is essential. There is a clear risk of malignancy after transplantation due to immunosuppression, and to prevent reactivation there is advice to not transplant within 2–5 years after definitive treatment. Urogenital abnormalities are relatively common among patients with CKD and a preoperative plan for how to deal with any relevant issues is critical; creation of alternative bladder conduits is reserved for only a few indications due to the potential morbidity of the surgical procedure.

Donor nephrectomy is a safe procedure with low morbidity and mortality, currently estimated at 3 per 10,000 cases. In the UK, a study of >2500 donors showed no perioperative deaths based on complete registry data, including 601 laparoscopic cases. The most common causes of death after living donation are pulmonary emboli, hepatitis, and cardiac events, so it must always be emphasized that there is a small but measurable risk which cannot be eliminated. Nonetheless, there is the potential for serious harm to be suffered by an otherwise healthy individual, having an operation that does not extend their own life. Living kidney donors need to understand the risks to themselves. The process of donor evaluation includes medical and surgical evaluation, psychosocial assessment, counselling, consent, and review of results with the multidisciplinary team. The medical evaluation should include a specific focus on personal risk for renal disease, or family history of renal disease, along with laboratory testing to evaluate renal function, risk of transmissible infection, and cross-sectional imaging.

Learning point Perioperative complications

Data from 14,964 living donors performed from 2008 to 2012 showed an overall incidence of 16.8% for any perioperative complication (Table 42.2).

Table 42.2 Perioperative complication rates

Complication	Rate
Clavien–Dindo grade II	8.8%
Clavien–Dindo grade III	7.3%
Clavien–Dindo grade IV	2.5%
Gastrointestinal	4.4%
Bleeding	3.0%
Respiratory	2.5%
Surgical/anaesthesia-related injury	2.4%

Data from Lentine KL, Lam NN, Axelrod D, et al. Perioperative complications after living kidney donation: a national study. *Am J Transplant*. 2016;16(6):1848–1857.

Transplant immunology

Multiple studies show that there is better graft survival in HLA-identical kidney transplants compared with HLA mismatched transplants. HLA proteins have a central role in immune recognition and defence against pathogens and cancer; they present self and foreign antigens to T lymphocytes. Matching HLA at three key gene loci has the greatest impact on renal transplant survival (*HLA-A*, *HLA-B*, and *HLA-DR*). As we inherit one copy of each gene from each parent, our potential degree of mismatch across these 3 loci is 0–0–0 (zero points) through to 2–2–2 (six points).

The compatibility of the donor and recipient blood groups is also checked. This is not a total barrier to transplantation but generally is only accepted in live donor situations and if the recipient has high levels of antibodies against the general population, making the likelihood of another match low. Desensitization requires specialist techniques such as immunoadsorption and/or plasma exchange.

For the cross-match test, or complement-dependent cytotoxicity test, donor cells are mixed with recipient plasma. A positive test indicates that a recipient would immediately reject a transplanted kidney from this donor, known as hyperacute rejection. Less reactive antibodies present in the recipient serum can be checked using flow cytometry, which is more sensitive and may therefore pick up antibodies that would not cause hyperacute rejection but may increase the overall risk of the transplant.

Expert comment Reducing immunological risk

In order to reduce the immunological risk of a transplant and reduce rejection rates, recipients receive immunosuppressing drugs. Immunosuppression medication is started at the time of transplantation and induction therapies with biological agents (antibodies) should be administered to all recipients. In patients at low immunological risk, this will generally involve an interleukin-2 (IL2) receptor antagonist. Lymphocyte-depleting antibodies may be considered for recipients at higher immunological risk, or for those at a lower risk if the intention is to avoid steroids. It is recommended that maintenance immunosuppression should normally consist of a calcineurin inhibitor and an antiproliferative agent (tacrolimus and mycophenolate being the first-line choices), with or without corticosteroids in low and medium immunological risk recipients.

Learning point Immunosuppressants

Different classes of immunosuppressants are all associated with common or rare but significant side effects. All are associated with increased risk of infections.

Antibodies

- Examples: basiliximab (anti-IL2 receptor), alemtuzumab (anti-CD52), antilymphocyte globulin.
- Side effects: lymphopenia (alemtuzumab), malignancy.

Calcineurin inhibitors

- Examples: tacrolimus, ciclosporin.
- Side effects: nephrotoxicity, diabetes, tremor.

Antimetabolites

- Examples: mycophenolate, azathioprine.
- Side effects: neutropenia, teratogenesis (mycophenolate).

Steroids

- Example: prednisolone.
- Side effects: hypertension, thin skin, weight gain, indigestion, diabetes.

Mammalian target of rapamycin (mTOR) inhibitors

- Examples: sirolimus, everolimus.
- Side effects: diarrhoea, mucosal ulcers, poor wound healing.

Transplant operation and perioperative care

The classical approach for kidney transplantation is to place the kidney in a retroperitoneal pocket lying on the psoas muscle and with the renal vessels anastomosed to the external iliac vessels end-to-side. This allows an extraperitoneal operation to be done, with the kidney lying in a good position for biopsy and close to accessible and straight blood vessels for anastomosis as well as the bladder.

A curved incision is made in the lower abdomen starting from the pubic symphysis and curving upwards and laterally, sometimes as high as the level of the umbilicus. The external oblique aponeurosis is cut along the line of the fibres, and the preperitoneal plane is entered. The peritoneal sac is then mobilized medially to expose the external iliac artery and vein. Care must be taken to protect the spermatic cord in males. The venous anastomosis is done first, typically end to side with Prolene® sutures, then the arterial anastomosis, to minimize the length of time that the external iliac artery is clamped. The clamps are then taken off to perfuse the kidney before the bladder is filled to do the ureterovesical anastomosis. The most commonly used method for this is the Lich–Gregoir technique, of extravesical anastomosis and a ureteric JJ stent is placed at this point to reduce the risk of urine leak.

In the immediate postoperative period, the patient is at risk of acute surgical problems as with any major abdominal surgery, such as bleeding or cardiorespiratory problems. Particular attention should be paid to the fluid balance status and the early function of the graft. Over 95% of live donor kidneys should function immediately and for renal failure recipients who are normally oligo-anuric, this will manifest as a sudden diuresis that necessitates aggressive fluid replacement. If this is not seen, then a cause must be sought. It may be as simple as a blocked catheter but urgent ultrasonography in recovery is recommended to assess for any ureteric, venous, or arterial problem. Delayed graft function is more common after deceased donor transplantation and typically is as high as 30% following DBD and 50% following DCD. It is defined in several ways, with the most common being the requirement for dialysis in the first week after transplantation. In the absence of a structural reason for poor urine output, the recipient continues with their normal dialysis regimen if possible until the kidney function reaches the level that dialysis is no longer needed. If there is persistently no renal function, then a renal biopsy should be considered to assess for any immune cause and a kidney biopsy every 7–10 days is recommended while there is delayed graft function.

Complications of renal transplantation

A critical element in the long-term success of renal transplantation is the treatment of early and mid-term complications such as vascular or urological problems, infections, and acute rejection. The most up-to-date data for kidney transplants in the UK show 1-year and 5-year graft survival of 94% and 87% for deceased donor kidneys, 98% and 92% for live donor kidneys, respectively.

The early graft function depends on a complex interaction of recipient, donor, and transplantation factors. Mechanical problems are usually the result of surgical complications that may require intervention; haematoma, urine leak, or lymphocoele contained within the retroperitoneal space can put a significant pressure on the graft and reduce perfusion. Acute renal vein thrombosis is a rare emergency that manifests as reduced urine output with a tender graft and haematuria and requires immediate exploration. Arterial thrombosis is also rare and may be related to a retrieval injury of the renal artery or dissection flap/recipient iliac artery injury. Arterial stenosis manifests as poor renal function in the setting of fluid retention and hypertension. Treatment options include angiographic balloon dilatation and surgical reimplantation or bypass.

Learning point Early, medium, and late complications of renal transplantation

Early (up to 7 days)

- Renal vein thrombosis.
- Haematoma/haemorrhage.
- Haematuria.
- Urine leak.
- Lymphocoele.
- Delayed graft function.

Medium (up to 12 months)

- Renal artery stenosis.
- Acute rejection.
- Calcineurin inhibitor toxicity.
- Ureteric stenosis.
- Infection.
- Recurrent disease.

Late (after 12 months)

- Chronic rejection and graft loss.
- Malignancy.
- Diabetes.
- Hypertension.

Ureteric stents are placed intraoperatively to reduce the risk of urine leak. However, they increase the risk of urine infection and therefore are removed cystoscopically after 2–4 weeks to balance the risk. Urine leak is usually due to a surgical complication or ischaemic necrosis of the distal ureter, which requires immediate repair. Ureteric obstruction typically presents a number of weeks after transplant and is related to ureteric ischaemia due to poor blood supply. It is treated by decompression of the renal pelvis by percutaneous nephrostomy, followed by a nephrostogram approximately 48 hours later and potentially antegrade stent placement if required. Sometimes these strictures are amenable to balloon dilatation, but if this is not suitable, then surgical reimplantation. This can be managed by anastomosing the transplant ureter to the recipient ureter, psoas hitch, or Boari flap.

Hyperacute rejection, within minutes of reperfusion, is now, thankfully, very rare. The systemic toxicity of a necrotic transplant in the early postoperative period can make recipients unwell with fever, tenderness, and there is a risk of transplant rupture necessitating graft removal. Despite a negative X-match test, recipients may develop antibodies against the graft after transplantation and experience antibody-mediated rejection. Acute (T-cell)-mediated rejection is more common than antibody-mediated rejection, and more readily treated. The highest incidence is in the first 3 months; it is diagnosed on transplant biopsy. First-line treatment of acute rejection is with pulsed intravenous methylprednisolone. If the rejection is steroid resistant, then other biological agents, such as alemtuzumab or antithymocyte globulin may be tried. Antibody-mediated rejection is treated with a combination of methylprednisolone and other therapies, such as plasmapheresis, intravenous immunoglobulin, or an anti-CD20 antibody (e.g. rituximab).

Due to immunosuppression, transplant recipients are at increased risk of infection. Donor-derived (transmitted) infections are rare, due to the thorough screening of donors prior to donation (Table 42.3). Bacterial infections in potential donors, as long as the organism is identified and treated appropriately, are not contraindications to donation.

There is the potential to reactivate infections that are latent within the recipient after the induction of immunosuppression. Diseases of this type include tuberculosis, herpes simplex virus, and varicella zoster virus. Vaccination and immunity/exposure status is therefore checked prior to transplantation and prophylactic medications started as early as possible after transplantation. Live vaccines are contraindicated after transplantation.

Table 42.3 Potential donor-derived infectious risks for transplant recipients, grouped by type

Potential infections	Examples
Viral	Herpesviruses (cytomegalovirus, Epstein–Barr virus) Hepatitis viruses (types C and C) Retroviruses (HIV, human T-lymphotropic virus)
Bacterial	*Staphylococcus* spp. *Pseudomonas aeruginosa* *Mycobacteria tuberculosis* Nocardia asteroids
Fungal	*Candida* spp. *Aspergillus* spp.
Parasitic	*Toxoplasma gondii* *Trypanosoma cruzi*

The risk of malignancy after transplantation is increased compared to the general population, due to the impact of immunosuppressing medication. Non-melanoma skin cancers are the most common cancers in renal transplant patients, followed by renal, bladder, and thyroid. Oncogenic viruses can play a role in the development of lymphoma and lymphoproliferative disease after transplantation. Post-transplant lymphoproliferative disorder is a malignancy primarily of B-cell origin and related to Epstein–Barr virus proliferation. It affects only 1–2% of kidney transplant recipients but is a life-threatening disease.

Despite improvements in immunosuppression and donor selection, a chronic deterioration in graft function and eventual progression back to dialysis is inevitable. This damage is a combination of immunological and non-immune effects resulting in interstitial fibrosis, tubular atrophy, and glomerular sclerosis. It is therefore important to identify and treat, or ideally prevent, the potential modifiable risk factors.

Learning point Risk factors for renal allograft damage

Following renal transplantation, modifiable risk factors for renal allograft damage and deterioration in function should be addressed. Non-modifiable risk factors are also described below.

Modifiable risk factors

- Calcineurin inhibitor toxicity.
- Ascending infection/sepsis.
- Hypertension.
- Hyperlipidaemia.
- Smoking status.
- Non-compliance with medication.

Non-modifiable risk factors

- Deceased donor.
- Older donor.
- Reperfusion injury.
- Delayed graft function.
- Acute rejection.
- Recipient ethnicity.
- HLA mismatch.

A final word from the expert

Renal transplantation is an expanding, exciting, and developing surgical field. Despite an increase in the number of transplants done, the waiting list continues to increase in many countries due to the rising numbers of patients with CKD. Attempts have been made to address this need by increasing the use of kidneys from donation after circulatory death, live donation, and by extending the criteria for acceptable brain death donors in terms of age or comorbidity. Research into new reconditioning technologies may further expand the potential donor pool. Many transplant recipients will need more than one transplant over their lifetime due to the still limited life expectancy of a transplanted organ. It is hoped that improvements in immunosuppression may address this particular issue by preventing chronic allograft nephropathy and return to dialysis.

Further reading

Gatz JD, Spangler R. Evaluation of the renal transplant recipient in the emergency department. *Emerg Med Clin North Am.* 2019;37(4):679–705.

Hadjianastassiou VG, Johnson RJ, Rudge CJ, Mamode N. 2509 living donor nephrectomies, morbidity and mortality, including the UK introduction of laparoscopic donor surgery. *Am J Transplant.* 2007;7(11):2532–2537.

Hagen SM, Lafranca JA, Steyerberg EW, ≥zermans JN, Dor FJ. Laparoscopic versus open peritoneal dialysis catheter insertion: a meta-analysis. *PLOS One.* 2013;8(2):e56351.

Kwong J, Schiefer D, Aboalsamh G, Archambault J, Luke PP, Sener A. Optimal management of distal ureteric strictures following renal transplantation: a systematic review. *Transpl Int.* 2016;29(5):579–588.

Lentine KL, Lam NN, Axelrod D, et al. Perioperative complications after living kidney donation: a national study. *Am J Transplant.* 2016;16(6):1848–1857.

Moers C, Smits JM, Maathuis MJ, et al. Machine perfusion or cold storage in deceased-donor kidney transplantation. *N Engl J Med.* 2009;360(1):7–19.

National Institute for Health and Care Excellence. Chronic kidney disease in adults: assessment and management. NICE guideline [NG203]. National Institute for Health and Care Excellence. 2021. https://www.nice.org.uk/guidance/ng203

NHS Blood and Transplant. Kidney transplantation: deceased donor organ allocation. Policy POL1 86/9. NHS Blood and Transplant. 2019. https://nhsbtdbe.blob.core.windows.net/umbraco-assets-corp/16915/kidney-allocation-policy-pol186.pdf

NHS Blood and Transplant. Organ specific report: kidney transplantation annual report. NHS Blood and Transplant. 2019. https://nhsbtdbe.blob.core.windows.net/umbraco-assets-corp/17289/kidney-annual-report-2018-19-november19.pdf

O'Callaghan J, Knight SR, Morgan RD, Morris PJ. Preservation solutions for static cold storage of kidney allografts: a systematic review and meta-analysis. *Am J Transplant.* 2012;12(4):896–906.

Ponticelli CE. The impact of cold ischemia time on renal transplant outcome. *Kidney Int.* 2015;87(2):272–275.

Shi X, Lv J, Han W, et al. What is the impact of human leukocyte antigen mismatching on graft survival and mortality in renal transplantation? A meta-analysis of 23 cohort studies involving 486,608 recipients. *BMC Nephrol.* 2018;19(1):116.

Sugi MD, Joshi G, Maddu KK, Dahiya N, Menias CO. Imaging of renal transplant complications throughout the life of the allograft: comprehensive multimodality review. *Radiographics.* 2019;39(5):1327–1355.

Summers DM, Johnson RJ, Allen J, et al. Analysis of factors that affect outcome after transplantation of kidneys donated after cardiac death in the UK: a cohort study. *Lancet.* 2010;376(9749):1303–1311.

Visser IJ, van der Staaij JPT, Muthusamy A, Willicombe M, Lafranca JA, Dor FJMF. Timing of ureteric stent removal and occurrence of urological complications after kidney transplantation: a systematic review and meta-analysis. *J Clin Med.* 2019;8(5):689.

UK Renal Association. Peritoneal dialysis in adults and children. Clinical Practice Guideline. UK Renal Association. 2017. https://ukkidney.org/sites/renal.org/files/final-peritoneal-dialysis-guideline667ba231181561659443ff000014d4d8.pdf

UK Renal Association. Post-operative care of the renal transplant recipient. Clinical Practice Guideline. UK Renal Association. 2017. https://ukkidney.org/sites/renal.org/files/FINAL-Post-Operative-Care-Guideline-1.pdf

UK Renal Association. Living donor kidney transplantation. Clinical Practice Guideline. UK Renal Association. 2018. https://ukkidney.org/sites/renal.org/files/Living-Donor.pdf

UK Renal Association. Vascular access for haemodialysis. Clinical Practice Guideline. UK Renal Association. 2020. https://ukkidney.org/sites/renal.org/files/vascular-access.pdf

Wilson C, Sanni A, Rix DA, Soomro NA. Laparoscopic versus open nephrectomy for live kidney donors. *Cochrane Database Syst Rev.* 2011;11:CD006124.

SECTION 14

Paediatric surgery

CASE

Recurrent urinary tract infections and non-neurogenic neurogenic bladder in children

Martin Skott

Expert commentary Imran Mushtaq

Case history

A 5-year-old girl with recurrent urinary tract infections (UTIs) was referred to our clinic. No problems were detected on antenatal scans, and she was potty trained at the age of 3–5 years. She had slight constipation, which was managed with laxatives.

Recently, she had been suffering from frequent daytime incontinence and occasionally night-time incontinence. Her mother described a classic history of withholding urination and urgency, although she had good sensation of bladder fullness. Mainly, she had been asymptomatic with no temperatures or dysuria. She reported a good fluid intake of 1.5 L per day. There was no relevant past medical history or family history of any significance. Pending further investigations, she was commenced on trimethoprim prophylaxis.

Expert comment UTI in children

UTI represents the most common bacterial infection in children.[1] In infants and children, the symptoms differ from those in neonates (Table 43.1). The incidence of UTIs varies depending on age and sex. In the first year of life, UTIs are more common in boys (3.7%), especially if they are uncircumcised, than in girls (2%). Later, the incidence changes, and about 3% of all prepubertal girls and 1% of prepubertal boys suffer from UTIs.[2]

Table 43.1 Presenting symptoms of UTIs at different ages

Symptoms	Neonates	Infants	Children
Icterus	+		
Sepsis	+		
Failure to thrive	+	+	
Vomiting	+	+	+
Fever	+	+	+
Diarrhoea		+	
Flank pain		+	+
Incontinence		+	+
Smelly urine		+	+
Lower urinary tract symptoms (i.e. frequency, dysuria, urgency)			+

It is essential to differentiate between lower UTIs (cystitis) and pyelonephritis (infections of the kidney parenchyma, with fever) because one-third of all pyelonephritis episodes will result in a parenchymal scar.

In community acquired UTIs, *Escherichia coli* is found in approximately 75% of the urine cultures. In contrast, in nosocomial UTIs, the most common organisms seen are *Klebsiella pneumoniae*, *Pseudomonas* spp., *Enterobacter* spp., *Enterococcus* spp., and *Candida* spp.[3,4]

Cardiovascular, respiratory, and abdominal examinations were normal with no evidence of faecal loading. The spine, lower extremities, and gait were normal and examination of external genitalia revealed normal anatomy.

Bladder function assessment showed a uroflow profile suggestive of abdominal straining with post-void residual urine of 30 mL and a reasonable capacity with a volume of 200 mL (estimated to be 188 mL). She voided eight to nine times per day, with episodes of dampness and urgency.

Clinical tip Bladder capacity

Several studies have shown that functional bladder capacity at different ages can be accurately estimated as a function of age with no differences in sex. For young infants, it can be expressed as[5,6]:

Bladder capacity (mL) = 38 + (2.5 × age (months))

For older children:

Bladder capacity (mL) = 30 + (age (years) × 30)

An ultrasound scan of the urinary tract showed both kidneys to be of normal size and echotexture, but with mild pelvicalyceal dilatation bilaterally. The bladder wall appeared slightly irregular and thickened, and a residual volume of urine was present post-void (Figure 43.1a). Diuretic renal scintigraphy using technetium-99m (^{99m}Tc) mercaptoacetyltriglycine (MAG3) with indirect cystography was suggestive of functional asymmetry (44% right side and 56% on the left side). Both kidneys and ureters demonstrated some stasis of tracer in the collecting system and ureters. There was no evidence of vesicoureteral reflux (VUR), though incomplete bladder emptying, on the indirect cystography (Figure 43.1b).

Learning point Residual urine

Residual urine is assessed by ultrasonography after a uroflow measurement. It is well known that healthy infants and toddlers do not fully empty the bladder every time they void, but should do so at least once during a 4-hour observation period.[7] Older children, however, are expected to empty their bladder to completion.

Expert comment Diagnostic workup

There is controversy about whether imaging studies should be performed after the first or after recurring episodes of UTI. In general, a maximum of two UTI episodes in girls and one episode in boys should trigger imaging studies. In terms of febrile UTI in infants, renal ultrasonography is strongly recommended as the first-line investigation.

Renal ultrasonography

Urinary tract imaging comprises of some form of renal and upper collecting system evaluation, usually renal ultrasonography and, selectively, voiding cystourethrogram (VCUG) and functional studies. As renal ultrasonography is not dependent upon renal function, it will detect both gross and subtle

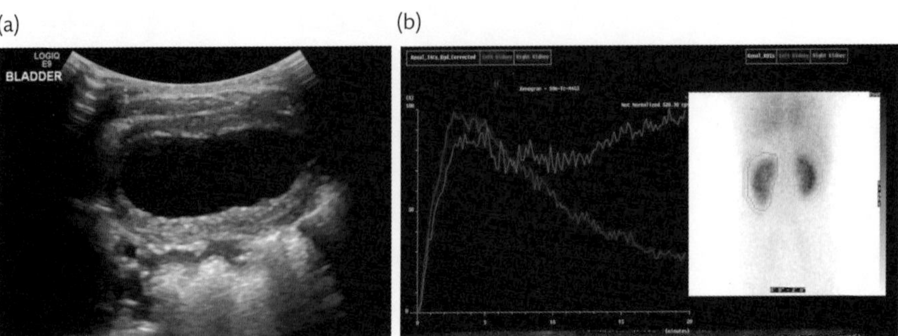

Figure 43.1 (a) Irregular and thickened bladder wall pre micturition. (b) Renogram which shows a functionally slight larger left kidney. No convincing evidence of renal scarring was noticed.

abnormalities of the urinary tract, including those that involve poorly functioning or non-functioning renal units. On the other hand, it is highly operator dependent and is not reliable to detect VUR.[8]

VCUG

A VCUG is still the gold standard to investigate VUR. The VCUG may be performed either with fluoroscopy and iodinated contrast medium or with nuclear imaging, but these studies give different information. A fluoroscopic VCUG can show urethral and bladder abnormalities and VUR. A radionuclide VCUG (usually ^{99m}Tc-MAG3) offers poor spatial resolution so anatomical details of the urinary tract and the degree of reflux may not be so easy to assess. The radionuclide VCUG can be performed using similar techniques as the traditional fluoroscopic VCUG with retrograde filling of the bladder with the radionuclide or indirect in which the radionuclide is injected intravenously and cleared from the kidneys into the bladder. VUR detection by either fluoroscopic or radionuclide VCUG is dependent upon the child voiding and being compliant.[9,10]

Nuclear renography (static)

Radionuclide scanning with ^{99m}TC dimercaptosuccinic acid (DMSA) can detect an area of acute renal inflammation and chronic scarring. It is the gold standard in the detection of renal scarring, and studies have shown a specificity and sensitivity for renal scarring up to 100% and 80%, respectively.[11] When combining DMSA with high-resolution computed tomography (single-photon emission computed tomography), a much better resolution, scar detection, and level of renal anatomic detail is possible.[12] On the other hand, if an assessment of renal parenchymal flow, function, and drainage is acquired, ^{99m}TC- MAG3 is superior to DMSA.

The patient's symptoms and findings on the ultrasound scan were suggestive of an overactive bladder (OAB), and therefore lifestyle modifications such as an adequate fluid intake of around 1.5 L a day without any bladder irritants (squash juices) were suggested. In addition, she was commenced on anticholinergic medication in the form of slow-release oxybutynin.

Expert comment OAB

OAB is the most common voiding dysfunction in children, occurring with a peak incidence between the ages of 5 and 7 years. OAB is thought to be caused by a delay in the maturation of inhibitors of non-voluntary detrusor contractions.[13] During bladder filling, detrusor contractions not centrally inhibited are recognized by the child as a sense of urgency, thereby prompting voluntary striated sphincter and pelvic floor contractions, and various holding manoeuvres such as leg crossing and attempts at external compression of the urethra.[14] Despite the holding manoeuvres, the child still may have leakage, mostly when tired, or at play when the child is distracted. Recurrent isometric contraction of the detrusor against a closed tightened sphincter causes progressive detrusor muscle hypertrophy, which will lead to decreased functional capacity and increased instability, perpetuating the vicious circle of OAB. It has been shown that anticholinergic treatment of OAB in association with a timed voiding regimen and adequate bowel management, significantly decreases the incidence of recurrent UTIs.[15]

After an interval of 6 months, the patient was reviewed in the clinic. A repeat bladder function assessment revealed that her post-void residuals had increased significantly. In addition, she had suffered two lower UTIs with mixed growth cultures, despite prophylactic antibiotics. The repeat ultrasound scan showed a significant increase in the bilateral hydronephrosis, the bladder was still thick-walled, but now with trabeculation and diverticula. She still had some ongoing problems with chronic constipation and day- and night-time accidents in between voids, despite regular voiding and practising a double voiding. The oxybutynin was stopped and, based on

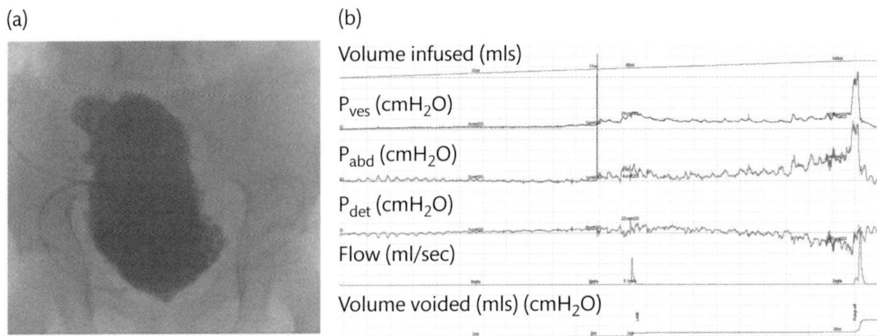

Figure 43.2 (a) Grossly trabeculated bladder. (b) Filling cystometry which shows some detrusor activity towards end fill associated with leakage (blue arrow). The voiding phase was characterized by maximum detrusor pressure (P_{det}) of 43 cmH_2O with associated abdominal straining.

the deterioration of the upper urinary tract, the possibility of a neuropathic element was considered.

A magnetic resonance imaging scan of her spine revealed no intraspinal abnormality. We then proceeded to cystoscopy, which confirmed an irregular, elongated, and grossly trabeculated bladder ('fir tree') (Figure 43.2a). A video urodynamic study showed reduced functional capacity bladder (180 mL) with some impaired compliance (a rise of 22 cmH_2O for 180 mL infused) (Figure 43.2b). Voiding dynamics revealed a dyscoordinated pattern and incomplete bladder emptying (residual of 20 mL). Fluoroscopy did not reveal any vesicourethral reflux, either during filling or voiding.

Learning point Invasive urodynamic investigations

If a suprapubic tube is inserted, a minimal delay of half a day is needed between tube placement and urodynamic testing. If a transurethral catheter is used, it must be as small as possible, since a large catheter can cause outflow obstruction.

The filling rate should be as physiological as possible, and the following can be used to calculate the filling rate: body weight (kg) divided by 4 and expressed in millilitres per minute[16] or as described by Hjälmås, as 5% of expected bladder capacity (mL) expressed in millilitres per minute.[6]

Bladder sensation can be challenging to assess in children. When filling exceeds expected bladder capacity, and no sensation is reported, it can indicate reduced bladder sensation.

In infants and children, any involuntary detrusor contractions observed before voiding can be considered pathological and are defined by an increase in detrusor pressure >15 cmH_2O above baseline.

Bladder compliance is the relationship between change in bladder volume and change in detrusor pressure:

$$\text{Compliance (mL/cmH}_2\text{O)} = \frac{\Delta\text{Bladder volume (mL)}}{\Delta\text{Detrusor pressure (cmH}_2\text{O)}}$$

Understanding bladder compliance is complicated in paediatric practice, as it tends to increase by age and the detrusor pressure can be affected by the rate of bladder filling. Furthermore, there are, at the moment, no reliable reference ranges available for bladder compliance in children. For this reason, a rule of thumb is that a detrusor pressure of ≤10 cmH_2O above baseline at expected bladder capacity for age is acceptable.[17] The clinical relevance of the pressure–flow relationship during voiding is unclear, as high pressures and interrupted flow are observed during voiding in children with normal lower urinary tracts.[18,19] However, detrusor sphincter dyssynergia is seen in neurogenic bladder disorders, characterized by a detrusor contraction concurrent with an involuntary contraction of the urethra and/or periurethral striated muscle leading to urinary flow interrupted during voiding.

Expert comment Non-neurogenic neurogenic bladder

The term non-neurogenic neurogenic bladder (NNNB) or subclinical neurogenic bladder and later Hinman syndrome, is presumably an acquired form of bladder sphincter dysfunction in children occurring after the age of toilet training.[20,21] The typical form includes (1) dyscoordinated voiding with day-and-night wetting and incomplete bladder emptying; (2) trabeculated bladder; (3) recurrent UTIs; (4) deterioration of the urinary tract with hydroureteronephrosis; (5) constipation and faecal soiling; (6) significant behavioural issues with frequent anxiety, depression, and familial integration disturbances; and (7) normal neurological physical examination and investigations.

The condition has all the clinical and urodynamic features typical of neuropathic bladder dysfunction, but no neurological pathology can be demonstrated on imaging, and it may be conceivable that the underlying neurological cause remains to be identified. In its severe form, the bladder sphincter dysfunction can cause full-blown bladder decompensation with day/night-time wetting, large postmicturition residual urine volumes, recurrent UTIs, and significant damage to the upper urinary tracts.

NNNB is believed to be an acquired pathology, but evidence of prenatal presentations has also been reported.[22,23] It is therefore likely that NNNB covers a wide range of disease, ranging from patients presenting early in childhood to those presenting at adolescence, and from children responding to limited detrusor sphincter physiotherapy and bowel management to severe NNNB which requires bladder augmentation and kidney transplant.[24]

Clean intermittent catheterization was attempted on several occasions, but the patient was very resistant and fearful. Therefore, a suprapubic tube (10-French Cystofix®) was placed temporarily, with clamp and release every 3 hours during the daytime and overnight free drainage. Following placement of the suprapubic tube, complete resolution of upper urinary tract dilatation and episodes of UTIs was observed. Subsequently, the suprapubic tube was replaced under general anaesthesia with a 10-French Foley catheter, which is changed every 10–12 weeks.

An up-to-date DMSA scan showed a functionally slight smaller right kidney (47%), but no definite focal defects were identified.

A final word from the expert

UTIs and incontinence are common problems referred to a paediatric urologist. In the majority of cases, the problem can be remedied with simple dietary modifications and/or anticholinergic medication. This case illustrates, however, that some children are at risk of progressing to more serious and irreversible upper and lower urinary tract pathology. This patient demonstrated concerning features at presentation of mild hydronephrosis and bladder wall thickening, which rapidly deteriorated over a short interval of 6 months to a classical Hinman syndrome. There is probably very little which could have been done to prevent this deterioration, and it is likely that on the basis of the current findings that the patient in the long-term, will need an augmentation cystoplasty with or without a continent cutaneous catheterizable channel.

References

1. Stull TL, LiPuma JJ. Epidemiology and natural history of urinary tract infections in children. *Med Clin North Am.* 1991;75(2):287–297.
2. Winberg J, Andersen HJ, Bergström T, Jacobsson B, Larson H, Lincoln K. Epidemiology of symptomatic urinary tract infection in childhood. *Acta Paediatr Scand Suppl.* 1974;252:1–20.

3. Magín EC, García-García JJ, Sert SZ, Giralt AG, Cubells CL. Efficacy of short-term intravenous antibiotic in neonates with urinary tract infection. *Pediatr Emerg Care.* 2007;23(2):83–86.
4. López Sastre JB, Ramos Aparicio A, Coto Cotallo GD, Fernández Colomer B, Crespo Hernández M; Grupo de Hospitales Castrillo. Urinary tract infection in the newborn: clinical and radio imaging studies. *Pediatr Nephrol.* 2007;22(10):1735–1741.
5. Holmdahl G, Hanson E, Hanson M, Hellström AL, Hjälmås K, Sillén U. Four-hour voiding observation in healthy infants. *J Urol.* 1996;156(5):1809–1812.
6. Hjälmås K. Urodynamics in normal infants and children. *Scand J Urol Nephrol Suppl.* 1988;114:20–27.
7. Jansson UB, Hanson M, Hanson E, Hellström AL, Sillén U. Voiding pattern in healthy children 0 to 3 years old: a longitudinal study. *J Urol.* 2000;164(6):2050–2054.
8. Preda I, Jodal U, Sixt R, Stokland E, Hansson S. Pediatric urology value of ultrasound in evaluation of infants with first urinary tract infection. *J Urol.* 2010;183(5):1984–1988.
9. McDonald A, Scranton M, Gillespie R, Mahajan V, Edwards GA. Voiding cystourethrograms and urinary tract infections: how long to wait? *Pediatrics.* 2000;105(4):E50.
10. Lebowitz RL. The detection of vesicoureteral reflux in the child. *Invest Radiol.* 1986;21(7):519–531.
11. Rushton HG, Majd M. Dimercaptosuccinic acid renal scintigraphy for the evaluation of pyelonephritis and scarring: a review of experimental and clinical studies. *J Urol.* 1992;148(Pt 2):1726–1732.
12. Björgvinsson E, Majd M, Eggli KD. Diagnosis of acute pyelonephritis in children: comparison of sonography and 99mTc-DMSA scintigraphy. *AJR Am J Roentgenol.* 1991;157(3):539–543.
13. Franco I. Overactive bladder in children. part 1: pathophysiology. *J Urol.* 2007;178(3):761–768.
14. van Gool JD, de Jonge GA. Urge syndrome and urge incontinence. *Arch Dis Child.* 1989;64(11):1629–1634.
15. Koff SA, Murtagh DS. The uninhibited bladder in children: effect of treatment on recurrence of urinary infection and on vesicoureteral reflux resolution. *J Urol.* 1983;130(6):1138–1140.
16. Abrams P, Cardozo L, Fall M, et al. The standardisation of terminology of lower urinary tract function: report from the Standardisation Sub-committee of the International Continence Society. *Neurourol Urodyn.* 2002;21:167–178.
17. Nevéus T, Gontard von A, Hoebeke P, et al. The standardization of terminology of lower urinary tract function in children and adolescents: report from the Standardisation Committee of the International Children's Continence Society. *J Urol.* 2006;176(1):314–324.
18. Yeung CK, Godley ML, Ho CK, et al. Some new insights into bladder function in infancy. *Br J Urol.* 1995;76(2):235–240.
19. Yeung CK, Godley ML, Dhillon HK, Duffy PG, Ransley PG. Urodynamic patterns in infants with normal lower urinary tracts or primary vesico-ureteric reflux. *Br J Urol.* 1998;81(3):461–467.
20. Hinman F, Baumann FW. Vesical and ureteral damage from voiding dysfunction in boys without neurologic or obstructive disease. *J Urol.* 1973;109(4):727–732.
21. Dorfman LE, Bailey J, Smith JP. Subclinical neurogenic bladder in children. *J Urol.* 1969;101(1):48–54.
22. Vidal I, Héloury Y, Ravasse P, Lenormand L, Leclair MD. Severe bladder dysfunction revealed prenatally or during infancy. *J Pediatr Urol.* 2009;5(1):3–7.
23. Jayanthi VR, Khoury AE, McLorie GA, Agarwal SK. The nonneurogenic neurogenic bladder of early infancy. *J Urol.* 1997;158(3 Pt 2):1281–1285.
24. Leclair MD, Héloury Y. Non-neurogenic elimination disorders in children. *J Pediatr Urol.* 2010;6(4):338–345.

44 Undescended testis

María S. Figueroa-Díaz and Kimberly Aikins

Expert commentary Imran Mushtaq

Case history 1

A newborn was referred with bilateral palpable undescended testes (UDTs) (Figure 44.1). He was born at term without any antenatal problems. He was reassessed at 3 months of age, when the left testis was in the scrotum and the right testis was in the inguinal region.

Learning point Incidence of UDT

A UDT affects 3–4% of boys at birth, and 1% at 3 months of age.[1] In a prospective cohort study in the UK, the incidence of UDT decreased from 6% at birth to 2.4% at 3 months.[2] Progressive descent of the testis can occur up to 3 months postnatally, this has been reported to be as high as 50–87%. For that reason, the position must be reassessed at that age and continued observation is needed because of the risk of recurrent cryptorchidism.[3] A UDT occurs in up to 45% of preterm male newborns;[1] 75–80% of UDT are palpable and 60–70% are unilateral.[4,5]

Clinical tip Physical examination

Physical examination must be done in a relaxed and warm environment. Abduction of the thighs contributes to inhibition of the cremasteric reflex, facilitating evaluation. Palpation begins lateral to the internal inguinal ring, moving the hand downwards following the inguinal canal, pushing the testis towards the scrotum. The other hand is employed to locate the testis, grasp it, and pull it downwards towards the scrotum, assessing tension of the cord and how far into the scrotum it can be pulled. Possible associated findings are hernia and hydrocele. The presence of penile abnormalities (hypospadias or micropenis) may indicate a disorder of sex development (DSD).

Learning point Classification of UDT

- **True UDT or cryptorchidism**: the absence of the testis in a normal scrotal position. The testis lies along the expected path of descent.
- **Ectopic testis**: the testis is in a location outside the normal path of descent, frequently upper inguinal, anterior to the external oblique muscle or, more rarely, in a perirenal, prepubic, femoral, perineal, or contralateral scrotal position.
- **Acquired cryptorchidism or ascending testis**: this refers to a cryptorchid testis that was previously a descended testis, previously described as retractile. The peak age is around 10 years of age and it has an incidence of 1–2%. A persistent fibrous remnant of the processus vaginalis is often present at surgery.
- **Retractile testis**: a descended testis that ascends easily due to the cremasteric reflex. Can be manipulated into the scrotum and when released does not retract immediately.

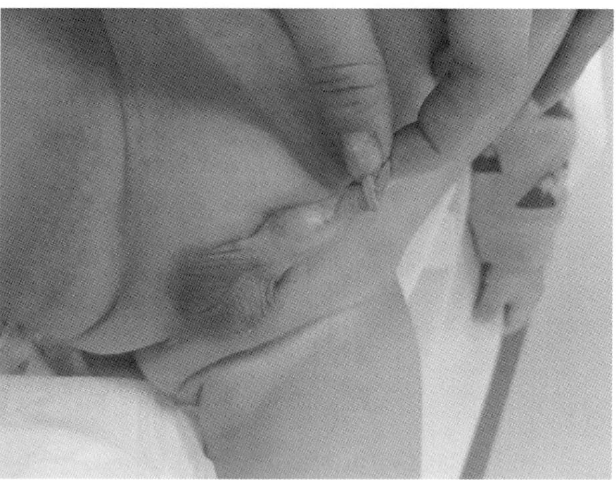

Figure 44.1 Flat scrotum in bilateral UDTS.

Learning point Effects of cryptorchidism

The scrotal environment is 4°C below the core body temperature. If a testis is not in a scrotal position, this can be associated with heat stress leading to progressive abnormalities in the biochemistry and physiology of the testis.

During the first year of life, the human testis undergoes important development, with neonatal germ cells (pluripotential gonocytes) differentiating into type A spermatogonia during the 'minipuberty period' (2–4 months). This period is characterized by gonadotrophic stimulation of testosterone production, an increase in Sertoli cell number, and production of inhibin B. Type A spermatogonia will slowly differentiate into type B spermatogonia, and by 3–4 years of age, they will further differentiate into primary spermatocytes, which will remain in this form until the onset of puberty. All these processes may be affected by heat stress in UDT. Which may inhibit the transformation into type A spermatogonia, reducing the number of stem cells for spermatogenesis. It may also inhibit the physiological apoptosis of the redundant neonatal gonocytes. The persistence of these pluripotential cells may lead to a carcinoma *in situ*.

This is the proposed cause of impaired fertility (present in up to one-third of cases of unilateral UDT and two-thirds of cases of bilateral UDT) and increased risk of malignancy (up to five to ten times) in a young adult with a history of UDT.[6]

At 6 months old, a right open groin orchidopexy was performed as a day case. At 6-month follow-up, both testes were equal in size and in a scrotal position.

Expert comment Hormonal treatment

Hormonal treatment with human chorionic gonadotropin or gonadotropin-releasing hormone is not routine practice due to low success rates (20%), a high risk of testicular re-ascent (20%), and concerns about their impact on spermatogenesis.[7–10] Actual management of UDT is surgical management.

Learning point Goals of surgical management

Optimize spermatogenesis

There is an inherent germ cell dysfunction in UDT which studies suggest is partially reversible by early surgical intervention.[11] The degree of dysfunction increases with bilateral involvement[12] and increasing age prior to surgery.

Testicular surveillance for malignancy

There is a five- to ten fold increased risk of germ cell tumours in UDT. Both seminoma and non-seminomatous tumours develop from Germ cell neoplasia *in situ* of the testis at a postpubertal age. There is emerging evidence of an additional increased risk of malignancy if orchidopexy is delayed.

A meta-analysis showed a relative risk of 5.8 if orchidopexy was done after 10–11 years of age.[13] A Swedish study showed the relative risk of testicular cancer in those who underwent orchidopexy before 13 years of age was 2.2 and this increased to 5.4 in those treated after 13 years of age.[14]

Evidence base The optimal age to perform an orchidopexy

International guidelines recommend surgery between 6 and 18 months of age for congenital UDT based on testicular biopsy results and testicular volume outcomes.[15,16]

Support for this approach

Effect on testicular growth and fertility

Several indexes of fertility have been examined, including testicular size, histology, semen analysis, and paternity rates.

Good-quality studies conclude that orchidopexy should be performed before 1 year of age. Comparative testicular biopsies demonstrate a decline in the number of germ cells and Sertoli cells between 9 months and 3 years of age.

Testicular growth is restored after early orchidopexy, at 9 months compared to orchiopexy at 3 years.[17]

A systematic review and meta-analysis in 2018 comparing outcomes following orchidopexy before or after 1 year of age, concluded that testicular volume was greater and there were more spermatogonia per tubule in infants undergoing orchidopexy before 1 year.[18]

Effect on malignancy

The risk of cancer is increased when orchidopexy is delayed beyond the first decade.

Anaesthetic considerations

Current evidence is controversial regarding the effect of general anaesthesia at an early age on neurodevelopment. An association has been found in animal studies, but the most robust studies in humans have not found an association.[19,20] Future research is needed to clarify this important issue.

Spontaneous descent

Spontaneous descent to the base of the scrotum is unlikely to occur in full-term males after 3 months of age, and 6 months of age in preterm babies. Surgery is indicated once failure of spontaneous descent is demonstrated on physical examination.

Surgical factors

Orchidopexy is safe in patients <1 year of age, and a 2018 systematic review and meta-analysis has shown that orchidopexy in small infants does not result in an increased atrophy rate.[18]

Case history 2

A 3-month-old infant was referred to the clinic with bilateral UDT and hypospadias. On physical examination, both testes are impalpable and there is a mid-penile hypospadias with chordee. Disorder of sex differentiation is suspected.

Expert comment Evaluation for DSD

- The association between non-palpable UDT and hypospadias requires complete evaluation for an associated DSD.
- DSD are detected in 15% of patients with bilateral UDT.

- Hypospadias associated with a unilateral impalpable testis should prompt the exclusion of ovotesticular DSD or mixed gonadal dysgenesis. Bilateral UDT with hypospadias may also represent a 46,XX baby with virilization due to congenital adrenal hyperplasia. In suspected congenital adrenal hyperplasia, hormonal and electrolytic analyses are performed urgently to obviate the potential adverse effects of an undiagnosed salt-wasting disease with a high risk of hypovolaemic shock due to cortisol insufficiency. Hypospadias is associated with cryptorchidism in 12–24% of cases.

The karyotype result is 45,X0/46,XY. Ultrasound demonstrates one gonad in the abdomen on the right, without any müllerian structures visible in the pelvis.

Learning point Impalpable testes

Impalpable testes account for 10–20% of UDT.

Possible clinical findings at laparoscopy include[4]:

- Absent/vanishing testis (15–45%)
- Intra-abdominal testis (25–50%)
- Extra-abdominal/canalicular impalpable testis (10–30%).

Clinical tip How is an impalpable testis managed?

Imaging is not routinely required, as it lacks the sensitivity and specificity to alter the need for exploratory surgery. It can be useful to confirm the presence of a suspected canalicular testis. See Figure 44.2.

Surgical approach

Examination under anaesthesia

Impalpability of the testes must be confirmed under anaesthesia; about 18% are palpable in the groin negating the need for laparoscopy.[21]

Diagnostic laparoscopy

- Examination of the deep inguinal ring: if closed and vas deferens and spermatic vessels are entering, a testicular remnant will be in the canal or scrotum. In these cases, an inguinal exploration may be performed.
- Determine patency of processus vaginalis: if patent, a testis is likely to be within the inguinal canal ('peeping' testis).

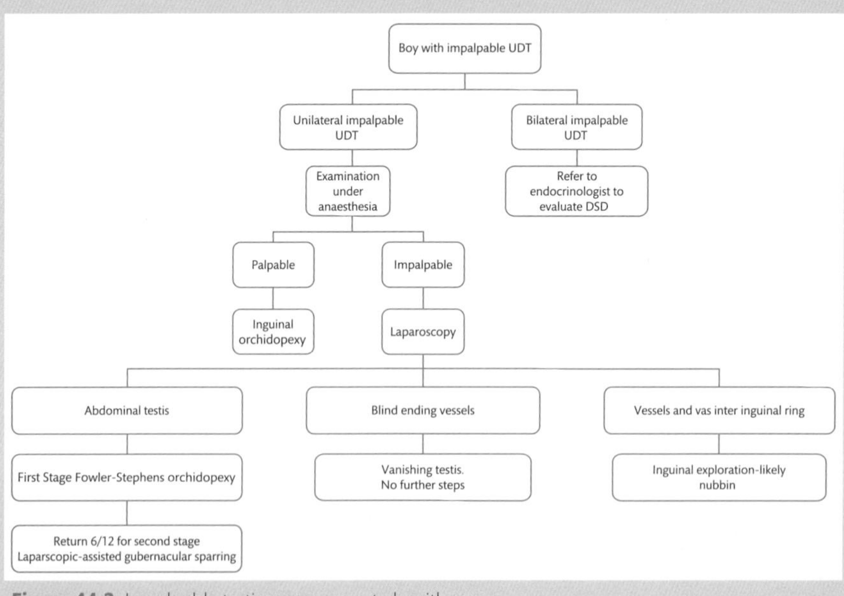

Figure 44.2 Impalpable testis management algorithm.

Intra-abdominal testis: plan definitive procedure

Fowler-Stephens orchiopexy: single/two-stage.

First stage: divide the testicular artery and vein to allow enhancement of the collateral circulation to the testes coming from the deferential vessels which supply the last 2 cm of the inner spermatic vessels.[22] The **second stage** must be done at least 6 months later. The testicle is mobilized on a flap of pelvis peritoneum overlying the vas, and brought down medial to the epigastric vessels and placed in a sub-dartos pouch in the base of the scrotum (Figure 44.3).

- A systematic review and meta-analysis conclude the success rate of laparoscopic two-stage Fowler-Stephens orchiopexy is 89%. Testicular atrophy occurs in 8%.[23]
- When one testis is impalpable, hypertrophy of the contralateral testis suggests that the impalpable gonad is absent, although this finding is not sufficiently reliable to avoid the need for laparoscopy.

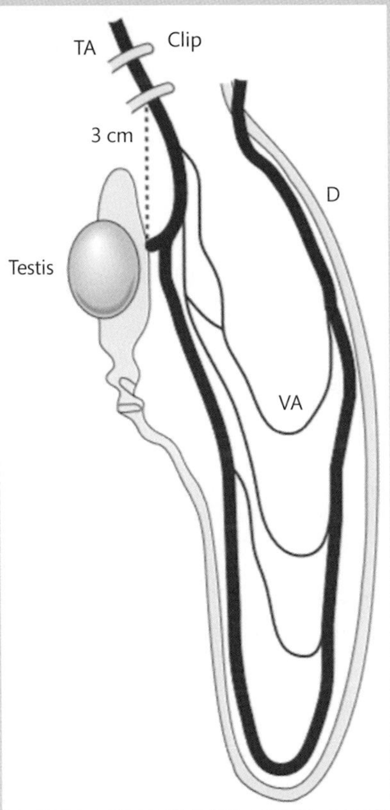

Figure 44.3 Fowler-Stephens procedure. TA, testicular artery; VA, vas artery.

Laparoscopic exploration findings

The right gonad is adjacent to the deep inguinal ring with vas and vessels (Figure 44.4), and on the left there is a streak gonad, a fallopian tube, and a rudimentary uterus. **Cystoscopy** demonstrates a normal-calibre urethra with an opening in the region of the verumontanum which leads to a large vagina-type structure with a cervix.

Diagnosis: mixed gonadal dysgenesis.

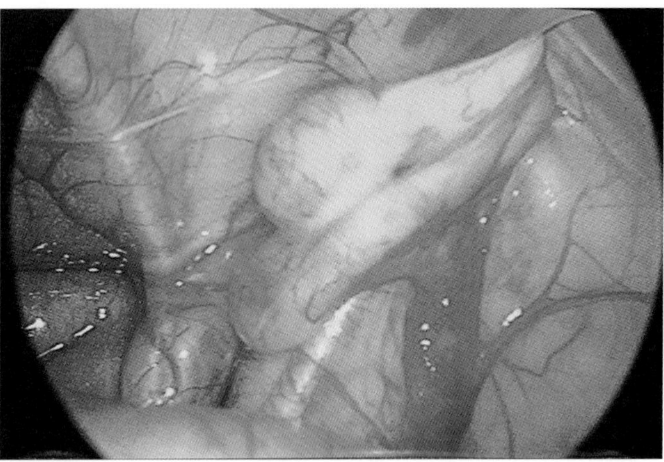

Figure 44.4 Right intra-abdominal testis close to the internal inguinal ring.

Learning point Mixed gonadal dysgenesis

- Mixed gonadal dysgenesis is a DSD caused by 45,X0/46,XY chromosomal mosaicism. It is the second-most common cause of ambiguous genitalia, after congenital adrenal hyperplasia. The phenotypic spectrum ranges from phenotypic females with Turner syndrome, to ambiguous genitalia, or even normal male genitalia.[24] Most of these patients have varying degrees of phallic development, urogenital sinus formation with labioscrotal fusion, and an undescended testis. In many of these patients, a rudimentary uterus, vagina, and fallopian tube are present.
- A streak gonad often is associated with ipsilateral müllerian derivatives. This occurs due to a failure in the local testosterone and müllerian inhibiting substance production which fails to cause müllerian duct regression.
- The external genital ambiguity arises due to inadequate *in utero* testosterone production.
- **Prognosis**: the normally descended or better testis can respond to gonadotropins and secrete testosterone in normal quantities at puberty, but this testis often lacks germinal structures, so these individuals are infertile.
- **Tumour risk**: gonadal tumours can occur in 15–35% of patients. Gonadoblastoma is the most frequent and has a low malignant potential. Dysgerminoma is the second most common. Germ cell tumours also occur in the testis and in the streak gonad, and therefore the latter should be removed. They have increased risk for Wilms' tumour and Denys–Drash syndrome (nephropathy, genital abnormalities, and Wilms' tumour).[25]
- **Management**: gender assignment, appropriate gonadectomy, and proper screening for Wilms' tumour.
  - Gender assignment should be done by an experienced DSD multidisciplinary team in discussion with the family. It is often based on the potential for normal function of the external genitalia and gonads. The likelihood of significant androgen imprinting is greater in association with a better-masculinized phenotype.
  - The streak gonad should be removed.
  - If the male gender is selected, which is often the case, the decision must be made between careful screening for tumours (physical examination and/or ultrasound scan) versus prophylactic gonadectomy and androgen replacement.

Studies of prenatal diagnosis of 45,X0/46,XY mosaicism have shown 90% have a normal male phenotype.[26] Some men may present later in life with gonadal dysfunction or testicular tumours.

Management

At laparoscopy, the streak gonad was removed. Histopathology reported a dysgenetic gonad without germ cells elements. The patient was brought to the DSD multidisciplinary team and in conjunction with the parents a male sex of rearing was chosen. The right testicle was brought to the scrotum by a Fowler–Stephens procedure. Hypospadias was repaired in two stages (Bracka technique). In respect to the müllerian remnants, they will be kept under observation. Often, they cause no problems but occasionally can cause post-micturition dribbling or urinary infection, particularly following the second stage of hypospadias surgery.

A final word from the expert

The management of UDT is no longer controversial and there is now sufficient evidence to support early orchiopexy before 12 months of age. The two-stage laparoscopic Fowler–Stephens orchiopexy has proven to be robust and reproducible for the intra-abdominal testis and should be considered in older children presenting with a high inguinal testis, where obtaining good length on the existing testicular vessels can be challenging. There should always be a high index of suspicion for DSD in children presenting with an impalpable testis and hypospadias. Urgent referral to an appropriate DSD team is strongly recommended.

References

1. Sijstermans K, Hack WW, Meijer RW, et al. The frequency of undescended testis from birth to adulthood: a review. *Int J Androl.* 2008;31(1):1–11.
2. Acerini CL, Miles HL, Dunger DB, Ong KK, Hughes IA. The descriptive epidemiology of congenital and acquired cryptorchidism in a UK infant cohort. *Arch Dis Child.* 2009;94(11):868–872.
3. Berkowitz GS, Lapinski RH, Dolgin SE, et al. Prevalence and natural history of cryptorchidism. *Pediatrics.* 1993;92(1):44–49.
4. Cendron M, Huff DS, Keating MA, et al. Anatomical, morphological and volumetric analysis: a review of 759 cases of testicular maldescent. *J Urol.* 1993;149(3):570–573.
5. Hadžiselimović F. Examinations and clinical findings in cryptorchid boys. In: *Cryptorchidism: Management and Implications*. Berlin: Springer Verlag; 1983:93–98.
6. Vickraman J, Hutson J, Li R, Thorup J. The undescended testis: clinical management and scientific advances. *Semin Pediatr Surg.* 2016;25(4):241–248.
7. Dunkel L, Taskinen S, Hovatta O, et al. Germ cell apoptosis after treatment of cryptorchidism with human chorionic gonadotropin is associated with impaired reproductive function in the adult. *J Clin Invest.* 1997;100(9):2341–2346.
8. Radmayr C, Dogan HS, Hoebeke P, et al. Management of undescended testes: European Association of Urology/European Society for Paediatric Urology guidelines. *J Pediatr Urol.* 2016;12(6):335–343.
9. Pyörälä S, Huttunen NP, Uhari M. A review and meta-analysis of hormonal treatment of cryptorchidism. *J Clin Endocrinol Metab.* 1995;80(9):2795–2799.
10. Cortes D, Thorup J, Visfeldt J. Hormonal treatment may harm the germ cells in 1 to 3-year-old boys with cryptorchidism. *J Urol.* 2000;163(4):1290–1292.
11. Feyles F, Peiretti V, Mussa A, et al. Improved sperm count and motility in young men surgically treated for cryptorchidism in the first year of life. *Eur J Pediatr Surg.* 2014;24(5):376–380.
12. Gracia J, Sánchez Zalabardo J, Sánchez García J, García C, Ferrández A. Clinical, physical, sperm and hormonal data in 251 adults operated on for cryptorchidism in childhood. *BJU Int.* 2000;85(9):1100–1103.
13. Walsh TJ, Dall'Era MA, Croughan MS, et al. Prepubertal orchiopexy for cryptorchidism may be associated with lower risk of testicular cancer. *J Urol.* 2007;178(4 Pt 1):1440–1446.

14. Pettersson A, Richiardi L, Nordenskjold A, et al. Age at surgery for undescended testis and risk of testicular cancer. *N Engl J Med.* 2007;356(18):1835–1841.
15. British Association of Paediatric Surgeons. Commissioning guide: paediatric orchidopexy for undescended testis. British Association of Paediatric Surgeons. 2018. https://www.baus.org.uk/_userfiles/pages/files/Publications/Commissioning%20guide%20for%20orchidopexy%20final%20v7.pdf
16. Chan E, Wayne C, Nasr A; FRCSC for Canadian Association of Pediatric Surgeon Evidence-Based Resource. Ideal timing of orchiopexy: a systematic review. *Pediatr Surg Int.* 2014;30(1):87–97.
17. Kollin C, Karpe B, Hesser U, et al. Surgical treatment of unilaterally undescended testes: testicular growth after randomization to orchiopexy at age 9 months or 3 years. *J Urol.* 2007;178(4 Pt 2):1589–1593.
18. Allin BSR, Dumann E, Fawkner-Corbett D, Kwok C, Skerritt C; Network Paediatric Surgery Trainees Research. Systematic review and meta-analysis comparing outcomes following orchidopexy for cryptorchidism before or after 1 year of age. *BJS Open.* 2018;2(1):1–12.
19. McCann ME, de Graaff JC, Dorris L, et al. Neurodevelopmental outcome at 5 years of age after general anaesthesia or awake-regional anaesthesia in infancy (GAS): an international, multicentre, randomised, controlled equivalence trial. *Lancet.* 2019;393(10172):664–677.
20. Sun LS, Li G, Miller TL. Association between a single general anaesthesia exposure before age 36 months and neurocognitive outcomes in later childhood. *JAMA.* 2016;315(21):2312–2320.
21. Cisek LJ, Peters CA, Atala A, Bauer SB, Diamond DA, Retik AB. Current findings in diagnostic laparoscopic evaluation of the nonpalpable testis. *J Urol.* 1998;160(3 Pt 2):1145–1150.
22. Fowler R, Stephens FD. The role of testicular vascular anatomy in the salvage of high undescended testes. *Aust N Z J Surg.* 1959;29:92–106.
23. Yu C, Long C, Wei Y, et al. Evaluation of Fowler-Stephens orchiopexy for high-level intra-abdominal cryptorchidism: a systematic review and meta-analysis. *Int J Surg.* 2018;60:74–87.
24. Johansen ML, Hagen CP, DeMeyts ER, et al. 45,X/46,XY mosaicism: phenotypic characteristics, growth, and reproductive function—a retrospective longitudinal study. *J Clin Endocrinol Metab.* 2012;97(8):E1540–E1549.
25. Drash A, Sherman F, Hartmann WH, et al. A syndrome of pseudohermaphroditism, Wilms' tumor, hypertension and degenerative disease. *J Pediatr.* 1970;76(4):585–593.
26. Hsu LY. Prenatal diagnosis of 45/46XY mosaicism: a review and update. *Prenat Diagn.* 1989;9(1):31–48.

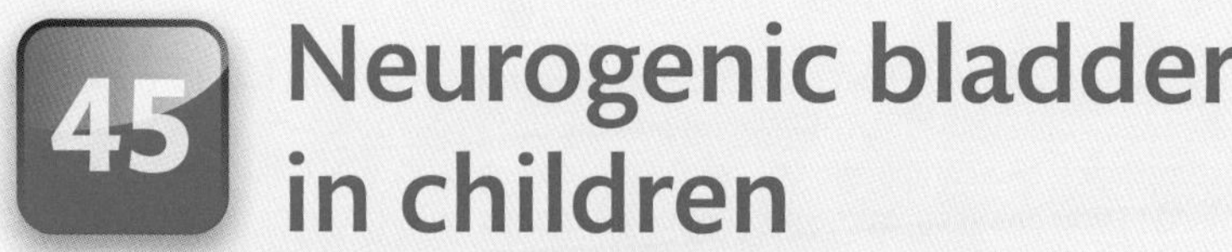

Neurogenic bladder in children

Sara Lobo and Kiarash Taghavi

Expert commentary Imran Mushtaq

Case history

A male baby was diagnosed at birth with a myelomeningocele (MMC) and underwent closure in the neonatal period. Shortly after birth he commenced clean intermittent catheterization (CIC) and antibiotic prophylaxis to minimize the risk of urinary tract infections (UTIs).

Learning point MMC and neurogenic bladder dysfunction

Neurogenic or neuropathic bladder is a heterogeneous condition that may result from a variety of underlying conditions affecting the central and peripheral nervous system. Although an initial decline in the incidence of myelodysplasia was seen following widespread folate supplementation, the incidence has stabilized over the past decade.[1] MMC remains the most common cause of congenital neurogenic bladder, and given the significant long-term morbidity and potential to impact neurological development, prenatal closure of the open MMC defect has been initiated in specialized centres. While fetal closure has been associated with an improvement in hydrocephalus and motor function[2], most recently the MOMS (Management of Myelomeningocele Study) has suggested fetal repair also improves aspects of bladder function.[3]

Neural tube defects result from the partial failure of tubularization of the neural plate. The extent and location of the non-tubularized neural plate determines the degree of paralysis.[4] Regardless of the neurological deficit, 25–30% of patients retain positive conus reflexes and among these a minority with low-level sacral or lumbosacral MMC have incomplete cord lesions with sensory and occasionally motor sparing.[5]

In patients with neurogenic bladder, normal voluntary control of voiding is often absent. Some artificial measures can be employed such as abdominal compression or straining, or CIC, whether via urethra or continent catheterizable channel.

As with acquired forms, congenital neuropathic bladder dysfunction is determined by the site of the cord lesion, albeit with the difference that an intermediate pattern of dysfunction is commonly observed (seen in 60% of patients with MMC). In suprasacral cord lesions, the conus medullaris is intact and so is the innervation of both the detrusor and external urethral sphincter (although isolated from higher centres). Conus reflexes are positive and detrusor contractility is enhanced. Often detrusor sphincter dyssynergia is present (dyscoordination between detrusor contraction and sphincter relaxation). In contrast, in sacral cord lesions, the conus medullaris is affected and consequently the innervation of the detrusor and external urethral sphincter. Conus reflexes are negative and detrusor contractility is absent. Some degree of external sphincter incompetence is always seen. Intermediate bladder dysfunction comprises a combination of detrusor hyperreflexia and some degree of sphincteric incompetence.[4,6]

Evidence base Secondary upper renal tract complications

Secondary upper renal tract complications including obstruction or reflux are prevalent in children with neurogenic bladder. Twenty per cent of children with a MMC are affected by the age of 2 years and 50% of boys are at risk of upper tract complications by puberty.[5] The most significant factors to predisposing to complications are febrile UTIs, vesicoureteric reflux (VUR), and bladder outflow obstruction (when associated with raised intravesical pressure due to detrusor overactivity (DOA), detrusor hypocompliance, or a combination of both). Renal damage and renal failure are among the most significant complications and treatment strategies are focused on maintaining renal function.[6]

Expert comment Natural history of neurogenic bladder malfunction and management challenges

For these patients, the therapeutic management is very challenging and many different protocols have been described. Our hospital protocol in the newborn period, following surgery for open spinal lesions, comprises regular and close monitoring by a paediatric urologist and neurosurgeon, administration of antibiotic prophylaxis with trimethoprim, and performing a bladder assessment by a urology specialist nurse at 6 weeks after surgical closure. If significant residual volumes are documented, commencing CIC may be advantageous (Figure 45.1). Therefore, not all patients benefit from starting early CIC.

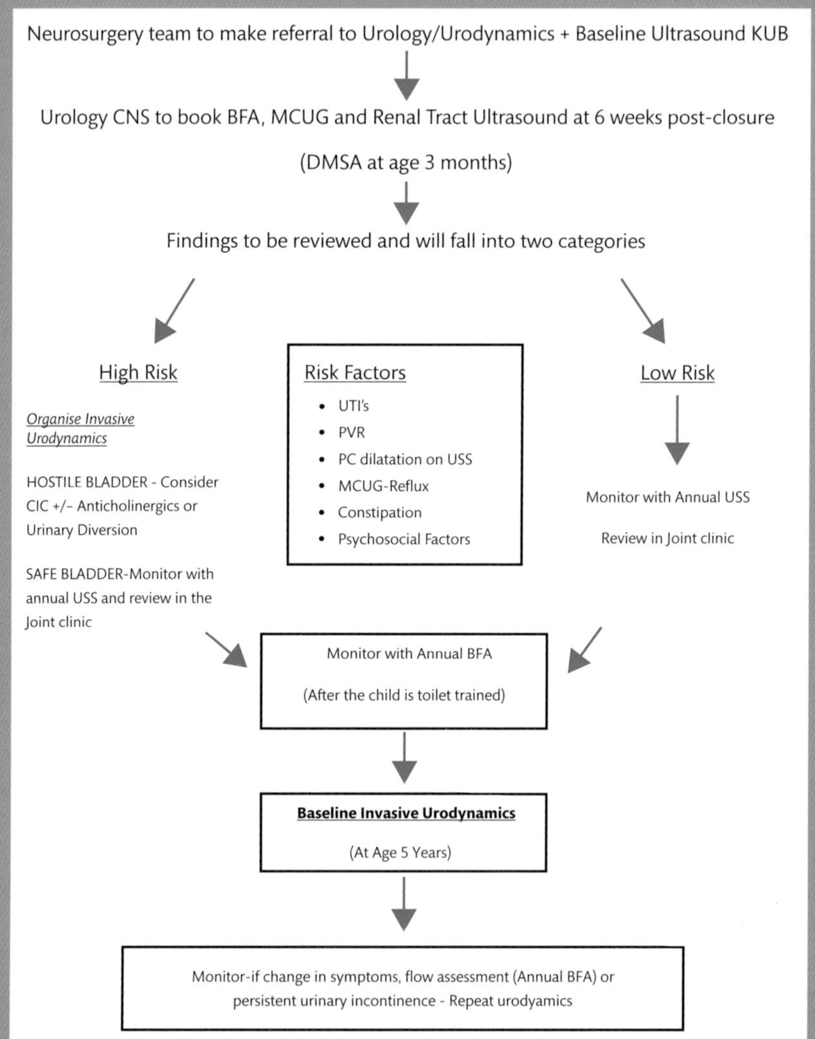

Figure 45.1 Protocol of MMC management in Great Ormond Street Hospital, London, UK. BFA, bladder functional assessment; DMSA, dimercaptosuccinic acid; MCUG, micturating cystourethrogram; PVR, post-void residual volume; USS, ultrasound scan.

Neurogenic bladder dysfunction can change with time, either in severity and/or the pattern of dysfunction. It is well known that the period of highest risk comprises the first 2 years, when around 30% of the 'safe' bladders become 'unsafe'. Puberty is also a period of risk when bladder dynamics can change.

Therefore, therapeutic management must be individualized and tailored to the patient's characteristics and abilities (age, sex, mobility—wheelchair vs no-wheelchair patients, spinal deformity, cognitive disorders, caregivers support, social circumstances).

Until 10 years of age the patient remained free of UTIs but reported frequent and significant urinary leakage between CIC which was performed 3-hourly during the daytime. He described intermittent dribbling exacerbated by coughing or standing. From the bowel management point of view, he was performing daily rectal washouts which were reasonably effective. At this point he was referred for specialist review and further investigation.

Clinical tip Managing urinary and faecal incontinence

During childhood before achieving puberty, many of these children can be managed with regular CIC performed via the urethra. In those cases where urinary leakage persists despite CIC and/or recurrent UTIs occur on antibiotic prophylaxis, different management is probably required.

The effects of spinal cord lesions on the rectum and anal sphincter are similar to those on the bladder and external urinary sphincter. Faecal incontinence may result from any combination of constipation, overflow incontinence, or sphincteric incompetence. The initial approach involves avoiding gross constipation by means of an appropriate diet or laxative medication, combined with retrograde enemas to ensure regular colonic emptying. If these measures are ineffective, an antegrade continence enema procedure could be considered.[3]

For a better understanding of the patient's clinical situation, new imaging studies were performed:

Ultrasound scan: the ultrasound scan showed a normal left kidney (measuring 9.5 cm on the long axis) with mild splitting of the calyces but no significant pelvicalyceal dilatation and a small scarred right kidney (measuring 7.7 cm, 5th centile for age) without pelvicalyceal dilatation. There was dilatation of both distal ureters, on the right measuring up to 10 mm in diameter and on the left up to 5 mm with a small-volume thick-walled bladder (Figure 45.2).

Micturating cystourethrogram (MCUG): bilateral VUR up to the level of non-distended collecting systems was documented in the MCUG performed. The bladder neck (BN) was incompetent with immediate leaking of contrast in the erect position. The bladder volume was approximately 200 mL when the patient stated he felt full (Figure 45.3).

Learning point Imaging investigation for neurogenic bladder

The options available to evaluate the neurogenic bladder and upper tracts include: ultrasound, fluoroscopy, nuclear scintigraphy studies, and urodynamic testing. There is current debate regarding the necessity and optimal timing of performing these studies, with the intention of minimizing radiation exposure and excessively invasive procedures in children.[2]

These studies provide a baseline for the structural and functional aspects of the upper and lower tract, can facilitate the diagnosis of hydronephrosis or VUR, and can help identify children at risk of upper urinary tract deterioration and impairment of renal function. In spina bifida patients undergoing MCUG assessment, the typical findings are of a spontaneously opened BN, elongation of the bladder, and abnormalities of the bladder wall (e.g. diverticula, trabeculae, 'fir tree' appearance).[6,7]

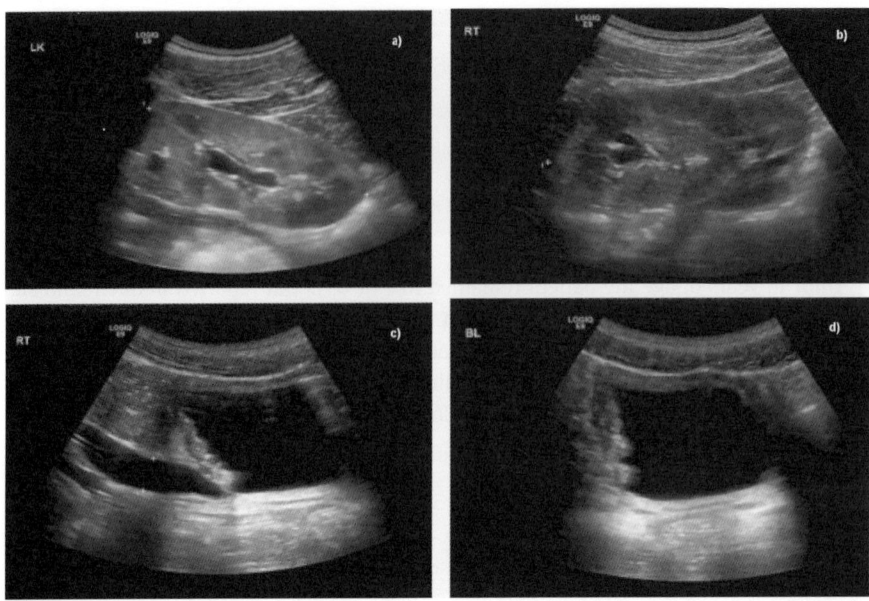

Figure 45.2 Ultrasound scan of the kidneys, ureters, and bladder. (a) Left kidney, transverse view; (b) right kidney, transverse view; (c) right distal ureter with bladder view; (d) bladder.

Dimercaptosuccinic acid (DMSA) scan: the renal DMSA scan reported the right kidney functionally smaller than the left, with multiple focal cortical defects (Figure 45.4). The differential function indicated the right kidney contributed 30% of overall renal function and the left kidney contributed 70%.

> **Learning point** DMSA
>
> DMSA scintigraphy is of value in patients with VUR or those experiencing febrile UTIs. Previous series of children with myelodysplasia have demonstrated rates of renal scarring or functional loss of 10–32% on DMSA nuclear medicine scans.[2]

Urodynamic study (UDS): the UDS showed a reduced functional capacity (200 mL, less than the expected bladder volume of 330 mL) with DOA (involuntary detrusor contractions during filling) (Figure 45.5).[7] There was a suggestion of hypocompliance

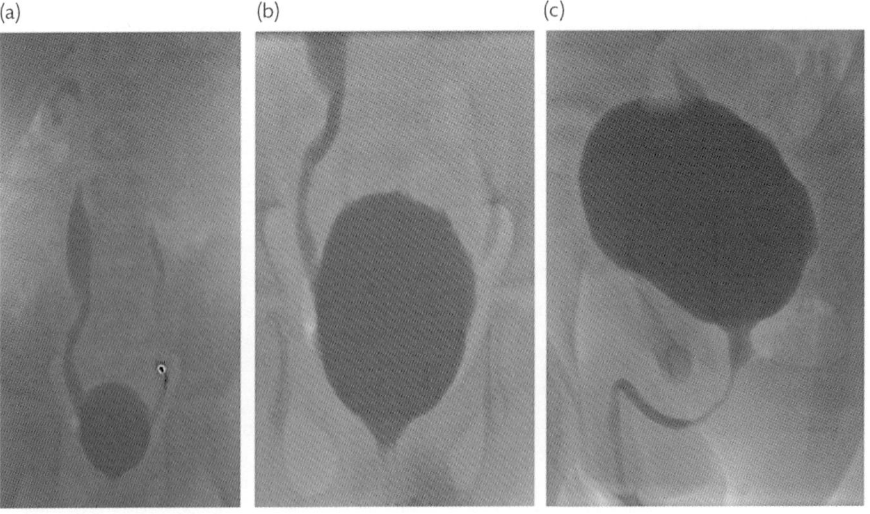

Figure 45.3 MCUG demonstrating VUR. (a, b) MCUG, anterior view; (c) MCUG, lateral view.

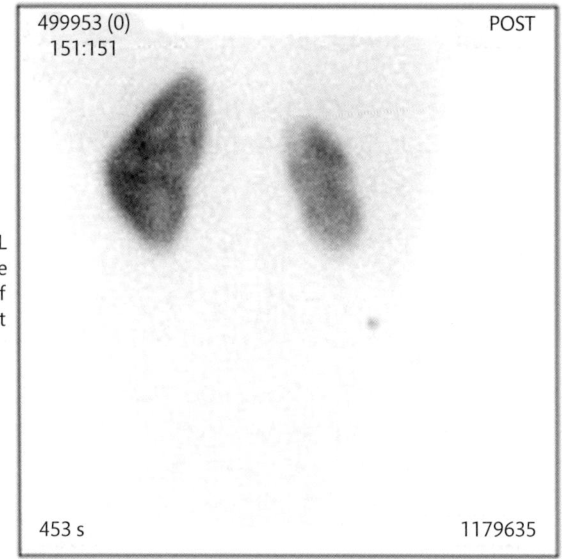

Figure 45.4 DMSA scan.

(pressure rise of 27 cmH_2O for 200 mL instilled, giving a compliance of 7.4) and leakage associated with DOA. Leak point pressure was low (< 30 cmH_2O around a urethral catheter) suggestive of outlet incompetence. The bladder emptied completely with CIC.

> **Learning point** UDS
>
> The bladder detrusor and sphincter are two components working in harmony to make a single functional unit. The bladder may be overactive with increased contractions, have reduced capacity or compliance, or be hypocontractile. The bladder outlet (urethra and sphincter) may be independently overactive causing functional obstruction.
>
> UDS abnormalities are present in >90% of patients with spinal dysraphism, demonstrating abnormal innervation of the bladder.[6] Invasive UDS provide the objective information necessary to understand bladder function including capacity, compliance, and outlet resistance, from which one can determine the need for augmentation with or without increasing outlet resistance to improve continence.[8]

> **Clinical tip** Bladder capacity
>
> Expected bladder capacity is calculated according to the following formula in children >12 months of age:
>
> Bladder capacity (mL) = 30 + (age (years) × 30)
>
> The expected bladder capacity for this child is 330 mL.
>
> In infants <12 months of age:
>
> Bladder capacity (mL) = weight (kg) × 7

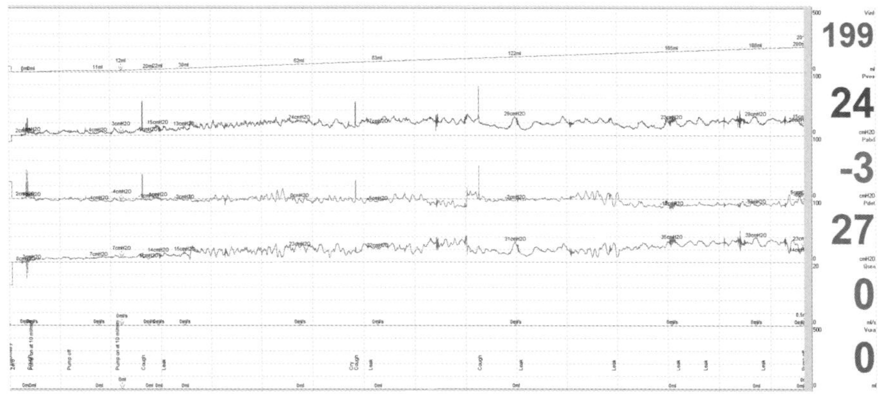

Figure 45.5 Video urodynamic study.

Expert comment Urodynamic investigations

Urodynamic investigations should be performed in a standardized manner to maintain quality of the data and to allow for comparison of results over time. The principal aim of any UDS assessment is to reproduce the symptoms while obtaining physiological measures in order to determine the pathophysiology underlying the symptoms. From the least to the most invasive assessment: (1) voiding diary, (2) uroflowmetry with post-void residual determination, (3) ward UDS, and (4) video UDS.[9]

Video UDS assessment provides a combination of anatomical and functional detail and for this reason is an essential assessment tool in complex cases where surgical intervention is being considered. Video UDS can be performed either via urethral catheter or suprapubic tubes, particularly in those cases requiring accurate evaluation of the BN.

Clinical tip Exclude UTI prior to UDS assessment

It is mandatory to exclude UTI prior to a urodynamic assessment. The presence of a UTI may invalidate the results as it results in abnormal bladder sensation (pain/discomfort during the investigation), DOA, and abnormal bladder compliance.

Reconstructive bladder surgery in the form of an ileocystoplasty and Mitrofanoff formation was performed. A BN sling was also completed to enhance bladder outlet resistance.

Evidence base Injection of botulinum toxin A

In neurogenic bladders refractory to antimuscarinic therapy, injection of botulinum toxin A into the detrusor can be an effective alternative treatment. Studies have demonstrated significant improvement in continence, bladder capacity, and compliance following multiple injections. This temporizing therapy effectively suppresses detrusor contractions for 6–9 months.[5] However, prospective controlled trials are scarce, and this type of treatment seems to be most effective in bladders with evidence of DOA. Hypocompliant bladders without obvious detrusor contractions are unlikely to respond to this treatment.

Children with treatment-resistant, reduced capacity bladder, DOA, and poor compliance will usually need surgical treatment in the form of bladder augmentation (ileocystoplasty).

Learning point Medical management with anticholinergics

Antimuscarinic therapy is the first-line medical therapy for neuropathic DOA. Initial treatment should consist of oral anticholinergic drugs in combination with CIC. Oxybutynin has proven to be cost-effective and efficacious and can be taken orally, intravesically, or transdermally.[5] Tolterodine, an alternative anticholinergic agent, is probably equally efficacious with a more favourable side effect profile.[4] Newer and more selective anticholinergics are being tested and undergoing clinical trials.

Learning point Bladder augmentation

When reconstructive bladder surgery is required, some issues must be considered. Although there is a poor evidence base supporting the use of one augmentation type over another (e.g. ileum vs colon), ileocystoplasty remains the preferred type. It is associated with less mucous production and less powerful intrinsic contractions compared to colonic. One must take into account several factors when incorporating bowel segments into the urinary tract. Reasonable renal function must be present as there will be urinary absorption from the bowel segment. It is imperative to preserve the terminal ileum in order to preserve vitamin B_{12} absorption and effective bile salt reuptake.[6]

The decision to proceed with augmentation surgery requires detailed preoperative education and preparation of the patient and family in order to ensure there will be good compliance with the catheterization regimen. Non-compliance or absence of regular CIC can lead to serious complications, such as UTIs, urolithiasis, and bladder rupture, and is associated with high morbidity and mortality.

The patient and family must be aware of several challenges that they will face in the postoperative period, such as mucous production that will require irrigation and the possible risk of malignancy which requires the need for a lifelong surveillance.[10,11]

Future directions Tissue engineering

Tissue-engineered grafts designed to replace the urinary bladder is the desired future of reconstructive urology. The ability to construct complex histological structures resembling the bladder wall with integrated autologous of epithelial, neural, and muscle components offer a superior treatment over currently available solution. However, there are still many clinically relevant issues that need to be resolved and optimized: sterilization of tissue-engineered constructs, biomaterial-associated thrombosis, risk factors for abscess formation/infection, graft adaptation for robotic or laparoscopic implantation, and impact of ageing on the regenerative capacity of human urinary tracts since all preclinical trials are planned on young, and large animal models.[12,13]

Learning point BN procedures

The treatment of sphincteric incompetence remains challenging. Marginal degrees of incompetence may benefit from alpha-adrenergic agonists, but patients with a paralytic pelvic floor will need BN surgery to achieve continence. The surgical options include periurethral/BN injections with a bulking agent (e.g. Macroplastique® or Deflux®), BN sling procedure, urethral lengthening procedures with creation of flap valve (Young–Dees–Leadbetter, Tanagho, and Mitchell techniques), artificial urinary sphincters, and BN closure.[4,5]

Variable success rates are reported regarding the sling procedure in males with neuropathic sphincter incompetence.[5,14] One of the techniques described is the opening of the pelvic diaphragm laterally, left and right, from the abdominal wall, to create a pathway that can be bluntly dissected for the sling around the BN. Autologous fascial tissue remains the material of choice in patients who may need a tighter sling and to avoid the use of synthetic material. The procedure comprises the exposure of rectus fascia and raising a strip of fascia that is then used to encircle the BN.

Expert comment Surgical option

For this particular case, the surgical option of a sling procedure for the BN was chosen. The reason for this was the advantage of representing a less radical procedure than closure of the BN, preserving the patency of the urethra and maintaining the option of urethral CIC.

A subject of debate is the amount of tension that is required on the sling. In the past, regulating tension by measuring urethral and leak point pressures was attempted but without encouraging results.[5] Currently, sling tension is determined by measuring the ability to pass a relatively large Foley catheter through the BN.

It has been shown that puberty does not adversely affect sling suspension of the BN, both in boys and girls, with no additional risk of obstruction based on prostate growth.[5] The erectile function of the penis is preserved after a sling suspension.

The postoperative period was uneventful and the patient was discharged from hospital after 7 days. Both the suprapubic and the Mitrofanoff catheters remained on continuous drainage, with daily irrigation of saline to ensure patency and to prevent mucus accumulation. After 3 weeks of drainage, the patient returned to hospital for clamping of the catheters, catheterization training, and removal of the suprapubic tube.

Future directions Minimally invasive surgery

The advent of minimally invasive surgery and robotics has provided novel and challenging approaches for reconstructive surgery of the lower urinary tract. Complex reconstructive procedures that have been performed including bladder augmentation with or without appendicovesicostomy and BN sling procedures. Gundeti et al. reported the first completely intracorporeal robotic laparoscopic augmentation ileocystoplasty and Mitrofanoff.[15]

Learning point Follow-up of children with neurogenic bladder

At birth, the majority of patients have normal upper tracts, but nearly 60% will develop upper tract deterioration due to increased detrusor filling pressures either with or without reflux. The leading cause of death later in life for these children is renal failure which underscores the importance of proactive management.[16] Table 45.1 illustrates a follow-up protocol from the Swedish National Programme.[17] A further significant area for development is the transition of care from paediatrician to adult services.[18]

Table 45.1 Swedish national protocol for follow-up of children with neurogenic bladder disorders

Age	Cystometry	MCUG	Ultrasound of kidneys	Kidney function	DMSA, renography	Glomerular filtration rate
Newborn	X	X	X	S creatinine		
1 month				U analysis		
3–6 months	X			S creatinine U analysis	DMSA scintigraphy	
12–18 months	X		X	S creatinine U analysis Cystatin C U osmolarity		X
>18 months, yearly	X		X	S creatinine analysis Cystatin C U osmolarity Blood pressure	Renography every third year	X[1]

S, serum; U, urine. Urine osmolarity by 1-desamino-8-d-arginine vasopressin (DDAVP) test; X[1], every third year when renography.
Adapted from Wide et al.[17]

A final word from the expert

There is no doubt that regular follow-up and timely intervention can prevent or at least delay the onset of upper tract deterioration in children with MMC. Most paediatric centres have established multidisciplinary teams to deliver this standard of care, with locally agreed follow-up protocols. Many patients will still require reconstructive surgery and lifelong follow-up. Developing a robust transitional care model remains a significant hurdle for many centres specializing in the care of spina bifida.

References

1. Lloyd JC, Wiener JS, Gargollo PC, Inman BA, Routh JC. Contemporary epidemiological trends in complex genitourinary anomalies. *J Urol.* 2013;190(4):1590–1595.
2. Sturm R, Cheng E. The management of pediatric neurogenic bladder. *Curr Bladder Dysfunct Rep.* 2016;11:225–233.
3. Clayton DB, Thomas JC, Brock III JW. Fetal repair of myelomeningocele: current status and urologic implications, *J Ped Urol.* 2020 Feb 1;16(1):3–9.
4. Thomas D, Duffy P, Rickwood A. *Essentials of Paediatric Urology*. 2nd ed. London: Informa Healthcare; 2008.
5. Jong T, Chrzan R, Klijn A. Treatment of the neurogenic bladder in spina bifida. *Pediatric Nephrol.* 2008;23(6):889–896.
6. Esposito C, Guys JM, Gough D, Savanelli A, eds. *Pediatric Neurogenic Bladder Dysfunction: Diagnosis, Treatment, Long-Term Follow-Up*. Heidelberg: Springer; 2006.
7. Snodgrass WT, Gargollo PC. Urologic care of the neurogenic bladder in children. *Urol Clin N Am.* 2010;37(2):207–214.
8. Bauer SB, Nijman RJ, Drzewiecki BA, Sillen U, Hoebeke P. International Children's Continence Society standardization report on urodynamic studies of the lower urinary tract in children. *Neurourol Urodyn.* 2015;34(7):640–647.

9. Chapple C, MacDiarmid S, Patel A, et al. *Urodynamics Made Easy*. 3rd ed. New York: Churchill Livingstone Elsevier; 2009.
10. Smith J Jr, Howards SS, Preminger GM. *Hinman's Atlas of Urology Surgery*. 3rd ed. Philadelphia, PA: Elsevier Saunders; 2012.
11. Husmann D. Long-term complications following bladder augmentations in patients with spina bifida: bladder calculi, perforation of the augmented bladder and upper tract deterioration. *Transl Androl Urol.* 2016;5(1):3–11.
12. Adamowicz J, Pokrywczynska M, Van Breda SV, et al. Concise review: tissue-engineering of urinary bladder; we still have a long way to go? *Stem Cell Transl Med.* 2017;6(11):2033–2043.
13. González R, Ludwikowski B. Progress in pediatric urology in the early 21st century. *Front Pediatr.* 2019;7:349.
14. Dean G, Kunkle D, et al. Outpatient perineal sling in adolescent boys with neurogenic incontinence. *J Urol.* 2009;182(4):1792–1796.
15. Barashi NS, Rodriguez MV, Packiam VT, Gundeti, MS. Bladder reconstruction with bowel: robot-assisted laparoscopic ileocystoplasty with Mitrofanoff apendicovesicostomy in pediatric patients. *J Endourol.* 2018;32(Suppl 1):119–126.
16. Woodhouse CR. Myelomeningocele: neglected aspects. *Pediatric Nephrol.* 2008;23(8):1223–1231.
17. Wide P, Mattsson G, Mattsson S. Renal preservation in children with neurogenic bladder–sphincter dysfunction followed in a national program. *J Ped Urol.* 2012;8(2):187–193.
18. Hettel D, Tran C, Szymanski K, Misseri R, Wood H. Lost in transition: patient-identified barriers to adult urological spina bifida care. *J Ped Urol.* 2018;14(6):535. e1–535.e4.

Haemorrhagic eschar of the glans: a case study in the myriad manifestations of urethral pathology

Emily Decker and Kevin Cao

Expert commentary Peter Cuckow

Case history

A healthy 8-year-old male presented with dysuria and ballooning of a non-retractile foreskin. He was diagnosed with balanitis xerotica obliterans (BXO) and received a circumcision followed by a course of 0.1% Betnovate® ointment.

Learning point Circumcision and BXO

Circumcision is one of the oldest and continuously practised surgical procedures in the world.[1] Phimosis is the inability to retract the foreskin. The separation of prepuce from glans is completed in 90% of boys by the age of 3 years[2] and 99% of boys have a retractile foreskin by age 16 years (see 'Clinical tip' box on phimosis).[3,4] The concern of whether this phimosis requires treatment results in high numbers of unnecessary referrals.[5] Pathological phimosis, where there is palpable thickening and preputial scarring preventing both retraction and protraction of the foreskin, is one of a few absolute medical indications for circumcision.[1] There are no objective data to suggest that physiological phimosis proceeds more readily to a pathological phimosis.

Expert comment Physiological phimosis

While reassurance and watchful waiting is adequate for the vast majority of boys with physiological phimosis, the question for physicians is when intervention may be appropriate. While it is true that a very small number of boys will become retractile late in adolescence or young adulthood, a good time point to consider intervention is during puberty, where a phimotic prepuce may impact psychosocial development. Sensitive questioning in this regard should be employed to investigate these factors at this age.

Clinical tip Phimosis

The typical appearance of a healthy physiologically phimotic prepuce is shown in Figure 46.1. Note the 'puckered' tip appearance on gentle retraction. It is not uncommon for there to be redness at the tip and ballooning of trapped urine during voiding, which generally improves with development.

Expert comment Non-retractile foreskin

Nearly all boys will become retractile at some point in their childhood or adolescence. While the majority are retractile in the first few years, an additional number will become so each successive year of age. Comparisons between children by parents or by children themselves are often the originating source of anxiety about phimosis. For the majority, reassurance is the best solution.

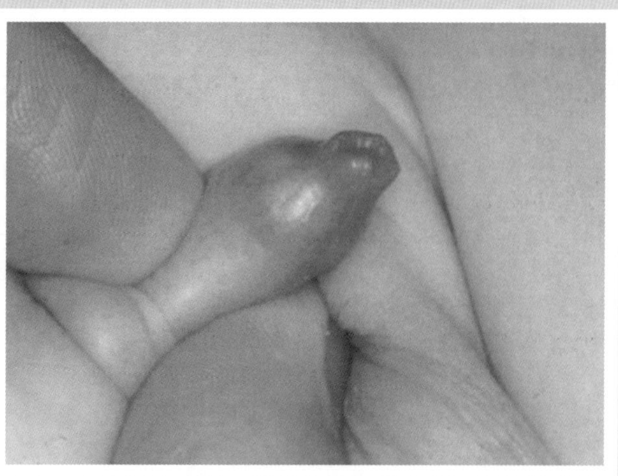

Figure 46.1 Appearance of a physiological phimosis.

Expert comment Indications for circumcision

The two 'absolute' medical indications for circumcision are BXO and recurrent balanoposthitis. Clinicians should become familiar with the appearance of the former as it is under-recognized. Balanoposthitis—oedema and erythema of the prepuce and glans—is likely overdiagnosed, being confused for the frequent and mild tip redness seen in many phimotic boys.

Learning point BXO

BXO, sometimes referred to as lichen sclerosis, is the hyperkeratinization of the epidermis, with T-cell lymphocytic infiltration and loss of skin elasticity (Figures 46.2 and 46.3).[6,7] It presents with tight white scarring of the foreskin, with white plaques visible on the prepuce and glans underneath. In severe cases, the urethral meatus can be involved, as can the distal urethra. The most common symptoms reported are phimosis, ballooning of the foreskin during micturition, dysuria, or recurrent balanitis.[7] BXO is rare in children <5 years old, with incidence being reported as 5–6%.[5] Typical age of presentation is 9 years old.[8] Many theories have been hypothesized for underlying aetiology, none have proven correct. Symptoms such as preputial ballooning and dysuria can both be found in physiological phimosis; the key for clinicians is to recognize from examination the differences between the two conditions. In the former, symptoms generally improve as phimosis recedes, while in BXO, no improvement can generally be expected.

Histology of BXO reveals hyperkeratosis, lamina propria thickening, and diffuse fibrosis with lymphocytic infiltrate (Figure 46.2). Traditionally, diagnosis is clinical and confirmed on histology. Circumcision has been the mainstay of treatment and is the best course to prevent recurrence. Longer-term complications following circumcision for BXO include recurrence, meatal stenosis, and urethral strictures.

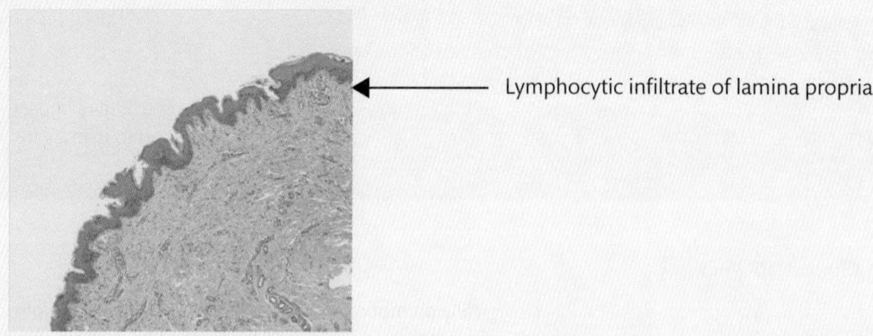

Figure 46.2 Histology of BXO.

Clinical tip BXO

Note the two classic features of the prepuce affected by BXO. The white ring of 'scarred' tissue reflecting dermatological changes and the 'blunted' appearance of the prepuce when gently retracted (e.g. no puckering is seen). The prepuce is unable to be retracted or protracted (Figure 46.3).

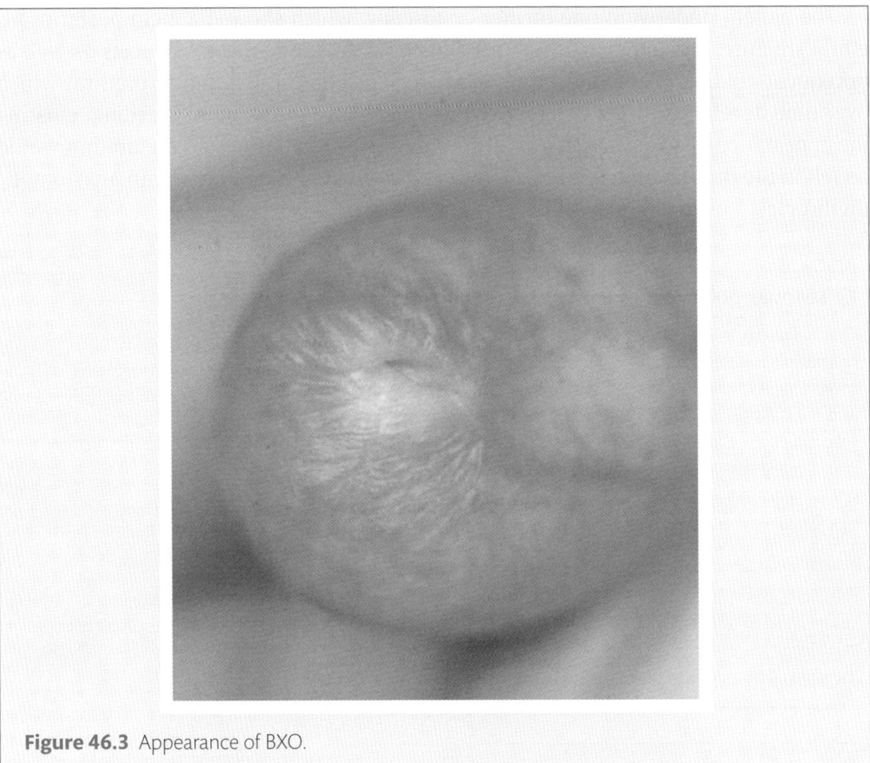

Figure 46.3 Appearance of BXO.

In this patient, the symptom of dysuria persisted. Intermittently, he noted an eschar forming at the end of the penis, which would dislodge when voiding. As time progressed, the eschar would need to be peeled off before he could urinate. He underwent an examination under anaesthesia, cystoscopy, meatoplasty, and biopsy 15 months post circumcision. Biopsy showed non-specific inflammation but no BXO. Postoperatively, he was instructed to apply 0.1% Betnovate® to the meatus and distal urethra using an 8-French (Fr) meatal dilator, which continued for 5 months.

The patient subsequently underwent four further cystoscopies and a urethral meatus biopsy over 4 years as he developed terminal haematuria without resolution of his previous symptoms. Histology repeatedly showed chronic inflammation, without malignancy, infection, or BXO. At one cystoscopic examination at age 14, a bulbar urethral stricture was noted, which was dilated to accommodate a 14 Fr cystoscope from 9.5 Fr. He was also reviewed by a paediatric dermatologist who prescribed fusidic acid ointment (Fucidin®) followed by Dermovate® with no change in symptoms.

At age 15, the patient was referred for a second opinion. He described a pain made worse when voiding frequently and he consequently developed a habitual tendency to withhold urine. This behaviour had in fact predated the initial BXO diagnosis.

Expert comment Monitoring for post-circumcision complications

It has been debated how best to monitor for post-circumcision complications in patients with BXO. Abnormal urinary stream can be common in the early recovery period in addition to the reality that many of these patients have contended with an abnormal stream for many years prior to surgery. A more sensitive marker is the need for straining when voiding which should prompt urgent assessment.

The patient underwent one further cystoscopy, which showed a 2 cm posterior urethral stricture. It is likely that high-pressure voiding due to meatal stenosis as well as infrequent voiding resulted in an inflammatory reaction in the bulbar urethra, which over time developed into a stricture. This would cause intermittent bleeding, creating the appearance of an eschar as it coalesced at the meatus. Pain from the urethra would be felt in the distal penile urethra. He will return in the near future for an anastomotic urethroplasty using an inlay of buccal mucosa.

Learning point Meatal stenosis

Narrowing of the urethral meatus, meatal stenosis, is a cited long-term complication of both circumcision and BXO. The risk following circumcision overall is low (0.7%) but much greater in patients with BXO, up to 20%.[9] Typical symptoms include initiation dysuria and high-velocity, narrowed, upwards diverging urinary stream.[10] Treatment options include meatal dilatation or meatoplasty.[11]

Learning point Causes and diagnosis of urethral strictures

Urethral strictures in children are rare and usually associated with trauma, specifically pelvic fracture or straddle injuries.[12] In children, the bladder and prostate sit higher than in adults and therefore are more prone to disruption during trauma. Other causes include infection, post-hypospadias repair, and meatal stenosis. Urethral strictures are rarely thought to be purely congenital in origin. One series records a bimodal pattern of presentation, with those presenting under the age of 1 year typically being investigated for bilateral antenatal hydronephrosis.[13]

By contrast, in adults, the most common causes of strictures are iatrogenic, such as prolonged catheterization during acute illness or idiopathic.[14] This epidemiological picture has changed from 30 years ago, where a common cause included urethritis from sexually transmitted infection.[14]

Diagnosis of stricture can be made on retrograde urethrography; however, incomplete filling or limited studies due to discomfort can give spurious results.[12] Direct visualization through cystourethroscopy can also underestimate the degree of stenosis due to hydrostatic pressure stenting the urethral walls at the time of procedure.

Learning point Management of urethral strictures

Management of strictures can be complex, with one series having 30% of patients with failed interventions, and a further 11% requiring re-do repair following urethroplasty.[15]

Surgical options for management include direct visual internal urethrotomy, excision and primary anastomosis, or urethroplasty. Posterior urethral strictures, usually in the context of trauma, are better suited to urethroplasty, rather than the minimally invasive urethrotomy, following a period of suprapubic urinary diversion.[12]

For anterior urethral strictures in adults, direct visual internal urethrotomy (DVIU) is a treatment option, especially for short (<2 cm) strictures.[16] With a success rate of 55%, the authors of that series advocate one single attempt at DVIU; there is concern that this technique may exacerbate the underlying scar formation thereby lengthening strictures.[17] Similar outcomes with DVIU are noted in children.[13]

By comparison, excision and primary anastomosis has a success rate up to 98%.[16] The exception lies in the subgroup of congenital strictures; these appear to respond well to DVIU without stricture recurrence.[13]

Expert comment Urethra passage

It is important for clinicians not to compartmentalize the urethra into unconnected distal and proximal components. The nature of the urethra as a passage, is to transport both physiological and pathological fluids, discharging them distally but also translating pressure from obstructions proximally.

Conclusion

Concerns of the foreskin can cause much work for primary and secondary care alike; the vast majority of concerns relate to physiological phimosis and reassurance is usually sufficient. Absolute indications for circumcision include pathological phimosis, of which BXO is an uncommon cause in paediatrics. Strictures are rare in children and can be complex to resolve but it is important to recognize the linear nature of the urethra: what one sees at its distal end can be an indicator of proximal disease.

A final word from the expert

The penis and foreskin generate a great deal of anxiety for patients and doubly so for their parents. This is reflected in the number of referrals for foreskin-related concerns to a paediatric urology clinic, the vast majority of which will be diagnosed with physiological phimosis and reassured. The success of said reassurance is to some extent dependent on expectations of circumcision. We would generally advocate two things. The first is to steer families away from comparing male siblings as the prepuce develops differently in each child and second, for clinicians to avoid where possible medicalizing cases of physiological phimosis. This can be harder said than done with the temptation to reschedule 6-monthly or yearly appointments to monitor the situation. This can be a rather frustrating experience for families and clinicians as the prepuce often shows little to no change between appointments, nudging clinicians towards advocating for intervention. If possible, it may be better to set out expectations, describe the symptoms of balanoposthitis, and warn parents of new-onset ballooning or dysuria where previously not present as an indicator for BXO. In the absence of these, it may be better to lengthen appointment intervals or aim to reschedule them nearer to puberty.

When concerning symptoms are present, such as in the case of this boy, we would encourage clinicians to think of the urethra as a single unit, with signs of disease generally transmitted along its length in either direction.

References

1. Yardley IE, Cosgrove C, Lambert AW. Paediatric preputial pathology: are we circumcising enough? *Ann R Coll Surg Engl.* 2007;89(1):62–65.
2. Gairdner D. The fate of the foreskin: a study of circumcision. *BMJ.* 1949:2(4642):1433–1437.
3. Liu J, Yang J, Chen Y, et al. Is steroids therapy effective in treating phimosis? A meta-analysis. *Int Urol Nephrol.* 2016:48(3):335–342.
4. Oster J. Further fate of the foreskin. Incidence of preputial adhesions, phimosis, and smegma among Danish schoolboys. *Arch Dis Child.* 1968;43(228):200–203.
5. Boksh K, Patwardha N. Balanitis xerotica obliterans: has its diagnostic accuracy improved with time? *JRSM Open.* 2017;8(6):2054270417692731.
6. Jayakumar S, Antao B, Bevington O, et al. Balanitis xerotica obliterans in children and its incidence under the age of 5 years. *J Paediatr Urol.* 2012;8(3):272–275.
7. Celis S, Reed F, Murphy F, et al. Balanitis xerotica obliterans in children and adolescents: a literature review and clinical series. *J Paediatr Urol.* 2014;10(1):34–39.
8. Rickwood AMK, Hemalatha V, Batcup G, et al. Phimosis in boys. *Br J Urol.* 1980;52(2):147–150.
9. Morris BJ, Krieger JN. Does circumcision increase meatal stenosis risk? A systematic review and meta-analysis. *Urology.* 2017;110:16–26.
10. Persad R, Sharma S, McTavish J, et al. Clinical presentation and pathophysiology of meatal stenosis following circumcision. *Br J Urol.* 1995;75(1):91–93.
11. Das S, Siva H, Tunuguntla GR. Balanitis xerotica obliterans—a review. *World J Urol.* 2000;18(6):382–387.
12. Priyadarshi R, Mohd A, Manmeet S, et al. Post-traumatic urethral strictures in children: what have we learned over the years? *J Paediatr Urol.* 2012;8(3):234–239.
13. Banks FC, Griffin SJ, Steinbrecher HA, et al. Aetiology and treatment of symptomatic idiopathic urethral strictures in children. *J Pediatr Urol.* 2009;5(3):215–218.
14. Lumen N, Hoebeke P, Willemsen P, et al. Etiology of urethral stricture disease in the 21st century. *J Urol.* 2009;182(3):983–987.

15. Helmy TE, Sarhan O, Hafez AT, et al. Perineal anastomotic urethroplasty in a pediatric cohort with posterior urethral strictures: critical analysis of outcomes in a contemporary series. *Urology.* 2014;83(5):1145–1148.
16. Hillary CJ, Osman NI, Chapple CR. Current trends in urethral stricture management. *Asian J Urol.* 2014;1(1):46–54.
17. Fenton AS, Morey AF, Aviles R, et al. Anterior urethral strictures: etiology and characteristics. *Urology.* 2005;65(6):1056–1058.

CASE

47 Vesicoureteral reflux in children

María S. Figueroa-Díaz and Alexander Cho

Expert commentary Imran Mushtaq

Case history

A male neonate was referred with an antenatal diagnosis at 31 weeks' gestation of bilateral hydronephrosis (right anterior–posterior diameter (APD) 21 mm and left APD 17 mm) with a distended bladder.

He was born at term via vaginal delivery with normal APGAR (Appearance, Pulse, Grimace, Activity, and Respiration) scores. His initial serum creatinine level was elevated at 102 µmol/L. A urethral catheter was inserted soon after birth to aid bladder drainage.

The ultrasound scan (USS) on day 4 confirmed the right kidney had a stretched cortex with bright echogenicity. The right APD was 12 mm with a tortuous ureter measuring 19 mm proximally and 17 mm distally. The left renal APD was 11 mm and the ureter measured 9 mm. The bladder wall was noted to be thick-walled (Figure 47.1). The spine USS was normal. A micturating cystourethrogram (MCUG) demonstrated a small-volume trabeculated bladder, vesicoureteric reflux (VUR) into a grossly distended right kidney (grade V), but no left-sided reflux. The urethra was noted to be normal (Figure 47.2).

Learning point Antenatal hydronephrosis

Antenatal hydronephrosis (ANH) is most commonly graded according to the APD of the renal pelvis[1]:

- Mild: 4 to <7 mm (second trimester); 7 to <9 mm (third trimester).
- Moderate: 7 to ≤10 mm (second trimester); 9 to ≤15 mm (third trimester).
- Severe: >10 mm (second trimester); >15 mm (third trimester).

There is uniform agreement that an APD >15 mm in the third trimester represents severe hydronephrosis.

Clinical tip Initial management of neonatal bilateral hydronephrosis

In a male neonate with antenatally diagnosed bilateral hydronephrosis and distended bladder, the condition of posterior urethral valves (PUV) needs to be excluded. Initial management, however, is the insertion of a urethral catheter and appropriate fluid management.

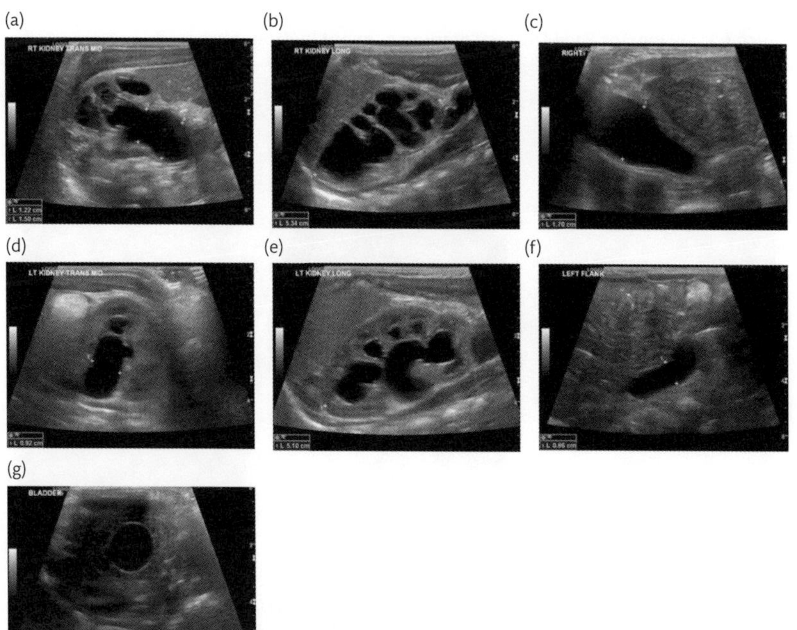

Figure 47.1 USS of the kidneys, ureters, and bladder. (a) Right kidney, transverse; (b) right kidney, longitudinal; (c) right distal ureter; (d) left kidney, transverse; (e) left kidney, longitudinal; (f) left distal ureter; (g) thick-walled bladder.

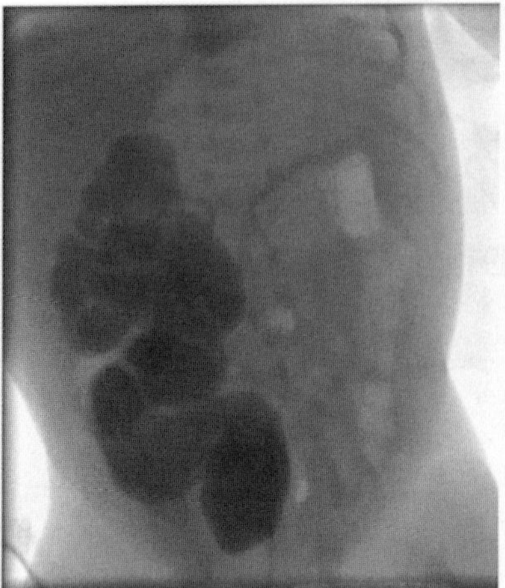

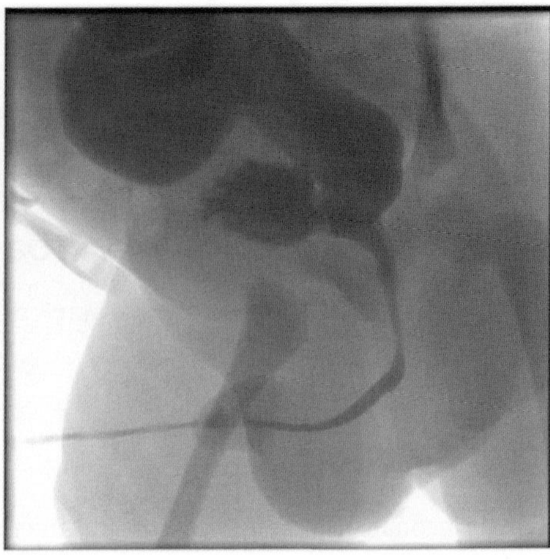

Figure 47.2 MCUG showing right-sided grade V VUR but a normal urethra.

Clinical tip Postnatal imaging

The first postnatal imaging study recommended is an USS. This should be performed after 48 hours of life to compensate for the initial neonatal dehydration and postnatal oliguria. An early USS may underestimate the severity of the hydronephrosis.

The distension of the urinary tract in the postnatal USS can be affected by the degree of bladder fullness and hydration. It is recommended that in the presence of urinary tract dilation, the patient should be rescanned after bladder emptying.

The Society for Fetal Urology grading system is commonly used for infant hydronephrosis and is based on the appearance of the renal pelvis, calyces, and renal parenchyma rather than the size of the renal pelvis (Table 47.1).

Table 47.1 Society for Fetal Urology grading of infant hydronephrosis

	Pattern of renal sinus. Splitting	Ultrasound variants
SFU grade 0	No splitting	
SFU grade 1	Urine in pelvis barely splits sinus	
SFU grade 2	Urine fills pelvis with/without major calyces dilated.	

Table 47.1 Continued

	Pattern of renal sinus. Splitting	Ultrasound variants	
SFU grade 3	SFU grade 2 and minor calyces dilated and parenchyma preserved.	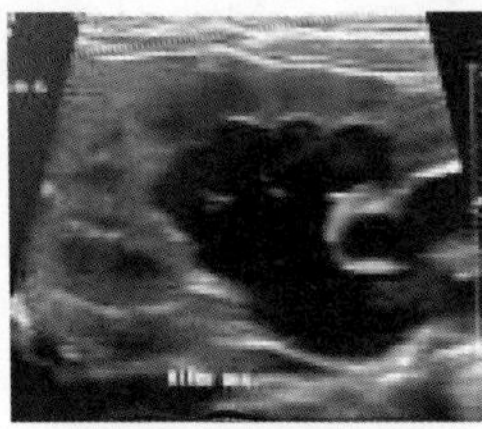	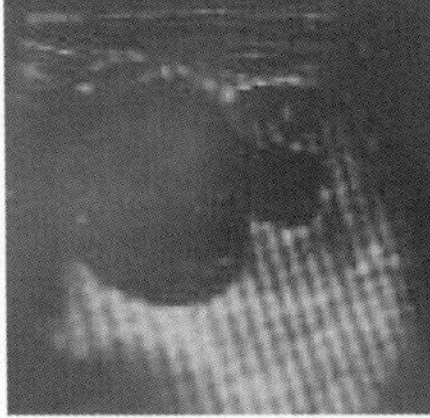
SFU grade 4	SFU grade 3 and parenchyma thin.	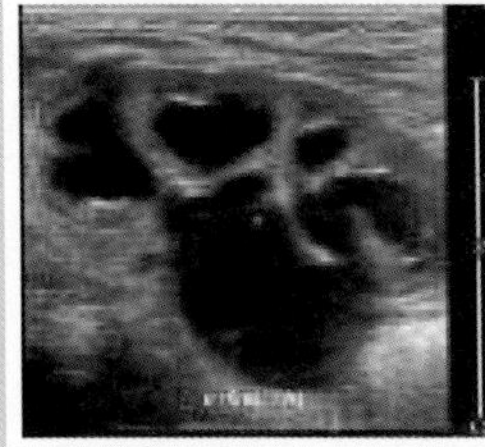	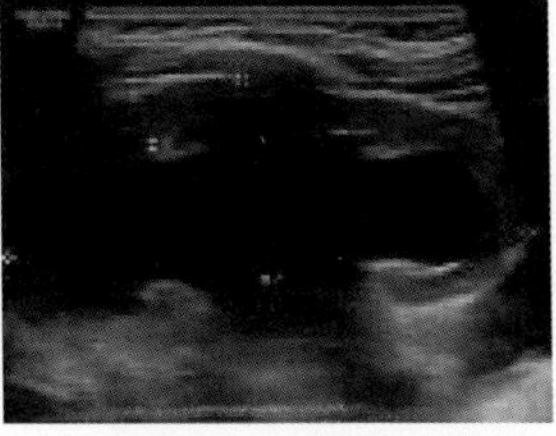

Adapted from Nguyen et al. *J Pediatr Urol.* (2014).[1]

Learning point Differential diagnosis

There are multiples aetiologies for ANH with the majority (50–70%) due to transient or physiological hydronephrosis with no clinical significance.[1] In those fetuses with mild ANH, 88.1% will have transient hydronephrosis. The incidence of any significant postnatal pathology is 11.9% for mild, 45.1% for moderate, and 88.3% for severe ANH.[2] The most frequent diagnoses are[1]:

- Transient/physiological: incidence 50–70%
- Ureteropelvic junction obstruction: 10–30%
- VUR: 10–40%
- Ureterovesical junction obstruction/megaureter: 5–15%
- Multicystic dysplastic kidney disease: 2–5%
- Posterior urethral valves: 1–5%
- Ureterocoele, ectopic ureter, duplex system, urethral atresia, Prune belly Syndrome, polycystic kidney diseases: Uncommon (<1%).

Learning point VUR

For an asymptomatic infant monitored for ANH, the estimated prevalence of VUR ranges from 10–15% if postnatally there is absent or mild hydronephrosis,[3] up to 40% if there are postnatal anomalies detected on USS including hydronephrosis, renal cysts, or renal agenesis.[4] A normal postnatal USS, therefore, does not exclude VUR. The grading of VUR is shown in Figure 47.3.

MCUG is the gold standard in the diagnosis of VUR. Reflux can occur during filling or voiding. Reflux during filling has been considered more severe because it occurs at low bladder pressures and this may be a poor prognostic sign for VUR resolution. There is a significant risk of urinary tract infections (UTIs) associated with the MCUG test and peri-investigation antibiotics are recommended.[5] Radionuclide studies for detection of reflux offer a lower radiation exposure than MCUG but the anatomical details demonstrated are inferior.[6]

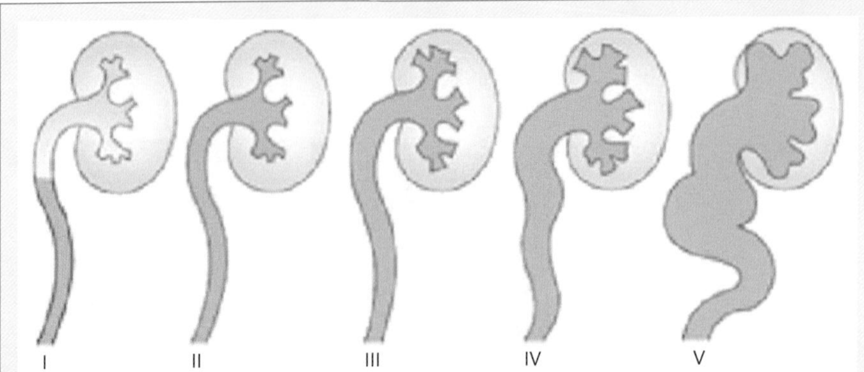

Figure 47.3 Classification of VUR based on the MCUG. (I) Reflux into a non-dilated ureter; (II) into the renal pelvis and calyces without dilatation; (III) mild to moderate dilatation of the ureter, renal pelvis, and calyces with minimal blunting of all the fornices; (IV) moderate ureteral tortuosity and dilatation of the pelvis and calyces; (V) gross dilatation of the ureter, renal pelvis, and calyces; loss of papillary impressions and ureteral tortuosity.
Adapted from Lebowitz RL et al. *Pediatr Radiol.* (1985).[7]

Incomplete bladder emptying was detected during a bladder function assessment that combined nappy alarms with residual bladder volumes detected by USS. Clean intermittent catheterization was initiated with oral trimethoprim prophylaxis. The patient's serum creatinine improved to normal levels corrected for age and weight.

Expert comment Primary versus secondary VUR

It is important to differentiate between the two types of VUR as their management differs significantly. This is demonstrated in this case study where the bladder seemed abnormal.

Primary VUR is due to a congenital abnormality of the antireflux mechanism at the vesicoureteric junction (VUJ) where the ratio between intramural ureter and its diameter is <5:1.[8] In **secondary VUR**, the VUJ is normal, but there is an abnormality of the bladder, bladder outlet, or urethra. Any obstructive bladder process, whether functional or anatomical, can produce high vesical pressures during storage and emptying that exceed the antireflux mechanism resulting in VUR.

The most common anatomical obstruction of the bladder in male infants is PUV. VUR is present in 48–70% of patients with PUV, but after PUV ablation, VUR resolution can reach 78%.[9] Functional causes of reflux must be excluded including a neurogenic bladder associated with spina bifida. When evaluating the patient, direct questioning must be made about constipation (and faecal incontinence if older), as well as an examination of the lumbosacral area. Spinal cord abnormalities can be excluded by spinal ultrasonography in young infancy or by a magnetic resonance imaging scan if older. The prevalence of bladder dysfunction in the VUR population varies and is seen in 18–52% of non-invasive investigations.[10] Abnormal micturition patterns without an indefinable neurological abnormality are important to identify. There is a spectrum of functional disorders known as 'dysfunctional elimination syndrome' with the most severe extreme labelled as 'non-neurogenic neuropathic bladder'. It presents both lower and upper urinary tract deterioration, but without evidence for neurological disease.

Expert comment High voiding detrusor pressure

Relevant to our case study, it has been reported that high voiding detrusor pressure in some infants with VUR may be related to inadequate relaxation of the external urethral sphincter.[11] In a normal immature bladder at infancy, maximum voiding pressure is higher than later in life. Asynchronous detrusor/sphincter activity is often noted characterized by a low bladder capacity, high voiding pressure, and overactivity during filling. The detrusor contraction with a closed urethral sphincter results in high bladder pressure and may lead to VUR depending on the competence of the VUJ. This dyscoordination is not considered a true neurogenic bladder because it is an immature bladder in maturation[12] and occurs more frequently in boys than girls.

Learning point Management of VUR

The primary goal of the treatment of VUR is prevention of febrile UTI and avoidance of renal damage. The management of VUR includes conservative management or surgical intervention which commonly comprises endoscopic correction or ureteric reimplantation.

Conservative management is based on the knowledge that VUR resolves spontaneously mostly in the younger patients with low-grade reflux due to the enlargement of the intravesical ureter and maturation of the antireflux mechanism. However, in high-grade reflux, spontaneous resolution is <25%[13] and when associated with bladder dysfunction this rate is further reduced.

Evidence base Continuous antibiotic prophylaxis

Continuous antibiotic prophylaxis (CAP) in the context of children with VUR is also much debated. A meta-analysis of randomized controlled trials concluded that CAP significantly reduced the risk of febrile and symptomatic UTIs. However, CAP increased the risk of UTI secondary to antibiotic-resistant bacteria and did not significantly impact the occurrence of new renal scarring.[14]

Supported by the European Society of Paediatric Urology, a safe approach would be to use CAP in most cases though decision-making would be influenced by risk factors for UTI (young age, high-grade VUR, status of toilet training, lower urinary tract dysfunction, female sex, and circumcision status) and parental opinion.[6]

At 1 month of age, following a culture-proven UTI, the patient was also started on overnight bladder drainage. A dimercaptosuccinic acid (DMSA) scan at 2 months of age showed 14% right kidney differential function. Due to difficulties with clean intermittent catheterization and overnight drainage, at 2 months of age, a diagnostic cystoscopy was undertaken that demonstrated a normal urethra and excluded PUV. A right-sided refluxing loop ureterostomy was formed and a circumcision was also undertaken.

Evidence base Circumcision to reduce the risk of UTI

The health benefits of routine newborn male circumcision remain controversial.[18] Less controversial is the role of circumcision in patients at high risk of UTI. The number needed to treat to prevent a UTI in a normal boy is 111 but in those with high-grade reflux, this number drops to 4.[19] When VUR is confirmed following ANH, circumcision reduces the incidence of UTI from 68% to 22%.[20]

Learning point Endoscopic correction

This minimally invasive approach consists of a cystoscopic subureteral injection of biocompatible bulking material to elevate the distal ureter and narrows the lumen which prevents VUR. The reflux resolution rate depends on the grade of reflux: grades I and II are 78.5%, and 51% for grade V. The success rate is lower in neurogenic bladder.[15] Endoscopic injection is safe, but a serious complication reported is VUJ obstruction in 0.1–5% of cases. It can present acutely or years later, highlighting the need for long-term follow-up.

Learning point Ureteric reimplantation

This approach has a high success rate of 92–98%, despite multiple described surgical techniques which have the principle of lengthening the intramural ureter. The most popular and reliable is the Cohen cross-trigonal reimplantation. Other alternatives are suprahiatal reimplantation (Politano–Leadbetter technique), infrahiatal reimplantation (Glenn–Anderson technique), or extravesical (Lich–Gregoir technique). Though ureteric reimplantation is safe and feasible in infants <1 year old,[16] there is still some apprehension due to concerns about iatrogenic bladder dysfunction.[17] This was not undertaken due to the concerns about causing worsening bladder dysfunction that could subsequently affect the much better functioning left renal unit.

Expert comment Urinary diversion

Endoscopic treatment was not undertaken in this patient due to concerns regarding the dysfunctional bladder with known reduced success rates in combination with high-grade VUR. The right-sided VUR may have been protective for the left renal system and therefore attempted correction of the right VUR may have compromised the left side without first resolving the bladder dysfunction. The authors feel that endoscopic treatment is safe to perform for high-grade reflux in isolation in the absence of bladder dysfunction and also concomitant VUR with obstruction.

The option of urinary diversion via a refluxing right ureterostomy was undertaken to allow VUR secondary to bladder dysfunction to be easily drained from the urinary tract and thereby avoid urinary stasis and reduce the risk of UTIs. Urinary diversion could also be achieved via a vesicostomy; however, the refluxing ureterostomy allowed continued bladder cycling and growth.

Expert comment Operative note: cutaneous loop ureterostomy

A transverse inguinal crease incision is made and the anterior abdominal muscles are split to gain access to the extraperitoneal space. The approach to the ureter is entirely extraperitoneal and the peritoneum is reflected medially. The obliterated umbilical artery is divided to demonstrate the ureter. The ureter is carefully mobilized, preserving the blood supply, so that the ureter can reach the skin. At times, the proximal ureter may need to be dissected and shorted to aid drainage if it is very tortuous and dilated; however, the surgeon must keep in mind the ureteric length required for later reconstruction.

The ureter is opened longitudinally to create the loop ureterostomy. The ureter is secured to the external oblique aponeurosis with a 6/0 absorbable suture with the proximal limb secured laterally. It is important to ensure a kink or stenosis is not created. The mucocutaneous anastomosis is undertaken with a 6/0 absorbable suture.

The ureterostomy is easily covered by the nappy, which makes it easy to handle.

Subsequent serial ultrasounds demonstrated decreased dilatation on the right side and no left-sided renal dilatation (Figure 47.4).

At 9 months of age, a non-invasive urodynamic study was performed but with some difficulty due to urinary leakage via the ureterostomy despite the placement of a balloon catheter to occlude the right VUJ. The study, however, demonstrated minimal post-void residuals (< 5 mL) but it was not possible to define bladder capacity.

A repeat DMSA scan performed at 17 months of age showed 10% differential function of right kidney (Figure 47.5).

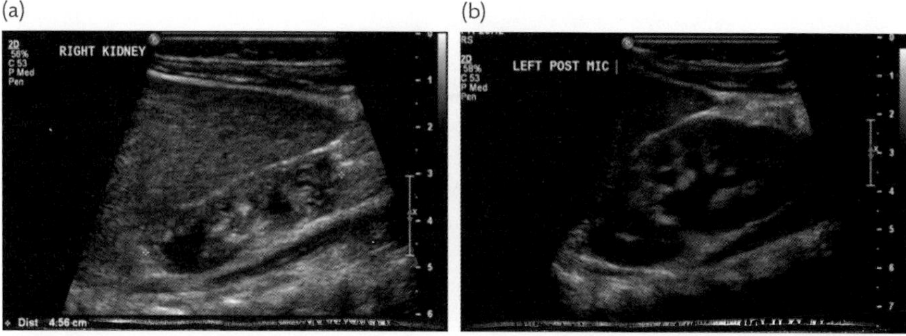

Figure 47.4 Postoperative renal USS showing (a) decreased dilatation in the right kidney, longitudinal; (b) no hydronephrosis in the left kidney, longitudinal.

At 19 months, an open right nephroureterectomy including ureterostomy closure was performed. At 3 years' follow-up, the patient remains well, without urinary prophylaxis and is UTI free. His estimated glomerular filtration rate is 86 mL/min/1.73m^2 and he has complete spontaneous bladder emptying as assessed by ultrasonography.

Expert comment Ureterostomy closure

The rationale for closure of the ureterostomy was based on the clinical stability of the patient with time and by demonstrating resolution of the immature infantile bladder with the urodynamic investigation that confirmed complete bladder emptying. The benefit of reconstructive surgery for the right dilated system with 10% function, including a ureteric reimplantation, did not outweigh the risks, therefore a more straightforward total right nephroureterectomy was undertaken. At the time of nephroureterectomy, it is important to remove the ureter as close to the bladder as possible to avoid any future problems with a refluxing ureteral stump.

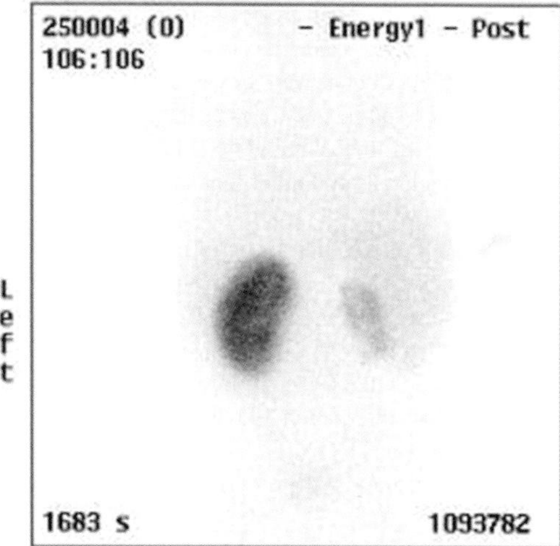

Figure 47.5 DMSA scan at 17 months showing a differential function of right 10% and left 90%.

A final word from the expert

This case is a good example of how sometimes we have to be innovative in our management. The conventional management of this infant would most likely have been endoscopic correction of the reflux once he reached an appropriate age. Due to the high grade of the reflux and the young age of the child, endoscopic correction was likely to fail and in fact may have resulted in worsening of the bladder dynamics and/or back pressure changes in the healthy left kidney. In this child, there was clear evidence of incomplete bladder emptying which was most likely related to the right refluxing system but in addition there could also have been a component of bladder immaturity/dysfunction. The initial management was with clean intermittent catheterization but when this became difficult, an alternative option had to be sought. Formation of a vesicostomy would be an option but this has the disadvantage of, at a later stage, not being able to accurately assess the bladder for capacity and efficacy of emptying. An elegant alternative to a vesicostomy is a refluxing ureterostomy. This system allows good decompression of the bladder, while still allowing for cycling of the bladder with urine from the contralateral kidney, a factor which may be important in maturation of bladder function. It is often seen that, over time, the quantity of refluxing urine from the ureterostomy reduces, probably due to a combination of maturation of the vesicoureteric mechanism but also due to linear growth of the child and changes in the angulation of the ureter at the level of the bladder. The parents witness the increased passage of urine per urethra and by occluding the ureterostomy with a Foley balloon catheter, one can make an objective assessment of bladder function. Once it is established that bladder function and emptying is adequate, one can then either close the ureterostomy, reimplant the refluxing ureter, or perform a complete nephroureterectomy as in this case.

References

1. Nguyen HT, Benson CB, Bromley B, et al. Multidisciplinary consensus on the classification of prenatal and postnatal urinary tract dilatation (UTD classification system). *J Pediatr Urol.* 2014;10(6):982–998.
2. Lee RS, Cendron M, Kinnamon DD, Nguyen HT. Antenatal hydronephrosis as a predictor of postnatal outcome: a metaanalysis. *Pediatrics.* 2006;118(2):586–593.
3. Phan V, Traubici J, Hershenfield B, et al. Vesicoureteral reflux in infants with isolated antenatal hydronephrosis. *Pediatr Nephrol.* 2003;18(12):1224–1228.
4. Zerin JM, Ritchey ML, Chang AC. Incidental vesicoureteral reflux in neonates with antenatally detected hydronephrosis and other renal abnormalities. *Radiology.* 1993;187(1):157–160.
5. Sinha R, Saha S, Maji B, Tse Y. Antibiotics for performing voiding cystourethrogram: a randomised control trial. *Arch Dis Child.* 2018;103(3):230–234.
6. Tekgül S, Riedmiller H, Hoebeke P, et al. European Association of Urology guidelines on vesicoureteral reflux in children. *Eur Urol.* 2012;62(3):534–542.
7. Lebowitz RL, Olbing H, Parkkulainen KV, et al. International system of radiographic grading of vesicoureteric reflux. International Reflux Study in Children. *Pediatr Radiol.* 1985;15(2):105–109.
8. Paquin AJ. Ureterovesical anastomosis: the description and evaluation of a technique. *J Urol.* 1959;82:573–583.
9. Priti K, Rao KLN, Menon P, et al. Posterior urethral valves: incidence and progress of vesicoureteric reflux after primary fulguration. *Pediatr Surg Int.* 2004;20(2):136–139.
10. Sillén U. Bladder dysfunction and vesicoureteral reflux. *Adv Urol.* 2008;2008:815472.
11. Chandra M, Maddix H. Urodynamic dysfunction in infants with vesicoureteral reflux. *J Pediatr.* 2000;136(6):754–759.

12. Sillén U, Bachelard M, Hermanson G. Gross bilateral reflux in infants: gradual decrease of initial detrusor hypercontractility. *J Urol.* 1996;155(2):668–672.
13. Weiss R, Tamminen-Möbius T, Koskimies O, et al. Characteristics at entry of children with severe primary vesicoureteral reflux recruited for a multicenter, international therapeutic trial comparing medical and surgical management. The International Reflux Study in Children. *J Urol.* 1992;148(5 Pt 1):1644–1649.
14. Wang HH, Gbadegesin RA, Foreman JW, et al. Efficacy of antibiotic prophylaxis in children with vesicoureteral reflux: systematic review and meta-analysis. *J Urol.* 2015;193(3):963–969.
15. Elder JS, Diaz M, Caldamone AA, et al. Endoscopic therapy for vesicoureteral reflux: a meta-analysis, I: reflux resolution and urinary tract infection. *J Urol.* 2006;175(2):716–722.
16. Jude E, Deshpande A, Barker A, Khosa J, Samnakay N. Intravesical ureteric reimplantation for primary obstructed megaureter in infants under 1 year of age. *J Pediatr Urol.* 2017;13(47):47.e1–47.e7.
17. Farrugia MK, Hitchcock R, Radford A, et al. British Association of Paediatric Urologists consensus statement on the management of the primary obstructive megaureter. *J Pediatr Urol.* 2014;10(1):26–33.
18. Earp BD. Do the benefits of male circumcision outweigh the risks? A critique of the proposed CDC guidelines. *Front Pediatr.* 2015;3:18.
19. Singh-Grewal D, Macdessi J, Craig J. Circumcision for the prevention of urinary tract infection in boys: a systematic review of randomised trials and observational studies. *Arch Dis Child.* 2005;90(8):853–858.
20. Evans K, Asimakadou M, Nwankwo O, et al. What is the risk of urinary tract infection in children with antenatally presenting dilating vesico-ureteric reflux? *J Pediatr Urol.* 2015;11(2):93.e1–93.e6.

SECTION 15

Urological radiology

Acute interventional radiology procedures in urology

Yousef Shahin

Expert commentary Steven Kennish

Case history

An 81-year-old male patient first presented with a 6-week history of rectal bleeding and change in bowel habit to the accident and emergency department. The patient was found to have a large fixed rectal mass on examination by the general surgeons. Following this, a computed tomography (CT) scan of the abdomen and pelvis confirmed the presence of a locally advanced rectal tumour infiltrating the prostate gland and the bladder in addition to a suspicious liver lesion. On magnetic resonance imaging (MRI) of the pelvis, the tumour was confirmed to be locally advanced and measured 3 cm in diameter. It was staged as T4N1M1 due to localized vascular invasion and confirmation of liver metastasis on liver MRI (Figure 48.1).

The patient was discussed at the multidisciplinary team meeting and started on neoadjuvant chemotherapy and radiotherapy. Follow-up CT scanning demonstrated tumour response with reduction in size. The patient underwent elective anterior pelvic exenteration, ileal conduit, and end-colostomy formation. Two months after the operation the patient presented with abdominal pain to the accident and emergency department. A CT scan of the abdomen and pelvis (urographic phase) showed a defect in the proximal posteromedial wall of the ileal conduit with contrast leaking out with an associated urinoma (Figure 48.2). The urinoma was drained by inserting an 8-French drain under ultrasound guidance.

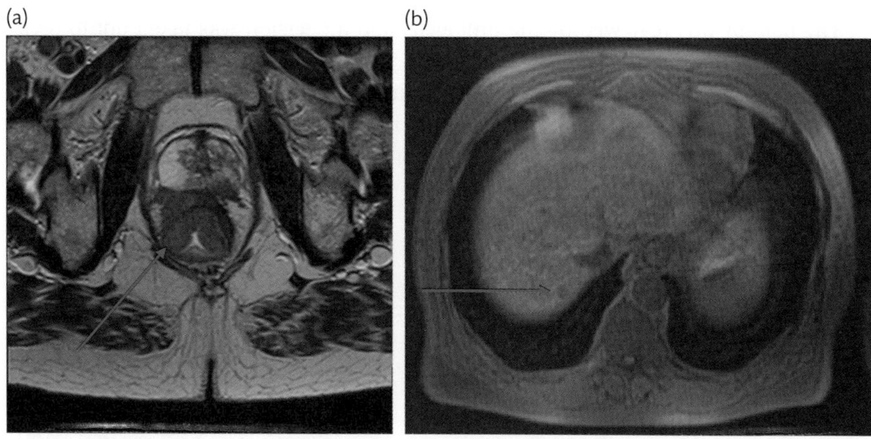

Figure 48.1 MRI of the abdomen and pelvis (axial) showing (a) locally advanced rectal tumour with invasion of the prostate; (b) single liver metastasis in the right lobe.

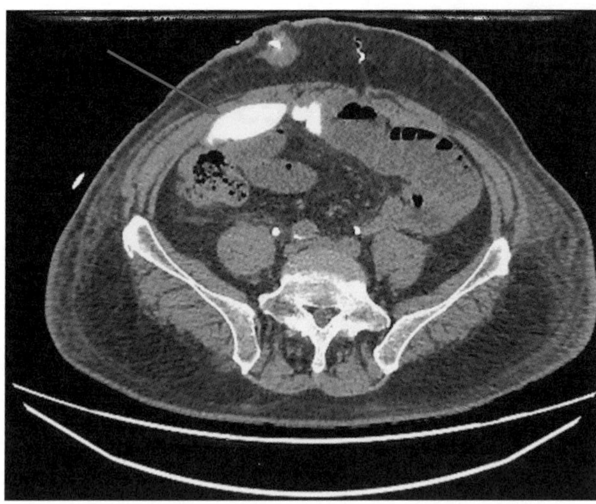

Figure 48.2 CT urogram showing a defect in the posteromedial wall of the ileal conduit and urinoma.

Learning point Pelvic exenteration and outcomes

Pelvic exenteration surgery for locally advanced rectal cancer is associated with variable outcomes. The operation is radical and involves the removal of most of the pelvic organs including the urethra, urinary bladder, rectum, and anus. The procedure leaves the person with a permanent colostomy and urinary diversion. In women, the vagina, cervix, uterus, fallopian tubes, ovaries, and, in some cases, the vulva are removed. In men, the prostate is removed.

In a recent multicentre study which included 1184 patients who underwent pelvic exenteration, the median overall survival was 36 months following R0 resection, 27 months after R1 resection, and 16 months following R2 resection ($p < 0.001$). Patients who received neoadjuvant chemotherapy had more postoperative complications (unadjusted odds ratio (OR) 1.53), readmissions (unadjusted OR 2.33), and radiological reinterventions (unadjusted OR 2.12). Bone resection (when required) was associated with a longer median survival (36 vs 29 months; $p < 0.001$). Node-positive patients had a shorter median overall survival than those with node-negative disease (22 vs 29 months, respectively). Multivariable analysis identified margin status and bone resection as significant determinants of long-term survival.[1]

Expert comment Ileal conduit and complications

Ileal conduit formation involves anastomosing both diverted ureters to a length of mobilized small bowel which is brought out of the abdomen as a stoma. It is among the most commonly performed procedures for urinary diversion, but attendant risks include anastomotic leakage and stricture formation as well as vulnerability to ischaemia and subsequent breakdown. Urinary diversion away from any leak allows healing while persistent urinary contamination leads to wound breakdown and urinoma formation with subsequent infection.

The patient was reviewed by the urologists and a decision was taken not to revise the urostomy due to the expected complexity of the procedure and patient frailty. In order to divert urine away from the leaking urostomy and allow the defect to close, the patient underwent bilateral nephrostomy insertion by interventional radiologists which was a challenging procedure due to non-dilated pelvicalyceal systems and the patient's inability to lie prone.

Clinical tip Percutaneous nephrostomy insertion

Percutaneous nephrostomy was first described in 1955 by Goodwin et al.[2] as a minimally invasive treatment for urinary obstruction causing hydronephrosis. It is now used in a wide variety of clinical indications in dilated systems to relieve urinary tract obstruction or non-dilated systems to provide urinary diversion away from distal leaks/fistula or to relieve lower urinary tract symptoms associated with bladder malignancy. The procedure is performed by interventional radiologists under ultrasound and fluoroscopy guidance with local anaesthesia and occasionally intravenous sedoanalgesia.

Indications

1. Relief of urinary obstruction.
2. Urinary diversion.
3. Access for endourological procedure.
4. Diagnostic testing.

Complications

Most case series report combined immediate major and minor complication rates of approximately 10%.[3,4] Immediate major complications include injury to adjacent structures, severe bleeding, or severe infection or sepsis and are uncommon. Injury to adjacent organs, most commonly the pleura or colon, is exceptionally uncommon when careful consideration is given to patient anatomy and periprocedural planning on CT and ultrasound scanning. Minor complications, including minor bleeding and transient low-grade fever post insertion, are more often seen and generally unavoidable in some clinical scenarios.

Late complications are mainly drain related such as displacement, blockage, and encrustation. Patients with long-term nephrostomy tubes will have these drains exchanged every 3 months to prevent blockage by encrustation.[5]

Expert comment Nephrostomy in a non-dilated system

Nephrostomy insertion is commonly undertaken for urinary diversion but can be challenging because the non-dilated target calyces are inherently very difficult to identify even with the most modern high-end ultrasound equipment.

If covering internal–external ureteric stents have been left in place by the surgical team, these can be utilized to retrogradely fill the pelvicalyceal systems with contrast to create target calyces visible to both ultrasound and fluoroscopy. If the stents have been removed prior to the discovery of a leak, other adjuncts include the intravenous administration of contrast to allow the draining renal collecting system to be visualized fluoroscopically and an intravenous diuretic with saline to create increased renal excretion and hopefully a visible calyx on ultrasound.

Retrogradely filling the conduit and ureters with contrast through a catheter is risky in the context of an ongoing leak or collection because of the risk of driving pyelovenous backflow and sepsis.

The patient was stabilized to allow time for antibiotic treatment and nutritional support in preparation for a laparotomy, revision of ileal conduit, small bowel resection, and end ileostomy. Unfortunately, the proximal aspect of the ileal conduit was too stuck down to access for revision surgery. Following this operation, he developed acute kidney injury and sepsis. A CT of the abdomen and pelvis showed a 7 × 12 cm pelvic collection. This was drained by interventional radiology under CT guidance (Figure 48.3) following which the patient improved clinically although renal replacement therapy (dialysis) was required.

A month later the patient presented with right-sided flank pain and had a CT scan which showed right-sided pyelonephritis. A nephrostogram showed a leak close to the ureteroileal anastomosis on the right and a stricture proximal to the ureteroileal anastomosis on the left (Figure 48.4). Blood and nephrostomy urine cultures grew *Klebsiella*.

Two weeks later, the right nephrostomy tube was not draining, and an unenhanced CT scan showed the nephrostomy tube to be displaced. A new nephrostomy tube was inserted on the same day by the interventional radiology team.

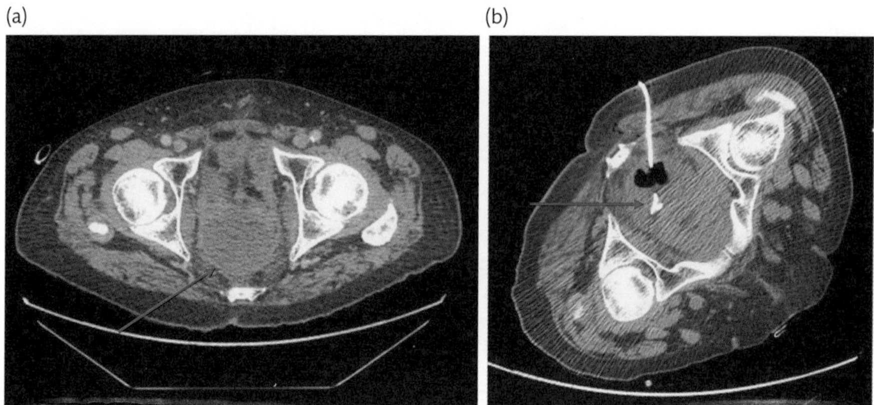

Figure 48.3 CT of the pelvis showing (a) pelvic collection; (b) CT-guided drainage of pelvic collection with the pigtail.

On a follow-up nephrostogram, contrast continued to leak into the pelvis from a point near the right ureteroileal anastomosis. This resulted in a persistent presacral pelvic collection. This was drained for the third time under CT guidance.

One week later, the patient underwent bilateral retrograde ureteric stent insertion by interventional radiology (Figure 48.5) utilizing an antegrade approach through the nephrostomies. This procedure helped to further divert urine away from the defective ileal conduit. The internal–external urinary stents negated the ongoing need for nephrostomy drains and are much better tolerated by the patient with drainage in to the stoma bag.

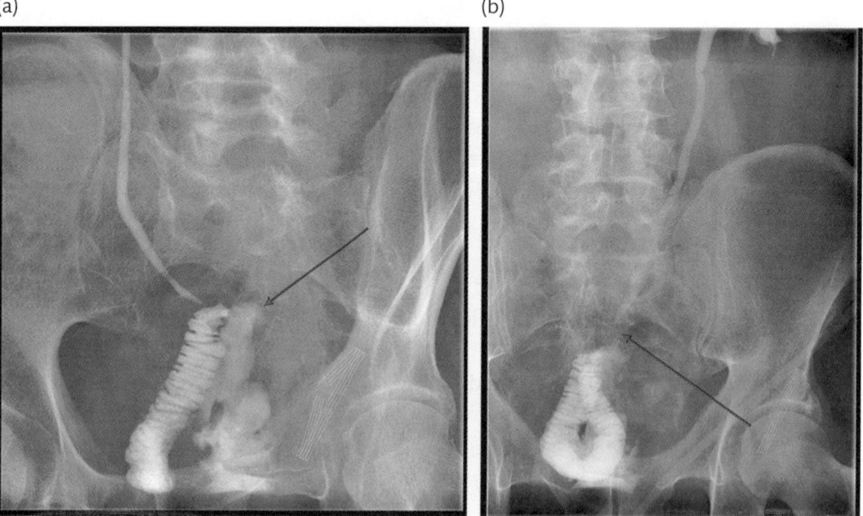

Figure 48.4 Nephrostograms showing (a) a leak close to the right ureteroileal anastomosis; (b) a stricture proximal to the left ureteroileal anastomosis. A CT scan on follow-up showed an ongoing pelvic collection measuring 3 × 6 × 11 cm which was drained a second time under CT guidance by interventional radiologists.

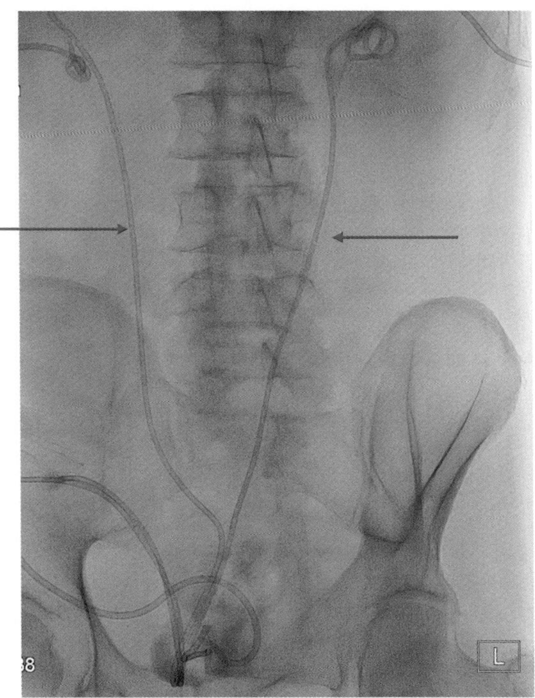

Figure 48.5 Static image during fluoroscopy showing bilateral retrograde ureteric stents.

A year later, the patient continued to have intermittent septic episodes and the small bowel stoma output was high. Following which, he had a laparotomy, reversal of ileostomy, and ileocolic anastomosis. In addition, the chronic pelvic collection was drained intraoperatively.

A solitary metastasis in the right lobe of the liver has increased in size on MRI follow-up, measuring 4 cm, and the patient underwent a liver resection (metastatectomy) as the lesion was not amenable to radiofrequency ablation due to its proximity to the diaphragm and the risk of potential thermal injury.

On the latest follow-up CT scan, the pelvic collection was found to be small and no further drainage was undertaken. The patient undergoes urinary stent exchange in radiology every 6 weeks.

Learning point Ureteric stents

Antegrade, retrograde, or internal (double J) stents are routinely placed by interventional radiologists.

Retrograde (transileal conduit) ureteric stent insertion

A retrograde stent is a catheter placed in patients who have undergone surgical treatment, such as cystectomy with ileal conduit formation in which it exits from the conduit and extends retrogradely to the renal pelvis.

It is estimated that 15% of patients develop complications in the form of a stricture at the ureteroenteric junction causing obstruction.[6–8] Treatment success of ureteric strictures and subsequent hydronephrosis by percutaneous methods can reach up to 100%. In addition, placement of retrograde transileal conduit stents can be successful in 90–95% of cases.[9]

A retrograde (transileal conduit) ureteric stent can be placed by an antegrade method if the patient has a nephrostomy *in situ* or by a retrograde approach, if not, through the stoma.

Retrograde placement of a retrograde (transileal conduit) ureteric stent technique

The ileal conduit is opacified by contrast that is allowed to reflux through the ureteroenteric junction leading to visualization of the ureter with success rates ranging from 14% to 86%. This can be performed by inserting a Foley catheter alongside an angle-tipped catheter in to the ileal loop. A guidewire is introduced through the catheter to access the ureteroenteric anastomosis and advanced up the ureter. The catheter is advanced into the renal pelvis and exchanged for a stiff guidewire. A catheter can then be advanced over the wire and its pigtail is formed within the renal pelvis. The distal end of the catheter can be cut to an appropriate length and left within the stoma bag for drainage.

Antegrade placement of a retrograde ureteric stent technique

The patient can be placed initially in a lateral oblique position or can be rotated from a prone position after obtaining initial access to the pelvicalyceal system. The renal collecting system is accessed under ultrasound guidance and contrast is injected, providing visualization of the urinary tract to the ileal conduit. A guidewire is advanced through the collecting system and manipulated using a catheter down the ureter and out the stoma. An angled-tip hydrophilic wire can be used. Once the wire is out through the stoma, providing through and through access, tension should be maintained on both ends of the wire and an antegrade or retrograde catheter can be advanced to allow guidewire exchange for a stiffer working wire to allow stent insertion through the stoma to form the pigtail within the renal pelvis. The wire can be removed once the catheter is adequately positioned. If there is a need to leave a covering nephrostomy then the wire can be pulled back to the renal pelvis and a nephrostomy tube can then be placed.

A final word from the expert

This patient required multiple interventional radiology procedures and the diversion of urine away from the postoperative pelvis allowed an attempt at a corrective laparotomy (although sadly this was only partially successful) and has allowed wound healing and a return to a relatively normal life for the patient at home.

Urinary diversion through the stents into the ileal conduit (urostomy) bag is much better managed by the patient at home than bilateral nephrostomy drains which impact heavily on the activities of daily living such as dressing and bathing. The risk of inadvertent nephrostomy tube displacement despite locking pigtail mechanisms, sutures and dressings can be up to 14.5%.[10]

Although better tolerated, ureteric stents draining in to a stoma bag can become encrusted by lithogenic urine and require regular exchanges every 2–3 months. Accidental displacement when changing the stoma bag is rarely complete and salvage via a retrogradely introduced guidewire under fluoroscopic guidance is usually successful. One of the few advantages of nephrostomies over stents draining in to a single stoma bag is the difficulty with the latter of recognizing reduced output from one or other kidney in the context of drain blockage or displacement.

Urinary leaks post cystectomy/pelvic exenteration and ileal conduit urinary diversion are uncommon (approximately 2%) but usually arise from the ureteroileal anastomosis and an early clinical presentation is a predictor for the need for adjuvant upstream urinary diversion with nephrostomies.[11] Ischaemic breakdown of the proximal ileal conduit itself is very uncommon but patient frailty and chemoradiotherapy are likely to have played a role.

Ultimately, if the surgeon is prepared to operate, the interventional radiologist should be prepared to provide all necessary support as required.

References

1. PelvEx Collaborative. Factors affecting outcomes following pelvic exenteration for locally recurrent rectal cancer. *Br J Surg.* 2018;105(6):650–657.
2. Goodwin WE, Casey WC, Woolf W. Percutaneous trocar (needle) nephrostomy in hydronephrosis. *J Am Med Assoc.* 1955;157(11):891–894.
3. Ramchandani P, Cardella JF, Grassi CJ, et al. Quality improvement guidelines for percutaneous nephrostomy. *J Vasc Interv Radiol.* 2003;14(9 Pt 2):S277–S281.
4. Zagoria RJ, Dyer RB. Do's and don't's of percutaneous nephrostomy. *Acad Radiol* 1999;6(6):370–377.
5. Dagli M, Ramchandani P. Percutaneous nephrostomy: technical aspects and indications. *Semin Intervent Radiol.* 2011;28(4):424–437.
6. Pappas P, Stravodimos KG, Kapetanakis T, et al. Ureterointestinal strictures following Bricker ileal conduit: management via a percutaneous approach. *Int Urol Nephrol.* 2008;40(3):621–627.
7. Alago W Jr, Sofocleous CT, Covey AM, et al. Placement of transileal conduit retrograde nephroureteral stents in patients with ureteral obstruction after cystectomy: technique and outcome. *AJR Am J Roentgenol.* 2008;191(5):1536–1539.
8. Tal R, Bachar GN, Baniel J, Belenky A. External-internal nephro-uretero-ileal stents in patients with an ileal conduit: long-term results. *Urology.* 2004;63(3):438–441.
9. Makramalla A, Zuckerman DA. Nephroureteral stents: principles and techniques. *Semin Intervent Radiol.* 2011;28(4):367–379.
10. Wah TM, Weston MJ, Irving HC. Percutaneous nephrostomy insertion: outcome data from a prospective multi-operator study at a UK training centre. *Clin Radiol.* 2004;59(3):255–261.
11. Farnham SB, Cookson MS. Surgical complications of urinary diversion. *World J Urol* 2004;22(3):157–167.

INDEX

For the benefit of digital users, indexed terms that span two pages (e.g., 52–53) may, on occasion, appear on only one of those pages.

Tables, figures, and boxes are indicated by *t*, *f*, and *b* following the page number

C

N

S

U